PROMOTING YOUR HEALTH

Walter D. Sorochan

San Diego State University

John Wiley & Sons, Inc.

New York   Chichester   Brisbane   Toronto

Production Supervisor—Jan M. Lavin
Designer—Rafael Hernandez
Cover Design—John Hite
Copyeditor—Ellen McElroy
Photo Researcher—Roberta Guerette—Omni Photo Communications
Photo Editor—Stella Kupferberg
Chapter Opening Photography and Collages—© Menschenfreud

Library of Congress Cataloging in Publication Data:

Sorochan, Walter D.
    Promoting your health.

Bibliography: p.
Includes index.
    1.   Health.   I.   Title.
RA776.S692   613   80-24347
ISBN 0-471-04681-7

Printed in the United States of America

10   9   8   7   6   5   4   3   2   1

The theme of this book is health promotion, which has always been a goal of health education. However, there has been considerable controversy over the process of promoting more and better health. Research shows that the traditional approaches of presenting the facts and letting people decide for themselves have not always been successful. Even though they are armed with information from a health class or book, most people still continue with their health-destructive habits. We assumed falsely that knowing about health would bring about behavior change and a constructive life style. Now we are aware that people may need to be shown how to promote their personal, family, and community well-being. They need to learn how to value their health and how to give high priority to optimal well-being in their lives. They also need to have a reason to change an old habit. It is for all of these reasons that this book was written with a focus on health promotion.

Traditionally, books in the health field have been treatment-oriented, much like the practice of medicine is today. That is, the information presented concerns curative approaches to health. The approach in this book breaks with this tradition. Instead, the focus is on health promotion and includes ways to attain and maintain optimal wellness. There is also emphasis on behavioral modification techniques that will help individuals to change deleterious habits and behaviors. To do so, however, they need to first be aware that they have a health problem or the makings of one. The self-assessment inventories, checklists, and other instruments at the beginning of each chapter can help the reader realize that he or she may be doing something wrong. Such awareness provides the rationale for making a change. Thus disease prevention and not disease treatment is the theme of this book.

Since many persons do have good health habits and values, suggestions are also given on how to maintain a positive healthy life style, which is in keeping with health promotion. To achieve this end, considerable time and effort have been put into getting up-to-date information on promoting well-being. Moreover, the information in each chapter supports the idea of promoting one's health.

Many chapters are unique. The opening chapter discusses the meaning and theory of health, topics seldom considered in other books. After 15 years of study and research into the significance and philosophy of health, in it, I bridge the relationship between well-being and its dimensions—not just levels of well-being—but fitness components, the basic human health needs, and life style. A person needs to have this background to make intelligent decisions and changes about health and life.

The second chapter makes readers aware of the many ways there are to monitor and assess health. Emphasis is placed on assessing all the dimensions of well-being, not just the physical.

Chapter 4 on social well-being is the only one of its kind in print. It discusses the basis for social well-being, why it is important for optimal well-being, and how to attain it.

Nutrition is everyone's business since everyone ingests food and drink. Nutrition is probably the most important behavior that determines our well-being. But not everyone eats balanced nutritious meals. Chapter 6 departs somewhat from the traditional treatment-health education approach and provides actual guidelines for assessing one's diet—ways to modify eating habits and nutrition information to help one make intelligent decisions about selecting foods to eat.

The final chapter, on health care services, makes practical suggestions on how to reduce medical expenses and what to do if sickness occurs. Going to the doctor or hospital when one is sick may be a most ineffective way to take care of an illness. The suggestions in this chapter reinforce those presented in the preceding topical chapters.

There is consistency in the format for all chapters. A brief introduction is followed by a self-assessment instrument. Assuming that the reader reacts to the self-assessment instrument, the interpretation of these reactions and additional topical information are presented as a reinforcement for change. Ways to modify one's behavior and where to go for help are complemented by suggested readings for those students seeking more information on the topic. Such a format promotes well-being in a practical and futuristically unique manner.

Although this book was written primarily as a textbook, persons of all backgrounds can benefit from it. I combined into a single presentation the inventories, health information, and suggestions for promoting optimal well-being. Although this has not been an easy task, it has been personally rewarding. My mission was not just to be different, or to reinvent another traditional health book. Instead, my aids, my publisher, and I have put together a useful and practical book to help people enjoy more and better health and live a long and fruitful life.

Walter D. Sorochan

ACKNOWLEDGMENTS

The initial spark for writing this book was provided by two persons. Charlie Ross, M.D., of Interhealth of San Diego and former president of The Society for Prospective Medicine, was the first to suggest that there was a need for a book on prospective medicine. This idea was shared with Wayne Anderson, health education editor of John Wiley & Sons, Publishers. After many months of deliberation and consultation with other health professionals, we concluded that there was a definite need for a text with a new approach—one that emphasized preventive medicine, and one that would promote health.

The research for the contents of the chapters began in earnest. My research assistant, Penny Pappas, became indispensible in running down articles, obtaining references, and assuming the role of secretary—as needed.

An old friend and health enthusiast, Milton Elliot, would react to an occasional chapter and point out what I had overlooked in exploring various topical ideas. Toward the end of the project, Beth Werker took charge of following up on acknowledgments and copyright permissions. Ethel Bender was just wonderful in typing my handwritten manuscript.

The original manuscript was revised several times. Special thanks are due to our reviewers: Marshall Kreuter, Bill Hettler, Ruth Ann Althaus, Kerry Redican, and Susan Brew. I am especially grateful to Ruth Ann Althaus for the dedication and time she gave to reviewing the various stages of the manuscript and her many suggestions for improvement.

A new book, like a new idea, needs to be tried out to see if it works. The manuscript was used as a text by my students at San Diego State University. I am most thankful to them for reacting to the inventories, the nutrition modification module, and to the content. Their comments and suggestions were most helpful in refining the manuscript.

Special thanks are due to the staff at John Wiley & Sons, Publishers: Ellen MacElree and Elaine Wetterau for a splendid job of editing; Jan Lavin for coordinating productions; and Stella Kupferberg for soliciting photos and the art work.

Finally, a special apology to all my friends and relatives who were somewhat neglected while I wrote this book.

W. D. S.

CONTENTS

Contents

PART A

INTRODUCTION

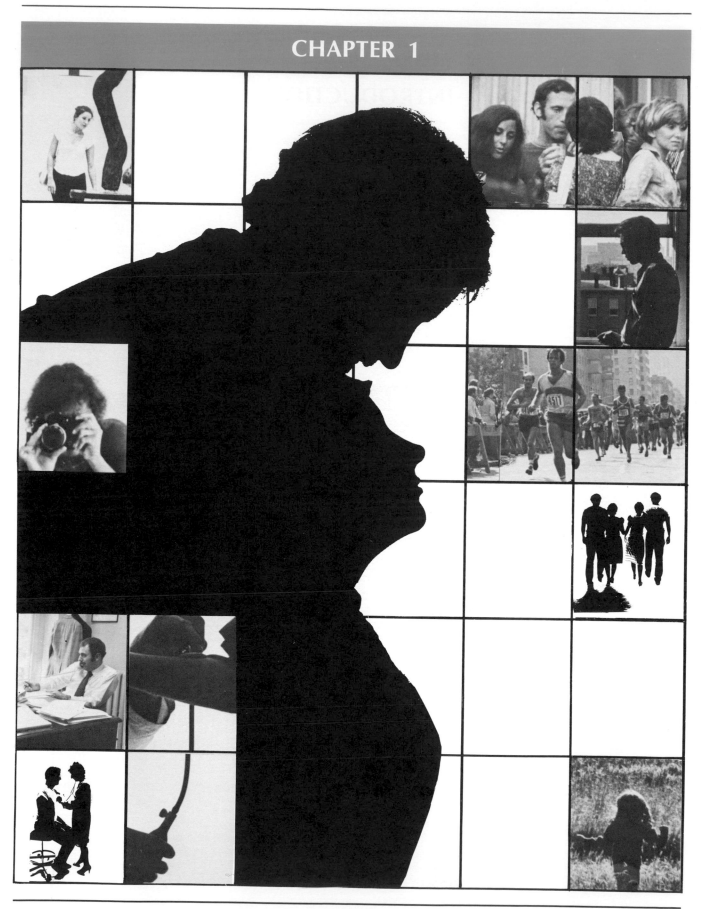

Are you really healthy or do you just appear to be healthy? How can you tell whether you have mimimum, average, above average, or optimal well-being? What influences and determines your personal well-being? Why do you need optimal health and not just average health? Does one need to be optimally well throughout life in order to live to 80, 100, or more years? Should you give higher priority and value to health in your life style? What can you do to attain optimal well-being or the maximum level of health possible? The answers to these and other related questions are discussed in this chapter, which will help you to interpret health and relate it to your style of living.

☞ LIFE-LINE-HEALTH VALUES GAME[1]

PURPOSE

1. To make you aware of the importance of conserving your well-being.
2. To make you aware of the relationship of life style (habits and behaviors) to optimal well-being.
3. To make you aware that optimal health is essential to accomplishing things in life.

DIRECTIONS

1. Draw a horizontal line across the paper. Mark it as a continuous scale, as illustrated in the accompanying figure.
2. Put a dot at each end of the line

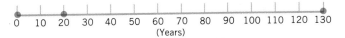

3. Over the left dot, put a "0". This represents your birth date.
4. Estimate your ultimate death (year) over on the right side. This dot should represent how long you wish to, or believe you will, live.
5. Place a dot on the line to represent your age now on the line between birth and death.
6. On the right side of your present age, plot five major goals you want to accomplish in your lifetime. Place them on the line as approximate dates. They might include some of the following:
   (a) Purchase a new car or airplane
   (b) Get married

[1] Adapted from Sidney Simon, et al., *Values-Clarification: A Handbook of Practical Strategies for Teachers and Students,* New York, Hart Publishing Co., 1972; and suggestions from Marshall Kreuter, Professor of Health Science, University of Utah, Salt Lake City, Utah.

(c) Purchase or build a home

(d) Have children

(e) Complete a Master's degree

(f) Complete a Ph.D degree

(g) Travel (e.g., Europe or Asia)

(h) Sell or write your first book

(i) Participate in your first big public event such as a golf or tennis tournament or a marathon

(j) Begin a new hobby or join a new club

(k) Become elected to political office (school board member, city mayor, etc.)

(l) Become president of a company

(m) Own your own business

(n) Become a millionaire

7. On the left side of your age scale, plot the "bad for health" habits or behaviors you have now. Many of these are listed in step 8.

8. Identify, in the following list, the lost years for each of your "bad for health" habits or behaviors. Lost years are those years that are lost because you die prematurely.

Self-Destructive Behaviors or Habits	*Lost Years*
(a) Smoking cigarettes (½ a pack or more per day)	−8
(b) Drinking alcohol (3 or more drinks per week)	−10
(c) Overeating (more than 2500 calories per day)	−5
(d) Eating excess fats in your diet (more than 20 percent per day of fats such as beef, pork, and cheese)	−5
(e) Eating lots of sugar (pastry, cookies, candy, ice cream, etc., during the week)	−8
(f) Using too much salt in your diet	−3
(g) Not exercising at least 3 times a week	−10
(h) Being overweight or obese	−10
(i) Having lots of stress in your life	−7
(j) Driving while intoxicated	−10
(k) Often handling firearms	−3
(l) Often working with or handling toxic chemicals	−3
(m) Often being depressed and unhappy	−5
(n) Often feeling lonely	−3
(o) Driving without using seat belts	−3

9. Total all the years that may be lost due to your bad habits. This value is the *total lost years*.

10. Subtract the total lost years from your projected age of death. This value is your premature death age.

11. Refer back to your life line and plot, in red, the age you will be when you die prematurely.

12. Identify all the goals that you will not be able to attain if you die prematurely. Do you have time to accomplish your major goal? What do you need to do in order to be able to fulfill your expectations? Which habits or behaviors do you need to modify or change? Do you need to give health a higher priority in your life?

DIFFICULTY INTERPRETING HEALTH

The meaning given to health arises from our experiences with exercise, play, sports, food, drinking at social parties, medication, drugs, fatigue, illness, disease, disability, and death. Since we live in a youth-oriented culture, our ability to perform and our personal appearance also symbolize health.

The American life style has many paradoxes about health and life-style behaviors, which add greatly to the confusion of interpreting health and giving it a high priority in our life. For example, a study of the cause of cardiovascular diseases reveals that eating a diet high in animal fat, refined sugar, white flour foods, and too much salt, combined with smoking cigarettes, being inactive, and having too much stress contribute to these diseases (see Figure 1.1). Although persons adopting these behaviors become more prone to heart attacks and premature death, our society does very little to prevent such persons from evolving self-destructive life styles and even allows public tax monies to help defray hospital-medical expenses of such terminal patients. Another example of this health–life style paradox is found in tobacco cigarette smoking. By just placing a warning label on all cigarette packages, we allow a ''dangerous-to-health'' consumer product to be sold. Doing so is contradictory to medical research, which has demonstrated that cigarette smoking is definitely hazardous to one's well-being. On the one hand, we say that it is one's right to smoke cigarettes, while on the other, we are alarmed at the high cost of hospital-medical care for those persons who have been smoking for 20 to 30 years and are now dying from emphysema, cancer, or heart disease. The public, the medical and health professions, and our political leaders are unable to accept the reality of many of our self-destructive life styles and realign national priorities toward a positive and constructive life style. Too many persons unwittingly allow mass media; doctors; the fast food and beverage industries; and other groups to manipulate their life styles, set goals for them, and even determine whether they will be sick or well. Many persons have become irresponsible in caring for themselves and maintaining their health; consequently, they live below their optimal health potentials and their best social-vocational accomplishments. They live less, have less, and die sooner.

LEVELS OF WELL-BEING

Perhaps one way to understand the meaning of health is to theorize about it. Such a theory should be multidimensional in nature, allow for fluctuations in the health-illness scale, provide for different aspects of health, and have the possibility of practical application for all ages and cultures. It should also account for the various kinds of health, illnesses, and diseases prevalent in our society.

Health can be conceptualized as levels of well-being. The interpretation of health as levels of well-being by the President's Commission on the Health Needs of the Nation (5:225), as gradations of health by Rogers (26), and

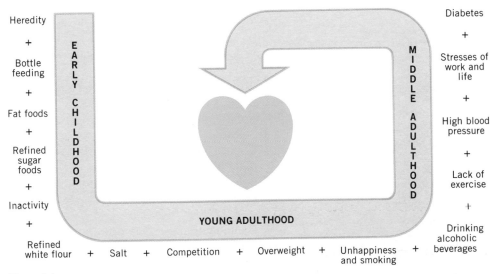

Figure 1.1
Cardiovascular disorders (CVD) are a consequence of life style. Many poor health habits are initiated in early childhood by parents. These habits become precursors to CVD and remain asymptomatic in early childhood, build up during adolescence and young adulthood, and then erupt in middle age (symptomatic).

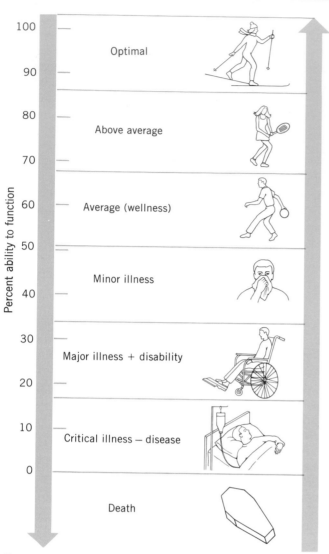

Figure 1.2

Levels of wellness. The levels of well-being extend from zero wellness at the bottom of a continuum to 100 percent optimal well-being at the other end. The arrows pointing up and down imply that one's level of well-being can change.

as levels of well-being by Dunn (4) and Hoyman (8:253) add reinforcement to such a conceptualization. *Well-being may be interpreted as a continuum, with optimal well-being at the top and death at the bottom of the stepladder* (see Figure 1.2). In between, we have gradations or levels of wellness. *Health is not a state, but a process.*[1] The word *state* implies a static and stable condition, whereas process implies constant adaptation or adjustment. Hence, being well, when symbolized by the stepladder idea (as shown in Figure 1.2), implies that one's level of well-being may fluctuate from time to time. *As a process, it is dynamic and ever-changing. Well-being is*

[1] The World Health Organization defines health as "Health is a state of complete physical, mental, and social well-being, and not merely the absence of disease or infirmity."

the integrated result of constant body changes and the whole of man adapting to his physical and social environments and being able to function socially. This rationale supports the thinking of health as well-being or levels of wellness. It accounts for the great variability of health found in the general population. Well-being obviously is a nebulous and abstract concept, one that is impossible to measure precisely or to define lucidly.

FITNESS COMPONENTS OF WELL-BEING

Although well-being cannot be measured at the present time, it can be theoretically identified by fitness components. These components are conceptualized in Figure 1.3 as physical, emotional, social, spiritual, and cultural fitness components. Each fitness identifies a different dimension of wellness.

The fitness components may be characterized by the following salient features:

1. Physical fitness (maintenance of body processes)
   (a) Efficient functioning of body systems and organs.
   (b) Ability to resist infections and communicable diseases.
   c) Freedom from disease, infirmity, or physical disorder.
   (d) Avoiding substances and experiences hazardous to optimal physical fitness.
   (e) Eating a variety and a balance of foods regularly.
   f) Overall minimum muscular strength.
   (g) Minimum cardiovascular-respiratory-muscular endurance.
   (h) Neuromuscular coordination, flexibility, and balance.
   i) Weight normal for body height, age, sex, and body density.
   j) Appropriate amount of body fat (adipose tissue).
2. Emotional (mental) fitness (feelings, thoughts, and self-identity)
   (a) Coping successfully with the stresses of daily living.
   (b) Being flexible in all social situations.
   (c) Feeling worthwhile and adequate as a person.
   (d) Feeling content and happy.
   (e) Feeling a sense of accomplishment and self-realization (success).
   (f) Facing up to and accepting reality.
   (g) Feeling worthwhile as a member of society by meeting the demands of life.
   (h) Having emotional stability.

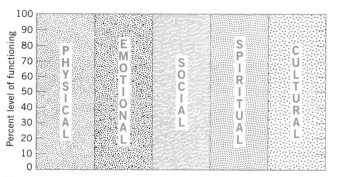

Figure 1.3

The fitness components of well-being. All fitnesses are interrelated and interdependent; that is, one affects the quality of all the others.

(i) Exercising self-discipline and self-confidence.

(j) Accepting responsibility for one's behavior and social roles.

(k) Feeling good about self and others.

(l) Having worthwhile hobbies and recreational interests.

(m) Being able to give, express, and accept love.

n) Having an adequate self-image.

(o) Having an identity structured by commitments.

3. Social fitness (interacting with others)

(a) Having a human approach to living and dealing with others.

(b) Setting up minimum moral standards of conduct (rectitude).

(c) Having ethical integrity in interpersonal relationships.

d) Wanting to share with others and to contribute to their happiness and welfare.

(e) Feeling responsible for others.

(f) Socializing by doing things with others and becoming involved with others.

(g) Cultivating close friends.

(h) Being able to make new friends.

(i) Being able to relate to people of all ages.

(j) Behaving in socially acceptable ways (morals).

4. Spiritual fitness (aspirations, ideals, and inner strength)

(a) Inner strength or energy acquired from social interaction, self-hypnosis, and so forth.

(b) Aspiring toward a safer and more abundant life for oneself and one's society.

(c) Aspiring toward "the better things in life."

(d) Feeling an awareness of a purpose in life and that living is worthwhile.

(e) Being able to appreciate aesthetics.

(f) Having ambition to achieve and to accomplish.

g) Being able to give way to creative imagination and to express creativity.

(h) Being able to set attainable goals and to experience the self-fulfillment of reaching them.

(i) Having the courage to face the unknown.

(j) Willing to take calculated risks.

(k) Feeling that what one does is worthwhile and appreciated by others.

5. Cultural fitness (identity with community)

(a) Feeling a sense of belonging ("rootedness") to a community.

(b) Responsible involvement in community affairs.

(c) Serving others as a public servant.

(d) Being a contributing member of society.

(e) Participating in cultural festivities and social functions, such as attending concerts and plays, and visiting museums. Cultural involvement would include music, art, dance, drama, and other aesthetic aspects of living wherein the talents and creativities of self and/or others may be publicly appreciated. One receives culture, as a passive spectator; one gives culture, as a performing musician or actor.

THE COMPLETE PICTURE OF HEALTH

Although these components of fitness have been exemplified as separate entities, they are normally undetectable as such; instead they are part of the whole and are interdependent. For example, physical fitness is conceived as the prerequisite for all the remaining fitnesses and is the easiest to identify. But it is not possible for a person with a high degree of physical fitness but a low social or a low spiritual fitness to have optimal well-being. Collectively, all five fitnesses complement each other synergistically and are responsible for contributing to a qualitative life style. Each expresses a different and distinct dimension of wellness.

The characteristics of each of the components of wellness reflect American values. Cultural and subcultural value differences would modify some of the characteristics of each of the components.

We can visualize health by using the vertical stepladder in Figure 1.2 as a symbol of wellness, with horizontal gradations. Consider the possibility of physical, emotional social, spiritual, and cultural fitnesses functioning as separate dimensions that would run up and down the stepladder of wellness as conceptualized in Figure 1.3. If

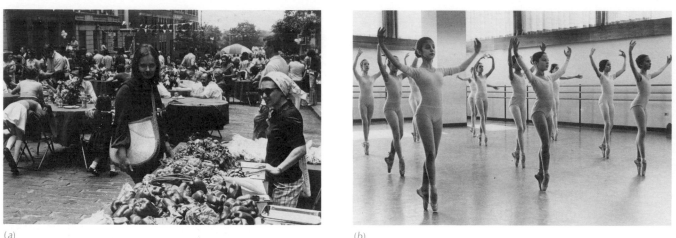

(a)   (b)

Figure 1.4
Examples of cultural well-being. *(a)* Block party where everyone participates socially. *(b)* Ballet classes where pupils will eventually perform for others.

each fitness could independently fluctuate up and down, then each fitness by itself could lower or raise one's level of wellness. This could also happen if two or more fitnesses collectively dropped into the middle or lower third of the wellness stepladder. Each fitness should be conceived as a two-directional conveyor belt, capable of moving up and down. With such mobility, it would have the ability to influence the other fitnesses, thereby lowering one's former level of total well-being, and consequently, one's potentials for self-actualization. The reverse would also be true.

DETERMINERS OF OPTIMAL WELL-BEING

Personal well-being is determined by four factors as shown in Figure 1.5 (8, 11, 15, 22):

1. Human biology (including heredity, physiological functioning of all organs and body systems, maturation, and aging).
2. Environment (food, air, water, soil, chemicals, people, microorganisms, and other living things).
3. Life style (behaviors and habits).
4. Health care organization (availability of health care—drugs, doctors, dentists, hospitals, etc.).

One's potentials for optimal well-being are genetically determined at birth. This endowment includes potentialities for our behavior and development throughout our lifetime. The ability to resist diseases, to fight infections, and to withstand stresses is largely due to genotypic makeup. Likewise, biochemical individuality plays a big role here (refer to Figure 1.6). Medical

research verifies such individuality: for example, metabolic enzymes may be lacking, causing a physiological disorder. Diabetes may occur when the Islands of Langerhans do not secrete enough insulin to metabolize carbohydrates. One becomes allergic to milk when the enzyme lactase is missing in the stomach to digest lactose in milk. We also inherit intellectual, creative, musi-

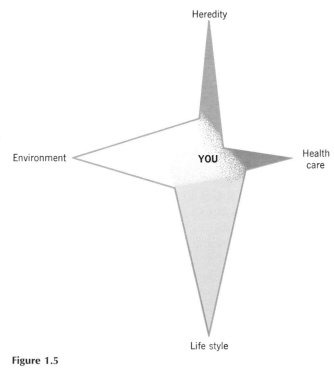

Figure 1.5
Determiners of optimal well-being. The length and width of each spike factor symbolizes the contribution of that factor to optimal well-being.

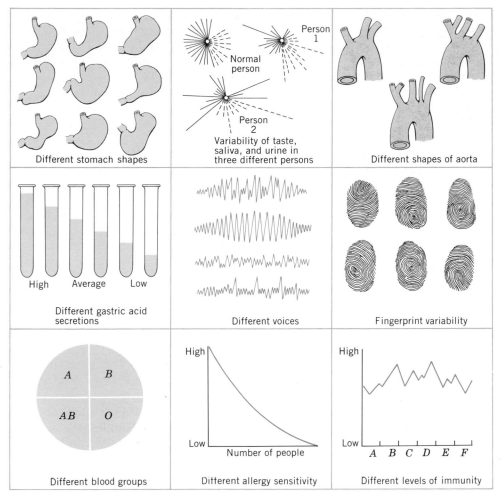

Figure 1.6

Examples of biochemical individuality. (Adapted from Roger J. Williams, "A New Brand of Nutritional Science," in *A Physician's Handbook on Orthomolecular Medicine*, Roger J. Williams and Dwight E. Kalita, eds., Elmsford, N.Y., Pergamon Press, 1977, p. 73; and Roger Williams, "On Your Startling Biochemical Individuality," *Executive Health*, Report Volume × 11, No. 8, May 1976, p. 8, Rancho Santa Fe, Cal., 92067.)

cal, artistic, athletic, and other potentials just as we do physical traits. Within these traits are potentialities for behavior, growth, optimal well-being, and longevity. We are unique and different from all others. What we are or can be and the kind of well-being we can enjoy is limited by our human biological makeup (refer to Figure 1.5).

The realization of our genetic potentials is dependent on the presence of minimal environmental conditions. The lack of vitamin C in the diets of sailors on sailing ships 300 years ago caused scurvy. Also, vitamin B–deficient diets caused beriberi and palegra. Insufficient iron in the body and diet causes anemia. Polluted air and excess noise are chemical stressors that create a greater demand on the human body for vitamins B_6, C, and E, and the mineral selenium. Polluted water can inhibit well-being by causing dysentry, cholera, and yel-

low fever. The chemical nicotine in cigarette smoke paralyzes the cilia in the bronchial tree, thereby allowing viral and bacterial infections to inhibit one's chances for optimal well-being. The lack of social involvement can make one feel lonely and unhappy. Our social environment molds our status and role in the group and plays a greater role than the physical surroundings in influencing our level of well-being.

Individuals cannot, by themselves, ensure that food, drugs, cosmetics, devices, water supply, and so forth are safe and uncontaminated; that the health hazards of air, water, and noise pollution are controlled; that the spread of communicable diseases is prevented; that effective garbage and sewage disposal is carried out; and that the social environment, including rapid changes in it, do not have harmful effects on health.

The most important determiner of optimal well-being

is one's life style. Life style includes decisions by individuals about habits and behaviors which affect their health and over which they more or less have control. As pointed out earlier, we cope with fulfilling our basic human health needs in many different healthy and unhealthy ways. Often, such coping and adaptation is destructive and hazardous to our well-being. We create and adopt bad habits as a way of coping with the emotional stresses of living. Smoking cigarettes, drinking beer or a cocktail, or several cups of coffee are examples of how we relieve tension. When repeated over a long time, these can become self-destructive behaviors. Most of our chronic and degenerative diseases, like heart disease, cancer, arthritis, cirrhosis, and depression, are self-induced. Most physical and emotional diseases and disorders are associated with behavioral influences that can be controlled by the individual. In general, personal decisions and habits that are bad, from a health point of view, create self-imposed risks. When these risks result in illness or death, the victim's life style can be said to have contributed to, or caused, his or her own illness or death. Because behaviors can be chosen, one's life style is the most important determiner of optimal well-being.

The organization of health care consists of the quality, quantity, arrangement, and relationships of people and resources in the provision of health care. It includes medicare practice, nursing, hospitals, nursing homes, medical drugs, public and community health care services, ambulances, dental treatment, and other health services such as optometry, chiropractics, and podiatry. Until now, most of society's efforts to improve health and the bulk of direct health expenditures have been focused on the health care organization. Yet, when we identify the present main causes of sickness and death in the United States and Canada, we find that they are rooted in the other three determiners of personal well-being listed on page 8.

Most medical care in this country focuses on treatment instead of prevention. Vast sums of money are being spent on treating diseases (like cancer and heart disease) that could have been prevented in the first place. Presently, there is very little medical care payoff for the average well person, since doctors spend most of their time treating sick people. For example, only about 15 percent of the population receives 85 percent of the medical attention (9). In summary, the organization of health care in general is the least important of the four determiners of optimal well-being.

There is overwhelming evidence (7,9,10,11,14, 15,17,22,27,28,30,33) that life style is the major determiner of well-being. One only has to review the longevity and wellness studies comparing Americans to the people living in Hunza land, the Himalayas and Vilcombaba, Ecuador, for instance, to realize that people living with right or proper life style attain a higher quality of wellness and are able to live well over the age of 100.

A 1974 research study at UCLA studied 7000 people and found that good habits of daily life were definitely related to health in general and longevity in particular (14:29). Adequate habits such as sleep and rest, not smoking, exercising regularly, eating moderately and regularly, and not being overweight, are cumulative habits extending life expectancy. The UCLA study concluded that humans who do almost everything wrong have an approximate average life span of 60 years. This is about half the human life expectancy of those humans who do everything right.

The UCLA study also concluded that five behaviors in the United States cause 80 percent of our health problems and diseases. (14)

1. Sedentary living.
2. Inadequate nutrition.
3. Smoking cigarettes.
4. Drinking alcoholic beverages.
5. Stress.

Eliminating or modifying these five behaviors ensures a high quality and quantity of health and contributes to longevity.

Realizing the magnanimous influence of life style on well-being, the Canadian government has spearheaded a national life style "fitness for Canadians" program. It is the only nationally sponsored and supported health program in the world that focuses on influencing wellness through a constructive life style.

In summary, life style (behaviors) and environmental influences are more significant than heredity and medical care in affecting one's well-being. Health is determined predominantly by the way one lives. One unconsciously adapts to a life style that predetermines either low-, average-, or high-level wellness and either a short, average, or long life expectancy.

LIFE STYLE AS A BASIS FOR WELL-BEING

One's life style evolves in an effort to fulfill one's needs. A person will be healthy if he or she fulfills most of the basic human needs. These needs are provided by life-support activities that keep us alive; they include exercising, eating, cleaning house, washing oneself, disposing properly of garbage and wastes, playing and socializing with friends, relaxing and resting, giving and receiving love, doing satisfying and worthwhile work, coping with problems of living, using safety devices and procedures to avoid injury and accidents, avoiding harmful food additives, and self-destructive substances such as cigarettes, coffee, soft drinks, and alcoholic bev-

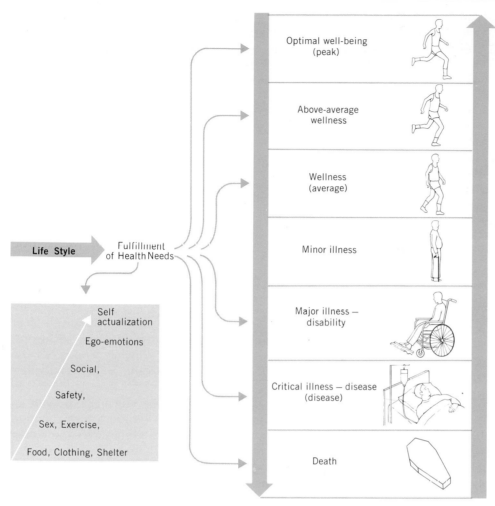

Figure 1.7
Illustration depicting relationships between life style, human health needs, optimal well-being, illness, disease, and death. Human health needs are those suggested by Maslow (physiological, safety, social, ego, and self-actualization). Maslow's needs have been translated by Sorochan as fitness components of well-being and are illustrated in Figure 1.3. Health, disease, and death are all a consequence of how human health needs are fulfilled. Needs, in turn, are fulfilled through life style.

erages. These examples are categorized by Maslow in his "Hierarchy of Human Needs." A person will be healthy if he or she fulfills most of these basic human needs. On the other hand, a person's life style may be characterized by self-destructive behaviors that may cause the person to become ill or disabled, or function at a lower level. These ideas are illustrated in Figure 1.7.

The idea of a right life style enhancing well-being is not a new one. Awareness of this possibility prompted Metchnikoff (3:141) at the turn of this century to suggest that there is a "right or proper style" of living that allows one to attain optimum health, thereby extending longevity. He called this mode of living "orthobiosis." It reflects how we conduct our lives each day, how we carry out the daily chores so essential to maintaining our

well-being. Orthobiosis implies constructive, responsible, abundant, fulfilling, purposeful, and prudent daily living as an individual and as a society.

In order to live properly, we must participate in constructive, life-sustaining behaviors. Selecting and discriminating among such behaviors requires values. Thus orthobiosis is characterized by behaviors, habits, and values. Values come into being when we need to interact with others. Values help us to set limits on what we can and cannot do. They help us to make decisions about health-related matters.

Orthobiosis is more important than health because health is a by-product of how we live. A right style of living is one that is constructive instead of destructive, salubrious instead of deleterious, healthy instead of sick,

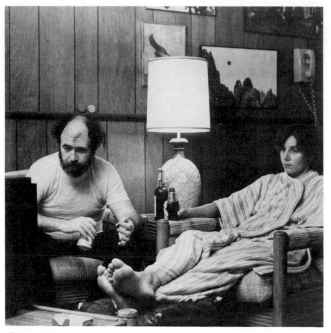

Figure 1.8

An example of a deleterious life style. What is wrong with this couple's life style?

adaptive instead of maladaptive, positive instead of negative, fulfilling and gratifying instead of frustrating, socially acceptable instead of socially rejectable, and worthwhile instead of worthless. A life style should provide opportunities for self-actualization. Obviously, one's life style needs a sense of balance and correctness for one to be an "orthobiot."

The obvious conclusion is that we all need to evolve a right or proper style of living early in life—the sooner the better. The ancient Romans chastised a man over 30 if he got sick, pointing out to him that he should have learned how to attain and maintain health. Being sick was a reflection of having failed to assume such responsibility early in life. So it should be with young people of college age today. The subsequent chapters of this book help you to assess the various dimensions of wellness, to "get your life style together," and to evolve a sound and rewarding orthobiosis. You should do everything you can to conserve your well-being now so that your present life style does not lead to chronic diseases in later life. Prevention is much less expensive and more rewarding than treatment of a health problem.

PURPOSE OF HEALTH

Health is a prerequisite for optimal living. One needs health to be able to earn a living, to study, to raise a family, to socialize with friends, and to actively participate in, and enjoy, music, sports, and other cultural arts. In-

deed, health touches every facet of living. There is no single element of political, economic, domestic, social, vocational, and professional life that does not require optimal well-being. Health, then, is a vehicle for accomplishment and achievement. It is essential for everyone.

PREVENTIVE LIFE STYLE

We stay healthy as long as our body organs and systems are able to function with ease in maintaining the body. When such functioning and/or maintenance is disrupted or interfered with, as by chemicals, stress, or bacteria, your body responds by activating your defense-alarm system. These responses or symptoms indicate that there is something wrong within your body or that there is something hazardous in the environment.

The body has a natural defense system to fight infection, illness, and distress. It is made up of (1) mechanical-chemical barriers, such as the skin, sweat cells, hair in the nose, cilia in the trachea, mucous secretions, saliva in the mouth, and tears; (2) white blood cells and megocytes inside the bloodstream; and (3) antibodies in the blood serum.

Nature has also provided the human body with an early warning system: nervous sensors to detect and to monitor hazardous conditions and substances, and their changes in the environment. These body sensors signal our defense system to prepare for battle, so to speak. For example, our eyes pick up light intensities and visual cues in the environment; our ears pick up irritating noise and air pressure changes; our nose picks up toxic odors; our mouth tastes potentially dangerous substances; our skin picks up pressure, texture, heat and cold variations, irritating chemicals, and dusts; and our semicircular canals detect our balance and orient us in space. Such a monitoring system sends continuous messages to the brain about our environment. When we are exposed to any of the aforementioned dangers, our body responds with signals, informing us that something is wrong— within our body, with how it is functioning, or with how it is coping with the life-threatening environment.

In addition to these outer body sensory diseases, our bodies also have internal, physical sensory organs for checking and regulating the internal body processes. These work much like a thermostat regulating the temperature in a house. A few examples of such blood-chemical regulatory mechanisms are the carotid sinuses in the neck, which check and regulate blood flow to the brain; the aortic bodies, which regulate blood flow to the aorta and arterial system; and the hypothalmus, which regulates moods of sadness and happiness, thirst, and hunger, the control of stress adaptation and glandular activities, and the maintenance of a constant body temperature, and the monitoring of chemicals, oxygen, and carbon dioxide in the bloodstream.

Your body continuously monitors your outer and inner body environments. When something is wrong or an inner body system malfunctions, the alarms are set off and the body defenses are set into motion. These warnings may include an array of any of the following (1;12;13;21;33):

1. Irritating eyes, squinting
2. Tears (burning or itching)
3. Hypersensitivity of the eyes to sunlight or strong light
4. Sneezing
5. Running nose
6. Stuffed-up nose
7. Coughing (throat irritation)
8. Ringing in ears
9. Discomfort in hearing or hearing problems
10. Earache
11. Itchy skin
12. Skin irritation
13. Fatigue
14. Stiff joints
15. Muscle spasms
16. Headache
17. Nausea (feeling sick or general discomfort)
18. Swollen glands
19. Fever
20. Nosebleed
21. Upset stomach
22. Vomiting
23. Flatulence (gas in colon)
24. Diarrhea
25. Constipation
26. Dizziness, vertigo
27. Inability to concentrate
28. Halitosis (bad breath)
29. Pain (e.g., side ache)
30. Feeling sad or depressed

These are your body's ways of telling you — warning you — that something is wrong within or outside your body, or that you have done something disagreeable or undesirable to your body. When you disregard your body's warnings and symptoms and allow them to persist, your body begins to feel uncomfortable and sick, to feel pain and to feel tired. More often than not, we take drugs to kill these feelings, thereby blocking off these sensory-monitoring devices. Drugs kill the pain but do not remove the cause of the problem. Anesthetizing these senses (as with alcohol, cigarette smoking, or antipain drugs) inhibits the body's ability to keep you healthy.

The most desirable way to cope with the early warnings of physiological discomfort and pain is to identify the initial cause that triggers the body alarms to go off. For example, a dust-allergic person should avoid working, visiting, playing, or living in dusty places. Such a person can relieve allergic symptoms by removing or trying to avoid dust. Similarly, a person who gets a headache should breathe some clean fresh air, get light-to-moderate exercise, and even lie down and sleep for several hours to relieve the physical tension causing the headache.

Dust as chemical substances in our external environment can cause the human alarm system to go off, so can an excess of chemical substances that we ingest or inhale. In most instances, one's liver will metabolize and detoxify these substances over a period of time. But the body needs time to do this and it is important to give the body the necessary time by resting and being inactive.

Although these few examples do not cover all the situations that trigger the body alarm system to go off, they do illustrate how we can listen to our body's warnings and how we can cope with pain, fatigue, discomfort, or nausea. The chapters that follow suggest many ways of coping with these health problems.

Further Readings

Dubos, Rene, *Mirage of Health,* Garden City, N.Y.: Doubleday, 1961.

Dunn, H. L., *High Level Wellness,* Washington, D. C.: Mt. Vernon, 1961.

Hoyman, H. S., "Our Modern Concepts of Health," *Journal of School Health,* September 1962, p. 253.

LaLonde, Marc, *A New Perspective on the Health of Canadians,* Ottawa, Canada: The Queen's Printer, 1974.

McKeown, Thomas, "Determinants of Health," *Human Nature,* April 1978, pp. 60–67.

Williams, Roger, *Nutrition Against Disease,* New York: Bantam Books, 1973.

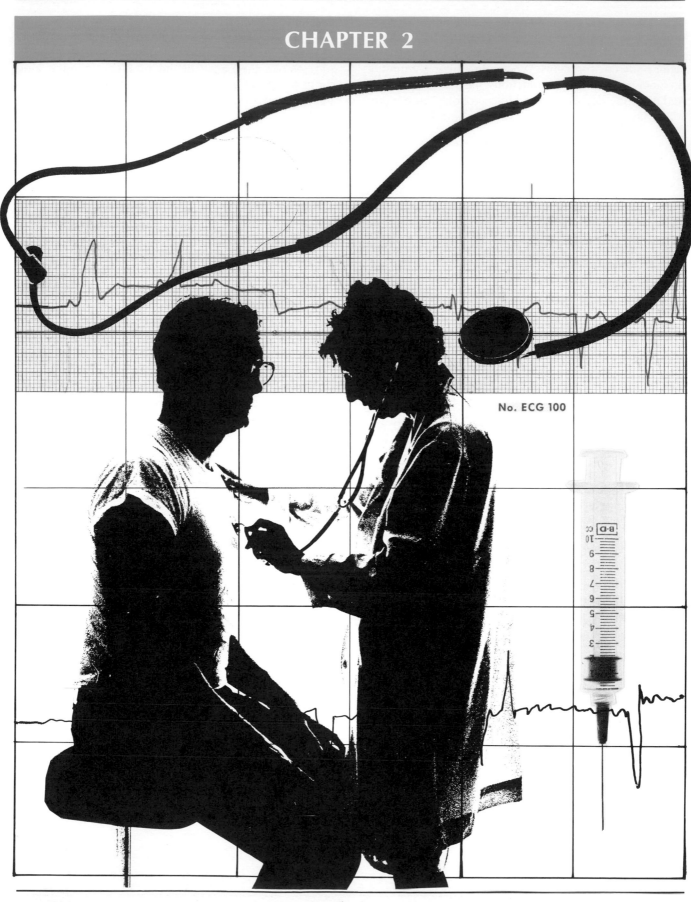

CHAPTER 2

No. ECG 100

A healthy person can be considered well when all five dimensions of his or her being are fulfilled optimally, and when he or she is free of disease or disability and is functioning optimally in society. One needs to get assurance that the potentials for optimal well-being exist. In the past, doctors gave a medical checkup or examination as a way of checking one's health status. Today, many doctors are questioning the value of annual physical examinations. An annual checkup in the past consisted mostly of a physical observation of the condition of the eyes, ears, nose, throat, mouth, skin, blood pressure, body reflexes, and breathing. Such a cursory examination did little to spot a hidden cancer, a heart disease, or other health problems that might be incubating. It neglected to analyze a person's diet and eating habits, drug use/misuse, alcohol intake, mood changes, and emotional and social problems, and other self-destructive behaviors that might contribute to early disease and premature death. Such physical examinations do not indicate one's level of well-being. Today, we have many sophisticated medical tests and technological devices, including the computer, that can analyze and instantly monitor physical well-being. Since well-being is a consequence of life style, we can also assess a person's life style and identify high risk habits and behaviors that, over a period of many years, are contributory causes to chronic diseases, disorders and disabilities, and early death. These diseases appear to incubate for 10 to 30 years before surfacing as a major disease or disorder.

This chapter will make you aware of what you can do to monitor and assess your health. The emphasis is on preventative medicine and keeping the well "you" healthy, not in treating you when you get sick or old.

☞ **SOCIAL READJUSTMENT RATING SCALE[1]**

DIRECTIONS Place a checkmark by the events listed in the Susceptability to Life — Change and Illness Scale that happened to you during the past year.

SCORING The value column opposite each life event gives it a numerically weighted value from 11 to 100. Total the values for all life-event changes you have experienced for a given year. This is your life-change score for the year.

[1] I am grateful to Dr. Thomas Holmes, Professor of Psychiatry at the University of Washington, for his reactions to this instrument and for granting his permission to adapt his Social Readjustment Rating Scale. Adapted from Thomas Holmes, and R. H. Rahe, "The Social Readjustment Rating Scale," Journal of Psychosomatic Research, 11:213–218, 1967.

Year

Life Event	Value	1980	1981	1982	1983	1984	1985	1986	1987	1988	1989	1990
Death of spouse	100											
Divorce	73											
Marital separation	65											
Jail term	63											
Death of close family member	63											
Personal injury or illness	53											
Marriage	50											
Fired at work	47											
Marital reconciliation	45											
Retirement	45											
Change in health of family member	44											
Pregnancy	40											
Sex difficulties	39											
Gain of new family member	39											
Change in financial state	38											
Death of close friend	37											
Change to different line of work	36											
Change in number of arguments with spouse	35											
Mortgage over $10,000	31											
Foreclosure of mortgage or loan	30											

		Year										
Life Event	Value	1980	1981	1982	1983	1984	1985	1986	1987	1988	1989	1990
Change in responsibilities at work	29											
Son or daughter leaving home	29											
Trouble with in-laws	29											
Outstanding personal achievement	28											
Wife beginning or stopping work	26											
Beginning or ending school	26											
Revision of personal habits	24											
Trouble with boss	23											
Change in work hours or conditions	20											
Change in residence	20											
Change in schools	20											
Change in recreation	19											
Change in social activities	18											
Mortgage or loan less than $10,000	17											
Change in sleeping habits	16											
Change in number of family get-togethers	15											
Change in eating habits	15											
Vacation	13											
Minor violations of the law	11											
	Total											

INTERPRETATION OF SCORES

Refer to the score range below to classify your life-change score.

Score Range	Interpretation	Susceptibility
300+	Major life change	Poor grades, major illness within year
250–229	Serious life change	Lowered resistance to diseases
200–249	Moderate life change	Depression
150–199	Mild life change	Colds, flus, occasional depression
149–0	Very little life change	Good health

Any great change—even a pleasant change—produces stress in human beings. That is the implication, at least, of a study recently reported to the American Association for the Advancement of Science by Dr. Thomas Holmes, Professor of Psychiatry at the University of Washington in Seattle. Furthermore, Holmes found that too many changes, coming too close together, often produce grave illness or absymal depression.

In the course of his investigation, Holmes devised a scale assigning point values to changes that often affect human beings. When enough of these occur within one year and add up to more than 300, trouble may lie ahead. In Holmes' survey, 80 percent of people who exceeded 300 became pathologically depressed, had heart attacks, or developed other serious ailments. Of scorers in the 250 to 300 range, 53 percent were similarly affected, as were 33 percent of those scoring up to 150.

A hypothetical example follows: John was married (50); as he had hoped, his wife became pregnant (40); she stopped working (26) and bore a son (39). John, who hated his work as a soap company chemist, found a better-paying job (39) as a teacher (36) in a college outside the city. After a vacation (13) to celebrate, he moved his family to the country (20), returned to the hunting and fishing (19) he had loved as a child, and began seeing a lot of his congenial new colleagues (18). Everything was so much better that he was even able to give up smoking (24). On the Holmes scale, these events total an ominous 323.

To arrive at his scoring system, Dr. Holmes assigned an arbitrary value of 50 to the act of getting married and then asked people in several countries to rank other changes in relation to marriage. For example, a person who thought that pregnancy represented a greater change than marriage was to assign to pregnancy a number higher than 50. To correlate change and health, Holmes kept a watch on 80 Seattle residents for two years and then compared their personal-change histories with their physical and mental ailments.

GENERAL OBSERVATIONS

1. A change in one's life is followed, about a year later, by associated health changes. Is this true of your life style?

2. Life changes tend to cluster significantly around health changes. Is this true in your case?

3. Academic performance (grade-point average) is inversely proportional to the amount of life change experienced. Was this true in your case?

4. Persons between 20 and 30 years of age display about 50 percent more life changes per person than those between 45 and 60, and twice as many as those over 60 years of age. Compare your changes to that of other persons of various ages and try to verify this research observation.

5. The greater the life change or adaptive requirements, the greater the vulnerability or lowering of resistance to disease, and the more serious the disease that does develop. Life-change events lower your body resistance to disease. Review your record of illnesses and relate them to life changes. This may be plotted on Graph 2.1. Also see the figures that follow the graph.

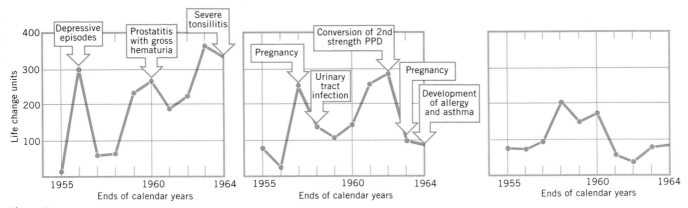

Figure B.

Examples of life change profiles over a 10-year period. These examples graphically illustrate a life crisis and major health change for three different persons. (a) A profile of a male's depressive episodes in 1956 coinciding with life crisis, whereas his episodes of prostatis in 1960 and tonsilitis in 1964 occured about 1 year after the appearance of the life crisis with which they were associated. (b) an example of multiple health changes associated with two life crises of major magnitude, and (c) a profile of a person who reported no major health changes during the past 10 years. (With permission from Richard H. Rahe, *Life Crisis and Health Changes.* U.S. Navy Bureau of Medicine and Surgery, February 1967, pp. 103-105, and from P. R. A. May and J. R. W. Wittenbern, eds., Psychotropic Drug Responces: Advances in Prediction, courtesy of Charles C. Thomas Publisher, Springfield, Ill. 1969, pp. 103 and 105.)

Consult with your health science instructor on how to minimize life changes in the future. Dr. Holmes suggests that physical and emotional illnesses may be prevented by counseling susceptible people not to make too many life changes in too short a time.

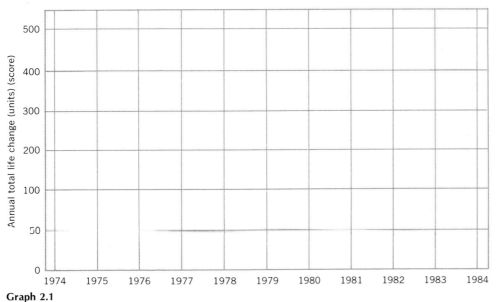

Graph 2.1

Profile of annual occurrence of total life changes over a period of 10 years. Plot your annual total life change score each year on this graph. Join the yearly plotted scores by a line. Doing this gives you a visual and analytical picture of whether you are experiencing many life changes and whether these changes relate to your illnesses during that time. Compare your profile to those in Figure 1.

☞ LIFETIME IMMUNIZATIONS RECORD

You should keep a lifetime record of all your immunizations and vaccinations. Ask your parents to help you.

DIRECTIONS   Opposite a disease that you have been immunized against, write the number of the month, date, and year you received the immunization in the appropriate age column.

Keep this record updated each time you have shots in the future, since time blurs total recall. Keep a similar record for all of your family members; this kind of information is often valuable for your doctor.

Consult with your local city or county Public Health Department for recommended immunizations and booster shots. These change periodically. With many people traveling internationally, it is important to record all the immunizations you have had.

Age When You Had Inoculation

Communicable Disease Infection	1–4	5–9	10–14	15–19	20–30	31–40	41–50	51–60	61–70	71–80
1. Cholera										
2. Colds										
3. Diphtheria										
4. Flu										
5. Malaria										
6. Measles (German)										
7. Measles (rubella)										
8. Mumps										
9. Pertussis (whooping cough)										
10. Plague										
11. Poliomyelitis (oral or trivalent)										
12. Smallpox										
13. Tetanus										
14. Typhoid fever										
15. Typhus										

16. Yellow fever											
17. Tuberculosis											
18.											
19.											
20.											

☞ PREVIOUS ILLNESS RECORD

PURPOSE

1. To help you keep a record of your previous illnesses, infections, surgery, medications, medical-psychiatric treatments and counseling, and your allergies.
2. To make you aware that previous illnesses, infections, medical-surgery, medications, and allergies limit and may affect your potentials for optimal well-being.

INTRODUCTION

An illness record is a vital part of your health-illness history.

Most of us find it embarrassing not being able to recall whether we were sick from measles, mumps, strep throat, or the age at which we were sick. Quite often our parents did not keep any family health records and, with the lapse of time, they cannot accurately recall such information. Such information (as part of family health records) may save your life in the future. Such information can be crucial in an emergency and can be very important even in a routine consultation, since it will help the doctor avoid prescribing a drug that may interact adversely with one that is already being taken. Its greatest benefit may be for your children as yet unborn. Genetic family counselors can make excellent use of such records.

A record of your previous illnesses, surgery medications, and allergies provides your doctor with a more complete history of your health. It may alert him to early symptoms in time to avert an advanced stage of a disease or resulting disability. Even common childhood disease should be recorded, since they sometimes have more serious—although rare—later effects.

Have your parents and family physician verify your illness records. Keep these records up to date. Your age when the disease first appeared is relevant to the form or severity of some disorders and should be recorded. It is also advisable to note your occupation at the time of an infection, since some occupations expose workers to environmental factors that affect health.

It is also important to note a history of good health—that is, freedom from infection, illness, allergies, and disorders.

The illnesses below may be identified or may have occurred in relationship when you:

1. Were treated by a physician, by your family, or by a friend.
2. Had consultation with a psychiatrist.
3. Visited a counselor.

4. Were hospitalized.
5. Were taking medication.
6. Visited a dentist.
7. Stayed home in bed.
8. Missed work or school because of illness.

DIRECTIONS: Identify each illness, allergy, and the like, that you have experienced in your lifetime by writing the dates when these occurred. Update these records whenever illness occurs and at regular intervals (at least once a year).

Illness (Disease)	*Date Illness Occurred*
A. Infectious Diseases	
Cold	
Influenza	
Mumps	
Measles (2-week)	
Measles (German-3 week)	
Polio	
Syphilis	
Gonorrhea	
Diphtheria	
Smallpox	
Chicken pox	
Rheumatic fever	
Malaria	
Mononucleosis	
Infectious hepatitis	
Rabies	
Yellow fever	
Strep throat	

Illness (Disease)	Date Illness Occurred
Scarlet fever	
Tetanus	
Tuberculosis	
Whooping cough	
Diarrhea (dysentery)	
Typhus fever	
Cholera	
Typhoid fever	
Plague	
Bronchitis	

Allergy	Date Allergy Occurred
B. Allergic Reactions	
Hay fever (pollen dusts)	
Ragweed	
Hives	
Foods	
Animals	
Poison ivy, poison oak, sumac, and the like	
Dust	
Feathers	
Molds	
Insect stings	
Fish stings	
Asthma	
Other	

Surgery	Date of Surgery	Physician
C. Surgery on Body		
Skin		
Tonsil (adenoids)		
Eye		
Ear		
Nose		
Throat		
Breast		
Lung		
Appendix		
Kidney		
Bladder		
Prostate		
Testicle or penis		
Uterus or vagina		
Bone		
Joint		
Blood vessels		
Brain		
Hernia (rupture)		
Hemorrhoid (piles)		
Stomach or intestine		
Colon or rectum		
Gall bladder		
Other		

Treatment	Date of Treatment	Physician
D. Medical-Drug Treatment or Surgery		
Hernia		
Leukemia		
Cancer		
Hodgkins disease		
Syphilis or gonorrhea		
Breast cancer		
Cervical cancer		
Heart disease		
Stroke		
Varicose veins		
Anemia		
Diabetes		
High blood pressure		
Epilepsy		
Kidney disease		
Emphysema		
Arthritis or rheumatism		
Cataract (eye)		
Overweight (obesity)		
Gallstones		
Kidney or bladder infection		
Menstruation		
Other		

Treatment	Date of Treatment	Physician
E. Medical-Psychiatric Treatment-Counseling		
Headache		
Nervous breakdown		
Alcoholism		
Use of drugs		
Excessive worry		
Attempted suicide		
Depression		
Drug use		
Sexual difficulties		
Other		

Graph 2.2 is included to help you plot your systolic and diastolic blood pressures separately over a period of 10 years. By joining the annual plots, you can make a profile of your blood pressure and obtain a baseline average or norm for yourself.

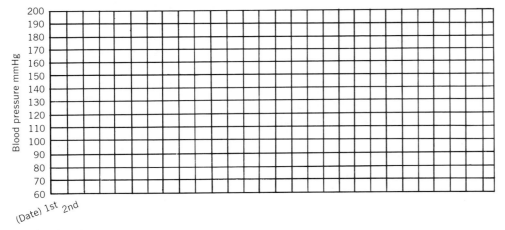

Graph 2.2

Comparison of systolic and diastolic blood pressures over a 3-month period for _____ (name), _____ (age), _____ (sex). The solid line (—) represents systolic blood pressure while the broken line (---) represents diastolic blood pressure. *Note:* This graph may also be used to record your blood pressure over a 10-year period or longer.

PHYSICAL EXAMINATION

Although many physicians are no longer advocating annual medical checkups, it is suggested that you get such an examination while in good health and before you are 25 years of age. You and your doctor can use this information as a baseline for future reference. For example, the doctor can compare your initial blood pressure and initial intraocular eye tension with what these would be at age 30, 40, 50, and so on, or this information about you in a healthy state may be compared to you in a possible diseased state later on in life. Such information could also be most valuable in establishing an individual norm for you rather than comparing you to a national norm. Establishing a base-line health reference should become an accepted medical practice in the future when the public and medical profession accept the concept of biochemical individuality (see Table 2.1).

Other baseline tests and health checks that may be performed at the same time as the medical checkup follow.

Chest X Ray. Most often the chest X ray is used to detect broken bones, lung cancer, and emphysema. If an individual smokes over one-half a pack of cigarettes daily and has been doing so for at least 10 years, then an X ray every 6 months may be in order. This may also be true of occupational workers. But for light smokers and nonsmokers, an annual chest X ray may be a waste of time and an unnecessary exposure to radiation.

Electrocardiogram (EKG). Most healthy persons do not need a routine EKG, which is a tracing of how the heart performs. It is much less expensive and easier to use blood pressure and serum/triglycerides as indicators of heart disease or hypertensive heart disease.

As with a chest X ray, one electrocardiogram should be taken while you are in good health and 18 to 20 years old for future reference. The best way to assess the cardiovascular system and its ability to cope with stress is to take the treadmill-EKG test. This test uses the treadmill to stress the heart while the EKG assesses the heart's ability to handle such stress.

Body Fat. Body fat is a more accurate indicator of health than body weight. Most physicians are unaware of this. The most accurate method of determining a healthy weight is to carefully assess body fat and not compare your body weight to a height-weight table. The percent of body fat may easily be predicted by a biannual pinch test. Females should consider themselves overweight if their waistlines are ¾ inch or more thick,

Table 2.1

Suggested Intervals for Health Evaluations[1]

Time	Frequency	Kind
Birth through 12 months	4–5 months	General physical
13 through 24 months	Every 6 months	General physical
Ages 2 through 4	Every year	General physical
Ages 5 through 18	Every 2-3 years	General physical, Nutrition, development, emotional well-being, hemoglobin + blood, blood glucose, and body fat
Ages 19 through 35	Every 4 years	General physical, gastric analysis/gastric acid, nutrition/diet, breast examination, emotional + depression, hemoglobin, baseline for blood tests (SMAC), health risk appraisal, pelvic test and Pap smear in women
Ages 36 through 45	Every 3 years	All of the above, and tonometry (glaucoma), and guaiac test (blood in stools)
Ages 46 through 55	Every 2 years	All of the above, prostoscopy or rectal examination in men and women, prostate exam in men, pelvic exam in women
Ages 56 and over	Every year or as recommended by doctor	All of the above

Source: Adapted from ''Planning for Health'' (Bulletin), Kaiser Permanente Medical Care Program, Spring 1978, p. 5.

and men $\frac{1}{2}$ inch or more thick; and both males and females should consider themselves obese if skinfold measures over an inch. A more precise skin-fold technique is suggested in Chapter 6.

Blood Pressure. Blood pressure is a popular indicator of well-being. Blood pressure is the force exerted against the walls of blood vessels by the blood flowing through them. This pressure is highest in the arteries and drops sharply in the smallest branches (arterioles) in the capillary areas and is lowest in the veins returning ''used'' blood to the heart. The pressure is constantly maintained by the pumping action (heartbeat) of the heart and by the constriction of the elastic walls of the arteries which maintain a constant blood pressure between heartbeats (see Figure 2.1).

Blood pressure in arteries is normally expressed in millimeters of mercury (mm Hg). The measurement consists of two numbers. The higher of the two is recorded during the heart's pumping stroke or systole and is called the systolic blood pressure. The lower number represents the actual pressure prevailing while the heart relaxes between beats and is called the diastolic pressure. Thus a measurement of 120/80 mm Hg means that the systolic pressure is 120 mm Hg, while the bottom figure of 80 mm Hg is the diastolic pressure.

There are numerous devices available to measure blood pressure. All of these work on the principle of the traditional sphygmomanometer, which has an inflatable cuff attached to a mercury meter.

Arterial blood pressure is affected by many conditions, such as emotions, increased rigidity or tension of the body, physical exertion or exercise, anxiety, emotional stress, meals, tobacco, bladder distension, drugs, climatic variation, and pain. It can occur in children, adolescents, and young adults. It is natural for systolic blood pressure to get higher in healthy older subjects until about 45 to 50, when it gets lower again.

Blood pressure, like blood and urine chemical values, is a personal value and is not fixed or constant. It is usually meaningless to compare your blood pressure to a national norm. There are many reasons for this rationale.

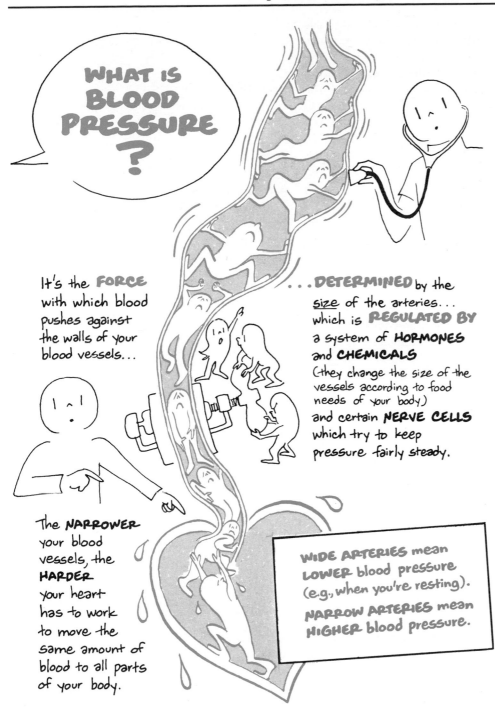

It's the **FORCE** with which blood pushes against the walls of your blood vessels...

...**DETERMINED** by the size of the arteries... which is **REGULATED BY** a system of **HORMONES** and **CHEMICALS** (they change the size of the vessels according to food needs of your body) and certain **NERVE CELLS** which try to keep pressure fairly steady.

The **NARROWER** your blood vessels, the **HARDER** your heart has to work to move the same amount of blood to all parts of your body.

WIDE ARTERIES mean LOWER blood pressure (e.g., when you're resting). NARROW ARTERIES mean HIGHER blood pressure.

Figure 2.1
Animated explanation of blood pressure. (Illustrations have been taken from "The Scriptographic Booklet," *You and Your Blood Pressure*, available from the Channing L. Bete Co., Greenfield, Mass. 01301. Copyright © 1975, Channing L. Bete Co., Inc. All rights reserved, reproduction in whole or in part prohibited without the express written consent of the Channing L. Bete Co., Inc.)

Blood pressure changes from minute to minute with what you do—it is affected by your internal and your external environments. Instead of comparing your personal values to a national or normal range, it is more meaningful to measure and record your blood pressure daily for a month or so (refer to Graph 2.2). By doing so, you can establish a normal range for yourself that may be used as a norm for you.

When recorded in a relaxed, resting young person, normal systolic pressure is around 120 mm Hg; normal diastolic pressure is around 80. This is written as 120/80. However, blood pressures somewhat above or below these values are also considered normal. For example, a blood pressure of 140/90 is within the normal range, whereas 150/95 is a little high. Systolic pressure tends to increase with age in healthy persons and in both sexes.

Many persons may record low blood pressure. Usually, it is considered an asset, placing less strain on the arterial system. Life insurance studies indicate that blood pressures below 110/70 are optimal for a long life span.

Physicians are more concerned about interpreting the bottom figure or diastolic instead of the systolic figure. Since diastolic pressure reflects the blood flow through arteries and capillaries, it reflects the pressure in the arteries when the heart is relaxed—between beats. Although 160/95 has been considered by most medical authorities as the cutoff point between normal and high blood pressure, many physicians are becoming concerned over a persistent elevation above 140/90. Insurance statistics clearly indicate that blood pressures above that level increase the chances of premature death. Thus, if a person's diastolic pressure (the bottom number) registers between 90 and 104 on three readings, one should suspect the possibility of hypertension. Systolic and diastolic blood pressures should be interpreted separately, since the conditions and circumstances causing each are different.

Tables 2.2 and 2.3 provide a guide for interpreting diastolic and systolic blood pressure. Refer to the inventory on susceptibility to cardiovascular disorders for an interpretation of the causes of hypertension or high blood pressure.

Emotional Well-Being. This is perhaps the most overlooked assessment, since depression and the inability to perform optimally in the job and society are probably greater health problems in this country than heart disease and cancer. You should identify your level of emotional well-being, including your tolerance to stress level, swings in moods, susceptibility to depression, the ability to cope with problems or crises of living, and the ability to function in society. Psychological health is just as important as physiological well-being. You should identify a baseline level of emotional well-being, and thereafter assess your emotional well-being as often as you and your doctor feel necessary. An emotional well-being inventory may be found in Chapter 3.

Holmes–Rahe Social Readjustment Rating Scale. This scale helps you to become aware that too many changes coming too close together can generate too much stress, resulting in grave illness or depression. Health changes tend to cluster significantly around life changes. Persons at age 20 display about 50 percent more life changes than they do after age 30. The greater the change in life,

Table 2.2

Guide to Interpretation of Diastolic Blood Pressure

140	
135	
130	**Severe Hypertension**
125	Organ damage is accelerated. Drugs can reverse
120	some effects and may prevent further damage.
115	
110	**Moderate Hypertension**
105	At 105 or above, drug treatment should begin.
100	**Mild Hypertension**
95	Drug treatment may begin. Have pressure
90	checked at least three times yearly.
85	
80	**Normal Blood Pressure**
75	Keep a record of them.
70	
65	

Source: With permission from *Consumer's Report,* October 1974, p. 735. Copyright © 1974 by Consumer's Union of the United States, Inc., Mount Vernon, N.Y. Note: When the heart is relaxed, between beats, the pressure in the arteries is known as the diastolic blood pressure. In the numerical fraction that expresses blood pressure—e.g., 120/80—the diastolic pressure is the bottom figure.

Table 2.3

Guide to Interpretation of Systolic Blood Pressure

CVD Risk Level	Systolic (Upper) Blood Pressure	Category
1	100 or less	Very low risk
2	101–120	Below-average risk
3	121–140	Average risk
4	141–160	Above-average risk
5	161–180	High risk
6	181–200	Very-high risk

Source: P. Kuhne, "High Blood Pressure," *Home Medical Encyclopedia,* London, Faber & Faber, 1960, pp. 57–58.

the greater the vulnerability to, or lowered resistance to, disease and illness. You should assess your life style changes once a year and keep a diary of this each year. (Respond to the scale at the beginning of this chapter.)

Heredity Checklist. You should identify the diseases and disorders that your relatives have had or died from. If your father, mother, sister, brother, or other relatives have or had a disease, there is a chance that you may have a genetic predisposition to it. Many diseases and disorders run in families. This information will also be useful for genetic counseling and predicting the chances of your children having diseases or disorders. Identify the incidence of hereditary disorders in your family before age 20. This checklist is included in Chapter 16.

Previous Illness-Immunization Record. Record all illnesses, as well as immunizations and surgery that you have each year. Such information should be part of your medical-health history. Unfortunately, since one out of every five Americans moves each year, such records are often lost or forgotten. Such information can be crucial in an emergency and can be very important in a routine medical-psychological consultation. Its greatest benefit may be for your children. The illness record may be found at the beginning of this chapter (Table 2.1).

Other Appraisals. Other baseline well-being appraisals are interspersed throughout the remainder of this book. Perhaps the most important baseline assessment of all is diet analysis and what you eat. Are you eating a balanced diet consisting of vitamins; minerals; amino acids; low fat intake; appropriate calorie food intake; low salt intake; and low or no refined sugar, refined white flour, and refined cereal products foods? You should assess your diet and eating habits once a year. This is more important than checking your weight.

Since the number one cause of death for college age persons is accidents, you should also assess your susceptibility to accidents in Chapter 12.

Biochemical Tests. Biochemical tests measure the amount of a chemical substance in blood or urine. These tests are usually performed as an aid in the diagnosis and management of various disorders and diseases. However, these tests can also be used to keep a well person healthy. Blood represents those nutrients actually absorbed from the digestive tract and made available to the cells. The lack of nutrients in the blood is a cue to their rate of absorption and utilization or the lack of one or both of these.

Biochemical tests are usually included in a battery of diagnostic tests in multiphasic screening programs. Multiphasic screening includes such assessments as cardiovascular, blood pressure and pulmonary functions, tuberculosis screening, the pap smear for cancer, and so on. Multiphasic screening has been used to screen masses of people in a community in an effort to identify persons unaware of a health problem, who may be incubating a disease.

Biochemical tests are used frequently to help diagnose an ill person. You should be acquainted with these tests so that you can understand not only the value of such tests in diagnosis and treatment, but also be able to communicate intelligently about test results with your physician.

Table 2.4 summarizes the normal values for each test and the diagnostic uses of a test.

Interpretation of Biochemical Tests. Biochemical tests measure the amount of a chemical substance in blood or urine. For example, when a sample of blood is analyzed for cholesterol, the minute amounts of cholesterol are identified in the sample weight or volume of blood. Thus we express the measurement of cholesterol in blood as milligrams of cholesterol in one deciliter (100 milliliters) of blood. This is usually expressed as milligrams percent or abbreviated as mg%. Since percent means parts per hundred by weight, we are expressing the amount of weight of cholesterol in a given volume of blood. Milligrams percent, then, is a unit of measure.

Table 2.4

Biochemical Values[a]

Chemical Substance	Normal Values	Diagnostic Purpose
1. Albumin[b]	3.2–4.5 gm% (fractionation)	Liver disease
	3.2–5.6 gm% (electrophoresis)	Malnutrition
	3.8–5.0 gm% (dye binding)	
2. Bilirubin[b]		Cirrhosis liver disorders
Direct	0.2–0.3 mg%	Gallbladder and pancreas disorders
Total	0.1–1.2 mg%	Excess breakdown of RBC jaundice
3. BUN[b]	8–18 mg%	Kidney function
(blood urea nitrogen)		Liver function (hepatitis, cirrhosis)
		Hypertension
4. Calcium[b]		Thyroid function
Ionized	4.2–5.2 mg%	Bone cancer
Total	9.0–10.6 mg%	Rickets malnutrition

Chemical Substance	Normal Values	Diagnostic Purpose
5. Cholesterol[b]		Atheroselerosis
Esters	65–75 of total	Arteriosclerosis
Total	150–250 mg%	Diet check, obesity
		Hypertension and stress
		Thyroid function
		Liver function
6. Creatinine[b,c]	0.6–1.2 mg%	Kidney function/disease
		Hypertension
7. Glucose[b,c]		Diabetes stress
Fasting	70–110 mg%[d]	Liver disease
Tolerance	70–110 mg%	Adrenal function
		Tumor in pancreas
8. LDH (WU)[b]		Liver damage (cirrhosis, hepatitis)
Lactic dehydrogenase		
9. Phosphorus[b]		Liver disease
(Alkali)	1.8–2.6 meq/l	Thyroid function
Inorganic[b]	3.0–4.5 mg%	Bone diseases
		Malnutrition
		Bright's disease
10. Sodium[b]	136–142 meq/l	Kidney function/disease
		Arteriosclerosis
		Adrenal gland function
		Diabetes
11. Thyroxine[b]		Thyroid gland function
Column	5.0–11.0mg%	
Murphy-Pattee	6.0–11.8 mg%	
12. TP[b]		Liver disease
(total protein)	6.0–7.8 mg%	Infection
		Malnutrition
13. Transaminases[b]		Liver disease (cirrhosis)
SGOT (serum glutamic (oxalacetic) (aspartic acid)	8–33 U/ml	Cardiac disease
		Pancreas function
		Bone tumor
SGPT (serum glutamic pyruvic) (alanine)	1–36 U/ml	Liver function (cirrhosis)
		Heart damage
14. Triglycerides[b]	10–190 mg%	Arterial diseases (arteriosclerosis)
		Malnutrition
		Lipid metabolism disorders
15. Uric acid[b]	Male 2.1–7.8 mg%	Gout, alcoholism, stress, adrenal gland function, liver damage in true toxemia of pregnancy
	Female 2.0–6.4 mg%	
16. VDRL[b]		Syphilis, infectious mononucleosis, collagen disease
17. Hematology		Blood diseases and disorders
Hematocrit		
Female	36–47 ml/100 ml	
Male	40–54 ml/100 ml	

Chemical Substance	Normal Values	Diagnostic Purpose
Hemoglobin		Anemia
Female	12.0–16.0 gm	
Male	14.0–18.0	
Red cell count (RBC)		
Female	4.0–5.6 millions/ul	Anemia
Male	4.5–6.5 millions/ul	Anemia
White cell count (WBC)		
Female	4.0–11.0 cells/ul	Leukemia, respiratory infections,
Male		stress
Prothrombin time	10–15 seconds	
		Clotting time
		Malnutrition
18. Urinanalysis (urine)		
(i) Glucose	1–15 mg%	
		Diabetes
(clinic test)		Thyroid function
(clinistix)		Liver function
(ii) Ketones		
(ketostix)		
(iii) Protein		Kidney function
(labstix)		
(iv) Microorganisms	10,000–100,000l/m	
		Kidney bladder infection
(v) Specific gravity	1.003–1.020	
		Diabetes
		Kidney function

[a] References consulted are those listed in the reference for this section. Averages range values are for combined population.
[b] Blood serum.
[c] Blood plasma.
[d] Normal values for glucose vary with postprandial time sequence.

Most biochemical tests use this unit of measure. Other measures, such as meq/1 or U/ml are similar units of measure.[1]

The interpretation of the results of a biochemical test is often based on why the test was taken. Such tests have traditionally been used to help a physican diagnose and treat a disease in a sick person. Biochemical values in such instances may be interpreted differently as compared to those values obtained from a well person. Instead of diagnosis or treatment, tests administered to well people are used to detect organ or body system malfunction, disorder, or disease. Such tests can be most useful in confirming that a person is well. As confirmations of good health, these tests can motivate health maintenance. On the other hand, a high cholesterol level may lead to assessment of life-style behaviors such as diet and situations creating stress. Those with elevated blood cholesterol would be wise to modify or change their eating habits and stress-coping behaviors. Obviously, biochemical tests provide a basis for assessing one's behaviors and life style. A course of action, such as behavior modification, should be prescribed as a follow-up to such tests.

Biochemical tests can be used in various ways. A review of these tests may provide further insight in interpreting such tests. Some tests have no significance other than to indicate diagnosis, for example, the glucose tolerance test. Should the result of such a test indicate the presence of diabetes, the test is of no further use in regulating treatment.

Many tests can be useful in following the course of a disease or in adjusting therapy. An example of the latter is the test for prothrombin time. In treatment with Dicumarol and similar drugs, tests for prothrombin time are performed daily to aid in prescribing the correct dose of the drug Dicumarol for the current day.

One should be aware that the origin of the test material does not always correspond to the organ or system

[1] meq/1 — milliequivalents per liter (a molecular amount reacting with an amount of something else); U/ml — international units per milliliter.

being examined. For example, a test may be performed on urine to obtain information on liver function.

Biochemical tests are also useful in diagnosing diseases of more than one organ or body system.

There is no standard or common approach to interpreting biochemical tests at the present time. Value ranges may vary within a person not only during a day, but also from day to day. Values have also been found to vary between populations or groups.

Values may vary according to age, sex, diet, drug intake, activity, geographic region, occupation, the presence of a disease or disorder, genetic factors, and the time of day that the blood or urine sample is taken. Thus interpreting test results on the basis of "normalcy" may be very misleading. Adding to the difficulty of interpretation is the kind of laboratory equipment and technology used to perform the test. A comparison of various biochemical normal values in various textbooks and laboratories reveals that normal values vary from laboratory to laboratory, depending on the equipment and diagnostic techniques used.

Before making judgment on individual test results, it is essential to check the normal values established by the laboratory performing the tests. The average values of one age group or region may not be applicable to another group. It is preferable to have each group compared against its own sample values and then examine such values for trends over a period of time. Thus, the values in this section are presented as a guide. Abnormal values on a test should always be confirmed by redoing the test.

In order to properly interpret a person's tests, it is suggested that he or she take a battery of tests while young and in good health. The tests should be repeated periodically. This procedure has the advantage of establishing baseline, normal biochemical values for the individual. These values can be compared from time to time and can be of great diagnostic aid when compared to test values obtained when life-style changes occur or when a person develops an illness.

Automated instruments are available for laboratory analysis of blood and urine samples. An example of such an instrument is the Autoanalyzer, referred to as the SMA (sequential multiple analysis).[2] The instrument is equipped with a printout mechanism that records 12 or more results on a graph form. A sample copy[3] of a graph-form printout, SMAC (sequential multiple analysis computerized) is included here (see Figure 2.2). The recording form includes light areas indicating normal ranges. A person's values for each test are plotted on the graph, thus making a profile that helps one to quickly interpret

[2] Autoanalyzer is a product of Technician Corporation, Tarrytown, N.Y.
[3] Courtesy of Interhealth, San Diego, Calif.

the results. The cost of doing a blood chemistry is relatively inexpensive if done by the Autoanalyzer. Costs range from $10 to $40.

Finally, a word of caution about interpreting values as norms. Nonmedical persons should let their doctor make the diagnosis and let him help with the interpretation of test results. The values in this section should be used as a guide and are not intended to license the college student to self-medicate and practice medicine.

It is hoped that the information in this section will provide the reader with the background to be able to communicate with medical-hospital personnel, to make better use of medical services, to become motivated to maintain optimal well-being, and to use the results of biochemical tests to direct intelligent self-behavior.

BIOCHEMICAL TESTS

Albumin. Albumin is a major component in blood proteins, and is found in blood and urine. It contributes to the balance of osmotic pressure between the blood and tissues. When this test is performed, along with the tests for globulin (A/G ratio) and total protein, liver, and kidney functions can be evaluated. See the section on "Total Protein."

Bilirubin. This is a product of the breakdown of hemoglobin. Since bilirubin is removed from the blood by the liver, this test is an important measure of liver function. Free bilirubin (indirect) is bound to albumin, a plasma protein. It is not soluble in water and hence cannot be excreted or tested for in the urine. It is a major contributor to the clinical signs of jaundice.

The direct form (conjugated bilirubin) is bilirubin which, through the action of the liver, has glucuronic acid or sulfate attached to the basic structure of its molecule. It is water-soluble and is therefore excreted in the urine unaltered. The direct or total form of bilirubin can be assessed by blood serum or urine sample tests.

Blood Urea Nitrogen (BUN). Urea is the chief end product of protein metabolism in the liver. Urea, a nitrogen-containing substance, is also a major excretory product of the kidneys. The test detects the nitrogen part of the urea in blood and helps to detect kidney damage and kidney disease.

Calcium. This mineral is essential to the formation of bony tissue, muscular activity, and blood coagulation mechanism.

Cholesterol. This is an alcohol derived from the breakdown of fats in the liver. Body cells also produce cholesterol in minute amounts. (Large amounts of cholesterol are also found in animal meats.)

Two types of cholesterol are looked for in biochemi-

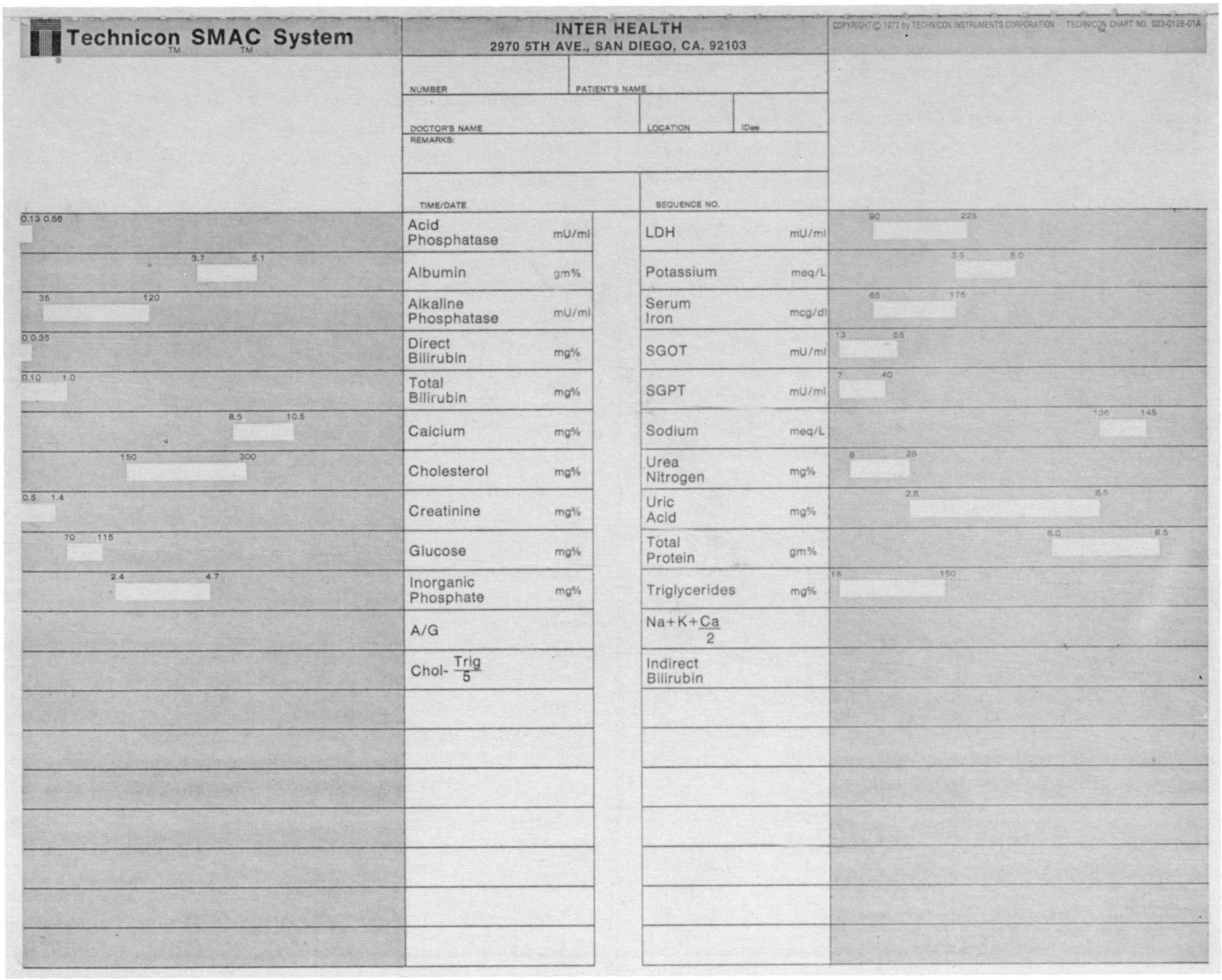

Technicon SMAC System ™ ™		INTER HEALTH 2970 5TH AVE., SAN DIEGO, CA. 92103			COPYRIGHT © 1973 by TECHNICON INSTRUMENTS CORPORATION TECHNICON CHART NO. 033-0128-01A
	NUMBER		PATIENT'S NAME		
	DOCTOR'S NAME REMARKS:		LOCATION	IDee	
	TIME/DATE		SEQUENCE NO.		
0.13 0.56	Acid Phosphatase	mU/ml	LDH	mU/ml	90 225
3.7 5.1	Albumin	gm%	Potassium	meq/L	3.5 5.0
35 120	Alkaline Phosphatase	mU/ml	Serum Iron	mcg/dl	65 175
0 0.35	Direct Bilirubin	mg%	SGOT	mU/ml	13 55
0.10 1.0	Total Bilirubin	mg%	SGPT	mU/ml	7 40
8.5 10.5	Calcium	mg%	Sodium	meq/L	136 145
150 300	Cholesterol	mg%	Urea Nitrogen	mg%	8 26
0.5 1.4	Creatinine	mg%	Uric Acid	mg%	2.5 8.5
70 115	Glucose	mg%	Total Protein	gm%	6.0 8.5
2.4 4.7	Inorganic Phosphate	mg%	Triglycerides	mg%	16 150
	A/G		$\frac{Na+K+Ca}{2}$		
	Chol- $\frac{Trig}{5}$		Indirect Bilirubin		

Figure 2.2

Sample copy of SMAC graph for recording results of automated biochemical tests. (Courtesy of Life Extens Institute Laboratory, San Diego, Cal., and Technicon Instruments Corporation, Tarrytown, N.Y., 10591.) (SMAC is the trademark of Technicon Corporation.)

cal tests. Cholesterol ester is the basic cholesterol compound modified at one position in the molecule to combine with other compounds. The free or uncombined cholesterol, plus the ester form, comprise total cholesterol. Thus, one test can be performed for the ester, and the other for total cholesterol.

Since the liver plays a prominent role in the metabolism and excretion of cholesterol, including its esterification, these compounds are tested for as part of liver function tests. The test results are also useful in assessing diet and stressful living.

Other organ interrelationships to cholesterol make it feasible to use the cholesterol test to assess bile function (free-form cholesterol is stored in the bile), and thyroid activity.

Creatinine. A protein (polypeptide) that is easily excreted by the kidney, creatinine is derived from the breakdown of muscle creatinine phosphate. An elevated blood creatinine level indicates a disorder of kidney function. This test complements the urea nitrogen test, since creatinine is produced by the body and excreted at a constant rate in the normal physiological state.

Glucose (Blood Sugar). A sugar found circulating in the blood, glucose is not present in normal urine. The burning up of glucose in muscles and organs is regulated by insulin. When there is not enough insulin in the body, the concentration of glucose in the blood increases, and vice versa. These two extreme metabolic disorders are forms of diabetes.

Since the amount of glucose in blood serum normally increases following a meal, it is important that the test be run only on fasting blood specimens.

Lactic Dehydrogenase (LDH). Lactic dehydrogenase are several enzymes found in blood serum and in several organs. They catalyze the reversible alteration between pyruvate and lactate. LDH is also present in nearly all metabolizing cells, but the highest concentrations occur in the liver, heart, skeletal muscles, and erythrocytes (red blood cells). Thus, damage to nearly any tissue can cause elevated serum LDH.

Phosphorus (Inorganic). A mineral whose function in the body is clearly related to that of calcium, phosphorus is essential in the storage and liberation of energy and in the intermediate metabolism of carbohydrates and lipids. Blood levels are measured in terms of phosphate ions (phosphorus combined with oxygen).

The test reflects physiological functions of many organs. The concentration may increase in severe kidney disease, hypoparathyroidism, and excessive vitamin intake; it may decrease in rickets, hyperparathyroidism, and certain kidney diseases.

Sodium. A mineral of extreme importance in maintaining water balance in the body. When taken in excess (as table salt in the diet) excess sodium is excreted by the kidney into urine. It has been implicated as a causative factor in cardiovascular disorders. Decreased sodium levels may occur in diarrhea, heat exhaustion, Addison's disease, and certain kidney disorders.

Thyroxine. The hormone thyroxine is made by the thyroid gland. This gland uses iodine in the synthesis of several hormones, one of which is serum thyroxine. Thyroxine regulates energy use, growth, and maturation.

Since iodine is bound to serum thyroxine, its concentration in thyroxine can be used to indicate the amount of thyroxine in serum. The test is used to study thyroid function.

Total Protein (TP). Proteins are nitrogen-containing compounds in the blood. Total serum proteins include fibrinogen, albumin, alpha globulin, and beta globulin, all of which are produced in the liver. Gamma globulin is derived from the lymphatic system. Albumin, the major component of blood proteins, contributes to the balance of osmotic pressure and, in addition, furnishes the building blocks for antibodies.

Proteins are measured by electrophoresis. This analytic procedure separates various proteins by means of an electric current that separates different proteins at various definite and characteristic speeds. After separation by electrophoresis, the relative amounts of various serum proteins can be determined.

Total protein levels decrease in cirrhosis and nephrosis, and increase in myeloma. Many other body functions affect the total protein concentration. This test is also useful in the diagnosis of kidney and liver function.

Transaminases (GOT and GPT). Transaminases are two enzymes in the liver that help to transfer the amino groups from one compound to another. These enzymes are also referred to as glutamic oxaloacetic transaminase (SGOT) and glytamic pyruvic transaminase (SGPT).

Transaminases are found normally in the heart, liver, muscles, kidney, and pancreas. Elevated serum levels are seen in disease conditions in which the transaminase leaks from the dead or damaged cells into the serum. Therefore, abnormal levels of GOT and GPT detected in blood serum may indicate tissue damage in the liver, and cardiovascular and muscle diseases.

Triglycerides. The triglyceride compounds are three molecule compounds of glycerol and fatty acids synthesized by the liver using dietary or other carbohydrates. These fat droplets are covered by a protein film. A large number of these fat droplets change the color of serum from straw-yellow to milky or creamy in appearance. Elevated serum triglycerides are now considered of greater importance than cholesterol in the etiology of arterial disease.

Uric Acid. This is an end product of metabolism of a class of compounds known as "purine bodies." Purines come mainly from cell muscles.

Elevated uric acid concentrations are found in gout, and elevated levels may also be found in conditions such as leukemia, pneumonia, toxemias of pregnancy, and severe kidney damage.

Serological Test for Syphilis (VDRL). The initials (VDRL) stand for venereal disease research laboratory test. The test measures body-building antibodylike substances, called reagins, which are made when the body is exposed to the syphilis microorganism *Treponema palladium*. Levels of reagin appear in the blood in increasing concentrations after the third week of exposure. The test identifies the number of reagins in blood serum. Prior to the third week, the serology test is negative.

A positive test indicates exposure to syphilis.

Hematology. This comes from the Greek word *haima*, meaning blood, and *logos,* meaning discourse, and refers to the study of blood. Blood is composed of a fluid called plasma (55 percent) and cells (45 percent). Blood cells are made up of white blood cells (leukocytes) and platelets (thrombocytes).

Red blood cells contain the red pigment hemoglobin, which helps in the exchange of oxygen and carbon dioxide.

By combining the red blood cell count, the hemoglobin concentration and the hematocrit test, one gets information about the size, capacity, and number of cells.

1. Hematocrit means "to separate blood." This is precisely what is done in the hematocrit test, for the cellular elements are separated from the plasma by centrifugation. The hematocrit indicates the number of red blood cells in the plasma.

2. Hemoglobin is the respiratory pigment protein found in red blood cells. Hemoglobin is made up of heme, an iron complex, and globin, a protein. It combines with oxygen and carbon dioxide, thus facilitating respiration.

Hemoglobin contains iron. Ample amounts of iron are essential for replacement of red blood cells (RBC). When there is interference or disruption of this replacement process, the RBC count falls and the hemoglobin level is reduced, producing anemia. This test measures the amount of hemoglobin in RBC.

3. Leukocytes or white blood cells (WBC) are a part of our disease defense mechanism. They function in phagocytosis.

4. Prothrombin time. Synthesized in the liver, prothrombin is an important factor in the coagulation of blood. When the liver is seriously damaged, the clotting time is prolonged because of inadequate production by the liver.

5. Red blood cells (erythrocytes) have a usual life span of about 120 days. By this time a cell has worn out and will be removed from circulation. Old red blood cells are broken down by liver and spleen cells. The hemoglobin content is further broken down and reused in making new cells.

Urinalysis. This is an analysis of urine. Kidneys filter excess wastes and substances from the blood. The excretory fluid, or urine, is the end result; its composition provides information about kidney function.

Routine urinalysis includes the observation of color, concentration, and acidity of the urine, along with a search for chemicals not normally present in urine, such as ketones, glucose, protein, blood, bile pigments, and microbes.

1. *Ketones.* Products of fat metabolism, ketone bodies are normally utilized by muscle tissue as a source of energy. However, if more than the normal number of fat bodies are metabolized by the body, the muscles are unable to utilize all the ketone bodies. The result is an increased concentration of ketones in the blood (ketosis), accompanied by increased concentrations of ketones in the urine (ketonuria).

Whenever fat is used as a major source of energy, ketone bodies accumulate and are excreted into the urine. A low-carbohydrate fad diet can also cause an accumulation of ketone bodies. These conditions may result in excess hydrogen ions in the blood, resulting in acidosis. The body attempts to compensate for this excess acid in the blood by eliminating it into the urine.

Another by-product related to ketone bodies is acetone. Under certain conditions, fatty acids are broken down and converted into a ketone body called acetone. Acetone is excreted by the kidneys. Acetone in the urine indicates a severe disorder of metabolism and is important in the diagnosis of ketosis.

2. *Color.* Normal urine ranges in color from pale yellow to deep gold, depending on the concentration of dissolved materials. Color deviations may indicate a pathological condition; for example, the presence of blood in urine imparts a red-cloudy, reddish-brown, or brown appearance.

3. *Glucose.* Urine contains virtually no sugar under normal conditions. However, glucose may occur in urine when high glucose levels in blood occur. The presence of sugar in urine should make one suspect diabetes mellitus.

4. *Protein (Albumin).* Both albumin and globulin may appear in urine during certain kidney malfunctions. A test for urine protein is probably the most important of urine tests to detect renal disease.

5. *Specific gravity.* This represents the amount of dissolved substances present in urine. This test is performed to assess the kidney's ability to eliminate normal waste products.

6. *pH.* Normal urine is slightly acid. A high acid (low pH) reaction is found in all forms of acidosis.

Hair analysis, just like blood and urine analysis, is another complementary aid in the diagnosis and analysis of body conditions. Although much skepticism has existed in the past about hair analysis, today hair analysis is in the same stage of medical acceptance as blood biochemical tests were 20 years ago. Its future appears promising. Many physicians are now using it as a diagnostic aid.

Hair analysis is done by numerous commercial laboratories in this country. There are accepted standards for obtaining a sample of hair, analytical techniques, and the interpretation of laboratory results.

Hair analysis gives a total physiological history of a person. Although hair itself is not required for sustaining life in humans, it is one of the first tissues to be affected in certain diseases, notably malnutrition. Since scalp hair grows at a rate of 0.37 to 0.45 mm each day, mineral analysis of hair therefore provides a continuous metabolic record summarizing what is going on in the body, including the presence of toxic metals. A hair specimen, which includes hair that is about 1 inch long and reflects growth for about two months, provides much more accurate information about mineral levels, nutrition, and body metabolism through time in general than do feces, urine, or blood analyses. Blood analyses are of limited use because they reflect only immediate nutrient levels (one to several days) and how they are absorbed and utilized in the body. Such a blood sample analysis may or may not reflect typical body occurrence from day to day. On the other hand, hair acts as a long-range recording filament of mineral intake, as well as the response to nutrient supplementation, therapy, and other past events in a person's life.

Thus, hair analysis may be very useful in (1) predicting early warning signs of degenerative diseases; (2) giving a time-trend analysis of body physiology; (3) giving a time-average that balances out highs and lows of a mineral; (4) reflecting dietary mineral intake; (5) predicting environmental exposure such as toxicity levels of heavy metals like lead and mercury, which, in turn, may cause hyperactivity and aggressiveness in children and adults; and (6) providing an educational motivational tool to encourage better health and eating habits, and greater safety in exposure to environmental levels of heavy metals. Although analytical techniques are quite accurate, their interpretation as an implication of health status is disputable.

A sample copy of a scalp hair analysis report is show in Graph 2.3.

It is noteworthy to mention that hair does absorb certain elements on its surface resulting from the use of certain cosmetic preparations and hair dyes (e.g., Selsun Blue hair shampoo contains selenium; certain hair dyes contain lead and copper). Also, cosmetic treatments of hair like permanent waving, bleaching, and hair straightening can damage the hair, making it more reactive to absorbing ambient metals. Obviously, analysis of hair subjected to the foregoing treatments would yield erroneous results. When scalp hair samples are thus contaminated, a sample of hair should be taken from the pubic region for analysis.

Interpreting the concentration of minerals in a hair analysis is a growing science. In order to interpret a hair analysis, one has to be aware that many functions of the body are under simultaneous control of antagonistic pairs of coenzymes so that dietary intake must consider functional opposites. For example, the ability of sodium to balance potassium and calcium, may be counteracted by toxic chemicals. Similarly, cadmium, a toxic metal found in welding fumes, blocks the functions of zinc but does not perform any of its functions.

Assessing Your Potentials for Optimal Well-Being

MineraLab, Inc.

CORPORATE OFFICE • 3106 DIABLO AVE • HAYWARD CA 94545 (415) 783-5622
22455 maple ct • hayward CA 94541 (415) 538-2322
409 massachusetts ave • acton MA 01720 (617) 263-3745

HAIR ANALYSIS REPORT

PERSONAL INFORMATION

NAME:

Sex	F	Hair Location	HEAD
Age	50	Hair Color, natural	
Ht.	5'4"	Hair Coloring	
Wt.	126	Shampoo	
Race		Bleach or Cold-Wave	
Occupation			

RETURN TO ADDRESS

**** SAMPLE ****

OFFICE INFORMATION

Batch-Sample	659 - 123
Control No.	195/57243
Date Rec'd.	10/25/79
Date Completed	10/26/79

NOTE: All minerals reported in mg%
(1 mg% = 10 ppm)

FOR MORE INFORMATION SEE REVERSE SIDE

SHADED AREA = REFERENCE VALUES

ESSENTIAL MINERALS

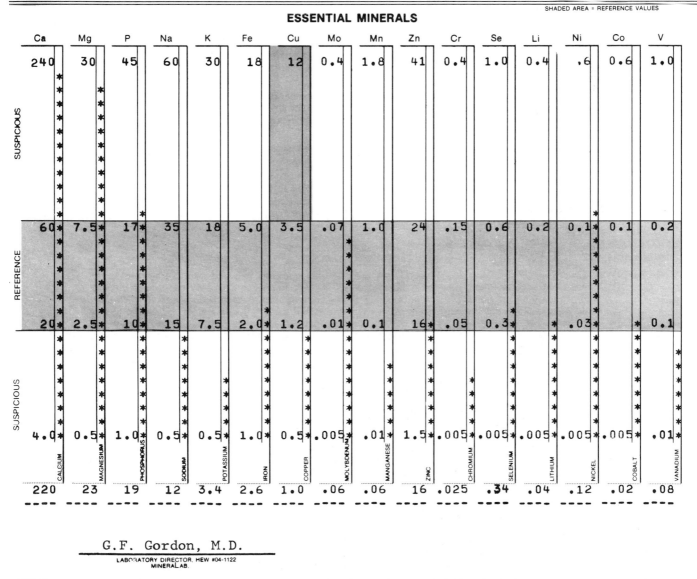

G.F. Gordon, M.D.
LABORATORY DIRECTOR, HEW #04-1122
MINERALAB.

39

Based upon functional relationships, minerals found in the human body fall into several groups:

1. *The electrolyte group* (sodium, potassium, and calcium) controls the intercellular and extracellular fluid volumes, the permeability of membranes, renal function, muscle contractibility, and neural excitability.
2. *The blood group* (iron, copper, zinc, cobalt, and molybdenum).
3. *The tissue group* (nickel, chromium, selenium, manganese, vanadium, sulfur, and magnesium) also act as electrolytes.

Health problems can arise when the ratio of minerals to each other is disbalanced. The best way to sort out these problems is to examine the ratio of one element to another, for instance, zinc to copper. Deviations from the ideal ratio of nearly 8 : 1 is a flag for potential dietary deficiencies or excesses of these two minerals. Another example is the desirable 1 : 1 ratio of calcium to phosphorus. The typical American diet is deficient in phosphorus, and a high ratio of 5 : 1 causes calcium to be leached out of bones, causing sclerosis. Thus, dietary deficiencies may somewhat be analyzed by hair analysis.

Heavy or poisonous metals (lead, mercury, and cadmium) interfere with specific metabolism of certain minerals. Hair tests are invaluable in revealing their presence and concentration. For example, lead interferes with the metabolism of iron, copper, zinc, and calcium. Thus, when an initial, heavy metal analysis is a basis for medical therapy, the effectiveness of such therapy may be monitored by additional hair tests at two- and three-month intervals.

It should be obvious that hair analysis may be most useful in health-profiling a person. The value of this test is dependent upon the quality of the laboratory, the physician's experience in its interpretation, and its integration with other test results. Hair analysis costs about $20. The art and science of hair analysis is still rapidly evolving.

HEALTH RISK APPRAISAL

Most of the major health problems that affect the quality and quantity of life in young and middle-aged adults, especially men, are influenced by the way they live. Violence—automobile crashes, drowning, and suicide, which are the major killers among the young—gives way to what have been called diseases of indulgence, such as heart attacks, lung cancer, chronic bronchitis and emphysema, and cirrhosis of the liver in middle age.

To reach old age in good health, we need to reduce the hazards associated with risky adventures, such as sky diving, car racing, car driving, boating, swimming, smoking, using alcohol and drugs, and eating. Although it is important to protect health by dealing with agents such as food, cigarettes, and cars, and with the environment—social, physical, and cultural—we need to focus on things that people can do to protect themselves. Infectious diseases, such as typhoid fever, diphtheria, and polio, were brought under control by preventive actions for the benefit of people—making their water safe or providing immunizations. Today, we need to motivate each person to take preventive measures to protect his or her own health and avoid or eliminate abuse of the body. Each person can do something about self-destructive habits and evolve a low-risk-to-health life style (see Figure 2.3).

Although the numerous ways (blood pressure, X rays, etc.) to monitor and manage your well-being have been discussed briefly, you should be aware that these by themselves may not be enough to help you or your physician analyze your present life-style habits and behaviors. It may be to your advantage to predict from your life style the chances of evolving future illnesses and diseases. Such predictive evidence could motivate you to change those behaviors and habits that are a high risk or precursors of future diseases for you. This can be done by either a computerized health risk (hazard) appraisal or by assessing your behaviors and habits by reacting to the inventories throughout this book. Such an appraisal can predict how long you may live based on your sex, age, and life style. It can also identify high-risk behaviors or precursors of natural or accidental death that may be changed or modified to improve the quality and quantity of your life. Such a preventive medicine approach is referred to as prospective or predictive medicine.

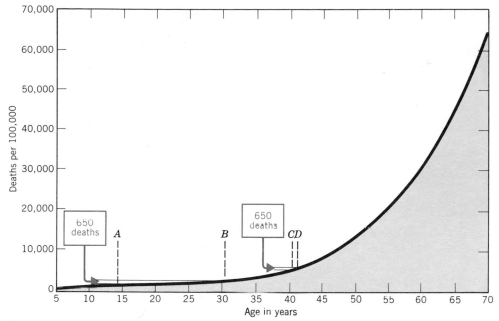

Figure 2.3

The value of behavior change. The risk of death is not constant. Young people die less frequently than older people. Death rates go up very slowly until about age 30 and much more rapidly thereafter. Thus, as you can see, a decrease in the death rate, say 650 deaths, as we get older represents the difference between the rate for people age 41 (point *D*) and those for people age 40 (point *C*). However, at the lower or younger end of the scale, a difference in deaths of that same number, 650, represents the difference between people age 30 (point *B*) and those of age 14 (point *A*). Thus, when one is younger, the achievable age could go from 30 to 14 by reducing the risk of death by 650; whereas at age 41, a similar size risk reduction will have much less effect, only 1 year, reducing the age to 40. To put it another way, we can affect our chances of living at almost any time in our lives, but the earlier we start, the greater will be the effect. (With permission of InterHealth, Inc.)

The salient features of prospective medicine are based on health–life-style risk (hazard) appraisal of the individual (see Figure 2.4). It includes getting a family genetic history; taking blood pressure; identifying emotional stresses; obtaining body weight; developing greater awareness of smoking-drinking and drug habits; analyzing diet and eating habits, driving behavior, and general physical activity; and performing biochemical analysis of blood and urine. Such personal background data reflect one's life style.

When these data are collectively analyzed by a computer, a printout displays, on a priority basis, the risk of death from the leading causes in this country in the next 10 years, according to sex and age, based on one's present style of living. Table 2.5 shows the major causes of death with their associated precursors. A *precursor* is any habit or influence that bears on the causes of death. For example, habits that influence the chances of developing arteriosclerotic heart disease (ASHD) include: high blood pressure, high cholesterol level, diabetes, exercise habits, family history of ASHD, smoking habits, and weight (see Figure 2.5).

The computer printout can alert doctors and you to the possible presence of diabetes, tumors, cancer, liver and kidney diseases, bone disorders, lung and heart diseases, malnutrition, stress-tension-depression, thyroid malfunctions, drug misuse, alcoholism and cirrhosis, and venereal diseases. High-risk habits and behaviors (precursors) would be identified and, as a follow-up, behavioral interventions would be recommended to lower or eliminate the self-imposed high risks to optimal well-being and longevity. Changes in life style or habits or the need for specific treatment would also be suggested where appropriate and you would be urged to consult your physician.

The emphasis in such a health appraisal is screening for health problems in well persons and not on treatment of sick persons. Such screening programs have uncovered a surprising number of persons walking around but unaware that they are already festering or incubating disabling or killing diseases. Young persons can do something about a future disease—they can stop it from incubating.

The values of a health-risk appraisal are many. One is detecting a health disorder early before it progresses into a disease state. Another is the savings in money because

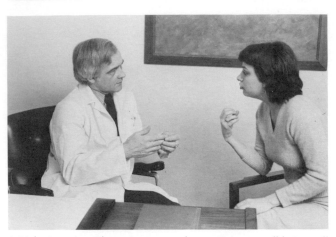

Initial orientation: The various ways of assessing your well-being will be explained to you.

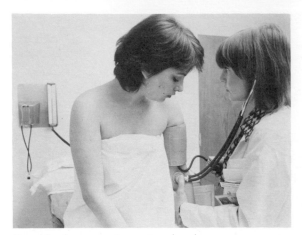

Your blood pressure is monitored and recorded.

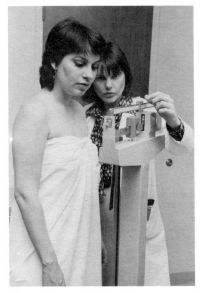

The traditional height-weight assessment.

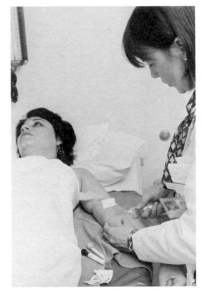

A blood sample will be taken to determine your blood count and levels of sugar, cholesterol and other substances.

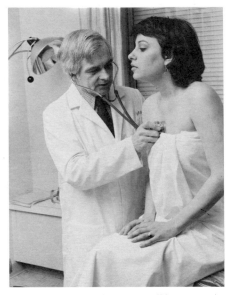

Your heart and lung functions will be assessed.

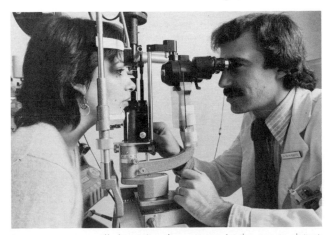

A tonometer test will determine the pressure in the eye to detect glaucoma.

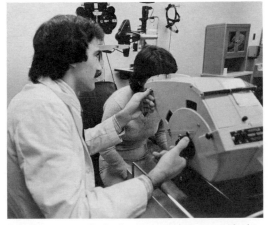

Other eye tests will also be given to determine whether you are color blind.

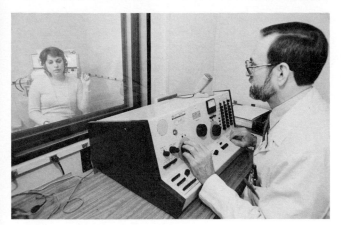

A hearing test will be given

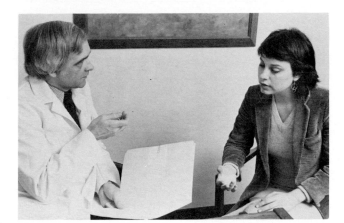

A follow-up meeting with your doctor or health appraisor. It can include results of your physical examination as well as identifying life style behaviors that increase risk of injury, illness, and death.

Figure 2.4
Some ways of assessing your health status. These tests could form a battery that may be part of health risk appraisal.

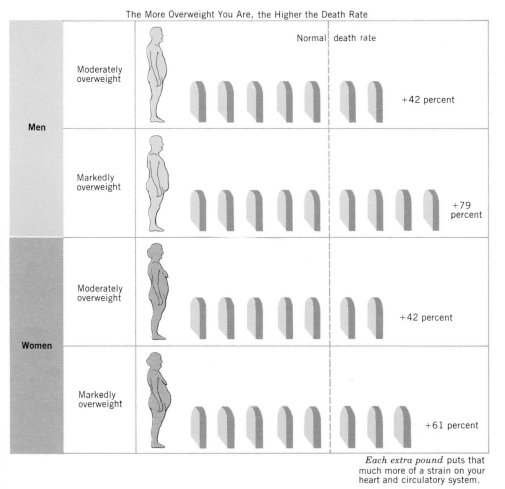

The More Overweight You Are, the Higher the Death Rate

Normal death rate

Men

Moderately overweight — +42 percent

Markedly overweight — +79 percent

Women

Moderately overweight — +42 percent

Markedly overweight — +61 percent

Each extra pound puts that much more of a strain on your heart and circulatory system.

Figure 2.5
An example of how weight loss can lower the risk of death.

Table 2.5
Causes of Death and Their Precursors

Motor Vehicle Accidents	Chronic Rheumatic Heart Disease
Alcohol habits	Murmur
Drugs and medication	Rheumatic fever
Mileage per year	Signs or symptoms: none
Seat belt use	Cirrhosis
Arteriosclerotic Heart Disease (ASHD)	Alcohol habits
Blood pressure	Diabetes
Cholesterol level	Family history
Diabetes	Weight
Exercise habits	Diseases of the Arteries
Family history of ASHD	Blood pressure
Smoking habits	Cholesterol level
Weight	Diabetes
Cancer of the Breast	Smoking habits
Family history	Emphysema
Self breast examination	Smoking habits
Cancer of the Cervix	Homicide
Economic and social status	Arrest record
Jewish	Weapons
Marriage or onset of intercourse	Hypertensive Heart Disease
Pap smear	Blood pressure
Cancer of the Uterus	Weight
Vaginal bleeding	Pneumonia
Cancer of the Colon and Rectum	Alcohol habits
Polyps	Bacterial pneumonia
Rectal bleeding	Emphysema
Ulcerative colitis	Smoking habits
Annual proctosigmoidoscopy	Suicide
Cancer of the Lung	Depression
Smoking habits	Family history of suicide
Cancer of the Stomach	Tuberculosis
Hypochlorhydria	Current X ray
	Economic and social status

Source: With permission from *Health Hazards* 1976, p. 22, Medical Datamation, Bellevue, Ohio.

it is less expensive to keep a healthy person well than to treat a terminal heart disease patient lingering in the hospital for 3 to 6 months. Becoming aware of an orthobiotic life style and learning to manage it in a constructive manner has its obvious rewards. Perhaps the greatest value of such an appraisal is that it motivates people to improve and maintain their health habits and modify, if necessary, their life styles.

A successful life is one that copes with the problems of living. Life itself is filled with adventure and risk taking. One needs to learn to recognize hazardous or destructive health risks and weigh them against the advantages of high risk. The best test of health and orthobiosis is whether you will live to be 100 or more years old. In order to have a chance of living to 100 or more years, one needs to lower the precursors, such as overeating,

being inactive, eating junk or refined-empty-calorie foods, smoking cigarettes, drinking alcoholic beverages, enduring excessive stress, and not getting enough rest and sleep. If these bad habits were reversed, then 80 percent of one's susceptibility to dying from the five leading causes of death would be eliminated.

BEHAVIOR MODIFICATION

Before you break a bad health habit, you need to feel a need for changing or modifying your health and life-style habits. To feel a need for change, most of us need information about our health and life style: that we are not as healthy as we should be, or that our present life style has high risks for future diseases, disorders, and premature death. We usually need to be made aware of this before making changes (see Figure 2.6).

Various tests, such as biochemical and hair analysis, and the health risk profile can be used to provide information about your health status and identify high-risk behaviors and habits. For those unable to obtain or use such procedures, numerous susceptibility inventories and checklists are included in each chapter. By responding to these, you can assess your susceptibility to a health condition and identify high-risk precursors operating now in your life style. By identifying high-risk precursors to, say cancer and heart disease, you can then try to lower your risk to cancer or heart disease by changing one or two habits first, and then one or two more several weeks later. You will find it easier to change one habit at a time. Ways of changing and providing reinforcements to help you do so are suggested in the chapters that follow.

High-risk habits and behaviors (precursors) that increase your chances of diseases, injuries, and premature death include:

1. Smoking tobacco and marijuana.
2. Overeating (too many calories).
3. Eating too many fat foods (beef meat and dairy products).
4. Not getting enough fiber in the diet.
5. Ingesting too much salt.
6. Imbalance of nutrients.
7. Lacking balance of nutrients in daily diet.
8. Ingesting refined white sugar (candy, chocolates, and canned foods).
9. Eating refined white flour products (pastry and bread).
10. Not exercising regularly.
11. Inability to cope with stress and relieve emotional-physical tension.
12. Persistent deep depression.
13. Misusing drugs to kill body pains and discomforts.
14. Drinking alcoholic beverages.
15. Drinking soft drinks.
16. Not using seat belts while driving or riding in automobiles.
17. Speeding excessively.
18. Riding a motorcycle.
19. Participating in high-accident-risk adventures, such as parachuting, gliding, scuba diving, and auto racing.
20. Receiving speeding or traffic tickets indicative of reckless driving.
21. Driving while drinking or taking drugs or medication.
22. Being arrested for crime or social disturbances.
23. Causing social disturbances.

BEHAVIOR MODIFICATION:

(Why people hesitate (resist) making changes in their life style).

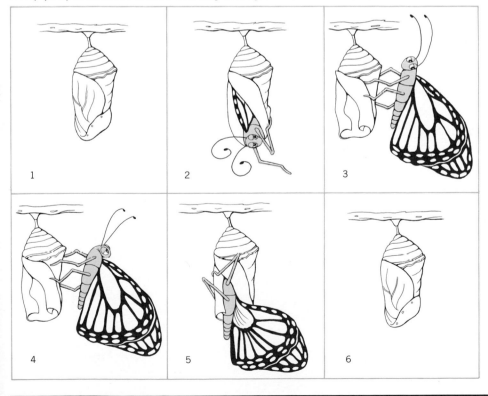

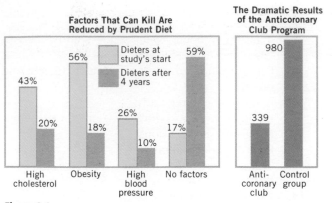

Figure 2.6

Examples of how health behavior can lower risk to illness, disease and premature death. Making changes in your life style can and does work. (With permission of George Christakis, ''An Anti-Coronary Club for Prudent Men.'')

24. Carrying a weapon (gun or knife).
25. Keeping an unsecured weapon in the home.
26. Driving while emotionally disturbed.
27. Being belligerent, rude, and inconsiderate.
28. Not getting enough rest and sleep.
29. Not having a pap smear test after age 25.
30. Inhaling polluted indoor and outdoor air.

Numerous commercial companies offer health appraisal screening and risk analysis. Should you wish to find out more about getting such an analysis, you may contact the following:

1. Database Acquisition for Student Health (DASH)
   Medical Datamation, Inc.
   Southwest and Harrison
   Bellevue, Ohio 44811

2. Interhealth
   2970 5th Avenue
   San Diego, Calif. 92103

3. Pacific Research Systems
   2222 Cornith Avenue
   Los Angeles, Calif. 90064

4. The Institute for Life Style Improvement
   University of Wisconsin
   Stevens Creek Foundation
   Stevens Point, Wis. 54481

5. Methodist Hospital
   Indianapolis, Indiana.

PART B

YOUR GENERAL WELL-BEING

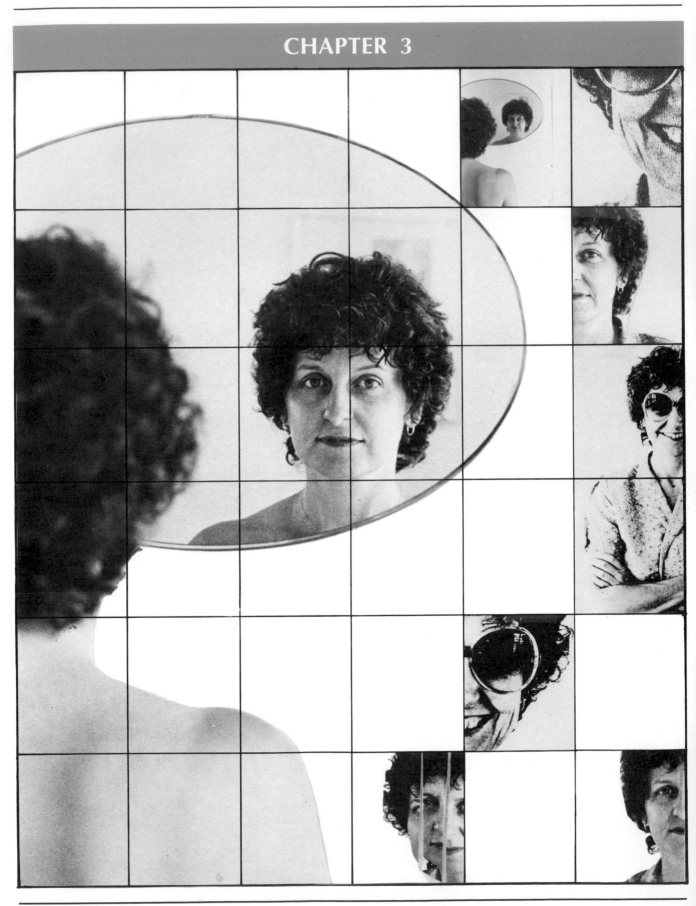

CHAPTER 3

EMOTIONAL AND SPIRITUAL WELL-BEING

Ever wonder why you cannot fall asleep sometimes? Or what brought on the last headache? Or why some people are more depressed than others? Why are some people more successful than others? Do successful people have better mental health than unsuccessful people? How can you maintain good emotional well-being? How can you overcome tension, insomnia, and depression? How can you feel better about yourself and others? And how can you become a more successful person? This chapter provides answers to all of these questions.

React to the self-assessment inventory that follows. First, it will help to make you aware of what emotional well-being is, and second, it will help you to appraise your own emotional well-being.

☞ EMOTIONAL WELL-BEING INVENTORY

PURPOSE
1. To make you aware of what emotional well-being is.
2. To help you to appraise your emotional (mental) well-being.

DIRECTIONS
This is not a test. As an inventory, it should be used to "take stock" of yourself.

React to each item and check the column that best describes, fits, or classifies you.

	Always	Often	Sometimes	Never
Section I ☐ *Thoughts*				
You:				
1. Worry a lot.				
2. Reject own shortcomings.				
3. Have values that bother you.				
4. Daydream.				
5. Lack self-confidence.				
6. Are dishonest with yourself.				
7. Are excessively moody.				

	Always	Often	Sometimes	Never
8. Mistrust or suspect others.				
9. Have difficulty concentrating.				
10. Are preoccupied with own problems.				
11. Fear failure.				
12. Set unrealistic goals for self.				
13. Are disinterested in college or job.				
14. Reject ideas or suggestions of others.				
15. Are restless.				
Subtotal				
Section II ☐ *Behaviors* Do you:				
16. Have accidents or injuries?				
17. Overeat?				
18. Smoke marijuana (pot) or take drugs or medicines with medical prescription?				
19. Smoke tobacco cigarettes?				
20. Drink coffee or soft drinks?				
21. Buy clothes you really don't need?				
22. Drink alcoholic beverages?				
23. Feel clumsy in sports or dancing?				
24. Commonly tease others?				
25. Lie to others?				
26. Cheat on others?				
27. Eat refined sugar (candy, cookies)?				
28. Stay away from classes or work?				
29. Break laws or college rules?				
30. Seek attention?				

	Always	Often	Sometimes	Never
31. Always want to be the life of the party?				
32. Put up a generally sloppy appearance?				
33. Argue with others or resist authority?				
34. Have problems with parents, teachers, friends, boss?				
35. Do things to get approval or reward?				
36. Talk too much?				
37. Drive your car fast?				
Subtotal				

Section III ☐ *Feelings*

Do you:

	Always	Often	Sometimes	Never
38. Feel uncomfortable with yourself?				
39. Feel sad or unhappy with life in general?				
40. Feel unworthy and unimportant (useless)?				
41. Feel physical tension?				
42. Feel unhappy with work or college?				
43. Feel guilty about yourself?				
44. Feel restless?				
45. Feel unhappy at home?				
46. Become easily upset?				
47. Become upset when others criticize you?				
48. Lack patience with others?				
49. Feel low in spirits?				
50. Feel depressed?				
51. Feel things don't turn out the way you want them?				
52. Feel others don't love you?				

	Always	Often	Sometimes	Never
53. Feel unable to be free to be yourself?				
54. Feel inadequate and awkward?				
55. Get headaches?				
56. Have difficulty falling asleep or sleeping soundly?				
57. Feel tired, worn out, or exhausted?				
58. Feel despair and hopelessness?				
59. Wish you were dead?				
60. Feel dissatisfied with life?				
61. Feel daily life is disinteresting?				
62. Feel overwhelmed with life?				
63. Feel lonely and alone?				
64. Feel others pick on you?				
65. Feel love-sexual unfulfillment?				
66. Feel jealous of others?				
67. Feel a need to prove yourself?				
68. Feel threatened by what others say when it does not agree with your views?				
69. Feel you have many mood changes?				
Subtotal				

Section IV ☐ *Actions or Adjustments*

Do you:

	Always	Often	Sometimes	Never
70. Solve problems of school and life successfully?				
71. Make changes in personal life?				
72. Do something about problems as they arise?				
73. Plan your activities and life?				
74. Have motivation to achieve?				

	Always	Often	Sometimes	Never
75. Accept responsibility for yourself and others?				
76. Enjoy having unusual or first-time experiences?				
77. Use logic in making decisions?				
78. Enjoy involvement with friends?				
79. Take part in a variety of interesting activities?				
80. Enjoy going to parties and social affairs?				
81. Take interest in others?				
82. Handle deadlines or assignments well?				
83. Take risks?				
84. Make good decisions?				
85. Work well with others?				
86. Get adequate sleep, rest, and exercise?				
87. Stay home a lot?				
Subtotal				

Section V ☐ *Body Image*

Do you feel satisfied about:

	Always	Often	Sometimes	Never
88. Your hair?				
89. Your eyes?				
90. Your ears?				
91. Your nose?				
92. Your mouth?				
93. Your teeth?				
94. Your voice?				
95. Your complexion?				

	Always	Often	Sometimes	Never
96. Your attractiveness?				
97. The size of your waistline?				
98. The size of your buttocks (seat)?				
99. Your height?				
100. Your weight?				
101. Your body movement and coordination?				
102. Your present level of physical fitness?				
Subtotal				

Section VI ☐ *Identities*

Have made commitment to self to:

	Always	Often	Sometimes	Never
103. Accept bad or good aspects of yourself?				
104. Stay slim and not be overweight or fat?				
105. Very particular about personal appearance?				
106. Shower or bathe daily or every other day?				
107. Get plenty of sleep and rest?				
108. Set aside a definite time for exercise each day?				
109. Attend a concert or play once a month or more often?				
110. Eat balanced nutritious meals each day?				
111. Strive to attain optimal well-being?				
112. Not to overeat?				
113. Strive to better and improve yourself?				
114. Not to smoke cigarettes?				
115. Have new experiences?				
116. Not to drink alcoholic beverages?				

	Always	Often	Sometimes	Never
117. Take risks?				
118. Deal with stress successfully?				
119. Interact with hobby twice a week?				
120. Attain goals?				
To others:				
121. Belong to at least one or more civic organizations?				
122. Have five or more close friends?				
123. Interact with close friend several times a week?				
124. Give and express love to another person several times a week?				
125. Make someone happy each day?				
126. Compliment someone each day?				
127. Make a new friend once a month?				
128. Accept bad and good aspects of friends?				
129. Participate in a social club once a month or more often?				
Sex role:				
130. Feel good about being a male/female?				
131. Enjoy being treated like a lady/gentleman?				
132. Enjoy being a mother/father?				
To family:				
133. Give love to dear one(s)?				
134. Want to get married?				
135. Are actually living with someone?				
136. Willing to raise (or are raising) children?				
137. Believe family comes first in life?				

	Always	Often	Sometimes	Never
Work or profession:				
138. Have a full-time, good paying job?				
139. Have (or are developing) special job skills?				
140. Never miss a day of work?				
141. Strongly believe in your work?				
142. Strive for self-improvement?				
Society and country:				
143. Believe in serving your country?				
144. Would die for your country?				
145. Believe this is best country to live in?				
Values:				
146. Feel your life is more important than that of friends?				
147. Feel your health is very important?				
148. Believe in honest conduct?				
149. Believe in personal integrity?				
Subtotal				

INTERPRETATION

Emotional well-being (mental health) may be identified by your thoughts (psychological) as in Section I, by your behavior (antisocial) as in Section IV, by body image in Section V, and by your identity in Section VI. The statements identifying each section are assumed to reflect the American "norm" or standard. You may interpret your scores for each section as follows.

SCORING FOR ALL SECTIONS

Rate your responses numerically by assigning a zero (0) to all of your checks (✔) in the "always" column, a one (1) to the responses in the "often" column, a three (3) to the responses in the "sometimes" column, and a four (4) in the "never" column. Add the scores for your subtotals.

Section I Thoughts

Interpretation: 28–45   *Positive, good, healthy level of well-being*
14–27   *Fair*
0–13   *Negative, unhealthy, low level of well-being, with indications of psychosomatic aberrations*

Section II Behaviors

Rate your responses in the columns as you did in Section I.

Interpretation   88   *Good, constructive, high level of responsible behavior*
22–43   *Fair*
0–21   *Poor, destructive, low level of irresponsible misbehaviors*

Section III Feeling

Rate your responses in the columns as you did in Section I.

Interpretation: 43–132   *Positive, healthy feelings*
23–42   *Fair*
0–22   *Negative, unhealthy feelings*

Section IV Actions or Adjustments

Rate your responses numerically in the columns as follows:

4   *Never*
3   *Sometimes*
1   *Often*
0   *Always*

Interpretation: 26–72   *Good, healthy, high-level adjustment*
13–25   *Fair*
0–12   *Poor, unhealthy, low-level maladjustment*

Section V Body Image

Give each check (✔) in the "satisfied" column a value of one (1) and a zero (0) for each check in the "dissatisfied" column.

Interpretation: 12–45   *Excellent*
8–11   *Good*
0–7   *Poor*

Section VI Identity and Commitments

Interpretation: 0–40   *Excellent*
41–60   *Good*
61+   *Poor*

Are you emotionally sick or emotionally well? This depends on what society interprets as normal and what it expects of you. Emotional well-being is not having poor mental health, being stupid, being insane, or having a sick mind. Instead, we should conceptualize it as (1) your thoughts, (2) your behavior, (3) your feelings, (4) your actions or adjustments, (5) your body image, and (6) your self-identity.

Scoring poorly or low on one response or several of them does not categorize you as having low emotional well-being or lacking it. What you should do is to consider each of these responses as symptoms. When you have many symptoms, they form an identifiable cluster or syndrome. You should or could suspect such a syndrome as indicating that you may have an emotional problem. You should verify your suspicions by taking the inventory again, rechecking your scoring, consulting with your family doctor, the campus counseling service, your church minister, or your health instructor. Read this chapter for more information.

Next to physical fitness, emotional fitness is the second most important component of well-being. The term *emotional well-being* is used in place of mental and psychological well-being. Emotional fitness refers to being able to successfully resolve problems and to cope with the stresses and crises of living in socially acceptable ways, so as to be able to function successfully within a culture. It reflects a person's subjective emotional or feeling states (22).

It is natural for most persons, when faced with a problem, to express initial concern and apprehension, and to feel some tension and nervousness about it! When such feelings are prolonged, they may lead to a building up of more tension and anxiety, possibly resulting in physical tension, headache, insomnia, fatigue, diarrhea, and/or depression. If these symptoms persist, they may give way to personality disorders that interfere with the ability to live comfortably with oneself and with other people. Those overwhelmed by the problem of living and lack of success often turn to self-destructive and antisocial behavior. How many persons lack good emotional well-being? The latest government statistics (11:80; 22; 47:12) estimate that between 20 and 30 million persons have serious emotional problems today and require some kind of medical care. However, these estimates may be merely the tip of the iceberg.

According to the 1977 President's Commission on Mental Health (47:12), "America's mental health problem is not limited to those individuals with disabling mental illness and identified psychiatric problems." It includes Americans who suffer from alcohol, tobacco, and drug misuse; obesity, overweight, and overeating; social isolation; gambling; sexual problems; poverty; discrimination; anger and hostility; the inability to be gainfully employed; anxieties and fears; and physical handicaps — all of which have a hidden shared commonality of emotional distress. Psychiatrist Roy Menninger (11:80) of the Menninger Foundation in Kansas projects that "if you add those who are adversely affected from time to time by what I term 'problems of living,' then as much as 70 percent of the population could be included."

Unfortunately, emotional disorders are largely overlooked and ignored in this country. Millions of Americans are unable to function at their best because of their reactions to these social problems.

EMOTIONAL WELL-BEING AND THE COLLEGE STUDENT

College students are in their late teens or early adulthood. Their many stresses are those of being away from home and friends; adjusting to a new social environment; making new friends; making decisions about sexual behavior and marriage; refining habits of personal well-being; managing personal finances; fulfilling classroom assignments and getting good grades; finding and holding a job; controlling the temptations to smoke, drink socially, and pop pills; setting realistic life goals; clarifying values; and structuring a self-identity. The major stress of college students is structuring a self-identity by assuming commitments to work or a profession, to friends and society, to a sexual role, to a family (marriage), to a set of values by which to live, and to self-care maintenance. This process of acquiring an identity has been going on for some time, and most college students will have clarified many of their commitments. However, a few commitments — as toward a job and family — may be delayed temporarily until after graduating from college. Because they have an incomplete identity, many college students are most vulnerable to self-destructive behaviors and poor health habits. They often do not eat properly, do not get enough sleep and rest, feel tired and exhausted, and feel uptight and tense. Such maladaptations may lead to viewing oneself as a failure, for they may experience numerous small failures. As a consequence, they may make bad choices, become irresponsible, exhibit deviant behavior, and have difficulty functioning in the classroom and in society. They are not mentally ill; instead, they are frustrated in not being able to attain a complete identity. Thus, acquiring a more complete and satisfying identity is a major emotional need of college students.

College students can anticipate more emotional stress upon graduation. Many will be distressed in not being able to find a suitable job. Others will become stagnant by the rapidity of social changes. The constant revision of moral standards, values, and social rules may leave many with a sense of being left out that may lead to an inability to function. They may go to work but be unproductive or work at a low level.

While in college, many will often look good but feel bad. They put on a facade, keep pace with the exterior, yet feel increasingly at odds with their self-inside. The young men may drive flashy cars and dress flashily; the young women may put on excess makeup and douse themselves with perfume — all to look attractive and sexually appetizing on the outside but be unable to relate to others and feel empty inside. They need to change their inner emotional makeup and not their exterior appearance. Overt behavior camouflages their ineptitudes and incompleteness as whole functioning persons.

These are a few of the emotional problems college students may experience. Often these same problems, if unresolved, may be carried into the adult vocational world.

CRITERIA OF EMOTIONAL WELL-BEING FOR ADULTS

From a consideration of the concept of emotional well-being or of emotional maturity, none of us consistently maintains or ever reaches ideal emotional well-being. We are all human; we make mistakes and have failures. We fumble the ball of life often. But most of us have (or should have) more successes than failures and nurture our emotional well-being, thereby allowing us to feel good about ourselves, about other people, to have the courage to cope with most problems of life, to accomplish many worthwhile things in life, and to experience happiness and contentment.

There are many theories about what emotional well-being is. Emotional well-being may be conceptualized as (1) thoughts (psychological), (2) behaviors, activities (interpersonal and antisocial), (3) feelings (emotions, moods, tensions), (4) adjustments (coping), (5) body or self-image (refer to Figure 3.1), and (6) identities. The characteristics of each of these dimensions for adults are summarized in Table 3.1. The characteristics, identifying positive and negative emotional well-being, were abstracted from many sources: Glasser (reality therapy and responsibility); Toffler (future shock); Erikson (socioemotional developmental states and identity); Maslow (valuelessness, and self-actualization); National Association for Mental Health (feeling good about self and others, and coping); Kaplan (adjustment); Caplan (coping with crises); Rucker and others (health as multivaried personality); May (man's search for himself); Rogers (values and self-worth); Selye (stress adaptation); Menninger (emotional maturity); and Gladstone (five stages of mental health). There are many interpretations of mental health. Most individuals need a practical model of emotional well-being, one that they can relate to and apply to everyday living. With this in mind, the characteristics summarized in Table 3.1 were adapted into an emotional well-being inventory.

In responding to this inventory, keep in mind that emotional well-being is interrelated with physical, social, spiritual, and cultural well-being. Your emotional well-being may be partially expressed by physical symptoms, such as fluctuations in eating and sleeping patterns, gastrointestinal disorders, skin blemishes, headaches, and insomnia. Your emotions affect the other dimensions of well-being. Putting it another way, emotional well-being must be interpreted from a wholistic point of view and not just as a single and separate entity. The idea of conceptualizing emotional well-being into six components was done on a theoretical basis to simplify the concept and to illustrate how emotional well-being may be interpreted. In a living person, it is impossible to separate the psychic mind from the physical body.

Table 3.1

Characteristics of Emotional Well-Being for Adults

Characteristics	
Positive (Successful coping)	Negative (Unsuccessful coping)
I. THOUGHTS	
1. Don't worry	1. Worry a lot
2. Very little daydreaming	2. Daydream a lot
3. Not moody	3. Very moody
4. Trust others	4. Mistrust and suspect others
5. Concentrate well	5. Difficulty concentrating
6. Think of others (people-centered)	6. Think mostly of self (self-centered)
7. Confident of success	7. Fear failure often
8. Confidence in self-ability	8. Lack self-confidence
9. Interested in work	9. Disinterested in work
10. Set realistic goals for self	10. Set unrealistic goals for self
II. BEHAVIORS	
11. Control feelings	11. Lose temper often
12. Seldom get mad	12. Get mad quick and often
13. Help others	13. Bully others often
14. Seldom tease	14. Tease others often
15. Honest with others	15. Lie to others often
16. Seldom cheat	16. Cheat often

Positive (Successful coping)	Negative (Unsuccessful coping)
17. Seldom overeat	17. Overeat often
18. Seldom have accidents	18. Have many accidents
19. Seldom absent	19. Absent often
20. Obey laws or rules	20. Break laws or rules often
21. Seldom argue	21. Argue often
22. Accept authority	22. Rebel against authority
23. Neat appearance	23. Sloppy appearance
24. Seldom seek attention	24. Seek attention often
25. Seldom drink alcoholic beverages	25. Drink alcoholic beverages often
26. Do not smoke pot or tobacco	26. Smoke pot or tobacco
27. Participate and become involved	27. Withdraw from others or projects

III. FEELINGS

Positive	Negative
28. Feel glad often	28. Feel depressed or very sad often
29. Comfortable being alone	29. Feel lonely often
30. Feel happy	30. Feel unhappy often
31. Feel relaxed	31. Feel physical tension often
32. Seldom have headaches	32. Have headaches often
33. Sleep well	33. Cannot fall asleep
34. Have faith in life	34. Often hopeless in situation
35. Feel successful	35. Often feel a failure
36. Feel comfortable with others	36. Often feel uncomfortable with others
37. Feel like laughing	37. Often feel like crying
38. Tell another you like him or her	38. Hold back telling another you like him or her
39. Look forward to going to work	39. Don't feel like going to work
40. Feel full of pep and energy	40. Feel tired often
41. Glad others are successful	41. Feel jealous of others
42. Feel content	42. Feel restless
43. Feel worthwhile	43. Feel unworthy often
44. Feel good about self	44. Feel bad about self often
45. Feel good about others	45. Feel bad about others often
46. Look forward to new adventures	46. Feel afraid of new adventures
47. Feel life has meaning or a purpose	47. Feel life has no meaning or purpose
48. Feel confident about job	48. Lack confidence about job
49. Feel like living	49. Feel like committing suicide
50. Not hypersensitive	50. Hypersensitive

IV. ADJUSTMENTS

Positive	Negative
51. Make decisions	51. Unable to make decisions
52. Solve problems of life readily	52. Have difficulty solving problems of life
53. Plan ahead well	53. Unable to plan ahead
54. Solve problems as they arise	54. Postpone solving problems
55. Realistic about life	55. Unrealistic about life

Positive (Successful coping)	Negative (Unsuccessful coping)
56. Complete tasks and assignments	56. Unable to complete assignments
57. Doing things with others	57. Unable to do things with others
58. Take new risks	58. Avoid risks
59. Accept working for a living	59. Reject working for a living
60. Participate in competition	60. Avoid competition
61. Commit self to ideologies, profession, or roles	61. Noncommitment to ideologies, profession, or roles
62. Intimate with others	62. Avoid intimacy
63. Do productive work	63. Unable to do productive work

V. BODY IMAGE

64. Normal body weight	64. Overweight—need to lose weight
65. Accept body figure	65. Change body figure often
66. Accept facial appearance	66. Change face appearance and hair-do often
67. Eat stable diet	67. Diet to lose body weight often
68. Buy things as needed	68. Go on buying sprees often

VI. IDENTITIES

69. Maintain positive health habits	69. Neglect health maintenance

70. Commitment to others
  Belongs to groups or clubs
  Interacts intimately with dear freinds
	70. Lack commitment to others
	  Withdraws from social organizations
	  A loner

71. Commitment to sexual role
  Accepts or feels good about his or her sex
	71. Lack commitment to sexual role
	  Wants to change sex role
	  Feels uncomfortable being male or female

72. Commitment to family
  Establish intimate relationship with opposite sex
  Assume responsibility as father or mother
	72. Lack of family commitment
	  Avoid intimate relationship
	  Reject responsibility as father or mother

73. Commitment to work or profession
  Spends unlimited time at work
  Works more than 8 hours
	73. Lack commitment to work
	  Is selfish in giving time to work
	  Works only as long as he is paid

74. Commitment to society and country
  Participates in a political campaign
  Believes in a political economic system
	74. Lack commitment to society and country
	  Observes from sidelines
	  Rejects a political economic system

75. Commitment to values
  Places priority on values
  Lives by moral values
  Accepts law and order
	75. Lack commitment to values
	  Lives without moral values or lacks code of behavior
	  Rejects law and order

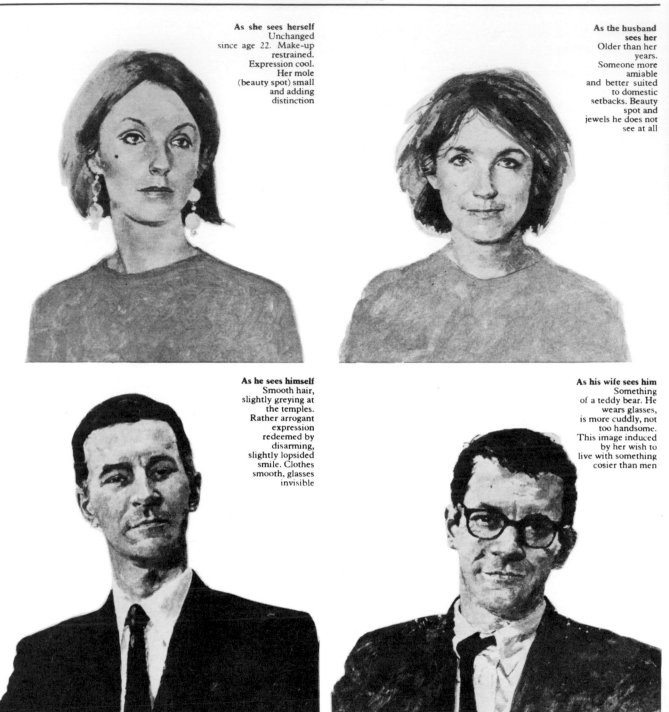

As she sees herself
Unchanged since age 22. Make-up restrained. Expression cool. Her mole (beauty spot) small and adding distinction

As the husband sees her
Older than her years. Someone more amiable and better suited to domestic setbacks. Beauty spot and jewels he does not see at all

As he sees himself
Smooth hair, slightly greying at the temples. Rather arrogant expression redeemed by disarming, slightly lopsided smile. Clothes smooth, glasses invisible

As his wife sees him
Something of a teddy bear. He wears glasses, is more cuddly, not too handsome. This image induced by her wish to live with something cosier than men

Aspects of identity: Self is a short word, yet it contains several groups of ideas concerned with inner identity and the outside world. An individual is aware of his identity as possessing continuity, which is to say that it remains essentially the same from day to day and is clearly related to the identity he recognised in his early life. A psychiatrist can only fully understand the relationship his patient has with others when the patient reveals his own conception of himself and the way in which this develops. The patient's conception is compounded of a variety of the views he has of himself and intuition and insight (not neces-

Figure 3.1

Perceptions of self image and how others perceive us.

As the camera sees her
She is 35, has good bone structure, carefully turned out but with an inhibited wary look. Jewels are smaller; the mole has a few fine hairs

As she thinks other people see her
Slightly tarty and cheap, and because she fears masculine approval she thinks any hint of it sharpens this public image and darkens the beauty spot

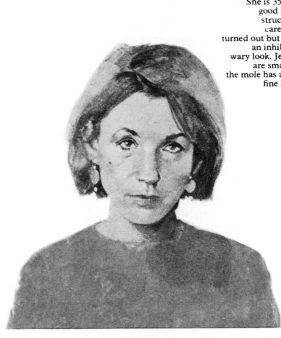

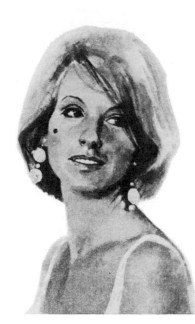

As the camera sees him
The camera shows a reliable, bespectacled conventional man, over 35

As he thinks other people see him
He thinks other people see him ageing and stooping. Not quite bright enough to get ahead on sheer merit, with superiors he stays very polite. Cannot understand why his friends do not mock him for his toadying

sarily accurate) into how members of his circle see him. The aspects of our inner selves revealed to us when we are in adversity differ from those that arise when we are in clover or in love. In different situations (singing in the bath; placating a boss who resembles an arrogant father) and different moods, al-

ternative notions come to the fore. If these drawings had been made on a day when the couple received good news or events had seemed to confirm or refute their feelings about themselves, the images would have been different. Together these ideas make up what people mean when they say 'myself'.

KINDS OF EMOTIONAL WELL-BEING (POOR AND GOOD)

The lack of emotional well-being (mental disorders and illnesses) takes many forms. Psychiatrists label the most severe as psychoses. These are associated with organic brain syndromes and with functional aspects of living. People are described as psychotic when their mental functioning is so greatly impaired that it interferes with their ability to meet the demands of ordinary life. This impairment often results from their inability to recognize reality, such as found in schizophrenia.

Neuroses, less-serious emotional disorders, are also more common than psychoses and cover a wide variety of emotional disabilities. Neurotic problems are exaggerations of feelings that we all have at various times (67:83). There is a desire to think or act in unacceptable ways while attempting to deal unsuccessfully with problems. The neurotic has a low energy level and has great difficulty in dealing with normal daily frustrations. Neurotic individuals tend to repress conflicts, while normal individuals try to maintain conflicts on a more conscious level.

The symptoms of emotional disorders are a consequence of an individual's coping with life in various degrees of success and failure. This has been referred to as the stress of living by Hans Selye. Often, an individual uses defense mechanisms (see Table 3.2) appropriately in coping with the stresses of living. These are usually socially accepted, although not always the ideal or desirable ways of coping. Persons using defense mechanisms are able to continue functioning in life and, more often than not, eventually substitute more appropriate coping methods for managing stress. Often they will acquire "hang-ups" or not so good coping mechanisms. These are often self-destructive habits and behaviors. Yet, in this day and age, most people manage to carry on a meaningful existence while harboring one or more hang-ups and further adapting to stress by using defense mechanisms.

STRESS

Stress is any action or situation that places physiological, social, or psychological demands upon a person (67:7). According to Hans Selye, the world's foremost authority on stress, stress can be either bad (distress) or good (eustress).

Some stress is necessary for optimal well-being, and a lack of it can be harmful. It seems that the absence of stress is itself a kind of distress. Few people would tolerate living an existence of "no hits, no runs, and no errors." For example, an athlete psyching himself up for competition creates tension and anxiety; in so doing, he outperforms the competitor who is emotionally flat. A certain amount of positive stress ensures top performance. Disasters and wars create stress in a population, forcing them to band together to survive and, in the process, building a spiritual will to live. Stress, then, is the very salt of life.

On the other hand, stress of the wrong kind, or too much of it, may be hazardous to one's well-being. Stress is productive as long as one does not push it past one's physiological endurance limit. Most persons are productive in the middle range of normal stress distribution. Prolonged or recurrent distress may cause numerous diseases and health disorders, such as heart disease, high blood pressure, ulcers, stomach cancer, skin blemishes, rheumatoid arthritis, diabetes, asthma, migraine headaches, chronic fatigue, inability to function, depression, and accident proneness (2:10;74:130–139). People often cope with distress by getting a headache, overeating, feeling sick, and so on. These disorders are referred to as psychosomatic.

Much distress and especially the psychosomatic symptoms of distress may be initiated and/or caused by artificial and chemical flavorings, colorings, and preservatives in foods, such as hot dogs, soft drinks, and ice cream (64:78); deficiencies of metabolic requirements for body cells or nutrient deficiencies; bacterial and viral infections; burns, bone fractures, and severe cuts; physical exertion or prolonged exercise; fear of failure, and so forth. That all such distresses are additive is suggested in Figure 3.1.

Perhaps the root base of all distresses may be the lack of adequate nutrition. The absence or excess of certain nutritional factors can impair mental health in certain persons (80:155). Nine vitamins have so far been identified as agents that help protect against mental disorders (81:162). They include adequate amounts of thiamine, niacine, B_6 or pyridoxine, B_{12}, biotin, folic acid, ascorbic acid, riboflavin, and panthothenic acid. In addition to the link between vitamins and emotional well-being, the minerals magnesium, iodine, potassium, copper, and lithium are necessary to maintain optimal, emotional well-being. Since amino acids are essential for minerals to be utilized in the body, they are also essential for emotional well-being. A rich sugar diet is a key contributing factor to emotional problems (79:111–112). Nutrition, although overlooked by most physicians, is obviously very essential to coping with stress and maintaining emotional well-being.

From studies on animals and people, Selye worked out a detailed sequence of behavior that he proposed as the generally applicable aftermath of stress. He (69;77:15) called such responses over a period of time a "general adaptation syndrome." Stress unfolds itself in three stages:

Table 3.2

Summary of Defense Mechanisms

Denial of reality	Protecting self from unpleasant reality by refusal to perceive or face it, often escapist activities like getting "sick" or being preoccupied with other things
Fantasy	Gratifying frustrated desires in imaginary achievements
Rationalization	Attempting to prove that one's behavior is "rational" and justifiable and thus, worthy of self- and social approval
Projection	Placing blame for difficulties upon others or attributing one's own unethical desires to others
Repression	Preventing painful or dangerous thoughts from entering consciousness
Reaction formation	Preventing dangerous desires from being expressed by exaggerating opposed attitudes and types of behavior and using them as "barriers"
Undoing	Atoning for and thus, counteracting immoral desires or acts
Regression	Retreating to an earlier developmental level involving less mature responses and usually a lower level of aspiration
Identification	Increasing feelings of worth by identifying self with a person or institution of illustrious standing
Introjection	Incorporating external values and standards into ego structure so that one is not at their mercy
Compensation	Covering up weakness by emphasizing a desirable trait or making up for frustration in one area by overgratification in another
Displacement	Discharging pent-up feelings, usually of hostility, on objects less dangerous than those that initially aroused the emotions
Emotional insulation	Reducing ego involvement and withdrawing into passivity to protect self from hurt
Intellectualization	Cutting off affective charge from hurtful situations or separating incompatible attitudes by logic-tight compartments
Sublimation	Gratifying or working off frustrated sexual desires in nonsexual activities
Sympathism	Striving to gain sympathy from others, thus bolstering feelings of self-worth despite failures
Acting out	Reducing the anxiety aroused by forbidden desires by permitting their expression

Source: With permission from James C. Coleman, *Abnormal Psychology and Modern Life,* 3rd ed., (Chicago: Scott, Foresman, 1964, p. 107.

1. *Alarm reaction.* Facing an alarm situation, the body undergoes chemical changes resulting in tension, uneasiness, and anxiety. The body is prepared instantly to fight or run away. A prolonged alarm response, or many small ones, leads to the second stage.
2. *Resistance.* The person functions to return to normal and builds resistance to new stimuli. If

severe stress continues, the person feels fatigued, restless, unable to sleep, loses interest in living, and body pains may set in.

3. *Exhaustion.* The body exhausts its fund of adaptation energy resulting in fatigue, insomnia, and depression.

The biochemistry of stress is illustrated in Figure 3.2: According to Bloomfield and Kory in their book *Happiness* (4:61), stresses waste energy in two ways:

First, people under stress require a significant amount of energy for stress data to remain locked in the memory banks but out of conscious awareness. Such repression consumes energy and is unproductive. Second, stresses contribute to the distress cycle in which energy is often wasted through disorganized thinking, alarm reactions, and unproductive actions. By triggering the stress response inappropriately, distresses drain energy in the same way that a physical illness does. The person caught up in the distress cycle expends large amounts of energy because he never gives his body a chance to recharge. His distress works like a constant drain on his "human" battery, even while he is sleeping. On the other hand, the person who gets onto the growth (coping) cycle can expend tremendous amounts of energy but never runs out because he is making use of his natural physiological recharging capacity.

Thus the human body is equipped not only to heal itself, but also to restore or recharge its energy fields biochemically.

The person who meets the pressures of life quickly and efficiently enjoys good emotional well-being and can function creatively in life. The opposite is true for the person who cannot cope with distress. Maslow (41) has pointed out that the most dynamic, creative, and fully healthy people in society enjoy substantially greater happiness than average individuals. Stress is a major factor behind the achievements of many great artists who deliberately expose themselves to stressful situations (72:34). Such persons do not get caught up in problems.

When a person encounters an extremely demanding situation, the first reaction is usually anxiety: a varying mixture of alertness, anticipation, curiosity, and fear that sets off a search for new information and solutions. The result can be more than the alleviation of anxiety. If one

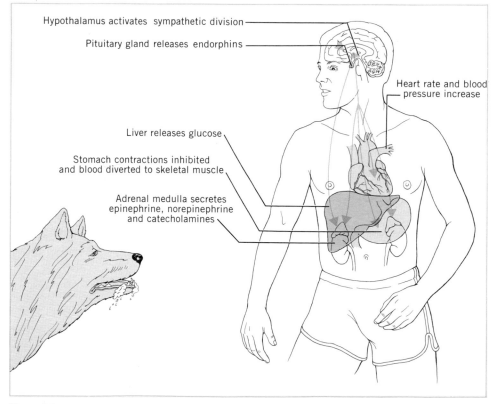

Figure 3.2

The physiological effects of stress. Upon seeing the dog, your brain interprets this as a danger and sends nerve stimulae by way of the sympathetic nervous system to the hypothalamus. The hypothalamus instantly sends messages to the vital defense parts of your body. In response, your heart rate increases, digestion is inhibited, blood flows to the muscles, and sugar is released from the liver. You are ready to fight or flee!

way is blocked, the individual may turn to another, possibly fusing two or more ideas or solutions, and the outcome may be very productive. It often seems that worthwhile art, important discovery, and inspired performance require the challenging good of stress.

But if anxiety mounts and success in a problem eludes the person, then less-welcome symptoms can appear. Anxiety may build to a state of overload, with information piling up faster than the mind can process it. With no apparent solution, the ability to improvise deteriorates and behavior regresses to simpler, more-primitive coping responses. Thus a cautious person, under distress, becomes more cautious, while a gambler will gamble, a fighter will fight, an eater will eat, and so on. In a crisis, most people fall back on the solution they know best to sustain pleasure and a good feeling. Often, we respond with socially acceptable defense mechanisms, such as rationalization and compensation (see Table 3.2), or with self-destructive behaviors like drinking beer and wine, popping pills, smoking, or overeating (refer to Figure 3.3). Those who are a failure in coping with stress often turn to less desirable alternatives wherein they can

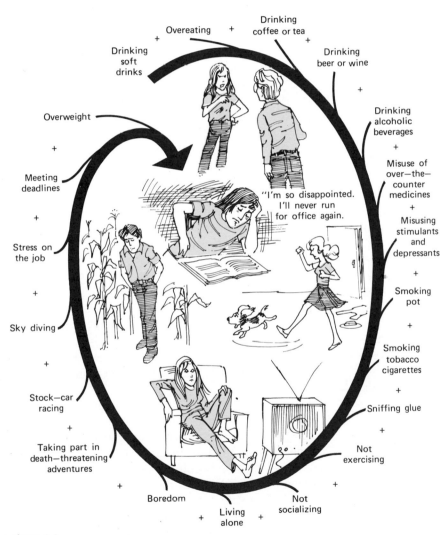

Figure 3.3

The inability to function optimally in society—an emergent and unrecognized health problem in the United States today. As a consequence of feeling uncomfortable about self and others, and having a poor self-image and an inability to make identity commitments, many young people and adults feel inadequate. To counter such feelings, they often turn to self-destructive life-style behviors (examples encircling illustrations). The self-destructive life-style behaviors and inability to perform in society are greater health problems today than chronic diseases. (With permission from W. D. Sorochan and S. J. Bender, *Teaching Secondary Health Science,* Wiley 1978, p. 465.)

attain immediate success and maintain the ego self-image balance. Thus responding to stress can result in learned responses that become permanent, poor coping habits and behaviors.

Most people under high pressure show less ability to tolerate ambiguity and to sort out trivia from the important (78). Their sense of judgment is poor; they are irrational in solving problems, tend to make continuous mistakes, and are unable to cope or function. Today, various degrees of this psychological paralysis appear to be a national symptom and problem. Thus too much stress all at once, or small stresses for too long, can impair one's total well-being. The late Margaret Mead (44), the world renowned anthropologist, pointed out that people who get sick are those who move too slowly and those who move too fast. People doing something have less anxiety and distress than those who do not.

When stress levels fall below their physiological endurance limit, people seek excitement in work and play as a substitute for inadequate eustress stimulation. Some go skiing, others drive fast cars or motorbikes, some go to sex or disaster movies, some play hockey or football, and so on. There are those who seem to thrive on constant stress. There is persuasive evidence (74:29) that many of those who reach the top in their vocation do so largely because they have learned how to manage stress and use it to advantage in themselves and others. They have fewer hang-ups, breakdowns, or heart attacks than middle managers and workers still further down the corporate ladder. Such successful persons are among many active stress (risk) seekers, and include many politicians, athletes, entertainers, scientists, and ordinary folk who find personal fulfillment in working under pressure, competition, danger, high risk, and/or the roar of the crowd. It is as though these stress workers have their own body hormones take the place of an addictive drug and enjoy getting "natural highs." Stress is a major positive factor behind the achievements of many great artists and persons. Instead of just dealing with the situation or problem on an adaptive basis, they deliberately use stressful conditions to achieve outstanding performances and feats, thereby attaining excellence in their endeavors.

Not everyone is capable of extending stressful situations into excellence and outstanding performances. Many psychologists now feel that learning to cope with stress, as well as manipulating stress for excellence, is a learned experience, much like learning to dress, drive a car, and walk (20). Society inadvertently structures physical and social environments for stresses of various kinds, as well as developing a basic personality. You can choose the stresses you want. You can learn how to cope with stress; your effort may be successful, somewhat successful, or unsuccessful.

Stress of any kind initially causes concern. If stress persists, the concern becomes anxiety. If stress continues, anxiety, in turn, may build up to the point that one disintegrates as a functioning person (mental breakdown). Such disintegration is accompanied by a feeling of chronic fatigue, emptiness, withdrawal, loneliness, and loss of identity. Anxiety can lead to depression, somatic disorders, and if unchecked, even suicide.

IDENTITY—THE CORE TO EMOTIONAL WELL-BEING

Lack of identity can cause psychological distress. A solid identity is the vital core of optimal emotional well-being. Although an identity should have been structured before entering college, a great many young adults are still in the developmental stage of doing so. Such delay may be reflected by confusion, emotional turmoil, rebellion, feeling a lack of belonging, rejection of social institutions, and the inability to function. Erickson (24:131) refers to this anomaly as identity confusion. Delay in structuring an identity may occur from a constant bombardment of many rapid changes, as well as inadequate parenting.

An identity is comprised of commitments to family, sex, friends and society, values, social institutions, work or profession, optimal well-being, and a dynamic and productive life style (24). These commitments to self and others evolve during childhood and extend into adulthood. They are the core to feeling secure and comfortable with oneself and others (52:22–23). Collectively, they let us know our station in society and life. Some of these commitments, like acquiring a sex role by accepting one's sex as well as choosing a socially acceptable pattern of sexual behavior, should have been structured long before entering college; others, like work and competency in work skills, may be acquired more fully after graduating from college.

Identity formation varies among individuals. Some find it easy while others find it difficult. Many may be successful in several commitments but have difficulty with one. Commitment is making a choice, believing in the choice, and then becoming loyally and continuously involved in that choice. It means becoming personally involved in a relationship and accepting its limitations: routine, materials, hours, personality, and accepting the bad and good in yourself and others. You care enough about the committed choice to give it your very best. If you do not give your very best, you are not really committed. We need commitments in our lives (52:23).

Commitment is the very core of constructive change, of personal growth, self-actualization, success, accomplishment, health, and happiness. It is vital to a sense of self (self-image) and to sustaining relationships with others. Only those with deep and sincere personal commitments are able to be honest and sincere with others, have a clear conscience, can take decisive stances about controversies, and can say yes or no to the demands of others. Commitment also stabilizes our values and provides an internal security so essential to evolving meaningful goals and a dynamic successful life style. Many college students develop half or partial commitments. For example, they work part time at a restaurant but hope to get a full-time job later on. They are making commitments by half steps, and this is acceptable as long as they do not become fixated in their part-time job.

It should be obvious by now that identity develops gradually out of successful identifications with others. Identity formation needs the reinforcements of love and self-worth through social acceptance and social involvements. The psychiatrist Glasser (29:14) has observed that people able to develop successful identities are those who have learned to find their way through love and self-worth. We all have attained numerous successful identities with the help of the home, school, and community. Schools and colleges, by offering opportunities for education, are thereby providing opportunities for the individual to feel and to become worthwhile. Families and friends give everyone a chance to give and to receive love. When young people lack commitments and are unable to develop identities through love and self-worth, they attempt to cope through deviant and/or self-destructive behaviors and withdrawal. These are maladaptive pathways that lead to a failure identity. Many persons are not mentally ill—they are frustrated in not being able to make commitments and attain a success identity. Lacking a good set of values by which to live, they make bad choices, become irresponsible, and have difficulty functioning in society. Although some distress is to be expected and most young people eventually develop an identity, many will be enduring an extended period of inability to integrate an identity, thus extending distress over a long period of time. Those experiencing extended commitment distresses can be most vulnerable to depression, withdrawal, apathy, and the inability to perform and function optimally in college, at work, and in society in general.

Identity confusion and disillusionment with life can occur when an individual assumes a role but cannot perform successfully in that role. Commitment to a job or profession is a good example of this. Although college students attend college in hopes of acquiring the necessary skills as preparation for work and life, many college graduates today are unable to find work suitable to their training, ability, and interest. An economic recession is only part of the reason for this. Perhaps a major reason is that our society is in a continuous state of many and rapid changes. Such changes cause our identities to also be in a state of transition. The old ways of doing things are suddenly displaced by new ways. Such changes bring new values that may conflict with traditional values. New values, in turn, create new roles and necessitate new identities. Thus updating an identity and refining an established identity is becoming an essential survival adaptation for people of all ages. Many middle-aged adults and graduating seniors may find their education and skills obsolete in the job market today and in the future. They may have to retool for new jobs every 10 years, instead of learning a trade once in a lifetime as their grandparents did. They may also do so in the interest of personal growth. They will have to acquire a new role, clarify this role, and search for meaning in their lives through a newly acquired role(s).

The key to forming an identity is to interact with society. Many college students still need to crystalize some of their identities. They may clarify or identity-test their commitments for various roles by starting a discussion or an argument with their classroom instructor, their friends, or by joining a sorority or fraternity, belonging to a campus club or organization, joining an athletic team, and so forth. By interacting in a group, they use others to help them clarify their social roles and social commitments. Self-identity develops gradually out of successfully using others as a ''clearing house'' for personal values, roles, and commitments. This is a natural process of acquiring a healthy identity.

ANXIETY

Anxiety results from the first or alarm stage of stress exposure. Anxiety is what we feel when our existence as selves is threatened. Our heart beats faster, breathing becomes more rapid, and one feels tense and uneasy. These physical symptoms should make us aware that an inner struggle is in progress. It is nature's way of letting us know that danger exists, or making us aware that some value we identify with our existence is being threatened (40:35). Much anxiety in our day comes from the threat of not being liked, being isolated, lonely, or cast off. Being hollow and lonely makes us vulnerable to anxiety. Anxiety also sets in when one does not know what role to pursue or what to believe in. Our individual anxiety is a basic confusion and bewilderment about where we are going (40:33).

Some anxiety is to be expected. It is natural for all of us to experience normal anxiety as we confront the various crises of life. Mild anxiety before an examination is normal. As long as we cope successfully with the crises, our anxieties dissipate, and we maintain a state of emotional balance. However, when our anxieties are allowed to build up and continue for a long time, then the anxiety becomes stressful. It disorients us, fatigues us, temporarily wipes out our knowledge of what to do, and who we are, and blurs our sense of reality (40:38). Needless to say, besides progressing into depression, an individual may also suffer from psychosomatic illnesses.

DEPRESSION

Depression is today the most prevalent of all psychic maladies in this country. It is so widespread that it has been called the common cold of mental disturbances (64:14). Like a cold, it can lead to more serious consequences, such as the inability to function socially or on the job, and suicide. Even the simplest chores seem monumental and pointless.

Depression is the last stage of reacting to stress. People usually describe it by such terms as feeling sad, low, down, blue, or discouraged, or they complain of emptiness and hopelessness, and not caring about anything. Such persons withdraw from their friends and relatives, and lose interest in recreation, in personal appearance, in health, in sex, and life in general. Unsuccessful in coping with the stresses of living, these stresses become so overwhelming that discomfort, anxiety, and tension are converted into chronic fatigue, exhaustion, and ineptitude, or depression. The somatic symptoms of depression—loneliness, emptiness, withdrawal, insomnia, restless sleep, early morning awakening, loss of appetite, compulsive overeating, melancholia, loss of self-esteem, misuse of drugs, fatigue, and body aches and pains with no organic basis—are all so common in everyday life that they often go unrecognized as symptomatic of depression. Thus you can slip into a mild or severe depression without even being aware of it.

There are many kinds of depression. Each suggests ways that depression may develop. People grieve or express emotional pain when they lose a loved one and they express their grief by mourning (talking, crying, walking alone, overworking, and so on.) Such mourning is a healthy way to relieve the built-up frustration and tension of grief. Mourning over the death of a loved one may result in a state of depression for 6 to 9 months, (refer to chapter 19 for more information on grief). Reactive depression follows the loss of something important in one's life, such as a house or car. Manic depression is characterized by recurrent states of depression and/or elation and may include wild spending sprees, sleeplessness, and grandiose schemes concerning business or world affairs. Women may experience depression (postpartum) following childbirth. The abuse of drugs, such as alcohol, barbiturates, or amphetamines, may also result in depression. Cyclic depressions may also occur

at certain times of a person's life, as during menopause, forced retirement, or during certain times of the year or season. Flash depressions occur when you experience despair over a sudden problem or quarrel with a friend.

Not all depressions are bad. A mild depression, in which one is sad, unhappy, and discouraged, but still able to function in life, may be an essential prerequisite to future development and adjustment. In this case, depression should be thought of as a healthy reaction if it results in positive coping with a problem and the person comes out of the depression in a few days. Thus it is quite natural to be depressed for a few days or even several weeks. Such a depression should be viewed as a "body alarm" signifying that all is not well in one's life.

Important facts to remember about a depression are:

1. It is an emotional disorder and not a form of mental weakness.
2. Anyone under sufficient strain can slip into a severe depressed state. It happens to one out of eight persons (15).
3. The depressed person is not sad or withdrawn by choice, nor can he get back to normal by using lots of will power or heeding the well-meaning urgings of friends and family.
4. It may be a natural defense gone awry, a kind of time out in the middle of a struggle with overwhelming odds (15).
5. It is a habit—a learned response to stress (80:72).
6. Some persons are more susceptible than others. Depressed persons have a family history of depression, and it may be hereditary (15).
7. It affects women twice as often as men.
8. Depression may be caused by a chemical hormone imbalance in the brain (15).
9. Most depression goes away in less than a year, whether you do anything for it or not (15).
10. Depressed persons need help in coping with life.
11. Nutrition can affect your moods and how you feel and act (64:67–77).
12. Most psychiatrists (90 percent) have been unsuccessful in treating depressed persons.
13. Many depressed persons have hypoglycemic conditions (64:93).
14. Alcoholics and drug users, due to overdose and drug intoxication, suffer from depression and are potential high-risk suicide candidates (64:197–198).
15. It is quite natural to be depressed for a short period of time (64:201). Usually such depressions run their course in a few days or weeks.
16. Depression is a most preventable emotional disorder.

17. Depression tends to follow predictable patterns:

Mild

feeling uncomfortable
restless sleep
concern about certain aspects of life
sorry
mild tension
mild headache

Moderate

loss of appetite or excess appetite
body tension
loss of interest in school, work, and friends
insomnia
fatigue
gradual withdrawal from customary activity
become disorganized in work, study, and
    home
abdominal pains
migraine headaches
feeling uncomfortable being around others
loss of interest in sex
difficulty concentrating on work

Severe

disregard for personal appearance
misinterpreting life experiences — making a big
    thing out of a small incident
blaming self
sense or worthlessness (lowered self-esteem)
chronic fatigue

LONELINESS — RELATED TO SOCIAL WELL-BEING

Millions of Americans lead lonely lives in spite of being in the company of their families and friends. Loneliness is a major sign of depression. It begins when a person starts to lose interest in his or her job, studies, and especially friends. Loss of interest may gradually progress to withdrawal from friends and relatives. When a person has these feelings, he or she also senses emptiness.

Often loneliness starts when a person lacks an inner conviction about his or her goals, feelings, or values. Lacking a sense of direction gives a feeling of inner void or emptiness. The natural reaction is to look around for some comfort and sense of direction from other people (40:24).

Loneliness affects one's self-esteem and self-identity. Human beings get their original experiences of being a self (identity) out of their relatedness to other persons (40:24). Their sense of reality evolves out of what others say to them and think about them (40:29). Compliments signify social acceptance and the pleasure of

being liked. Such positive ego experiences are most powerful in holding feelings of loneliness at bay. All persons, of all ages, need to be merged into the group and to be surrounded by social warmth. More important, one needs to establish meaningful relations with others as a way of fortifying against loneliness and feeling empty.

EMPTINESS

Emptiness is closely related to loneliness and the lack of close social ties. It is probably the chief distress symptom of depression today (40:14) and is interrelated to a lack of self-identity.

Emptiness is characterized by a person's not knowing what he or she wants, lacking clarity of feeling, and feeling powerlessness and vacuousness (40:14). One feels powerless to do anything effective about one's life or the world in which one lives; eventually the person may give up wanting, feeling, and trying. Such powerlessness and hopelessness eventually leads to painful anxiety and despair, immobilizes the person, and contributes to, or results in, depression.

Mayo, in his book *Man's Search for Himself* (40:17–18), theorizes that the great vulnerability of young people and adults in this country today to emptiness (loneliness, anxiety, and general depression) is that most Americans have become outer-directed instead of inner-directed. We do not strive to be outstanding or to excel (inner-directed) but instead try to "fit in" (outer-directed). Needing "positive emotional strokes," we let the crowd and the peer group choose for us, decide for us, and motivate us into action. Although we do things to please others, and in return get emotional ego strokes, we still become outer-directed. In essence, we lack inner strength or spiritual well-being.

Many young people of today have by and large given up the driving ambition to excel and to be at the top. Instead, they want to be accepted by their peers even to the extent of being inconspicuous and absorbed into the group. As empty or hollow persons, they become bored with life. They endure the monotony of their lives by an occasional "blowoff" or by identifying with someone else's "blowoff" (40:20). They cheer as spectators; they blow off steam at rock concerts and at weekend sprees ("nite fever"). A state of value and goal emptiness becomes a state of boredom and transcends into a state of futility and despair, and the lack of a will to function. They live as stagnant people, unable to function as their true selves. They work but sense little satisfaction from work; they socialize but cannot become intimately involved with others; they live but without direction; they lack quality and are unable to excel. They are unable to experience real happiness.

INSOMNIA

Insomnia, like headache, is also a symptom of depression. The body is saying that there is something wrong with the way you live. Taking a sleeping pill in order to be able to fall asleep does not cure insomnia. It provides a temporary holding action.

Insomnia is caused by (36:4–5):

1. Stressful situations—such as job stress or college, travel (jet lag), and being in unfamiliar surroundings
2. Physiological disorder—respiratory or gastrointestinal difficulties
3. Psychological distress—anxiety, feeling inadequate, depression, or neurosis.
4. Drug intake or withdrawal—alter sleep.

There are several drawbacks to taking sleeping pills. It is easy to build up tolerance for them—the longer they are used, the bigger the dose needed to get relief. This can lead to dependence and sometimes serious withdrawal symptoms when medication is stopped.

Ways to get a good night's sleep are:

1. Exercise regularly.
2. Do not go to bed on a full stomach.
3. Drink a glass of warm milk just before going to bed.
4. Avoid stimulants, such as coffee or tea. These keep you awake.
5. De-program yourself—develop a calming routine an hour or so before bed.
6. Change the bed you have from a soft to hard mattress, or vice versa.
7. Sleep in a cool room.
8. Go to bed when you are sleepy.
9. Psych yourself into sleeping:
   (a) Try to relax all the muscles in your body.
   (b) Find a comfortable lying position.
   (c) Take deep breaths and exhale, trying to relax.
   (d) Block out all the day's worries and forget about tomorrow.
   (e) Count from 0 to 100 slowly, breathing deeply, slowly, trying to relax and fall asleep.
10. Learn transcendental or some other meditation technique.

HEADACHE

Except for the common cold, headache is the leading reason Americans seek medical help. Each year more than 42 million persons suffer from a headache (30).

Some headaches may be part of the depression syndrome.

Most headaches are mild and usually self-induced. They are brought on by eating and drinking too much, stuffed-up sinuses, constipation, not enough sleep, overwork, and overstress. Headaches interfere with normal, happy, efficient living, often unnecessarily. A headache is nature's way of telling you that something is wrong in your body, that you are doing something wrong, or that you are exposing yourself to dangerous poisons. It is a warning that you are not living properly or of some serious condition.

In most cases, rest, sleep, exercise, proper diet, and sensible living will alleviate the headache. However, many suffer from severe and frequent headaches.

The three kinds of headaches (30) are:

1. Tension or muscle contraction—triggered by the stress of work, causing neck muscles to press against the sensory nerve cells, which, in turn, send pressure messages to the brain, where this is interpreted as a headache. Muscle contraction is a normal reaction to stress. As many as 9 out of 10 headaches may arise from prolonged contraction of the muscles of the neck and head (72:132). Such muscular tension is a readiness of the body to spring into physical action. If these muscles stay contracted for long periods without release, they too may produce pain, sending it up the back of the head, down the neck and over the shoulders (72:132). This is the most common of all headaches and may be caused by anxiety, overstress, and depression.
2. Inflammatory or traction—results from illness or injury, brain tumors, blood clots, strokes, eye infections, colds, flu, and toothache. Pressure and pulling on the blood vessels and nerves cause pain. Such headaches are relatively rare.
3. Vascular pain—results when body chemicals surrounding the cranial blood vessels cause them to dilate rapidly, stretching the pain-sensitive walls.
   (a) Migraine—the most common vascular headache. Migraine attacks its victims one to four times a month. Women are affected more often than men. Most first attacks occur when victims are in their teens or twenties, and seldom past 50. About a third of the victims have a premonition, or an "aura," before pain starts; this sensation is caused by vessel constriction preceding dilation. Migraines may be set off by tension—such as beginning a new semester, moving to a college, taking estrogen hormones, eating foods containing tyramine and similar substances

found in chocolate, some cheeses, most citrus fruits, onions, nuts, coffee, tea, pork, and alcohol; being exposed to carbon monoxide, and taking certain drugs.

(b) Cluster—the most painful vascular headache. The attacks come in bunches. Intense pain lasts from 30 minutes to 4 hours, causing one's eyes to tear and nose to stuff up; then the pain goes away, only to resume later. The attacks occur almost always in men, and often during sleep.

Relieving a Headache

Many people take an aspirin to relieve a headache. An aspirin merely masks the pain and does not locate or remove the cause. Learning to handle a headache, much like learning to swim and play a musical instrument, is a learned habit and often requires a good teacher. The following are ways of treating and preventing a headache:

1. Get prompt fresh air. Get away from possible undetected, odorless carbon monoxide, or other dangerous gas; or away from a crowded, overexciting, and tension-creating gathering.
2. Lie down and try to fall asleep.
3. Massage the neck muscles.
4. Apply heat from an electric pad to the neck muscles.
5. Apply heat from a shower to the neck muscles.
6. Eat a regular breakfast and other meals.
7. Get a light snack to avoid a hunger headache.
8. Assess your diet for a balance of nutrients.
9. Exercise regularly as a way of relieving stress, tension, and muscular tension.
10. See your family doctor to diagnose your headache.
11. Medication prescribed by your doctor should be taken as a last resort.
    (a) Muscle relaxant and tranquilizers for a muscle contraction headache.
    (b) Antibiotics for an infection-caused headache.
    (c) Special drugs to reduce a high blood pressure headache.
    (d) Decongestant for a nasal disorder headache.
    (e) Antihistamine for allergy headache.
12. Reassess all the habits and behaviors in your life style, including the chemicals found in foods, your car, work, and home environments for excess noise, gases, and chemicals. Identify the stresses in your life style that may cause tension to build up, give them priority, and try to eliminate the most stressful ones.
13. Learn transcendental or some other meditation technique.

HAPPINESS

Up to now, this chapter has dwelt on the negative aspects of emotional well-being. This should be balanced out by positive aspects—happiness is one of them. Happiness, like health and wealth, is not to be found at the end of the rainbow. No human desire is more fundamental than the search for happiness. Everyone aspires to it, but few know how to recognize or get it, much less appreciate it or keep it.

According to a University of California study (28), the happiest people are those with many resources, many successes, and many accomplishments. They have gained inner strength from many frustrations, blighted hopes, and losses of various kinds. In other words, positive (resources) and negative (deficit) stresses actually interact to enhance a sense of well-being. Middle age is generally considered to be the happiest time of life, probably because middle-aged persons have been able to more successfully fulfill their aspirations and basic health needs.

The happiest persons place great importance on peace of mind, clear conscience, friendship, affection, love of one's work, and enjoyment of nature. By contrast, the less happy seek happiness in thrills, excitement, acquiring money, travel, new clothes, new cars, and entertainment (28).

According to Pitirim Sorokin (28), a Harvard University sociologist, love is the most essential ingredient in happiness. Self-centeredness and unhappiness go hand-in-hand.

Happiness can be attained by finding out what one is best suited to do, and also finding the opportunity to do it. It also necessitates being free of distress or stress overload. Most people seek happiness incorrectly: they set happiness as a goal to strive for. Instead, they should evolve a life style wherein happiness ensues as a by-product, or as a concomitant or side effect of living. One needs to establish a minimum happiness (4:96–102), which occurs when one acquires the skills of adaptability, emotional stability, fulfillment of goals, many successes accruing from the completion of tasks, new experiences, the ability to relax, the ability to perform competently in one or more aspects of life, the expression of their creativities, the establishment of intimate relations with others, and high self-regard and image. A person can strengthen his or her baseline happiness by increasing the frequency of pleasurable experiences, and by dissolving deep-rooted stresses recorded in one's memory bank (4:109). Thus fundamental to good health and a dynamic personality is a minimum happiness. Many creative men and women have been free from neurosis, were able to work under immense pressures, and also lived happy and fulfilling lives.

There is a greater chance for happiness to occur if you have clarified your life goals and values, structured an identity, are able to accomplish many things successfully, explore and extend your creative abilities, and can love another human being. You should set up a goal to go after, and then strive to attain the goal. Happiness ensues as you successfully fulfill that goal and enjoy the pleasure of doing so. In order to enjoy happiness on a continuous basis, you should set up diversified goals in various dimensions of life on a continuous basis. Doing so ensures many little goal enjoyments, as well as a few big accomplishment pleasures. Happiness lies within you. To feel it, you must let it come out naturally. The easiest way to do this is to interact with others synergistically, doing good deeds, and loving others. The more successes and pleasurable experiences one attains, the greater the chances for happiness and optimal emotional well-being. Happiness unfolds more readily when a person is free from distress (4:5). Happiness is a consequence of doing and living, and as such, one can learn how to identify and appreciate it.

ACTUALIZING YOUR POTENTIALS

Actualizing, or developing and then using your talents, abilities, and potentials, is closely related to optimal emotional well-being. Most of us, as Maharishi (5:259) has pointed out "are like a millionaire who has forgotten his wealth and goes on begging in the street." This analogy implies that each of us has the natural capacity to gain access to his or her full creative intelligence and become a self-actualizing person. Those failing to do so limit themselves to less of the good and happy things in life. Regardless of your ability, you have more potential than you can ever fully develop in a lifetime. Just as you can perceive limitless opportunities in your external environment, so you must perceive limitless potentials within yourself as a person.

The door to actualizing your potentials is opened by fulfilling your lower and middle human health needs (see Figure 3.4). A lower need does not have to be completely satisfied before the next higher need emerges or is partially fulfilled. Thus the lower health needs — biological (food, clothing, shelter, sex), safety, social, and ego (emotional needs) — need to be fulfilled 40 to 85 percent before self-actualization can be attained (refer to Figure 3.5).

People who satisfy their basic health needs throughout their lives (especially in childhood and adolescence) develop exceptional powers to withstand present and future thwarting of these needs. They have a strong, healthy character-identity structure as a result of past satisfactions and pleasures, and can stand up to hatred, rejection, and the truths and realities of life (32:99). They develop resilience to stress, great inner strength, and are better able to cope with life.

Once the lower and middle health needs are fulfilled,

Figure 3.4 a through e
Examples of human needs.

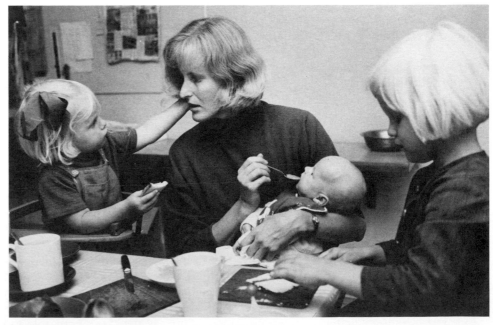

(a) People need food as as well as emotional understanding.

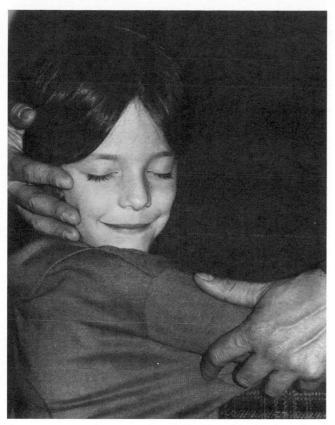

(b) Love is a strong human need. A child is being loved and comforted by her father. How often do you express love and affection to your family and friends?

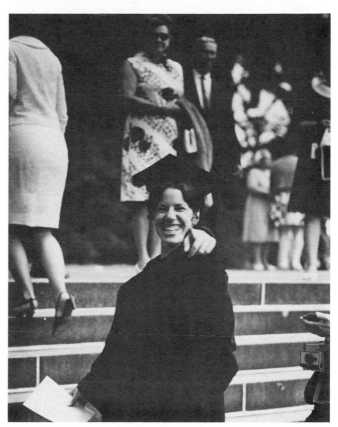

(c) Self-esteem is another middle human need that drives one to achieve and accomplish in life.

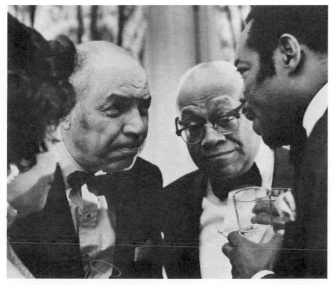

(d) People interacting with each other is an example of a middle human need—to socialize. Is socializing a good way to feel good about yourself?

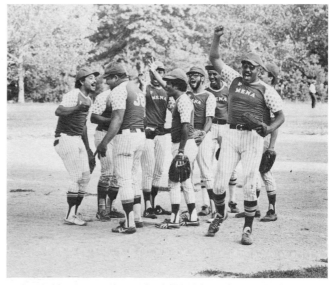

(e) Several human needs may be fulfilled through a single activity. By participating physically in the game of baseball, the players fulfill their social, spiritual, and physical needs.

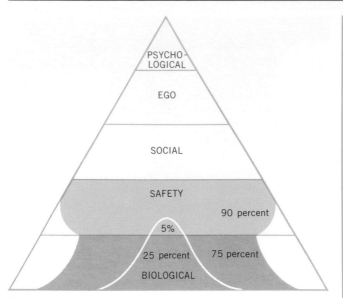

PSYCHO-
LOGICAL

EGO

SOCIAL

SAFETY

90 percent

5%

25 percent   75 percent

BIOLOGICAL

Figure 3.5
Fulfillment of higher needs is a gradual process by slow degrees. A need does not have to be satisfied 100 percent before the next higher need emerges or is partially fulfilled (Hountras, 32:100). For example, if the biological need is satisfied 75 percent, the safety need may emerge 90 percent, and so on.

one needs a positive attitude and commitment to optimal well-being and orthobiosis, and a desire to aspire to excellence instead of mediocrity. It is the person who also makes a commitment to self-improvement and excellence that most readily can become a self-actualizing person.

Excellence implies a desire for attaining the highest quality and doing the best that one is capable of—in college, in marriage, and in work. Striving for excellence reinforces one's sense of accomplishment and self-worth. More important, one derives numerous opportunities for pleasure, satisfaction, and happiness.

Attaining ever-spiraling heights of achievement and excellence contributes immensely to happiness and a healthy mind. You should examine your life style in light of this chapter and evolve a life style that fosters self-actualization (self-growth and optimal well-being).

BECOMING SUCCESSFUL

Success is the opposite of failure. Both affect our emotional well-being, and personality. The more successful a person is, the more confident, productive, active, and involved he or she becomes. Success leads to more success. The opposite is true of failure—failure identifies

with failure. Most people ''learn'' to fail early in life. Like all of our habits, both success and failure are learned responses to coping with life. Many persons are unsuccessful or partially so: They learn to live with failure, frustration, and apathy. They are low achievers in life. However, they can do something about their psychological state. They can take the initiative to change and to learn the art of being successful.

Success is the progressive realization of worthwhile predetermined goals. Success begins with a dream and an aspiration; then follows the process of acquiring the skills necessary to achieve the aspiration. In other words, you must set up personal life goals that you want to accomplish. This setting up of goals is inside you—it is not based on money, friends, or welfare. Successful people become successful first as persons by developing skills to cope with their personal life; then they develop successful skills in their work, profession, and business. To become more successful than you are now, you should start by evolving positive and constructive health habits and behaviors. Good habits save you time, organize you as a person, and help you to concentrate on your goals. It may help to pick out someone you know who has a positive approach to life, is a ''go-getter'', and observe his or her patterns of behavior. Copy the positive habits and practice them as skills until they become part of you.

Having competency in at least one skill helps bolster your confidence in striving for success in other avenues of life. Make yourself unique by knowing more about a given subject than any other person. Having expertise that no one else has gives you a head start on success. If you can perform with excellence and expertise in one skill or job, it, in turn, helps you to accept lesser ability in another job. Persons who have very little or no competency at all will find it very difficult to succeed in life. The secret is to be able to do at least one thing well while developing competency in other skills, thereby diversifying and actualizing one's talents and abilities.

People usually fail for three reasons:

1. They have a poor attitude. Most persons become discouraged and stay discouraged—afraid to try new adventures. They lack the motivation or desire to try, or they cannot follow instructions. They lack the desire to better themselves.

2. They lack the knowledge and the skill needed to make an intelligent decision, which, in turn, results in success. They act on partial or irrelevant knowledge. The greater the amount of information accumulated and analyzed, the greater the chances of success. Often they lack the skills that are based on adequate informa-

tion. Lack of information creates a fear of failure, fosters anxiety, and paralyzes one's ability to act.

3. They are unable to work diligently or are too lazy to do so. Success comes from hard work and not just luck or brains; work and more work results in success. All successful persons have learned to work hard and many long hours.

Successful people have the following positive habits and attributes: they have a strong commitment to their predetermined goals; they have high self-discipline; they are highly organized in daily life; they get up early and work late or many hours; they think and reason in their work; they perceive hang-ups and plan carefully; they are willing to sacrifice and trade off some pleasures of life for success; they experience many small and big accomplishments in life. They are also able to plan how to accomplish their goals; they have confidence in themselves and what they can accomplish; they have great determination to succeed; they are willing to take a chance; they relate well to other people; they make sound decisions; they tackle one thing at a time; they are honest and have integrity; they have an open mind about trying something new; and they develop a tolerance of possible failure. Successful people have experienced failure many times along the way, but their persistence eventually wins out. They have learned to see failure not as failure, but as a step toward ultimate success. Once they attain a few small successes, they structure a success pattern for future experiences. Success is a pleasant experience, and pleasure is perhaps the greatest reinforcement for success.

WAYS OF MAINTAINING EMOTIONAL WELL-BEING

There are many ways to make success more likely and to manage distress, headaches, tension, and depression. You should read the suggestions that follow and select those most relevant to helping you.

1. Eat a balanced diet regularly, one that contains adequate amounts of vitamins and minerals.
2. Cut down or eliminate refined sugar foods and drinks. Doing so regulates the blood sugar level, minimizes the risk of tooth decay and disease, and cuts down the risk of hypoglycemia (sugar addiction). The symptoms of hypoglycemia are weariness, nervousness, hypertension, anxiety, irrational behavior, and depression.
3. Exercise regularly: go jogging, run, or play sports. Exercising releases endorphins, which give one a "natural feeling good" high.
4. Surround yourself with happy, successful people.
5. Stop drinking alcoholic beverages, taking drugs, and eating junk foods. Drugs aggravate problems and let problems surface as self-destructive behaviors. Eating produces temporary relief from stress by releasing betaendorphins from the pituitary gland, giving a "temporary feeling good" at the risk of become overweight.
6. Stop smoking cigarettes.
7. Take a half-hour nap in the late afternoon, or whenever you need it. (The more demands you make upon yourself, the more sleep you will need.)
8. Have a change of pace in your work and life style so as to avoid getting stale.
9. Start a new hobby or interest every so often as a change of pace.
10. Take a holiday vacation three to four times a year, or as needed.
11. Take a brief vacation from work and your home, and socialize every weekend.
12. Avoid stress-producing persons and situations.
13. Be successful—learn to complete and finish projects that you start. This gives you a sense of accomplishment and success.
14. Relax—stretch the neck-back-shoulder-blade muscles. Most headaches and tensions will be relieved in 10 to 15 minutes by this procedure (refer to Figure 3.6).
15. Give yourself an annual emotional checkup, which should include the following (38:28):
    (a) What are your goals in life (or aspirations)?
    (b) Where are you going in your (1) personal life, (2) social life, and (3) professional life?
    (c) What are your priorities? Are your priorities now different from those of last year?
    (d) What are your ambitions?
    (e) What are your emotional needs (ego inflation)?
    (f) Do you have commitments to your job or profession? Do you find your work meaningful?
    (g) Do you take an annual vacation? Did you take a vacation this past year?
    (h) Do you participate in a hobby regularly? Do you have a new hobby?
    (i) Do you have several constant friends?
    (j) Do you have problems getting along with other people?

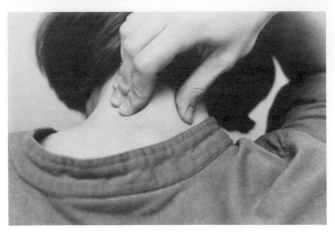

Relieve a stiff neck by positioning fingers over the trapezius muscle as shown. Gently massage up and down.

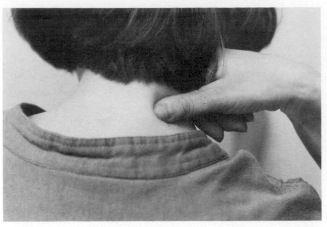

An alternative to massage is to locate the sensitive spot along the muscle and press that sensitive spot for about 10 seconds. Repeat two or three times.

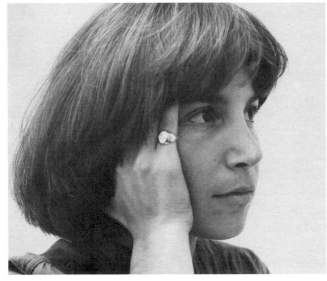

Exercise neck muscles by applying resistance with your hand while you slowly turning your head; then repeat to other side.

Figure 3.6
Suggested ways to relieve a tension headache.

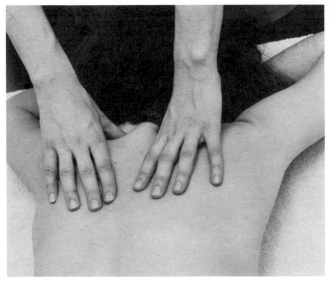

Press the balls of the thumbs down the muscles on either side of the spine from the neck to the lower back.

(k) Do you have mood changes?

(l) Are you able to cope with stress? How do you deal with stress? Do you freeze when the going gets rough? Do you get mad when things are not going well?

(m) Do you enjoy doing things? Do you get fun from accomplishing things?

(n) How do you relieve your tension and anxieties? Do you exercise regularly? Do you go to social parties often?

(o) Do you accept some frustration in life?

BEHAVIOR MODIFICATION TECHNIQUES

Try those that appeal to you.

1. Do easy simple household chores, such as making the bed in the morning, washing dishes after each meal, and cleaning up your room or home. Doing this regularly gives one a sense of accomplishment and success. Expand this to personal grooming and hygiene, and tackle bigger tasks, like fixing a leaky kitchen faucet or weeding the yard.

2. Learn to relax.
   (a) Sit quietly in a comfortable room.
   (b) Close your eyes, and breathe slowly and deeply.
   (c) Beginning at your feet and slowly progressing up to your face, tense your muscles and then physically relax all the muscles.
   (d) Breathe deeply and slowly through your nose. As you breathe out, say one . . ., in . . ., out . . ., one . . ., in . . ., out . . ., and so on. Continue for 10 to 20 minutes. Sit quietly for several minutes after you finish. Practice this technique several times a day. It will take several efforts before it becomes a habit. If thoughts distract you, ignore them, and always return to repeating the word *one*.

3. Identify your abilities, talents, and potentials. To do this, you may need to consult a job placement psychologist. Then, find a job or develop skills for a job that match your aptitude and innate ability, and satisfies your personality. Get a job that challenges your mental, emotional, and physical abilities. Convert stress into a positive force in your life.

4. Plan for happiness—set up big and small goals to accomplish. Happiness is a by-product of your successfully attaining those goals. Start with many simple goals (make your bed, wash the dishes, be nice to a friend) that ensure instant success, and then progressively tackle more difficult ones to attain bigger goals.

5. Analyze your life style and identify behaviors that are contributing to your emotional problem. Just as we learn good habits, as well as bad habits, we also learn to become depressed and feel hypertension. You may need the professional help of your health instructor, doctor, or a psychologist to be able to identify the bad habits and mistakes in your life style.

6. Make new friends or reestablish old ones and begin talking, interacting, and doing things with your friends and relatives. People need people, and people can make you feel better! Develop social habits—be with them and do things with them each day. Cultivate friends who are successful at all ages and both sexes, and who fulfill your social needs as a person.

7. Learn self-discipline and self-control.

8. Learn to concentrate.

9. Learn to grow or develop as a person according to your own internal health needs. Most people have been culturally brain-washed to grow according to arbitrary plans set up by society (52:14). Learn how to fulfill your own physical, emotional, social, spiritual, and cultural needs.

10. Stop playing social games at dances, parties, and social gatherings. Be honest with yourself and others. Relate to others in intimate, sensitive, and honest ways instead of as a flighty and transparent bumblebee. Be yourself and learn to relate to others by establishing communication, identity, equality, and trust (52:19). Above all, be aware that most of your opportunities for personal growth lie in the unfamiliar (41:90–92).

11. Learn to solve problems—avoid becoming an option glut (52:21) in an effort to resolve stress and life crises. Option gluts bounce from yoga, to astrology, to biofeedback, to encounter groups, to Billy Graham, to Jesus Freaks, and so on, in an attempt to reestablish self-identity and relieve stress. They never really learn to handle crises this way. Instead, they should learn how to solve problems:
    (a) Temporarily cope with the immediate crisis —this is merely a delay tactic giving you a breathing spell until you are ready to face the crisis head-on. Ways of coping, according to Menninger (47), in his book *The Vital Balance,* are (1) using drugs, alcohol, or tranquilizers, (2) working, (3) smoking, (4) eating, (5) blaming others, (6) crying, (7) cursing, (8) laughing it off, (9) watching TV, or (10) going to a movie. These ways of coping can give us the momentary assurance we need to gather our strength to solve the problem or crisis.
    (b) Solve the problem in the meantime:
       (1) Recognize and accept your problem.
       (2) Get all the facts—gather information about the problem.
       (3) Analyze the problem: the cause, symptoms, and possible solutions.
       (4) Interpret facts in the light of your and societal values.

(5) List alternative solutions.

(6) Select the best alternative.

(7) Take action on the chosen alternative.

12. Ways to deal with crises and stress:

(a) Your attitude toward the crisis is very important. How you perceive the crisis is more important than what you see as the crisis.

(b) Find out your stress-crisis potential. Some of us can handle stresses better than others. We have different personal, social, family, and economic resources with which to help us deal with crises.

(c) Distinguish between stress precipitated by external events (catalytic crises) from those provoked by internal causes (recognition crises). Inner stresses and crises have been building for a long time.

(d) Deal with one crisis at a time. If you have more than one crisis to handle, give priority to the most disturbing and important one.

(e) Do not panic.

(f) Discover the crisis question:

(1) Can I live without my divorced husband or loved one?

(2) Can I bring more positive changes into my life now?

By exploring such crisis questions, you can better understand and anticipate the changes ahead and dissipate the psychic effects of a crisis.

(g) Explore the crisis:

(1) How can I break through the crisis?

(2) What do I need to do to change?

(3) How can I change?

(h) Do not make snap judgments or look for immediate solutions. Perceive short-range and long-range consequences.

(i) Find someone who cares and who can listen to you.

Air out the crisis with your dear friend. There is no need for secrecy in your time of greatest need. By talking to him or her, you can defuse your anxiety, and clarify some of your confusion and hurt. Only you can solve your crisis, so talk; advice, although cheap, should be considered as fact-finding and stress-relieving. Clues can be obtained from other people by asking them how they handled their own crises.

(j) React to the Social Adjustment Rating Scale to determine whether you are experiencing too many changes or making too many decisions all at one time. Reorder your priorities and goals so you can cut down on the changes and just cope with several changes and/or circumstances.

(k) Try something new. It helps to "shift gears" into your new self.

13. Work on your commitments. Establish them—clarifying and establishing your commitments will solidify your self-identity and greatly dissipate stresses and crises.

14. List life changes you can expect and approximately when these should occur. Opposite each change, indicate what you can do to prepare for it. Each change can be an opportunity for growth, and each adversity can be turned to an advantage if you are prepared to handle it and are willing to meet the challenge (52:24).

15. Use stresses and crises as a way to grow and become a better person. Accept a crisis as a positive omen instead of a crippling disaster. Crises are a normal and inevitable part of human existence. Learn to handle crises in a positive way. Crises, like puberty, marriage, and divorce, are psychophysiological crises, full of stresses of developing as a person, can be thought of as making a transition from one level into a more meaningful self-developmental level (52:36). Out of every crisis comes the chance to be reborn, to reconceive yourself, to choose change that fosters growth and self-fulfillment.

16. Become involved in something big—a community, campus, or political or health cause. Doing so and being actively involved in such a project brings a chance to explore yourself, attain personal fulfillment, and add meaning to life. Active involvement in a worthwhile cause gives you a chance to give yourself something larger than you, and it gives you a spiritual mission in life. We all need it. Your campus or local newspaper carries a list of groups and organizations that you can identify with.

17. Learn to manage yourself (52:236–237). If you do not, then by default, circumstances or other people will manage you. Take a stand on life, yourself, and others by being able to say yes or no. Take charge of your personal life. Never put yourself into the hands of another. Seek advice, counsel, and accept criticism, but in the end, make up your own mind. This way you control your own destiny.

18. Try Transcendental Meditation (TM) (4:39–40) as a way to develop will power and indulge in natural body highs. During the practice of the TM technique, a person gains a state of physical

rest deeper than sleep, while the brain and nervous system begin functioning in a way more integrated and orderly than usual. This state of unique physiological ease and order literally bathes all of a person's stresses in very deep relaxation, thereby exposing them to the full intensity of the body's regenerative and purifying mechanisms. Dipping the body and mind in this exceptionally deep rest twice a day for about 20 minutes permits the whole backlog of stresses to begin dissolving naturally and automatically. The TM technique is easy to learn, works immediately, requires no special postures, and does not involve a change in religion, belief, or life style. You must learn it from a teacher and not a book.

Research supports the observation that the TM program improves every aspect of a person's life (4:46–50)—improves self-regard; increases intelligence; improves the capacity for intimate contact; decreases depression; decreases hostility; improves ability to handle aggression; increases psychological well-being; decreases the use of alcohol, cigarettes, tranquilizers, sleeping pills, and other drugs; reduces high blood pressure; improves asthmatic conditions; and fosters increased resistance to disease. Although Erhard Seminar Training (EST), Silva Mind Control, biofeedback, and other techniques are practiced for psychological-emotional maintenance and growth, there is very little scientific research to validate the benefits these programs claim to produce (4:86). However, research does support the TM program.

19. Give priority to the things you do each day and to the goals you set up in your life. One way to do this is to make a priority list on paper and check off each thing you accomplish. Doing so gives you a sense of accomplishment and a feeling of success each day.

20. Learn to develop willpower (inner strength or spiritual well-being). Willpower is necessary to attain success in all avenues of life. Some people refer to it as the spiritual aspect of life and health. Willpower can be absorbed from association with those who have it, or it can be developed just like physical strength is developed—from exercising. One way is by physical endurance activities: run a time trial in the half-mile. Repeat several days later, trying to better your previous time trial by a few seconds each time. After several weeks of training and running, try running a longer distance, like the mile. Improv-

ing your performance each time out increases your physical endurance and "psychic" willpower and leads to success. All persons can develop an inner strength or "psychic" willpower.

21. Learn to get natural highs from life instead of food highs from overeating food, or chemical highs from ingesting drugs and alcoholic beverages. Glasser (29) refers to this as *positive addiction*. It is inner or spiritual strength. Positive addiction is a state of mind, an aura, an ecstatic state of mind. One transcends from a conscious to a subconscious state of mind. The result is a sense of good feeling that is unrelated to anything. It is a mental spin-out into transmeditation and develops spiritual strength. According to Glasser, there are three ways to attain highs:

(a) Through *drugs*—shooting heroin into the bloodstream gives an instant high.

(b) Through *physical exercise,* such as long-distance jogging and running. A cross-country runner has to train for two or more months to attain peak physical condition before his physical body is capable of running at a fairly fast pace and a long distance before the mind spins-out into a natural high. This peak experience is similar to the instant high obtainable from drugs. The runner gets into a kind of self-hypnotic trance, and his body senses (eyes and ears) block out all external stimuli. He lets the mind drift freely in almost a dream state while continuing to run.

(c) Through *yoga and transmeditation*—learning the skill of meditation and developing mental control.

Time is an important difference in these three ways of attaining highs. Taking drugs is instant, but artificial, short-lived, addictive, and eventually an unfulfilling and frustrating "high" experience. A physical high takes two or more months to acquire. The prerequisite for a physical high is a very high level of physical fitness, running long distances, and running for longer than half an hour. In order to continue experiencing natural highs, the runner must continue to stay physically fit; hence the feelings he gets from such experiences become positively addicting. He needs to exercise to feel good. Transcendental meditation takes longer to master and acquire than the other two techniques. Although many persons practice meditation, it is doubtful that they have mastery and control of the mind and body as would an experienced yogi.

Where To Go For Help

Most persons with emotional problems and illnesses do not have to be hospitalized. They need help, the kind of help we all need from other people (67:69). A person who develops emotional problems frequently does not have the normal supportive resources that many of us can draw on: a stable family unit, friends, and colleagues. Most persons needing help or therapy have very few and/or bad relationships with others. People need people for their mental health.

Depending on the severity of the emotional problem or crisis, you can seek help from:

1. Friends.
2. Parents.
3. Teachers.
4. Family doctor.
5. Campus health center.
6. Local Department of Public Health or local Department of Human Services.
7. Nearby hospital.
8. Self-help groups (local chapters are listed in the telephone book):
   (a) Recovery Inc.
   (b) Neurotics Anonymous.
   (c) Emotional Health Anonymous.
   (d) Gamblers Anonymous.
   (e) Parents Without Partners.
   (f) Child Abuse.
   (g) Police department.
   In these organizations people with similar crises meet on a regular basis to talk about possible ways to resolve and cope with their problems.
9. Crises, hot or HELP lines—suicide prevention (numbers listed in the local telephone directory)
10. Paraprofessional aid (69:154ff):
    (a) Pastoral counseling (local church directory).
    (b) Alcohol and drug counseling (hot lines).
    (c) Encounter groups and sensitivity groups (help people to overcome alienation or emotional distance from others).
    (d) Training groups (T-groups train people to help others).
    (e) Parent effectiveness training (teach parents how to deal more effectively with their children).
    (f) Sex therapy and marriage counselors.
    (g) Transcendental meditation (TM) (help people learn to relax and gain mental control).
    (h) Erhard systems training (EST) (teach people how to help themselves).
    (i) Silva Mind Control (help people learn to relax and gain mental control).
    (j) Reality therapy (persons learn to assume responsibility for all their sick and healthy actions).

Write for information to:

1. American Psychiatric Association
   1700 Eighteenth Street, N.W.
   Washington, D.C. 20009
2. American Psychological Association
   Office of Professional Affairs
   1200 Seventeenth Street, N.W.
   Washington, D.C. 20036
3. National Institute of Mental Health
   Public Inquiries Branch
   Division of Scientific and Technical Information
   5600 Fishers Lane
   Rockville, Md. 20852
4. Mental Health Association
   1800 Kent Street
   Arlington, Va. 22209
5. Recovery Inc.
   116 South Michigan Avenue
   Chicago, Ill. 60603
6. Neurotics Anonymous
   Room 426, Colorado Building
   1341 G Street, N.W.
   Washington, D.C. 20005
7. Huxley Institute for Bio-Social Research
   1114 First Avenue
   New York, N.Y. 10021
8. Gamblers Anonymous
   National Service Office
   P.O. Box 17173
   Los Angeles, Calif. 90017
9. Parents Without Partners
   7910 Woodmont Avenue
   Bethesda, Md. 20014
10. National Society for Autistic Children
    3063 31st Street
    Huntington, W.V. 25702
11. American Association of Suicidology
    274 West 20th Avenue
    San Mateo, Calif. 94403
12. National Migraine (Headache) Foundation
    2422 W. Foster Avenue
    Chicago, Ill. 60625
13. American Association of Sleep Disorders Center
    University of Cincinnati Sleep Disorder Center
    Christian R. Holmes Hospital
    Eden and Bethesda Avenues
    Cincinnati, Ohio 45219

Further Readings

Cheraskin, E., and W. M. Ringsdorf, *Psychodietetics,* New York: Bantam Books, 1976.

Glasser, William, *Positive Addiction,* New York: Harper, 1976.

Howard, K., and Martha E. Lewis, ''Does Your Personality Invite Disease?'' *Science Digest,* December 1972, pp. 30–32.

O'Neill, Nena, and George O'Neill, *Shifting Gears,* New York: Avon Books, 1975.

Remsberg, Charles, and Bonnie Remsberg, ''Exercise to Help You Relax,'' *Reader's Digest,* May 1978, pp. 65–71.

Ross, Harvey M., *Fighting Depression,* New York: Larchmont Books, 1976.

Tonner, Ogden, and Time-Life editors, *Stress,* Alexandria, Va.: Time-Life Books, 1976.

CHAPTER 4

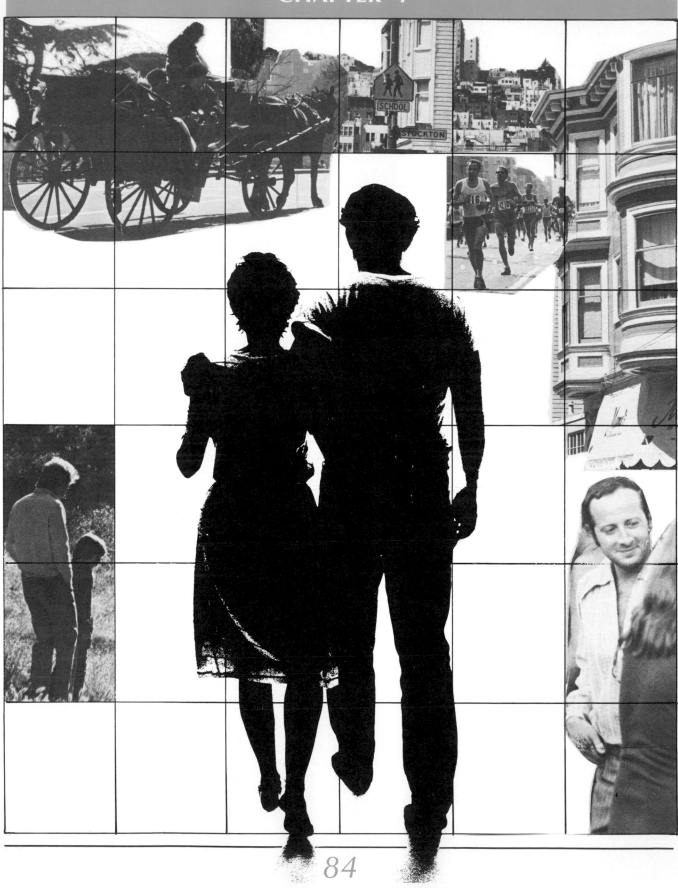

SOCIOCULTURAL WELL-BEING

People need people. This is just as true today as it was during the caveman days when cavemen banded into human packs to hunt, to protect themselves from enemies, and to comfort each other. Even animals, such as buffaloes, baboons, and wolves; insects such as ants and bees; and even small microorganisms such as bacteria, band together socially for survival. The need for interaction among people is greater than ever today, but many of us are experiencing difficulty in fulfilling our social needs. This chapter explores the nature of social well-being, how a lack of it affects human development and well-being, and how humans can fulfill this basic need.

Before reading this chapter, assess your sociocultural well-being by reacting to the inventory that follows.

☞ SOCIOCULTURAL WELL-BEING INVENTORY

DIRECTIONS: Circle the number opposite the statement that best fits or describes your involvement, interaction, or feeling.

		Your Responses		
	Past Week	Past Month	Past 3 Months	6 months or Longer (Never)
A. Family—relatives When did you last:				
1. Visit with your parents?	4	3	1	0
2. Your family or relatives last visit you?	4	3	1	0
3. Visit with your grandparents?	4	3	1	0
4. Visit with your uncles or cousins	4	3	1	0
5. Get a compliment or encouragement from your parents or in-laws?	4	3	1	0

	Your Responses			
	Past Week	Past Month	Past 3 Months	6 months or Longer (Never)
6. Feel happy or comfortable with your family?	4	3	1	0
7. Visit your brothers or sisters?	4	3	1	0
8. When did your brothers or sisters last visit you at your home?	4	3	1	0
9. When were you sexually satisfied with your loved one?	4	3	1	0
B. Close friends				
When did you last:				
10. Have a special boyfriend or girlfriend?	4	3	1	0
11. Talk to your professor?	4	3	1	0
12. Visit your friend's home?	4	3	1	0
13. Your friends last visit your home?	4	3	1	0
14. Telephone your friends?	4	3	1	0
15. See five or more of your best friends?	4	3	1	0
16. Write a letter to a friend?	4	3	1	0
17. Share an intimate feeling or secret with a friend?	4	3	1	0
18. Have a party with your friends?	4	3	1	0
19. Discuss politics, nuclear power plants, etc., with your friends?	4	3	1	0
20. Play cards, games, checkers, back-gammon, etc., with friends?	4	3	1	0
21. Make or meet a new friend?	4	3	1	0
22. Have lunch or a drink with a friend?	4	3	1	0
23. Get a compliment from a friend?	4	3	1	0
24. When were you last invited to a party?	4	3	1	0

	Your Responses			
	Past Week	Past Month	Past 3 Months	6 months or Longer (Never)
25. Visit with a friend you have known at least 6 to 12 years?	4	3	1	0
C. Work or classes				
When did you last:				
26. Have a steady job?	4	3	1	0
27. Have a good paying job?	4	3	1	0
28. Get a compliment from your boss?	4	3	1	0
29. Get a compliment from your classmates or co-workers?	4	3	1	0
30. Get a compliment from your professor?	4	3	1	0
31. Enjoy attending classes or working?	4	3	1	0
D. Community or campus				
When did you last:				
32. Vote in an election?	4	3	1	0
33. Attend a political rally?	4	3	1	0
34. Attend a special lecture or seminar?	4	3	1	0
35. Attend a sports event (baseball, football, etc.)?	4	3	1	0
36. Attend a social club function?	4	3	1	0
37. Attend a professional meeting?	4	3	1	0
38. Perform as an entertainer (singer, actor)?	4	3	1	0
39. Display your hobby or share it with others?	4	3	1	0
40. Hold office in a club or organization?	4	3	1	0
41. Attend a church service?	4	3	1	0
42. Attend two or more clubs or organizations?	4	3	1	0

E. Other special events				
When did you last:				
43. Play a sport for fun with others?	4	3	1	0
44. Exercise with others (jogging, bicycling, etc.)?	4	3	1	0
45. Go dancing (discoing)?	4	3	1	0
46. Go to a play or concert?	4	3	1	0
47. Visit the zoo, art gallery, museum, etc.?	4	3	1	0
48. Celebrate a national holiday (such as July 4th)?	4	3	1	0
49. Attend a county fair, parade, or picnic?	4	3	1	0
50. Share your hobby with others?	4	3	1	0

SCORING
Step 1. Add all the checks in each of the four columns.
Step 2. Total the four columns—this is your score.

      Range: 120–200   Very good to excellent
               100–119   Above average
                50–99   Fair to average
                 0–50   Poor

INTERPRETATION

Read this chapter to interpret the five parts of this inventory. Identify the part(s) that you are weakest in. Refer to the suggestions at the end of this chapter on ways to improve and maintain your social well-being.

Social well-being is characterized by interpersonal interactions and involvements with others (e.g., visits, telephone conversations, and doing things with close friends and neighbors). These involvements include intimate relationships with family members and relatives, neighbors, close friends, and interactions with co-workers, and church and professional acquaintances. The quality of such relationships, such as how well one is getting along with others, is an important part of optimal social wellness (see Figure 4.1). Most persons have about 10 "dear" friends that they can confide in and share their bad and good experiences with (8:22).

The matrix of such social interactions and involvements of a few persons extends into a network of social participations and involvements in the community. As one reaches 30 years of age and has begun a family and home, one usually starts to take an active interest in the betterment of the community and furthering one's vocational or professional growth. One becomes more civic-minded. Such involvements are expressed through memberships in clubs, and activities in work, church, professional, and political organizations (see Figure 4.2).

One may interact with 50 to 100 persons in a professional meeting one day and become one of 50,000 spectators at a football game the next day. Without realizing it, one strives for cultural wellness when one "attends" social community functions and cultural festivities such as athletic events, dramas, operas, concerts, parades, and political rallies as a spectator or observer, and also when one "performs" as an athlete, actor, musician, political campaigner or public office holder. To attain cultural well-being, one must give of oneself to others—by sharing one's talents or being willing to provide service. In addition, one must also take, appreciate, or receive the talents and services of others as a spectator or member of the audience. Most young people and adults are receivers or takers. If one does not balance out the community interaction of "giving and taking," and mostly takes, then one will feel only partially fulfilled and will lack a real commitment to his or her community.

Thus cultural well-being reflects an identity commitment with the community, whereas social well-being reflects interrelationships with friends and acquaint-

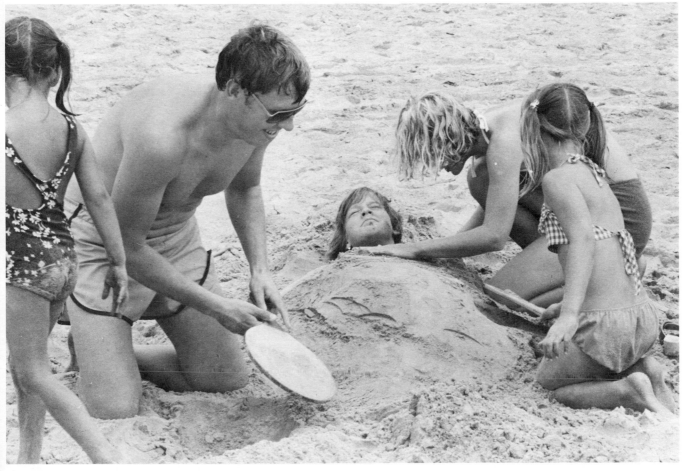

Figure 4.1a
Playing on the beach is one way to fulfill one's need to do things with others.

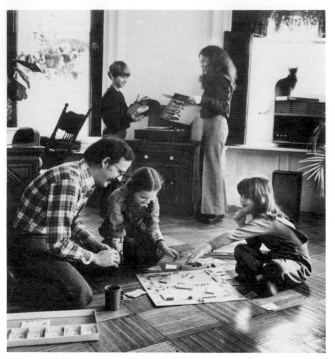

Figure 4.1b
We learn to socialize and to fulfill the need to interact with others at home. Family members can be your very best friends and can provide much affection, emotional comfort and joy. A good family life can enrich you as a person.

ances. Those establishing commitments to both friends and community will feel a sense of belonging, rootedness, and a sense of "community." Such feelings contribute to emotional and spiritual well-being.

Researcher Cathy Donald, and her associates (8) at the Rand Corporation in 1978 concluded, after a thorough review of the literature and research on social and cultural well-being, that (1) most researchers refer to both social and cultural well-being by the single term *social well-being,* and (2) most researchers identified social well-being under five role and activity categories (8:23):

1. *Family and close relatives*—number of activities or contacts, relationships and involvements. Relating intimately to a loved one through sex and emotions is an important part of social well-being.
2. *Close, intimate friends and acquaintances* —number of activities, involvements, and personal interactions. These interactions include sharing intimate feelings and secrets, seeking help in times of crises, solving problems, and talking with or having telephone conversations or doing things with them on a daily basis.
3. *Work*—performing on the job and satisfaction with the work itself, and interacting with co-workers.

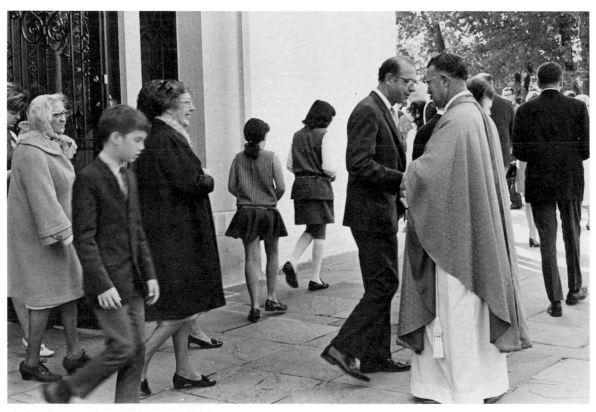

Figure 4.2
Attending church is an important way to socialize for many people.

4. *Community*—participation in and belonging to various social-recreational clubs, organizations, church groups, and political and civic groups.

5. *Other social phenomenon*—recreation that may or may not involve interactions with other persons, such as attending athletic events, discos, plays and dramas, rituals and ceremonies, musicals and concerts, and dances; and visiting places like zoos, art galleries, and museums.

Attaining and maintaining social well-being is dependent on continuous and regular interactions with others of all ages on a daily basis. It means sharing time, things, and possessions, experiences, and yourself with others in a variety of social, recreational, and leisure activities. One develops continuous commitments that include caring for and loving others, contributing to their happiness, welfare, and general well-being, feeling responsible for them, and functioning socially in the community.

Social well-being begins between two or more family members in the home, or two persons living together. It includes satisfactory, intimate personal sexual relationships. Since the family is the smallest social unit, it stands midway between the individual and society (12:168). A well family perpetuates well individuals, resulting in well communities and healthy cultures. The opposite is also true. Families are the training grounds for structuring the many essential social skills in children and adolescents, while the community and friends provide the social reinforcement for rooting and grafting such skills.

GENERAL BENEFITS OF SOCIAL WELL-BEING

The benefits of social well-being are many and are interrelated with physical, emotional, and spiritual well-being. Suicide rates are lower in communities where people actively interact in social activities and have a stake in the community (8:2). Socially healthy persons are more able to cope successfully with the day-to-day challenges and crises of life. They have fewer psychosomatic, emotional disorders, physical problems and illnesses. Socially fulfilled persons are able to become more successful as persons and are more able to perform optimally in most adventures of life. Perhaps the most important benefit of social interaction is emotional-spiritual fulfillment (see Chapter 3). Such fulfilled persons are more likely to participate in community activities, to become involved in the community and, hence, acquire cultural well-being (see Figure 4.3). They would be more apt to conform to the moral codes of society (8:2–3) so that there is less crime and violence in a healthy community.

There is no doubt that community (cultural) well-being influences the individual (8:2). Many of our personal problems are the result of not having enough close friends. Society acts as a personal support system for the individual. It not only provides feedback about oneself, and how one is doing (8:4), but also provides the "ego massage" so vital for feeling good.

VALIDITY OF SOCIAL WELL-BEING

The importance of social involvement for healthy human development and social functioning has been substantiated by many researchers (3;8;16;18;34;37). They have found that physical isolation has profound effects on the psychological disposition of isolated animals and human beings. Any change in the social environment works a change in the individual. Social isolation decreases the environmental or sensory stimulation, thereby producing subtle biochemical fluctuations in the brain and nervous system, and, in turn, changes in mental-emotional processes.

The outward manifestation of these biochemical changes have been recorded many times in animals. As an example, researchers of the Regional Primate Research Center at the University of Wisconsin studied isolated monkeys (34) and found that 6 months of social isolation resulted in seemingly permanent, abnormal social, sexual, and maternal behaviors. Isolated monkeys show severe persistent psychopathological behavior similar to those of autistic children (37). For example, young monkeys separated from their mothers showed signs of hyperactivity (excessive vocalizing), followed by periods of depression. An analysis of the brain of these animals revealed that major biochemical changes do accompany separation. Likewise, mice kept alone in cages and allowed no physical or social contact with other mice developed classic symptoms of depression (37). They reacted violently and aggressively to their renewed social contacts. An analysis of the brains of isolated mice revealed that their brains had lost much of the capability to metabolize glucose. Thus biochemical changes induce social and psychological changes. Social withdrawal and isolation appears to slow down the turnover and release of chemicals (neurotransmitters) in the brain. The researchers (37) felt that similar reactions could also take place in lonely or isolated and withdrawn human beings, since the biochemistry of mice and humans is very similar.

Research with humans supports the research done on animals. It has long been known that infants will not thrive if their mothers are hostile or even merely indifferent. For example, 90 percent of infants in Baltimore orphanages and foundling homes in 1915 died within a year of admission, in spite of adequate physical care

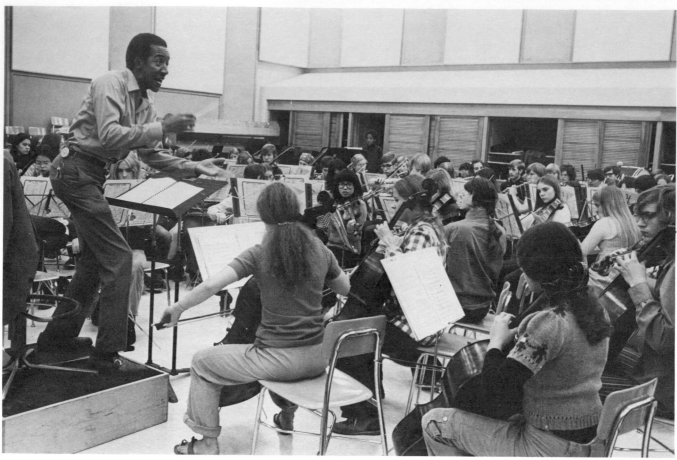

Figure 4.3
Playing in an orchestra is a good way to socialize and make friends. Such experiences are also emotionally fulfilling and contribute to spiritual well-being.

(17). The reactions of orphans to an adverse emotional-social environment stifled their growth rate. Emotionally deprived children (lacking contact with parents and adults) stop growing and lose the will to live. Pediatricians (17:149) have observed that when normal contact between mother and infant is disrupted, diarrhea in the child becomes more prevalent and muscle tone decreases, resulting in a psychological disturbance marked by anxiety and sadness. The stomachs of depressed and withdrawn children secrete less hydrocholoric acid thus impeding digestion. On other hand, acid production increases when they are angry, talking, or actively relating to parents or objects. Such children quickly respond to the attention they receive from the hospital staff, begin gaining weight, and attain emotional stability. These changes were unrelated to any change in food intake. Doctors felt that the enrichment of the child's social environment, not the diet, was responsible for the normalization of growth.

A relationship between physiological deficiency and deprivation dwarfism in human babies has been observed at the Massachusetts General Hospital for nearly 20 years (17). Parentally rejected babies, because of stunted growth, were found to be suffering from an emotionally induced pituitary deficiency. Also, the loss of appetite in adolescents, due to adverse interpersonal relations with parents (anorexia nervosa), can also stifle physiological growth (17). Adolescent girls having parental difficulties may stop menstruating. The adverse social climate of the home disrupts pituitary hormones that, in turn, control ovarian function (17). In summary, the observations about emotional deprivation of infants, children, and adolescents reflect the vital importance of daily social interaction.

WHY COLLEGE STUDENTS NEED SOCIAL WELL-BEING

Friends, professors, co-workers, family members, and acquaintances help all persons to clarify and get a self-identity. Erickson (15:59) perceives identity as developing gradually out of successful identifications during childhood and adolescence. The psychiatrist, Glasser, (19:14) believes that those who have had the support of their parents and friends, and who have received love and a sense of self-worth, are better able to develop successful identities than those who were deprived of love and self-worth. Since the identities of many college students are in the formative stages, they use their peer friends, professors, and relatives as a testing ground for values. While playing, discussing, and arguing about controversial topics, they clarify their personal value systems. People use others in society as a value yardstick or reference point. Needless to say, values are essential for making sound decisions, for guiding one's behavior, and for cementing relationships and involvements.

Friends and others soothe our egos and bolster our achievement status (28:82). College students need emotional and spiritual support during examination time, when term papers are due, and when they receive grades. They need to know whether what they are accomplishing meets social standards and expectations. Compliments and social recognition for achievement in the classroom give the emotional and moral support to carry on and to face the next semester. Thus individual endeavors in the college and business world are enhanced by good social relationships.

People socialize through *dating,* parties, and group activities. Although people date for many reasons, most do so to feel good emotionally and to clarify their identity. Dating is a basis for identifying friends with common interests and goals and may eventuate in love and marriage. Being in demand as a date or being popular is prima facie evidence of social acceptance. High self-appraisal follows such acceptance and low self-feeling results from failure to date. Continuous dating gives one the sense of social acceptance and popularity that is prolonged into establishing wholesome relationships with the opposite sex (see Figure 4.4). When dating becomes a romantic involvement, one's ego is instantly bolstered by the affectionate responses of another. Thus college students may fulfill much of their need for emotional and social well-being through dating while married persons are able to do so through marriage.

Friends are essential for other reasons. We need them to *fortify our sense of security and belonging to the group or community* (culture) (see Figure 4.5). Friends verbally and emotionally make us feel good. We need friends as confidants—to share our troubles with, and to help us solve the problems of living (2, 29, 35). This is especially important during times of crises when we desperately need comfort through moral and emotional support (29). When under emergencies and stress, interpersonal behavior deteriorates the most (18:36). One begins to see oneself as a special person entitled to special consideration. When upset, one often uses one's

depression or anger as a means of forcing friends, teachers, or the family to take notice of the problem and to give one special attention and understanding. Thus one's relationships with friends and others can deteriorate most often when under emotional stress. Interacting with others is most essential in maintaining an emotional balance. While providing moral and emotional support, friends indirectly also give us a spiritual lift. Thus a wholesome and supportive social environment allows us to survive crises. Indirectly, it protects us from illnesses and emotionally related disorders.

Caplan (6) suggests that one needs to feel socially adequate in order to feel emotionally well. For example, you need competency in a skill while working. Having the skill garners the social recognition that you are good, worthwhile, and important. Social "strokes" from co-workers are essential to feeling successful and feeling good. Caplan suggests that one needs to develop and use many social skills in order to feel socially adequate.

Studies (1, 24) of the cultures of people living past the age of 100 reveal that octogenarians have developed dependent social life styles. The people in Abkhasia, in the Georgian Soviet Socialist Republic, derive great emotional security and fulfillment from a variety of continuing ritual and kinship relationships that involve lifetime obligations. They toast the accomplishments of everyone while eating a meal that lasts socially for 3 to 5 hours (24:108). By working on collective farms, the elders interact with relatives and friends on a daily basis. They get social recognition for doing useful work, and their community makes them feel needed. A similar social-work relationship was observed among the people living in Vilcambamba Ecuador, by the author in 1973. Persons of all ages in Vilcambamba interacted as a group while working in the fields, while walking on the road on a Sunday, or while playing volleyball. These people do things together.

History supports the importance of social involvement in work to well-being. History books abound with stories about the impact of social changes brought about by the industrial revolution, and the profound effect these changes had on the emotional, spiritual, and social well-being of man. Machines deprived people of a sense of fulfillment from creatively participating on the job in group activities. Failure to satisfy this emotional-social involvement resulted in smoldering despair, boredom, listlessness, and alienation. The technological era has had a similar dehumanizing effect on us. An excess of comfort goods, and the change from physical work in social settings to a computer technology makes many men and women feel social isolation and a loss of worthiness. The social environment of jobs has become very temporary, which has resulted in a loss of identity, loss of friends, and loss of emotional prestige and ego.

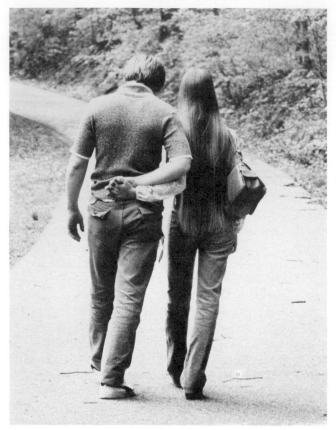

Figure 4.4a
Social dating may lead to a couple falling in love and marriage.

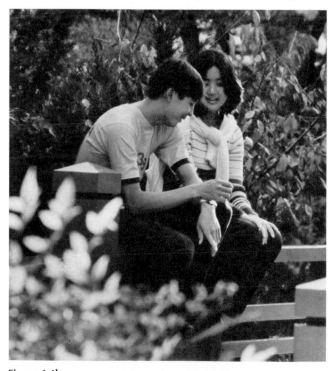

Figure 4.4b
Dating is a good way to socialize and fulfill your social needs.

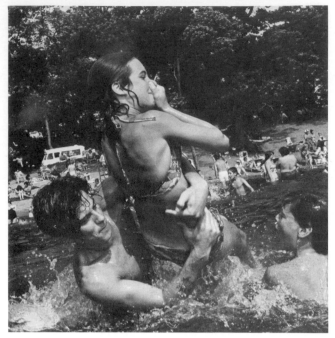

Figure 4.4c
Dating can be a way of getting to know each other by sharing a variety of experiences.

Able to only partially fulfill their social and emotional needs through work, many people now find their work less meaningful. They lack a sense of job and social commitment, and hence, have lost an important segment of their identity. Such work consequences have a carry-over effect on how we relate to others outside work environments (3:146;30:30). Toffler (36:78) feels that loss of job commitment breeds a loss of commitment to friends and community.

Although most persons today lack total job commitment, they fulfill their social needs by developing close buddy-type relationships on the basis of common interests. They join the ski club in the winter or a dance club, and form friendships that are changed rapidly as the interest in the group or activity changes (36:94). Because of this, much of the social activity of individuals today is described by Toffler (29:94) as "search behaviors"—a relentless searching for new friends to replace those who are either no longer present or who no longer share the same commitments. This turnover impels us to seek a very large pool of acquaintances; from this large pool we select a few dear friends. Thus while searching for friends by attaching ourselves to cults, organizations, and groups, we also search for ways to clarify our identities. Continuous searching reflects an inability to fulfill social-emotional needs, causing continuous stress, and the resultant overstimulation, fatigue, and additional distress.

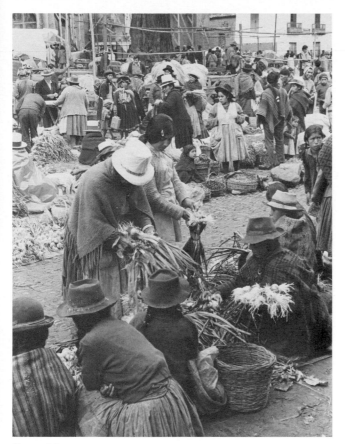

Figure 4.5

An example of how people in other cultures fulfill their need for socializing. The Peruvian women use the market place to socialize—a very important daily or weekly event for them.

In the past, people in permanent work and social settings derived emotional satisfaction and mental equilibrium, not only from their jobs, but from intimate association with the church, rituals, ceremonies, funerals, and with holiday celebrations (9:180). Today most of these socializing experiences have been displaced by massive rock concerts where most persons, as strangers, experience meaningless relationships. Rituals, ceremonies, and political rallies have been displaced by impersonal, temporary politics on television. Television displaces intimate social experiences and contributes to personal isolation, withdrawal, and social deprivation. We tend to live alongside city neighbors we seldom know, with little commitment to them or the local neighborhood. Although in very close physical contact, many of us have become isolated and lonely strangers.

College students leave behind old role expectations and old myths of the self upon entering college and engage in a range of experiences in new styles of friendships; student life; and special vocational, recreational, and leisure interests. They enter a period of transition into early adulthood, which Levinson (25) projects as extending from about age 20 to 30. He perceives young people of this age testing an adult life structure that provides a viable link between the valued self and the adult society. Chances are that you will refrain from making strong commitments until you have explored all the options for friendships, jobs, marriage, and so forth. At the same time, you will gradually evolve a stable life style—settle down, become more responsible, and make something of yourself. You will unify your self-identity. While endeavoring to do all this, you will need the support of your friends and society.

Everyone progresses at his or her own rate in evolving a comfortable and meaningful life style. While doing so, a few young persons will lead a transient life and capriciously change jobs, residences, and relationships. They create a loosely knit life style without stability or roots. Others will structure a mixture of stability and change, and make some commitments while postponing others. Still others will make strong commitments at the outset and build what they hope will be an enduring life-style structure. A few will become overwhelmed by the pressures of prestige-bearing success and try antisocial means to attain success.

It is not uncommon for young men and women attending college to flirt with deviance. While many will relate to revolutionary groups and attend counterculture meetings in their search for self-identity, they hold back from total commitment to such experiences. They may smoke pot or attend a Marxist meeting but withhold commitments to both as a way of life. Although they may deviate in one sense, realistically they keep the door open to future social-cultural commitments. Most will try to "settle down" by age 30 and seek a life of greater order and more stable attachments and commitments. Social support is vital for such a smooth transition into responsible adulthood during this time.

Social well-being recharges our psychic, spiritual, and total well-being. Having friends and acquaintances compliment us on how we look and how well we perform is an essential ego builder and status reinforcer. It gives us a sense of involvement—that someone cares, that we do have a place in society, and that we do belong with others in a community. It is only when we get such feedback from society that we can place a value on how important it is for us to do certain things. This feedback, in turn, clarifies and molds our values, strengthens our commitments, and gels our self-identity.

You can also use such social feedback to strengthen constructive health habits and behaviors. It is a lot easier not to smoke cigarettes, not to eat sugar products, and to exercise regularly when your friends do the same. Friends are your best medicine and therapy.

WAYS TO INCREASE YOUR SOCIAL SKILLS

Interpersonal skills that will help you to socialize include:

1. Developing communication—speaking, writing, body language; being able to carry on a conversation.
2. Developing work skills and cooperating with co-workers.
3. Being a good listener.
4. Becoming a good confidant—being prepared to receive and to share intimacies and secrets.
5. Being considerate of others and their feelings.
6. Having empathy for others.
7. Identifying with the interests of others.
8. Having good manners, tact, courtesy, and diplomacy—social grace.
9. Having sports skills—developing competency in two or more sports.
10. Having hobby competency—being skilled in at least one hobby.
11. Having art skills—in painting, ceramics, etc.
12. Having musical or dramatic skill.
13. Having dancing skills—in a variety of ballroom and social dances.
14. Having card and board game skills, such as bridge, monopoly, canasta, backgammon, black jack, checkers, and chess.
15. Staying physically fit, attractive, neat and clean.
16. Being able to comfort and care for others.
17. Being able to cook and keep house.
18. Being able to overlook faults and weaknesses in others.
19. Finding something nice to say about a person, even though you may not like the person.

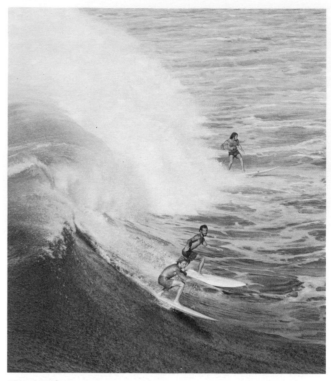

Figure 4.6b
Participating in a sporting event with friends can provide a lot of emotional fulfillment and allow for socializing. The three surfers share a lifetime sports experience that they can talk about in the future.

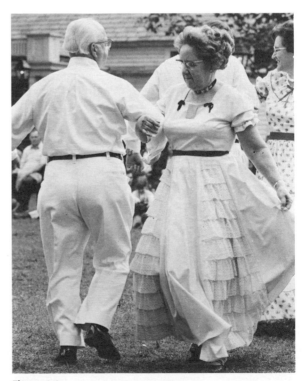

Figure 4.6c
Dancing is an excellent social activity for all age groups.

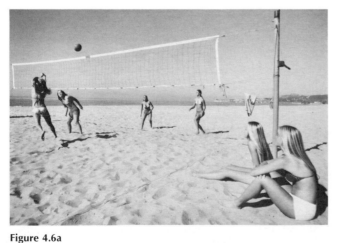

Figure 4.6a
Playing sports (volleyball) contributes to one's physical, emotional and social well-being.

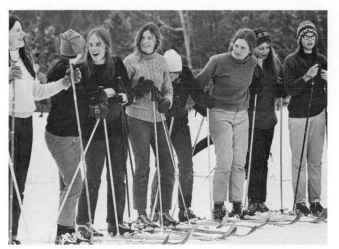

Figure 4.6d
Skiing is another way of socializing.

20. Sharing ideas, feelings, work, play, and possessions.
21. Showing others you appreciate them.
22. Smiling and displaying a pleasant and cheerful disposition.
23. Willing to try new adventures and meet new people.
24. Meeting people enthusiastically.
25. Having self-discipline and emotional control.
26. Being able to entertain onself.
27. Having moral values and rectitude.
28. Being able to initiate activities and assume responsible leadership.

These skills will help you to be more socially acceptable to others. They will make you a more interesting and likable person. Essential social well-being evolves from having personal skills to communicate, interact, and relate to persons of all ages. You should also have friends of various backgrounds and interests. Friends need to be cultivated each day—much as plants need to be watered each day.

WAYS TO MAINTAIN SOCIOCULTURAL WELL-BEING

College students are more fortunate than other persons in having a campus setting in which to fulfill their social needs. Going to classes, parties, and special events on or near the campus provides daily opportunities to interact with friends, as well as make new friends. The key is direct participation and involvement.

Here are a few ways to help you to socialize—choose several to accomplish each week. Start with those that appear easiest to you and progress to the more difficult. Record your personal reactions, as well as those you have attempted (39):

1. Introduce yourself to a new person in class each day.
2. Try to talk to your instructor at least once a week.
3. Invite someone who is going your way to walk with you or share a ride.
4. Ask someone new to have lunch, or a refreshment, with you once a week.
5. Ask someone to study with you.
6. Volunteer to work with another person on an assignment.
7. Ask someone you don't know very well if you can borrow 10 to 20 cents for a phone call, or to buy an apple. Arrange to pay the person back.
8. Invite someone every 2 weeks to accompany you to an inexpensive special event—like going to an art museum, or a noon-hour concert, or to just walk on the beach.
9. Find out the name of someone (opposite sex) in your class or social club. Call him or her on the phone and ask about the latest class assignment or coming event.
10. Go to a cafeteria and smile at the first three people who look at you. Strike up a conversation with at least one person of the same sex.
11. Sit down beside a stranger in a cafeteria and strike up a conversation.
12. Strike up a conversation with whoever is near you while you stand in line at a grocery store, bank, or movie.
13. Sit down beside a person of the opposite sex who looks interesting while on a bus, in a lounge, in class, or elsewhere. Strike up a conversation.
14. Ask several persons for directions, and strike up a brief conversation with one of them.
15. Converse with two or more strangers while jogging, running, or swimming.
16. Look for someone who needs help in your class or dormitory and offer to help.
17. Organize and throw a small party. Invite at least one person you do not know well but would like to get to know better.
18. Share your problem with another person and seek his or her advice.
19. Say "Hi" to five new people today. Smile and try to provoke a smile and a "Hi" from them.
20. Strike up a conversation with a person you would like to date. Establish rapport with the person before asking for a date.

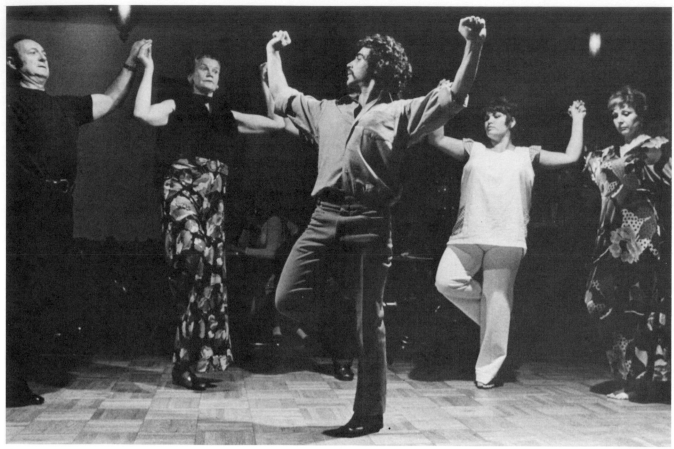

Figure 4.7
Trying a new first-time novel experience, like dancing the Greek folk dance Zorba, can be an enriching social experience.

21. Ask a new person to go running or jogging with you.
22. Ask a new person to help you with your hobby.
23. Ask a new person to show you how to do something new, such as a new dance step.
24. Do something thoughtful for a friend or someone you would like to meet.
25. Make a list of topics you can discuss with a stranger. Carry the list with you for quick reference.
26. Strike up a conversation with a young child at least once a day, and also with an older person. Share something with them.
27. Start volunteer work.
28. Borrow something, like a cup of honey, from your neighbor as an excuse to meet him or her.

BEHAVIOR MODIFICATION TECHNIQUES

A few suggestions for changing some aspects of your life style so as to improve your opportunities for sociocultural well-being are given here. Begin by responding to the inventory at the beginning of this chapter (if you have not done so yet).

Sociocultural well-being is structured by five role-activity categories. Identify the categories you are weakest in and try to strengthen these categories. This is especially important if you scored 100 points or less in the inventory. Try changing some of the ways you interact and relate with others. A few suggestions for improving each category follow:

Categories A and B (Family-Relatives)

If you do not visit very often with your friends and relatives, then you should begin doing so at least once a week. Visit in person a close friend or relative at least once a week. Find an excuse to visit, have lunch, watch TV, go dancing, go to the movies, or go for a walk.

Many places and activities lend themselves to socializing. Some of them are listed here. Which ones appeal to you?

1. Family or home.
2. Work.
3. Sports events—as spectator or participant.
4. Theater—as a member of the audience or a performer.
5. Musical concerts—as a member of the audience or a performer.
6. Parties and picnics.
7. Assemblies.
8. Parades.
9. Birthday parties.
10. Dances.
11. Special holiday celebrations like July 4, Halloween, Valentine's Day, Labor Day, etc.
12. Special awards.
13. Community meetings.
14. Evening and day classes.
15. Hiking.
16. Political rallies.
17. Recreational activities.
18. Vacationing.

Category C (Work or Classes)

Do your co-workers or boss, classmates or professors, compliment you one or more times a month about your studies or work? If not, then you should try to improve the quality of your work and make a deliberate effort to strike up a conversation with your boss, professors, co-workers, and classmates. Try going to social functions when they will be in attendance and become more gregarious.

Category D (Community or Campus)

Assess your cultural involvement a minimum of once a month as a performer or participant in campus-community activities, such as attending sports events, political rallies, special lectures or seminars, clubs or church, and so on. Plan to do something "cultural" with your friends or relatives.

Category E (Other Special Events)

Identify special events that you do not participate in. Plan to participate in one of these events one or more times a month on a regular basis.

Where to Go for Help

1. Campus counseling service.
2. Health education instructor.
3. Local YWCA or YMCA.
4. Local church groups.

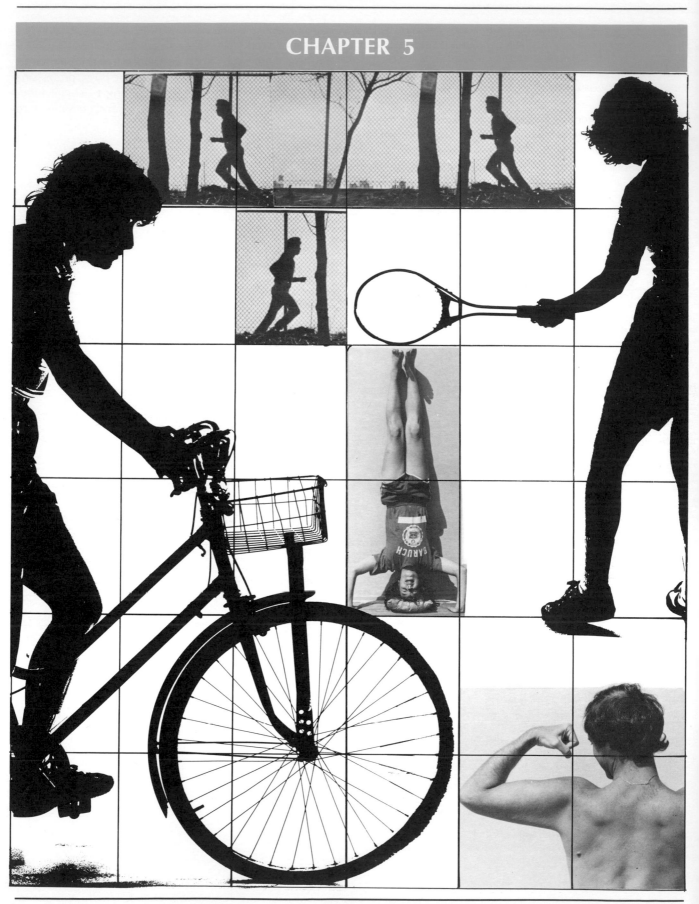

What is physical fitness? Many people define it as the capacity to carry out every-day activities (work and play) without excessive fatigue and with enough energy in reserve for emergencies. Those who subscribe to this definition are probably not as physically fit as they should be. Why? Because physical fitness refers to more than just energy for work and play. It is the capability of the heart, blood vessels, lungs, and muscles to function at optimal efficiency. Optimal efficiency means the capacity not only for enthusiastic and pleasurable participation in work, daily tasks, and recreational activities, but also for prevention of cardio-vascular disorders, obesity, and other health problems.

In this chapter we will be examining the components of physical fitness and the numerous benefits of physical fitness for emotional and physical health. The main focus of the chapter will be on the type of fitness program that provides benefits for all systems in the body and on how you can tailor-make your own fitness pro-gram for lifelong good health. Your fitness program can be inexpensive, require very little, if any, facilities or equipment and can be independent of what others do.

Find out just how fit you really are before reading this chapter.

☞ WHAT IS YOUR PHYSICAL FITNESS LEVEL?

Here are two ways to determine how physically fit you are: the 12-minute test and the 1.5-mile test.

THE 12-MINUTE TEST

If you already feel that you are in poor shape, do not take this test, as it may be too taxing. If you feel that you are physically fit but would like to determine your level of fitness, follow these steps:

1. Find a track of clearly defined length (440-yard outdoor track, 220-yard indoor track) or make one of your own up to 2 miles long.
2. Dress comfortably (shorts and running shoes). You should abstain from smoking or eating for 2 hours prior to test.
3. Bring a watch with a second hand to mark the time accurately. You can keep the time yourself or have a friend keep it for you.
4. Warm up with 5 to 10 minutes of calisthenics.
5. Start the watch and start running. Keep track of the number of laps you run. Mark the spot where you finish at the end of 12 minutes. Record the dis-tance you ran.

6. If your breath gets short while running, walk for a while until it comes back; then run some more. Keep going for the full 12 minutes. When you are through running, be sure to ease down afterward—walk around rather than sit down on the ground.
7. Use Table 5.1 to determine your fitness level.

Table 5.1

12-minute walking or running test
Distance (miles) Covered in 12 Minutes

Fitness Category		Age (years)					
		13–19	20–29	30–39	40–49	50–59	60+
I. Very poor	(men)	<1.30 miles[a]	<1.22	<1.18	<1.14	<1.03	<.87
	(women)	<1.0	< .96	< .94	< .88	< .84	<.78
II. Poor	(men)	1.30–1.37	1.22–1.31	1.18–1.30	1.14–1.24	1.03–1.16	.87–1.02
	(women)	1.00–1.18	.96–1.11	.95–1.05	.88– .98	.84– .93	.78– .86
III. Fair	(men)	1.38–1.56	1.32–1.49	1.31–1.45	1.25–1.39	1.17–1.30	1.03–1.20
	(women)	1.19–1.29	1.12–1.22	1.06–1.18	.99–1.11	.94–1.05	.87– .98
IV. Good	(men)	1.57–1.72	1.50–1.64	1.46–1.56	1.40–1.53	1.31–1.44	1.21–1.32
	(women)	1.30–1.43	1.23–1.34	1.19–1.29	1.12–1.24	1.06–1.18	.99–1.09
V. Excellent	(men)	1.73–1.86	1.65–1.76	1.57–1.69	1.54–1.65	1.45–1.58	1.33–1.55
	(women)	1.44–1.51	1.35–1.45	1.30–1.39	1.25–1.34	1.19–1.30	1.10–1.18
VI. Superior	(men)	>1.87	>1.77	>1.70	>1.66	>1.59	>1.56
	(women)	>1.52	>1.46	>1.40	>1.35	>1.31	>1.19

Source: With permission from Kenneth H. Cooper, *The Aerobics Way,* New York: Evans, 1978, p. 88.
[a] < Means "less than"; > means "more than."
NOTE: Other means of field testing, treadmill, and detailed instructions regarding the administration of the 12-minute running test can be found in the appendix of *The Aerobics Way* (pp. 277 and 280–283).

Having identified your physical fitness level or category, you can begin to prescribe an exercise program for yourself. (Such programs are described in this chapter.) The same 12-minute test can also be used to assess the progress you are making toward improved physical fitness. By testing yourself periodically (every 2 weeks or so), you can observe your improvement. The test will also help to motivate you to continue to exercise regularly.

THE 1.5-MILE TEST

Fitness expert Kenneth Cooper (1970) has suggested that a run of at least 1.5 miles, or at least 12 minutes, is necessary to determine whether a person is in peak condition. He worked with Air Force personnel to develop both the 12-minute and the 1.5-mile tests. Once again, you need not take the test if you already consider yourself to be in fitness category I or II.

For the 1.5-mile test, follow these steps:

1. Find an area to run in that has clearly defined distance markings. Determine the number of laps or how far you will have to run to reach the 1.5-mile point.
2. Dress comfortably.
3. Bring a stopwatch or a watch with a second hand so that you or a friend can keep track of your time.
4. Warm up with 5 to 10 minutes of calisthenics.

5. Start the watch and start running. If you feel yourself short of breath, slow down to a walk until your breath comes back, and then run some more.

6. When you reach the 1.5-mile mark, stop running and record your time. Be sure to ease down from your run by walking around for a while. Do not sit or lie down immediately after the run.

7. Use Table 5.2 to determine your fitness level.

Table 5.2

1.5-Mile Run Test Fitness Categories
Running Time (minutes) for 1.5-Mile Distance

Fitness Category		Age (years)					
		13–19	20–29	30–39	40–49	50–59	60+
I. Very poor	(men)	>15:31 miles[a]	>16:01	>16:31	>17:31	>19:01	>20:01
	(women)	>18:31	>19:01	>19:31	>20:01	>20:31	>21:01
II. Poor	(men)	12:11–15:30	14:01–16:00	14:44–16:30	15:36–17:30	17:01–19:00	19:01–20:00
	(women)	18:30–16:55	19:00–18:31	19:30–19:01	20:00–19:31	20:30–20:01	21:00–21:31
III. Fair	(men)	10:49–12:10	12:01–14:00	12:31–14:45	13:01–15:35	14:31–17:00	16:16–19:00
	(women)	16:54–14:31	18:30–15:55	19:00–16:31	19:30–17:31	20:00–19:01	20:30–19:31
IV. Good	(men)	9:41–10:48	10:46–12:00	11:01–12:30	11:31–13:00	12:31–14:30	14:00–16:15
	(women)	14:30–12:30	15:54–13:31	16:30–14:31	17:30–15:56	19:00–16:31	19:30–17:31
V. Excellent	(men)	8:37–9:40	9:45–10:45	10:00–11:00	10:30–11:30	11:00–12:30	11:15–13:59
	(women)	12:29–11:50	13:30–12:30	14:30–13:00	15:55–13:45	16:30–14:30	17:30–16:30
VI. Superior	(men)	< 8:37	< 9:45	<10:00	<10:30	<11:00	<11:15
	(women)	<11:50	<12:30	<13:00	<13:45	<14:30	<16:30

Source: With permission from Kenneth H. Cooper, *The Aerobics Way,* New York: Evans, 1978, p. 89.

[a] < Means ''less than''; > means ''more than.''

NOTE: Detailed instructions regarding the administration of the 1.5-Mile Run Test can be found in the appendix of *The Aerobics Way* (pp. 282–283).

BASIC COMPONENTS OF PHYSICAL FITNESS

There are five *major* components of physical fitness: muscular strength, muscular endurance, flexibility, balance, and cardiovascular-respiratory endurance and efficiency (see Figure 5.1).

Muscular Strength

A prerequisite to all other aspects of physical fitness, muscular strength is the capacity of a muscle to exert proximal force against a resistance. Muscular strength is built through the exercising of specific muscles, as by weight lifting and calisthenics.

Muscular Endurance

The capacity of a muscle to exert a force repeatedly over a period of time is called muscular endurance. It is the ability to apply strength and sustain it. Muscular endurance is developed by exercizing muscles and gradually taxing them for longer and longer periods.

Flexibility

The optimal range of movement around body joints, flexibility is developed and maintained by regular exercise of all parts of the body. Particularly good exercises are those that involve the bending and stretching of muscles in the legs, arms, thighs, back, waist, and neck.

Balance

Balance is the ability to maintain bodily equilibrium in some fixed position. To develop a good sense of balance, one needs muscular strength and endurance, as well as practice.

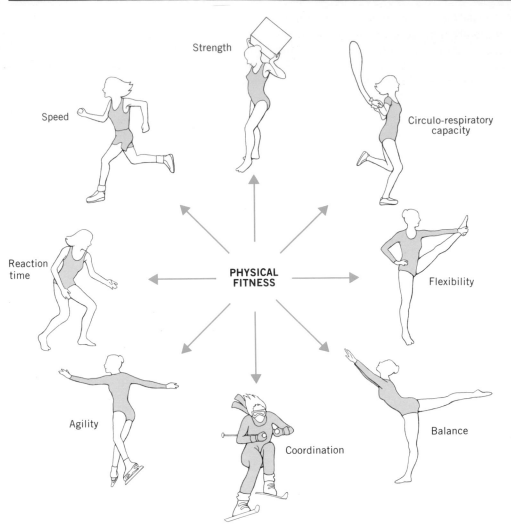

Figure 5.1.
Physical fitness is composed of many components.

Cardiovascular-Respiratory Fitness

The most essential fitness component is cardiovascular-respiratory fitness. It is the ability of the heart, blood vessels, and lungs to deliver nutrients and oxygen to the tissues and to remove wastes as quickly and efficiently as possible. This type of fitness is developed and maintained through regular whole-body movement over an extended period of time, such as occurs with running, swimming, and bicycling.

Other elements of fitness, such as speed and agility, are less important for everyday living. They are valuable in certain sports and activities, but they are not essential to optimal health.

Keep in mind that physical fitness is an essential prerequisite for optimal well-being (see Chapter 1). Before you can have emotional, social, and spiritual well-being, you must have physiological fitness.

THE BENEFITS OF PHYSICAL FITNESS

Why go to the trouble of exercising everyday? What is the value in being physically fit? Can't one live a long and healthy life without purposely including physical activities in one's daily schedule? The fact is that physical fitness *can* lengthen your life and improve your health (see Table 5.3). Furthermore, it can improve your appearance and even your emotional health. The benefits of a regular fitness program are so numerous that we will be able to examine only a few of them here (see Table 5.4).

The most valuable aspect of regular high-level exercise is its contribution to the health of the cardiovascular system. In regular exercise, the large leg and body muscles put stress on the heart and arteries, thereby forcing them to work and to be fit. Another way to keep

Table 5.3

Deaths[a] per 100 Men by Degree of Exertion

Age	No Exercise	Slight Exercise	Moderate Exercise	Heavy Exercise
40–49	1.46	1.17	1.12	1.00
50–59	1.43	1.17	1.06	1.00
60–69	1.91	1.64	1.19	1.00
70–79	2.91	2.03	1.45	1.00

Source: E. C. Hammond and L. Garfinkel, "Coronary Heart Disease, Stroke, and Aortic Aneurysm," *Archives of Environmental Health,* 19, August 1969, p. 174.

[a] From coronary heart disease.

NOTE: Data are based on a study of more than 1 million men and women followed over a 6-year period.

the arteries elastic and young is to vary the tempo of the workout. For example, by accelerating—and then taking short rests between exercise bouts and allowing the pulse rate to drop from 150 to 120 beats per minute, and then with exercise to raise it to 150 beats or more per minute—you force the arteries to dilate and constrict and become stronger and more elastic. It is this arterial elasticity that keeps your blood pressure around 120/80. Thus the cardiovascular system is the most important body system to take care of.

If you maintain a healthy heart and arteries, then all the other body systems and organs will be automatically aligned into physical fitness. Thus the faster and more efficiently the cardiovascular system transports the blood to the muscles, the better the physical fitness level. So, if you want to improve and maintain the physical fitness level of your body in general, then concentrate on improving your cardiovascular system. As the saying goes "You are as young (old) as your blood vessels." The aerobic way of exercising utilizes exercises that keep the cardiovascular system physically fit.

People who exercise regularly have a slower heart rate, lower blood pressure, better circulation and oxygen supply to all parts of the body, and lower blood cholesterol and triglyceride levels than those who do not exercise. Maintaining a high level of physical fitness is therefore a major method of preventing the number-one killer of Americans: heart disease.

Physical fitness also helps to combat obesity. Regular exercise helps regulate the appestat center that controls appetite. Exercise does help somewhat in using up calories as shown in Figures 5.2 and 5.3. Other health benefits of exercise include increased lung capacity, the alleviation of menstrual disorders, reduced fatigue, better sleep, firmer muscle tone, and ability to recover quickly from bodily injuries and illnesses.

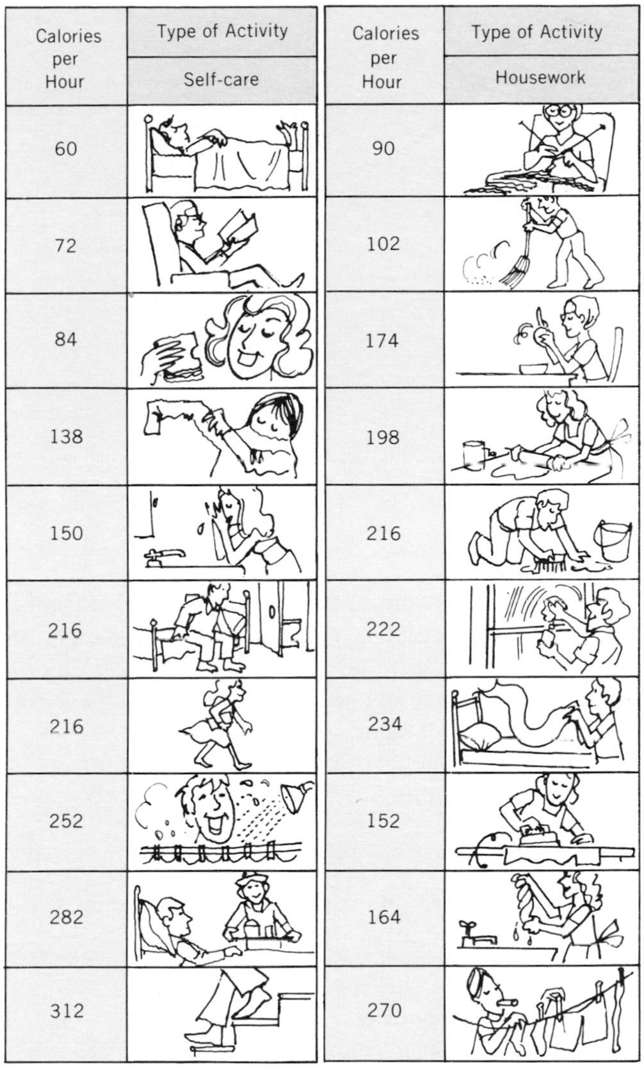

Calories per Hour	Type of Activity — Self-care	Calories per Hour	Type of Activity — Housework
60		90	
72		102	
84		174	
138		198	
150		216	
216		222	
216		234	
252		152	
282		164	
312		270	

Figure 5.2.

Calorie expenditures for different kinds of activities. (Adapted with permission from Justice J. Schifferes and Robert J. Synovitz, *Healthier Living,* New York: John Wiley & Sons, Inc., 1979, p. 163.)

Regular exercise is also a boon to physical appearance. Exercising all parts of the body firms up muscles at the waist, hips, thighs, arms, and stomach, helping you to retain an attractive and youthful figure throughout life. Exercise is also beneficial to the skin and helps in maintaining a clear and healthy-looking complexion. Furthermore, posture improves with regular exercise. Exercise slows down the aging process and keeps you looking young longer.

Finally, a fitness program can improve your emotional health in a number of ways. Physical activity relieves tension and stress, which allows you to be more efficient in your work and more relaxed in social inter-

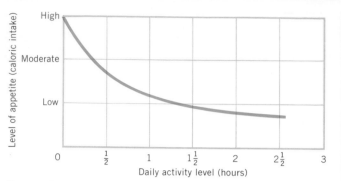

Figure 5.3.

The effect of exercise on appetite. We tend to eat less food when we exercise one-half hour or more each day. Physical activity does affect the appestat. (Adapted from Jon N. Leonard, J. L. Hoffer, and N. Pritikin, *Live Longer Now*, New York: Grosset, 1974, p. 197.)

actions. Regular exercise gives you a general feeling of well-being and alertness that permeates your other activities. Also, the fact that you are actively contributing to your optimal well-being enhances your self-concept and increases your self-esteem.

Many other benefits of prolonged physical fitness are summarized in Table 5.4.

Table 5.4

Summary of Benefits of Prolonged Physical Fitness

1. Improves physical appearance
2. Enhances popularity
3. Cements social relationships
4. Improves your personality
5. Improves your posture
6. Slows down the aging process
7. Relieves tension
8. Helps fight or control depression
9. Helps you to sleep more soundly
10. Helps to maintain emotional stability
11. Enables you to better adapt to and cope with the stresses of life
12. Enables you to work more efficiently
13. Provides greater stamina for everyday activities and emergencies, and allows you to recover more quickly from fatigue
14. Regulates (tunes up) all body systems and organs
15. Redistributes blood to all parts of body
16. Improves oxygen supply to all parts of body
17. Maintains sound muscle tone throughout the body
18. Alleviates dysmenorrhea (painful menstruation due to blood pooling in pelvic area)
19. Helps with process of childbirth (strengthens the uterus and the muscles)
20. Provides a greater supply of blood to the brain, making you more alert mentally
21. Prevents heart disease, stroke, cancer, and arthritis
22. Regulates or lowers blood cholesterol and triglyceride levels
23. Strengthens the heart muscle and keeps arteries elastic and young
24. Lowers high blood pressure
25. Decreases blood clotting time
26. Increases red blood cell mass and blood volume
27. Promotes regular bowel movements and prevents constipation
28. Speeds recovery from illness and injury
29. Helps you to survive (prevent accidents and injuries)
30. Regulates appestat (in hypothalmus), thereby regulating overeating, moods, emotions, and body weight
31. Depresses hunger
32. Aids digestion
33. Increases high-density lipoproteins
34. Reduces skin infections
35. Increases or improves sexual activity
36. Increases endorphins

TYPES OF EXERCISE

There are four major types of exercise, each with its particular effects and advantages: isometrics, isotonics, anaerobics, and aerobics (see Figure 5.4).

Isometrics

Exercises that tense muscles without producing movement, while demanding little or no oxygen expenditure, are called isometrics. For example, pushing against opposite sides of a door jamb, or making a fist and tensing your fist and lower arm would be considered isometric. Isometric exercises are capable of increasing the size and strength of individual skeletal muscles, but they have no significant effect on overall health. They do not increase cardiovascular-respiratory efficiency. At best, isometrics affect the skeletal muscles only.

Isotonics

Examples of isotonic exercises, which tense muscles to produce movement but make little demands for oxygen, include calisthenics and weightlifting, as well as such mild participant sports as shuffleboard, bowling, archery, and horseshoes. These exercises are preferred over isometrics because they exercise muscles over a range of motion. Thus they increase flexibility and firm up muscles. Principle muscle groups to exercise through isotonics are the back, abdominal, arm, shoulder, neck, and leg muscles. None of the isotonic exercises condi-

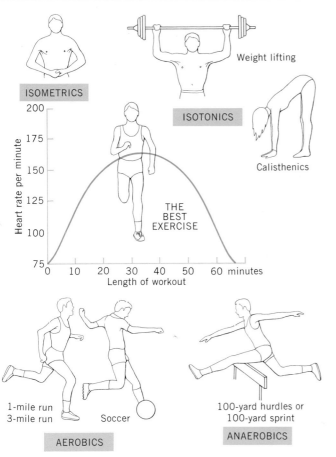

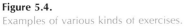

Figure 5.4.
Examples of various kinds of exercises.

tion the heart, lungs, or blood vessels, since they are usually done for a very short time.

Anaerobics

Exercises that demand a lot of oxygen but are over too quickly to produce a definite training effect (i.e., a positive change in cardiovascular-respiratory functioning) are called anaerobics. They fall into two classes: (1) those that demand reasonable amounts of oxygen but are cut short voluntarily, and (2) those that demand exorbitant amounts of oxygen and are cut short involuntarily. Examples of the first type include running a short distance, swimming a few laps, or walking up a flight of stairs. Examples of the second include wind sprints, interval training 100-yard and 220-yard sprints, swimming races, and bicycle sprints. These exercises demand so much oxygen in so short a time that the heart and lungs cannot supply it, thus creating an "oxygen debt" that must be paid by stopping and "catching your breath." Although such activities are good for building up speed, they are not complete in developing overall physical fitness.

Aerobics

Exercises that demand sufficient oxygen and last long enough to produce a definite training effect—a measurable improvement in the functioning of the cardiovascular and respiratory systems—are called aerobics. The value of aerobics was indicated in Kenneth Cooper's 1968 book, *Aerobics,* and since its publication, thousands of people around the world have taken up aerobic exercise programs. Examples of aerobic programs include running a mile in less than 8 minutes, swimming 24 laps (600 yards) in less than 15 minutes, cycling 5 miles or more in less than 20 minutes, playing soccer (not American football) for 60 minutes, and playing handball or racquetball for 35 or more minutes. All these activities must be done regularly, at least three or four times a week, for a fitness-training effect to be achieved. They must be built up to gradually over many weeks, as we will see later in the chapter.

All aerobic programs involve endurance activities. They demand oxygen without producing an intolerable oxygen debt, so they can be continued for long periods. Aerobics provide all the major benefits to physical health, appearance, and psychological well-being mentioned earlier in the chapter. For example, they create the kinds of physiological changes that help to insure against heart attack and disorders of the blood vessels. They improve your body's capacity to bring in oxygen and to deliver it to cells in all body tissues. At the same time, your heart grows stronger, pumping more blood with fewer strokes, the blood supply to your muscles improves, and your total blood volume increases. As oxygen consumption increases, the capacity for endurance increases. Thus aeorbic exercise proves to be the most valuable kind you can do, both for your body and your overall optimal well-being.

WHAT EXERCISE IS BEST?

What kind of exercise program will produce the desired training effects? Cooper suggests that your activity program, if limited to 12 to 20 minutes a day, must be vigorous enough to produce a sustained heart rate of 150 beats or more per minute. That is, for a training effect to take place, you must participate in an activity that accelerates your heart rate to 150 beats or more, and you must continue to exercise with the heart at a working steady state of 150 beats or higher (refer to Figure 5.5). If the exercise is not vigorous enough to produce a sustained heart rate of 150 beats but is still demanding oxygen, the exercise must be continued longer than 20 minutes; the total period of time depends largely on the oxygen consumed.

But how can you figure out your heart rate while you

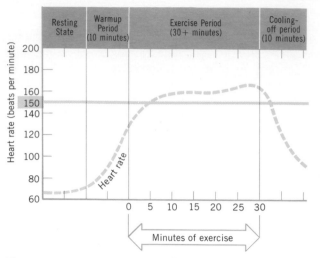

Figure 5.5.

Example of desirable exercise training pattern. Changes in heart rate are contrasted during periods of rest, warm-up, exercise activity and cooling off. A good warmup will prepare the cardiovascular system for more strenuous activity. A good exercise program is one that accelerates the heart rate up to 150 beats or more per minute and sustains this heart rate for up to 30 minutes or longer three or more times a week.

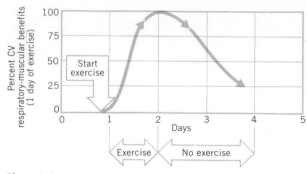

Figure 5.6a.

The effect of one day's exercise on all body systems over a 4-day period. Exercise-fitness benefits degenerate quickly; most of the benefits are lost by the third day of nonactivity.

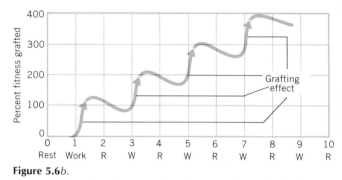

Figure 5.6b.

Grafting effects of continuous and regular exercising on the body. New muscle strength is grafted (added on) onto old strength. It pays to exercise regularly a minimum of every second day. The grafting effect is greatest in the early or beginning phase of an exercise program; the effect is less as one's fitness improves.

are exercising? By measuring various exercises for the amount of oxygen they require and by studying the heart rates of thousands of men and women engaged in aerobic exercises. Cooper has worked out a point system that eliminates the need for you to keep track of your heart rate; that is, Cooper awards points for exercises for certain types and duration. The more vigorous and sustained the exercise, the more points it is worth. For example, running 1 mile in less than 8 minutes is worth 5 points, running 1 mile in 8 to 10 minutes is worth 4 points, and running a mile in 10 to 12 minutes is worth 3 points.

According to Cooper, to achieve and maintain a training effect, men must earn 30 points a week, and women 24 points. Thus one could choose a 5-point activity (such as running a mile in under 8 minutes) and do it six times a week (for men), or a 4-point activity and do it six times a week (for women). With Cooper's point system, you do not need to measure your pulse constantly. Instead, the system tells you whether your exercise is strenuous enough for a training effect to take place.

How often should you exercise? Can you earn all 30 or 24 points in one day and then just exercise once a week? According to Cooper, you must exercise at least three or four days a week, or every other day. Training effect benefits start dropping off when you do not exercise at least every other day (see Figures 5.6a and 5.6b). Cooper prefers to exercise at least five or six days a

week, although he urges that people following an aerobics program rest at least one day a week (6).

What activities are the best aerobic exercises; that is, which provide the greatest training effect? In general, the best aeorbic activities are running, swimming, soccer, cycling, walking, stationary running, handball and racquetball, rope jumping, and basketball (see Table 5.5).

ESTABLISHING YOUR OWN FITNESS PROGRAM

There are a number of physical fitness programs available that can provide you with the exercise you need to ensure optimal fitness for your body systems. You should be cautious of any program, however, that promises you will lose pounds and feel better by only exercising a few minutes a week or that lasts for only a few short weeks, after which you will be "totally fit." Fitness involves a lifetime commitment to regular workouts—there are no shortcuts.

Table 5.5

Aerobics Point System Equivalents. Alphabetical listing of Activities Yielding Two Points.

Activity	Duration and/or Distance
Basketball	14 min
Cycling	2 miles in 6–8 min
Fencing	20 min
Football	20 min
Golf	12 holes (no motorized carts)
Handball	14 min
Hockey	14 min
Lacrosse	20 min
Rope skipping	8 min (continuous)
Rowing (2 oars)	12 min (20 strokes per min)
Running—walking	1 mile in 12–14$\frac{1}{2}$ min
Skating (roller or ice)	30 min
Skiing	20 min
Soccer	20 min
Squash	14 min
Stationary running	7$\frac{1}{2}$ min at 450–525 steps per min
Swimming	250 yards in 4–6 min
Tennis (singles)	1$\frac{1}{2}$ sets
Volleyball	30 min
Walking	2 miles in 29–40 min
Wrestling	5 min

Source: Adapted from *Aerobics* by Kenneth H. Cooper, M.D., M.P.H. Copyright © 1968 by Kenneth H. Cooper and Kevin Brown. Reprinted by permission of the publisher, M. Evans and Company, Inc., New York.

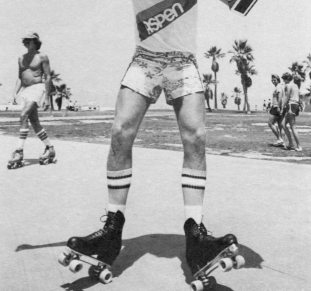

Figure 5.7
Roller skating—a new fitness fad.

Before you begin any program of regular vigorous exercise, be sure to see your doctor for a checkup. Tell your physician of your exercise plans to make sure that they are compatible with any health conditions you may have. Conditions that limit strenuous exercise include obesity, heart irregularities, high blood pressure, diabetes, kidney disease, and lung diseases.

What should you include in your exercise program? A balanced program exercises all the large skeletal muscles in all parts of the body. The muscles in the fingers and arms, the shoulder-joint area, the stomach, the legs, and the back should be involved. Strengthening the stomach muscles firms them up, preventing a "pot belly" in later life. Similarly, strengthening the back muscles would avoid backaches and back troubles in middle age. Generally, vigorous activity of the aerobic kind (running, cycling) does not exercise all these major muscles. So your exercise program should include regular calisthenics that are designed to stretch your muscles, make your joints and muscles flexible, and strengthen all your body muscles.

Most important for lifelong health is including regular vigorous activities in your exercise program. Although there are a number of approaches to this type of exercise, we will focus on what has become the most popular exercise program of all time: Kenneth Cooper's aerobics.

BEGINNING YOUR AEROBICS PROGRAM

Before starting an aerobics program, you will need to determine your fitness level. You can do so by taking either the 12-minute test or the 1.5-mile test described at the beginning of the chapter. If you feel that you are in poor physical condition, you need not take the test; in fact, it may be too hard on you.

Once you have classified yourself in a fitness category, you can choose a fitness program from many outlined in Dr. Cooper's books. He has developed programs for walking, running, cycling, swimming, stationary running, handball, racquetball, squash, basketball, soccer, hockey, stationary cycling, stair-climbing, and rope skipping. You should choose an activity that is compatible with your interests, your life style, and the facilities available to you.

Dr. Cooper's programs are broken down into several different age groups. We have space here to cover only the basic information for men and women under age 30. If you are over 30, you should consult Cooper's *The Aerobics Way* (1977) for programs geared to your age.

The object of aerobics is to earn exercise points and to gradually work up your weekly points until you reach the maintenance level (30 points for men, 24 points for women). If you fall into fitness category I, II, or III, you should begin exercising at a level of 1 to 9 points a week. In *The New Aerobics* (1970), Cooper offers programs that begin with a six-week "warm-up" period before you actually begin to earn points. If you are in category I, it is probably safest to begin this way. If you are in category II or III, you may want to go directly to a program that begins earning you points. Tables 5.6 through 5.10 outline basic 12-week programs for four

Table 5.6
Zones of Physical Fitness. (Most persons can be classified into one of these three zones. Behavioral characteristics are included to help classify persons.)

Behavioral Characteristics Who?	Discomfort Zone Unfit	Twilight Zone Semifit (Most Persons)	Comfort Zone "The Fit"
Signs when exercising	Distress Discomfort Pain (e.g., side ache) Tire quickly No will power Give up quickly Feel bad while exercising No endurance	Occasional discomfort Some self-discipline Some will power Some self-control Some endurance	Feel good Feel comfortable No pain Enjoy activity Pleasantly exhausted Good endurance Lots of will power Good self-control Addiction to exercise "Natural high"
Weight loss	None	1–3 pounds per week (gradual loss)	Weight controlled
Body figure	Overweight, obese	Moderate	Trim and slim
Use sleeping pills and medication	Often	Sometimes	No need
Insomnia	Often	Sometimes	Seldom—if ever
Tension and stress	A lot Difficulty handling stress	Fair amount ?	None—handle stress well
Control appetite and overeating	Unregulated hypothalmus Eat junk foods and overeat	Hypothalmus is flustered or confused Eat junk foods	Regulates hypothalmus Do *not* overeat Refrain from junk foods Do not drink alcohol or smoke
Emotional-psychic attitude	Poor Negative attitude toward life	Moderate Some negativism—take easy way out	Excellent Positive attitude toward life
Length of training *Transition*—based on exercising 3–4 times a week training effect	2–3 weeks or more	4–6 weeks Most persons get stuck here	2+ months of training to attain this zone

major activities. Cooper stresses the fact that the point levels are what you should try to reach by the *end* of the week—you should start gradually and work toward the full point value after a few days. Furthermore, you should not be a slave to the points. If you reach a plateau at, say 15 points a week, do not worry about it. Eventu-

ally you will be able to work your way up the point ladder. Most importantly, do not try to "get ahead" of the program. Even if you feel you can make 30 points the first week, take it easy and gradually work toward that total when it is scheduled to come up in the program.

Table 5.7

Walking Exercise Program (under 30 years of age)

Week	Distance (miles)	Time Goal (min)	Frequency per Week	Points per Week
1	2.0	35:00	3	9
2	2.0	34:00	3	9
3	2.0	33:00	3	9
4	2.0	32:00	4	12
5	2.0	31:00	4	12
6	2.0	30:00	4	20
7	2.0	29:00	4	20
8	2.0	28:00	4	20
9	2.5	34:00	4	26
10	2.5	33:00	4	26
11	3.0	42:00	4	32
12	3.0	41:00	4	32
	or			
	2.5	33:00	5	32.5

Source: From *The Aerobics Way,* p. 95, by Kenneth H. Cooper, M.D., M.P.H., Copyright © 1977, by Kenneth H. Cooper. Reprinted by permission of the Publisher, M. Evans & Co., Inc., New York, N.Y. 10017.

Table 5.8

Running Exercise Program[a] (under 30 years of age)

Week	Distance (miles)	Time Goal (min)	Frequency per Week	Points per Week
1	2.0	32:00	3	9
2	2.0	30:30	3	9
3	2.0	27:00	3	15
4	2.0	26:00	3	15
5	2.0	25:00	3	15
6	2.0	24:30	3	15
7	2.0	24:00	3	21
8	2.0	22:00	3	21
9	2.0	21:00	3	21
10	2.0	19:00	3	27
11	2.0	18:00	4	36
12	2.0	<17:00	4	36
	or			
	2.5	<22:00	3	34.5

Source: From *The Aerobics Way,* p. 95, by Kenneth H. Cooper, M.D., M.P.H., Copyright © 1977, by Kenneth H. Cooper. Reprinted by permission of the Publisher, M. Evans & Co., Inc., New York, N.Y. 10017.
[a] Start the program by walking, then walk and run, or run, as necessary to meet the changing time goals.

Table 5.9

Cycling Exercise Program (under 30 years of age)

Week	Distance (miles)	Time Goal (min)	Frequency per Week	Points per Week
1	2	9:00	3	1.5
2	2	8:00	3	4.5
3	3	10:45	3	9
4	3	10:00	4	12
5	4	15:00	4	18
6	4	14:30	4	18
7	5	18:30	4	24
8	5	18:00	4	24
9	5	17:30	5	30
10	6	22:30	4	30
11	6	22:00	4	30
12	6	21:30	4	30

Source: From *The Aerobics Way,* p. 96, by Kenneth H. Cooper, M.D., M.P.H., Copyright © 1977, by Kenneth H. Cooper. Reprinted by permission of the Publisher, M. Evans & Co., Inc., New York, N.Y. 10017. *Note:* During the first 6 weeks, warm up by cycling slowly for 3:00 min before attempting the specified distance and time. Cool down by cycling slowly for 3:00 min at the conclusion of exercise.

Table 5.10

Swimming Exercise Program (under 30 years of age)

Week	Distance (yards)	Time Goal (min)	Frequency per Week	Points per Week
1	300	12:00	4	0
2	300	10:30	4	0
3	300	10:15	4	0
4	500	20:00	5	0
5	500	18:00	5	0
6	500	17:00	5	0
7	200	4:00	5	8.35
8	300	6:00	5	12.5
9	400	8:00	5	16.65
10	500	10:30	5	20.85
11	600	12:30	5	25
12	800	15:30	4	30.68

Source: From *The Aerobics Way,* p. 96 by Kenneth H. Cooper, M.D., M.P.H., Copyright © 1977, by Kenneth H. Cooper. Reprinted by permission of the Publisher, M. Evans & Co., Inc., New York, N.Y. 10017.

Periodically through your 12-week program, you may want to retake the 12-minute or 1.5-mile test to assess where you are. Generally, the number of points you earn each week correlates with your level of fitness, as listed in Table 5.11.

Table 5.11
Classification of Physical Fitness

| Category | Fitness Points | |
	Men	Women
Very poor	<1	<1
Poor	1–14	1–9
Fair	15–29	10–23
Good	30–50	24–40
Excellent	>50	>40

Before you begin any aerobics program, there are a few preparations you should make. First of all, you should dress correctly (see Figure 5.8). If you are running, for example, your most important investment will be a pair of running shoes that will help cushion your feet from the shocks of contact with hard surfaces and help to prevent such problems as ankle sprains, calluses, and foot disorders. You will need to dress loosely for freedom of movement. By all means avoid rubber suits or heavy clothing designed to make you perspire heav-

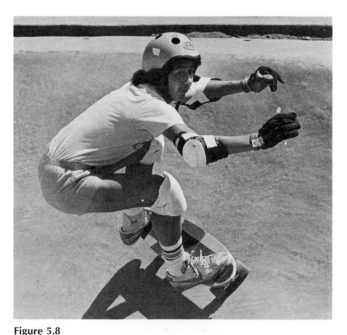

Figure 5.8
Skateboarding—a new Olympic sport? Is this skater dressed safely?

ily. These suits interfere with the body's cooling system by preventing perspiration from evaporating.

Second, you should avoid exercising within 90 minutes after a large meal. After a meal, blood flow is rerouted from your muscles to the digestive system for a while, and you need that blood flow for your muscles during exercise. Furthermore, you should drink plenty of liquids, as the body loses a great deal of water when you participate in vigorous exercise.

Before starting your regular aerobics run, walk, or swim, always spend at least 10 minutes warming up. Warm-up exercises should include those that stretch muscles throughout the body, but they should not be so vigorous as to wear you out before your regular aerobics activity begins. Warm-ups are important because they are safeguards against cramps, sprains, and strains, and they condition the heart and blood vessels for more vigorous exercise. Equally important is devoting 5 or 10 minutes to cooling down after your aerobic exercise. If you run for two miles, for example, do not sit down or lie down at the end of the run. Instead, walk around slowly for at least 5 minutes. If you swim, walk up and down along the pool's edge when you finish your workout. Cooling down helps to prevent nausea, cramps, and faintness because your blood is not allowed to pool in your legs and feet. Cooling-off exercises keep the blood circulating and allow the cardiovascular-respiratory-muscular systems to deprogram from a working state to a resting state. You should not go directly to a shower or sauna after an aerobics workout.

Finally, if you develop distress symptoms, such as shortness of breath, side aches, or nausea, while working out, do not continue. If you are running, slow down and walk for a short distance. Allow yourself to return to normal. If you experience such discomfort regularly while working out, or if your pulse rate does not return to normal within 10 minutes after an aerobics session, you have probably taken on too strenuous a program for your level of fitness. You will have to ease up in your program until your body is ready for more strenuous activity.

MAINTAINING YOUR AEROBICS PROGRAM

If you fall into category IV, V, or VI, or if you have completed a 12-week basic aerobics program, you are ready for a regular maintenance program that will give you your necessary number of points per week. During the 12-week program you need to stick to one type of exercise, but once you have reached at least 30 points a

Table 5.12

Three Suggested Maintenance Programs

Exercise	Distance	Time	Frequency	Weekly Points
1. Running	1–½ miles	12 min	Mon., Wed., Fri., and Sun.	32
2. Walking	1–½ miles	25 min	2 times per day 4 days per week	16
Handball or racquetball		30 min (not counting breaks)	Mon., Wed., and Fri.	15
3. Cycling	3 miles	11 min	2 times per day 5 days per week	30

week for men or 24 for women, you can vary your activity program. Choose any combination of activities; as long as they add up to your minimum number of points per week, and as long as you do them at least every other day, you can be assured of optimal physical fitness.

Three possible maintenance programs are listed in Table 5.12. Or you could build an exercise program combining several activities, based on your life style, interests, climate, and so on. You might run 1½ miles two days a week, play handball for 30 minutes one day, swim 600 yards another day, and go bicycling 5 miles on a fifth day, and earn 30 points for the week.

For more alternative activities and for detailed point values for each activity, see Kenneth Cooper's *The Aerobics Way*. This book also provides point values for such activities as golf, rowing, tennis, badminton, dancing, skiing, skating, volleyball, and fencing. Main-

tenance programs designed specially to follow the 12-week programs are presented in Tables 5.13 through 5.16. They offer several combinations of duration, distance, and frequency to choose from in order to maintain minimum fitness points.

Whatever fitness program you decide on, remember that physical fitness is a lifelong process. If you stop when you reach 30 points in Cooper's program, for example, you will not remain "physically fit." You have to maintain your fitness program for the rest of your life—and your life will most likely be longer and richer because of it. Keep in mind that the reason for exercising is to stay healthy. Staying healthy means not only freedom from colds and flu, but the ability to reduce the risk of heart disease and cancer, sleep well, feel good, and function optimally on the job and in social interactions. The more physically fit you are, the greater your potential for optimal well-being.

Table 5.13

Walking Maintenance Program

Distance (miles)	Time Requirement (min)	Frequency per Week	Points per Week
2.0 or	24:01–30:00	6	30
3.0 or	36:01–45:00	4	32
4.0 or	48:01–60:00	3	33
4.0	60:01–80:00	5	30

Source: From *The Aerobics Way,* p. 129, by Kenneth H. Cooper, M.D., M.P.H., Copyright © 1977, by Kenneth H. Cooper. Reprinted by permission of the Publisher, M. Evans & Co., Inc., New York, N.Y. 10017.

Table 5.14

Running Maintenance Program

Distance (miles)	Time Requirement (min)	Frequency per Week	Points per Week
1.0 or	6:41–8:00	6	30
1.5 or	10:01–12:00	4	32
1.5 or	12:01–15:00	5	32.5
2.0 or	16:01–20:00	4	36
2.0	13:21–16:00	3	33

Source: From *The Aerobics Way,* p. 129, by Kenneth H. Cooper, M.D., M.P.H., Copyright © 1977, by Kenneth H. Cooper. Reprinted by permission of the Publisher, M. Evans & Co., Inc. New York, N.Y. 10017.

Table 5.15

Cycling Maintenance Program

Distance (miles)	Time Requirement (min)	Frequency per Week	Points per Week
5.0	15:01–20:00	5	30
or			
6.0	18:01–24:00	4	30
or			
7.0	21:01–28:00	4	36
or			
8.0	24:01–32:00	3	31.5

Source: From *The Aerobics Way,* p. 129, by Kenneth H. Cooper, M.D., M.P.H., Copyright © 1977, by Kenneth H. Cooper. Reprinted by permission of the Publisher, M. Evans & Co., Inc., New York, N.Y. 10017.

Table 5.16

Swimming Maintenance Program

Distance (yards)	Time Requirement (min)	Frequency per Week	Points per Week
600	10:01–15:00	6	30
or			
800	13:21–20:00	4	30.5
or			
900	15:01–22:30	4	36
or			
1000	16:41–25:00	3	31

Source: From *The Aerobics Way,* p. 130, by Kenneth H. Cooper, M.D., M.P.H., Copyright © 1977, by Kenneth H. Cooper. Reprinted by permission of the Publisher, M. Evans & Co., Inc., New York, N.Y. 10017.

BEHAVIOR MODIFICATION TECHNIQUES

If you are in poor physical condition, you can evolve a good exercise program by referring to the section on "maintaining your aerobic program." You need to begin exercising and making a commitment to workout regularly. You should also be motivated to exercise and get into a routine that breaks old inactivity habits and behaviors. Here are a few suggestions to help you structure and establish a regular weekly exercise pattern:

1. Initially measure and record, each month thereafter, your physical body size-weight, body fat, waistline, and upper arm and thigh girths. Compare them each month for changes.
2. Exercise the same time each day.
3. Get proper clothes for exercising (shorts, T-shirt, running shoes, etc.)
4. Establish fitness and exercise goals for yourself. Such goals should allow for progression, improvement in physical fitness, and success in feeling good about exercising regularly. For example, you should move from a very poor fitness to a poor fitness classification in about a month. Your next goal should be to improve from poor to a good fitness level by the third month. Keep revising your goals until you get into the excellent or superior classification. Thereafter you can establish other goals, like running in a 6-mile run.
5. Plot your daily and/or weekly achievements (your fitness points as well as distance, time trial, or both) on Graph 5.1. Doing this allows you to instantly analyze your performances and progression from week to week. It also gives you a good idea of your fitness level and provides an incentive to continue with your fitness program.
6. Add variety to your fitness program. Such a variety, as detailed earlier in this chapter, helps to overcome the mental boredom of doing a routine.
7. Clarify for yourself a philosophy of exercising, physical fitness, well-being, and life style. You should not just run to win a race or improve your fitness level. Instead, you should exercise to maintain physical fitness so that you will keep all of your body physically fit, feel better, maintain good health, and strive for optimal well-being. See Table 5.4 to review the benefits of prolonged physical fitness.
8. Exercise near where you live so that you do not

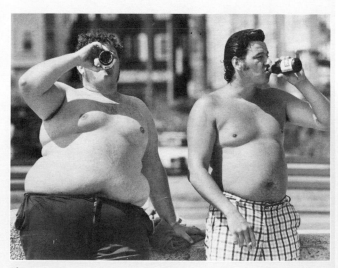

Figure 5.9

Inactivity and social drinking often can displace physical fitness. The lifestyles reflected by the behaviors of the two men and their physiques tell one a great deal about the physical fitness states of the two men.

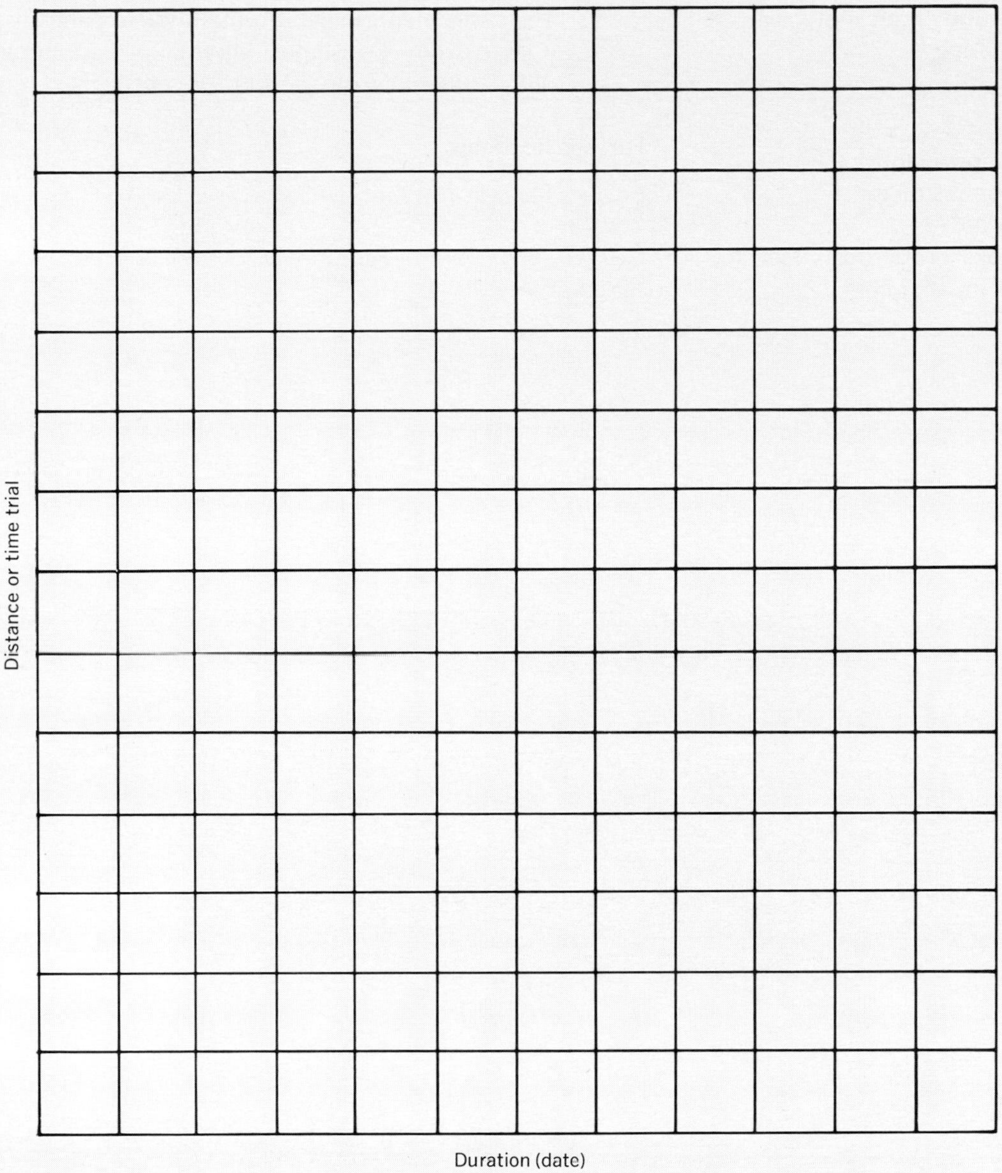

Distance or time trial

Duration (date)

GRAPH 5.1

Profile of your physical fitness. This graph helps you to keep a record of your physica fitness test over a period of time. By plotting your performances on this graph and joining the plots each week for 3 months, you can get a visual profile of your fitness level and also your progress in attaining and maintaining it. Or you can keep a profile of your physical fitness progress for a year.

There are no designated units on the vertical column on the left side of the graph. You should use units that are part of your physical fitness test (e.g., the distance covered in a 12-mile jog-run test, or time for the 600-yard or mile distances).

need to travel. This allows you greater opportunity to exercise and also allows you to shower after the exercise.

9. Exercise with someone if possible. Having a companion makes it more fun and adds a social dimension to exercising. But do not become overly dependent on the companion should

he or she not be able to exercise with you all the time.

10. Participate occasionally in a special athletic or sports event in which you can self-test your improved state of physical fitness in the presence of your friends. This allows you to get social recognition and compliments from your friends

and relatives, one of the motivations we all need to continue exercising.

Where to Go for Help

1. Your health education instructor.
2. Your physical education instructor.
3. Your local YMCA or YWCA.
4. Kenneth Cooper's books on aerobics (see the references at the end of this chapter).
5. The consumer booklet "Adult Physical Fitness." (Order from Consumer Information, Center–088–F, Pueblo, Colo. 81009; 70 cents).

Further Readings

Cooper, Kenneth H., *The Aerobics Way,* New York: Evans, 1978.

Getchell, Bud, *Physical Fitness-A Way of Life,* 2nd ed., New York: Wiley, 1979.

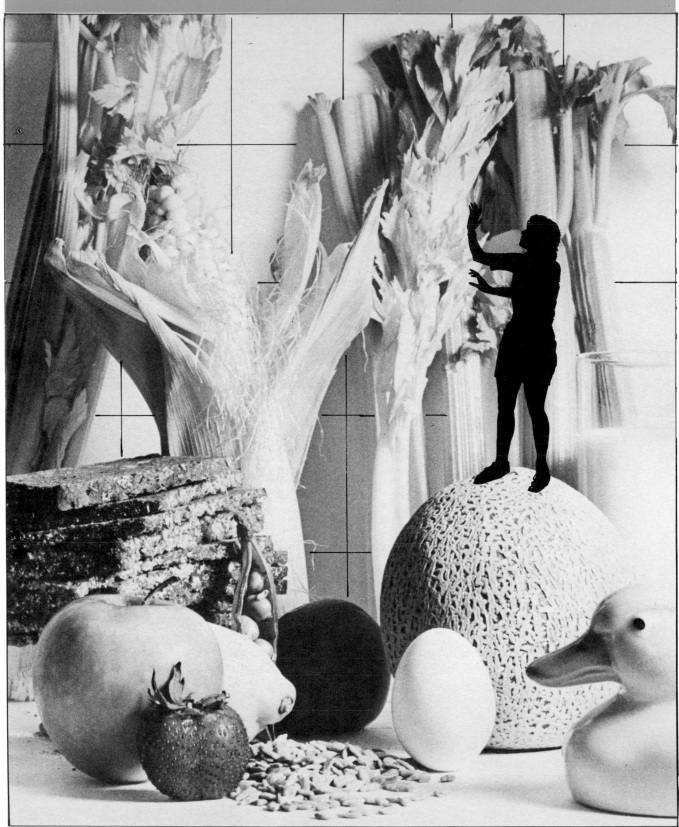

CHAPTER 6

NUTRITION

Debbie, a college freshman, had the following dinner: a big glass of Coca-Cola, two servings of French fries, a medium-sized hamburger on a white bun, a small lettuce salad with blue cheese dressing and lots of salt and pepper, and a single scoop of pistachio ice cream.

Was this a nutritious meal?
Will Debbie become what she eats?
What vitamins and minerals did she get from this meal?
Was her meal too high in fats?
Was this a balanced meal? If not, then what should she eat in the future?
If she eats this kind of diet for over 20 years, will she become fat and overweight? Or will she be predisposed to cancer, arthritis, acne, heart attack, and dental caries?
Was this meal deficient in vitamin C?
Does she need to supplement her meal with vitamin and mineral pills?

These and other questions related to diet and health are answered in this chapter, which provides you with the information you need in order to eat properly for optimal well-being. A behavior modification module to help you access your own diet and eating habits is included at the end of the chapter.

☞ NUTRIENT DEFICIENCY INVENTORY

(Do I need to take vitamin-mineral supplements?)

DIRECTIONS   Circle the answer in one of the four columns that best identifies you.

Health Behavior or Eating Habit	Always	Often	Sometimes	Never
1. Eat raw carrots	10	7	2	0
2. Ingest mineral oil as laxative	10	7	3	0
3. Boil vegetables (cabbage, beans, peas, etc.)	25	15	5	0
4. Eat beefsteak, hamburger, and roast pork	25	18	5	0
5. Eat white refined sugar and sweets (candy, ice cream, and chocolate bars)	40	30	10	0

Health Behavior or Eating Habit	Always	Often	Sometimes	Never
6. Eat refined white flour pastry (cookies, pies, puddings, etc.)	40	30	10	0
7. Eat French fries, fried chicken, etc.	40	30	10	0
8. Eat canned or processed foods	20	15	5	0
9. Drink cola drinks (other soft drinks) (1 or more 6-oz container)	40	30	7	0
10. Drink coffee or tea (1 or more cups per day)	40	30	7	0
11. Drink alcoholic beverages (3 to 5 drinks per week)	20	15	5	0
12. Smoke tobacco or marijuana cigarettes	50	35	10	0
13. Work in a cigarette smoke-filled room	30	20	5	0
14. Live in an air-polluted community	40	30	10	0
15. Use or work with pesticides or are exposed to paint, gasoline, or other fumes	30	20	5	0
16. Work in a noisy place	30	20	5	0
17. Experience work-caused emotional stress	60	45	10	0
18. Have colds, flu, or other infections	20	10	5	0
19. Take prescription drugs or medication (e.g., aspirin or sleeping pills)	40	30	8	0
20. Use birth control pills	15	10	3	0
21. Take laxatives or antacids	20	15	5	0
22. Get upset stomach or diarrhea	30	20	7	0
Subtotal	+	+	+	
Total				

CLASSIFICATION

Score Range	Need for Nutrient Supplements	Corrective Action
500–675	Very high	1. Take multinutrient supplements
		2. Eat a more-balanced diet
300–499	High	3. Change your life style
100–299	Moderate	1. Reassess your eating habits
		2. Reassess your life style
		3. If above reassessments still indicate moderate need, then take some supplements
0–100	Low	1. Eat a more-balanced diet

INTERPRETATION

Your responses to the Nutrient Deficiency Inventory is a very quick way to determine whether you might be deficient in vitamins and minerals. Confirm the results of your reaction to this inventory by analyzing your daily diet for vitamin, mineral, and amino-acid (protein) intake at the end of this chapter. Compare this analysis to the Recommended Minimum Daily Allowances (RMDA) in Table 6.12.

If this comparative analysis indicates that your diet is deficient in a few or many nutrients, then you should substitute foods rich in these nutrients. Second, follow up this substitution of foods by assessing your life style. Identify those daily habits and behaviors (e.g., how you cook foods, smoking cigarettes) that may be depleting or destroying nutrients, interfering with their absorption, or requiring nutrient amounts greater than the RMDA by referring to Table 6.12. Alter your high-risk circumstances before taking nutrient supplements. Try out your alternative habits for about a month or longer. Do you feel better? Reassess your diet—Are you getting enough nutrients from the food you eat? The procedures for making this diet assessment and suggestions for making habit changes are presented as a guide in the latter part of this chapter.

When the above priority suggestions fail to make you nutrient-sufficient, you should consider taking nutrient supplements. But before you do, read the remainder of this chapter so that you may become better informed about the nutrients your body needs and the best food sources of those nutrients, and then be able to decide for yourself.

WHAT IS FOOD?

Food is the basis of life and good health. It is essential for the body's growth, maintenance, and repair of tissues, and the regulation of body processes; it also provides the energy to perform or function adequately in society. Food is made up of seven major chemical substances called nutrients. These include carbohydrates, fats, amino acids (proteins), vitamins, minerals, fiber, and water. Most foods contain a mixture of these substances; hence foods fulfill more than one function. For example, practically all foods contain mixtures of all three energy nutrients (fats, carbohydrates, and proteins), although they are sometimes classified by the predominant nutrient. A protein-rich food, such as beef, actually contains a lot of fat, as well as protein, while a carbohydrate-rich food, such as corn, also contains fat and protein. Scientists have now identified about 50 different chemical substances in foods that are essential to sustaining life. These are summarized in Table 6.1. Although nutrient deficiency may appear only in a single organ or body system, the deficiency affects the entire body. Similarly, all the nutrients need to be present in the proper amounts in order for them to be utilized effectively and in order for the body to stay healthy. Thus ingesting a daily balance of these nutrients not only provides the energy for the body, but also prevents serious health problems, such as obesity, heart disease, diabetes, cancer, depression and emotional disorders, colds, allergies, and other disorders.

Different foods furnish different amounts of nutrients. Whether we do obtain adequate amounts of these nutrients from the foods depends on many factors. The foods we eat need to be broken down in the digestive system into minute particles so that they can be absorbed into the bloodstream, circulated through the body, and used by each individual body cell. This breakdown process is referred to as digestion and takes place in the mouth, stomach, and small and large intestines (see Figure 6.1). Techniques of food preparation, such as fermentation, and cooking, can affect the breakdown processes in various ways. On the one hand, cooking makes some of the nutrients in vegetables more readily digestible (carotene in carrots); on the other hand, cooking can destroy water-soluble vitamins.

Table 6.1

List of Essential 50 Nutrients[a]

Nutrient	Kinds of Nutrients
1. Water	
2. Fats	Essential linoleic acid
	Nonessential
	saturated
	unsaturated
3. Carbohydrates (CHO)	Simple CHO
	monosaccharides (sucrose) e.g., sugar
	disaccharides (fructose) e.g., honey
	Complex CHO
	polysaccharides (starch) e.g., whole unrefined grains, vegetables, and fruits
4. Proteins	Essential amino acids (incomplete proteins)
	histidine phenylalanine
	isoleucine threonine
	leucine tryptophan
	lysine valine
	methionine
	Nonessential amino acids (complete proteins)
	alanine hydroxyproline
	aspartic acid proline
	cystine serine
	glutamic acid tyrosine
	glycine

Nutrient	Kinds of Nutrients	
5. Vitamins	B-complex	
	B₁ (thiamin) → B_1 (thiamin)	choline
	B_2, G (riboflavin)	inositol
	B_3 (niacin)	lipoic acid
	B_5 (pantothenic acid)	(hioctic acid)
	B_6 (pyridoxine)	H (biotin)
	B_{12} (cyanocobalamin)	PABA (p-amino
	*B_{13} (orotic acid)	benzamine acid)
	*B_{15} (pangamic acid)	
	B, M, U (folic acid)	
	C (ascorbic acid)	
	*P (bioflavonoids) (related to vitamin C)	
	A (retinol)	
	D (folacin)	
	E (tocopherol)	
	K (prothrombin)	
6. Minerals	Calcium	Manganese
	Chlorine	*Molybdenum
	*Chromium	Phosphorus
	*Cobalt	Potassium
	Copper	*Selenium
	Fluorine	Sodium
	Iodine	*Sulfur
	Iron	*Vanadium
	Magnesium	Zinc
7. Fiber	Undigestible carbohydrate	
	Cellulose	
	Hemicellulose	
	Lignin	
	Pentosans	
	(Bran)	

[a] This table lists officially and unofficially recognized nutrients. Official ones are those recognized by the U.S. National Academy of Sciences. Unofficial nutrients* are those recognized by scientists and nutritionists in foreign countries but not so by the U.S. National Academy of Sciences. Prior to 1980, scientists in foregin countries conducted much more research on nutrition and health than in the United States. *Note:* The following elements have been found to be essential for laboratory animals since 1970, but human requirements are unknown: nickel, silicon, and tin.

OUR EATING HABITS

The American life style is not at all conducive to sound nutritional habits and optimal well-being. Most of us eat a variety of foods in an attempt to ensure a balanced daily diet. By doing so, we assume that the foods we eat contain adequate amounts of vitamins, minerals, and other essential nutrients that our bodies need. Unfortunately, this is not always the case. Instead, malnutrition—in the form of vitamin, mineral, and micro-nutrient deficiencies—is commonplace these days. This has been verified by numerous nutritional surveys. The first recent extensive nutritional survey made by the U.S. Department of Agriculture (USDA) in 1965 revealed that only 50 percent of American households had diets rated as "good" as those based on USDA standards (54:17). A follow-up study by the Public Health Service in 1970 of the eating habits of American people revealed gross vitamin and iron deficiencies (42:67, 54:17). Surveys also show that some teenagers

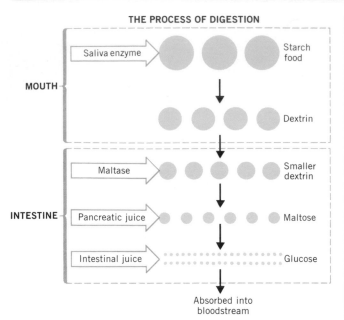

THE PROCESS OF DIGESTION

MOUTH

Saliva enzyme → Starch food

Dextrin

INTESTINE

Maltase → Smaller dextrin

Pancreatic juice → Maltose

Intestinal juice → Glucose

Absorbed into bloodstream

Figure 6.1.

Digestion breaks down large molecules of starch into smaller ones. Eventually, the small molecules (e.g., glucose) pass through villi in the walls of the small intestine into the bloodstream.

have food intakes that fail to supply the Recommended Daily Allowances (RDA) for most of the minerals (42:116). Numerous vitamin C deficiencies have been found among the 18 to 25 age group and in the elderly (42:162). Our food habits are continually changing for the worse and are more responsive to social, cultural, economic, and television influences than to the real nutritive needs of human bodies. These changes are summarized in Table 6.2 Americans of all ages are not eating foods that contain enough quantities of certain vitamins, minerals, amino acids, and other nutrients. A well-fed, nonhungry person is not necessarily a well-nourished person. We appear to be eating a lot of calories but not adequate amounts of vitamins and minerals.

In the decades since the Basic Four Food Groups Guide was developed, the amount of nutritional knowledge, food supply patterns, health conditions, and behavioral life style patterns has changed. People are less active physically; obesity and overweight is very common; and more people than before die from nutrition-related diseases. In 1976 and 1977, the U.S. Senate Select Committee on Nutrition and Human Needs (67) considered the evidence linking the health status and

Table 6.2

Dietary Changes in the United States 1900–1980: Many Nutrient Foods of the Past Have Been Displaced by Refined and/or Empty Calorie Foods

Old Diet (1900–1940)	Today's New Diet (1980)
1. Home-cooked	Processed TV-dinner foods and fast-food restaurant meals
2. High complex starch (CHO) diet (peas, potatoes)	Refined sugar (sucrose) and low starch diet
3. Whole grain cereals	Refined sugar cereals
4. Fresh vegetables	Frozen or canned vegetables
5. Fresh vegetables	Beef meats
6. Fresh fruits as dessert	Sugar desserts
7. Water	Beer or wine
8. Milk	Soft drinks
9. High-fiber diet (bran and fresh vegetables)	Low-fiber diet (refined cereals, breads, and pastry)
10. Natural food taste	Additives and colorings
11. Fresh fruit	Canned fruit and juices
12. Fresh potatoes	Processed potatoes (French fries)
13. Some sugar	Great amount of refined white sugar
14. Butter	Margarine
15. Low-fat intake	High-fat intake
16. Low-salt diet	High-salt diet
17. Adequate calories	Excess calories

Source: Walter Sorochan from review of related literature.

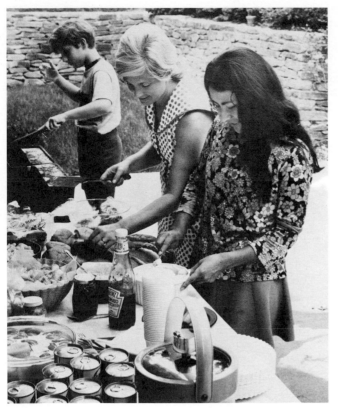

Figure 6.2

Eating is a social experience. We copy both good and bad eating habits from our parents. We develop preferences for foods early in life. These help structure eating habits that are often difficult to break.

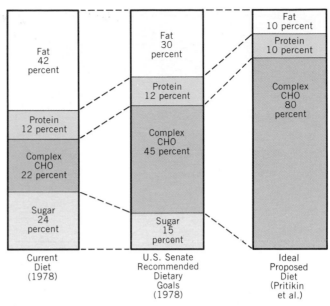

Figure 6.3.

Comparison of current diet with the U.S. Senate recommendations of 1978 to that of the ideal proposed diet of Pritikin and others. Three big changes are summarized in this comparison: fat intake should be reduced from 42 to 10 percent, complex CHO increased from 22 to 80 percent; and sugar reduced from 24 to 0 percent. (Adapted from the U.S. Senate Select Committee on Nutrition and Human Needs, Dietary Goals for the United States, Washington D.C., December 1977.)

dietary intake of the American public. On the basis of this study, and the testimony of experts, the committee concluded that 6 of the 10 leading causes of death, accounting for half of all deaths in the United States, are linked to diet (heart disease, stroke, arteriosclerosis, cancer, cirrhosis of the liver, and diabetes). Faulty diet appears to account for about half of all deaths. The committee's recommended dietary changes and goals are summarized in Figure 6.3. The general conclusions of this study are that Americans eat too much fat, too much beef meat, too much refined sugar products, and too much salt; and do not eat enough fresh green leafy vegetables, fruits, and fiber. The average American also ingests more calories than needed.

Our eating habits contribute to many of our nutritional deficiencies. Perhaps the major reason for such deficiencies is that our eating habits have become dependent on convenience-processed foods, such as frozen TV dinners, canned foods, hot dogs and French fries, soft drinks and beer, and an overwhelming variety of refined snack foods, such as cookies, potato chips, ice cream, popcorn, and so on.

Processed foods are rich in sugar (see Table 6.5) and–or salt (see Table 6.8) and have lost many of their nutrients. Processed refined white flour, for example, loses most of the 22 nutrients that unrefined whole grain flour has (73:36). Although breads and cereals are often enriched by the return of vitamin B_1, B_2, and niacin, the other 12 essential vitamins are not returned (54:22). Whereas only 10 percent of foods in grocery stores in 1940 were convenience foods, today 55 percent of foods in super markets are convenience foods (42:142;61). The real danger of poor choices, poor eating habits, and nutritional deficiencies in children and college-age students is not just malnutrition, overweight and obesity, but poor consumer-eating habits that may initiate and incubate chronic diseases early in life. The abundance and availability of processed foods has contributed to many persons eating nutrient-deficient diets.

In addition to eating nutrient-deficient foods, we often deplete nutrients in the body by eating foods containing chemicals that preserve, sweeten, and make foods more attractive. The over 2000 food additives, perservatives, coloring agents, sweeteners, dyes, drugs, and other chemicals that may find their way into our bodies (6:185; 15:166; 52:162) are detoxified by the liver. The

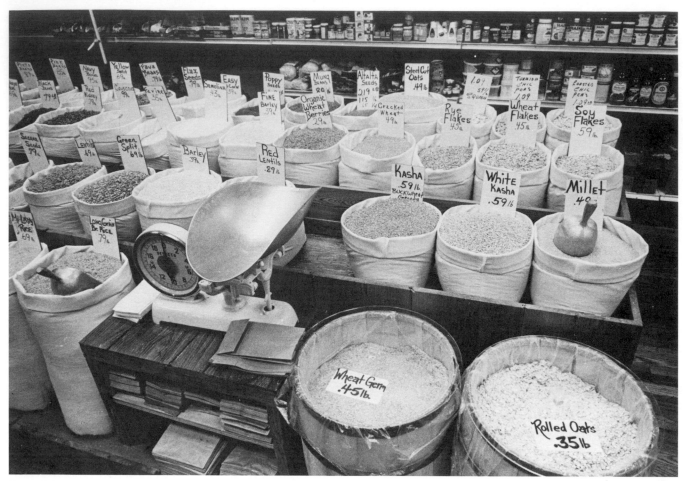

Figure 6.4
The popularity of health food stores reflects people becoming more health conscious and more concerned about eating foods that are unadulterated and that contain adequate nutrients.

liver uses vitamins, minerals, and amino acids to synthesize enzymes that detoxify these ingested chemicals. The more chemical preservatives ingested, the greater the liver's demand for additional vitamins, minerals, and amino acids. When these are lacking in the daily diet, liver function slows down and one usually feels fatigued and functions suboptimally.

There is mounting support for the claim that many of our health problems and diseases originate in vitamin and mineral deficiencies, and/or the eating of too many of the wrong foods (3;4;6;13;15;18;20–25;26; 31;35;36;39;42;44;53–58;60;63–72). Table 6.3 summarizes the benefits from improving our diet on a national basis.

The answer to the management of heart disease, cancer, obesity, diabetes, arthritis, emotional disturbances, allergies, and other diseases may very well be through new kinds of nutritional life style approaches.

In summary, many of us select and eat foods that do not provide adequate amounts of essential nutrients. We also eat far more than is necessary to relieve hunger. We need to give our body cells the nutrients they need and not eat foods that gratify our egos.

A glance at Table 6.1 should make you aware that your body needs seven major essential nutrients. Thus your daily diet should be prepared and eaten with this in mind. It is doubtful that selecting foods and eating a diet based on the traditional four food groups will provide one with all the essential nutrients that the human body needs.

The remainder of this chapter provides information about six essential nutrients: proteins, fats, carbohydrates, vitamins, minerals, and fiber. The reasons why your body needs these nutrients, the best sources of them, and the eating habits that will not destroy these nutrients are also discussed.

Table 6.3
Magnitude of Benefits from Improving Diet in the United States

Health Problem	Magnitude	Potential Savings from Improved Diet
Heart and vasculatory	Over 1 million deaths in 1967	25% reduction of deaths
Respiratory and infectious	141 million work days lost in 1965–1966; 166 million school days lost	15–20% fewer lost days
Mental health	5.2 million people are severely or totally disabled; 25 million have manifest disability	10% fewer disabilities
Early aging	About 49.1% of population have one or more chronic impairments; 102 million people	10 million people without impairments
Reproduction	15 million with congenital birth defects	3 million fewer children with birth defects
Arthritis	16 million afflicted	8 million people without afflictions
Dental health	One-half of all people over 55 have no teeth; $6.5 billion public and private expenditures on dentists' services in 1967	50% reduction in incidence, severity, and expenditures
Diabetes and carbohydrate disorders	3.9 million overt diabetic deaths in 1967; 79% of people over 55 with impaired glucose tolerance	50% of cases avoided or improved
Osteoporosis	4 million severe cases; 25% of women over 40	75% reduction of disability
Obesity	30 to 40% of adults; 60 to 70% over 40 years	75% reduction of obesity
Alcoholism	5 million alcoholics; $\frac{1}{2}$ are addicted; annual loss over $2 billion from absenteeism, lowered production and accidents	33% reduction in alcoholism
Eyesight	48.1% or 86 million people over 3 years wore corrective lenses in 1966; 81,000 became blind every year; 103 million in welfare	20% fewer people blind or with corrective lenses
Allergies	22 million people (9%) are allergic; 16 million with hayfever asthma; 7–15 million people allergic to milk	20% of people relieved; 90% of those allergic to milk
Digestive	About 20 million incidents of acute condition annually; 4000 new cases each day; 14 million with duodenal ulcers	25% fewer acute conditions; over $1 billion in costs
Kidney and urinary	55,000 deaths from renal failure; 200,000 with kidney stones	20% reduction in incidence and deaths
Muscular disorders	200,000 cases	10% reduction in cases
Cancer	600,000 persons developed cancer in 1968; 320,000 persons died of cancer in 1968	20% reduction in incidence and deaths
Improved growth and development	324.5 million work days lost; 51.8 million people needing medical attention and/or restricted activity	25% fewer work days lost
Improved learning ability	Over 6.5 million mentally retarded with I.Q. below 70; 12% of school age children need special education	Raised I.Q. by 10 points for persons with I.Q. 70–80

Source: This table was compiled from information presented by Dr. Edith Weir of the Department of Agriculture to the United States Select Committee in Nutrition and Human Needs, and Reported in *Dietary Goals for the United States,* 2nd ed., Washington, D.C.: U.S. Government Printing Office, December 1977, pp. 73–74. The Weir data was for 1967.

  Health benefits from better nutrition would include: 250,000 fewer deaths from heart disease and stroke; 150,000 fewer deaths from cancer; death rates for unborn children, infants, and mothers giving birth cut in half; 250 million cases of respiratory infections cut in half; substantial reductions in mental illness, arthritis, allergies, alcoholism, dental problems, diabetes, obesity, and other health problems; improved learning ability, personal appearance, and extension of life span. The Gross National Earning power of this country would increase, as would the income of each worker. Overall, we would be saving billions of dollars.

PROTEINS

Protein-rich foods are excellent sources of most of the essential nutrients. When digested in the stomach and small intestines, proteins are broken down into about 22 amino acids, which are absorbed from the intestine into the bloodstream and carried throughout the body. Amino acids may be linked together in a great variety of ways to form various protein substances in the body. The role of protein in the diet is not to provide human body proteins but to supply the essential amino acids from which the body can make its own protein substances. Many protein foods are also rich sources of the B-complex vitamins and minerals.

Amino acids are the building blocks of life. The liver and other parts of the body use amino acids to synthesize enzymes, hormones, hemoglobin in red blood cells, nuclear cells [deoxyribonucleic acid (DNA) and ribonucleic acid (RNA)], and structural tissues such as muscles, skin, hair, and nails. Amino acids are also used by mammary glands to synthesize human milk, while muscles synthesize ATP (adenosine triphosphate), which converts glycogen in muscles into energy. Various amino acid proteins in the blood regulate the exchange of water between tissue cells and surrounding body fluids, and the water and acid-base balance as a whole. A prolonged low level of protein intake depletes the protein content of blood plasma. This results in an inefficient supply of nutrients to the cells and inefficient removal of cellular waste products. Persons experiencing such disorders suffer from swollen and puffy ankles and tissues or nutritional edema. A severe deficiency of protein in the daily diet results in the disease kwashiorkor,* which affects brain development in infants.

The protein intake of the average American exceeds the Recommended Daily Allowance of 46 grams of protein per day by 45 percent (44:29). This surplus of protein cannot be immediately used by the body, and the excess is converted into fat or energy.

More important than the surplus protein intake is the lack of quality in the proteins we consume. Protein foods are classified as complete and incomplete proteins. A complete protein contains all nine essential amino acids, which the body cannot synthesize (see Figure 6.5). The essential amino acids and their daily requirements are summarized in Table 6.4. Those foods low in one or more of the essential amino acids are incomplete proteins. In general, animal proteins (meats, egg, cheese,

* Kwashiorkor is a disease resulting from the absence of animal or vegetable proteins in a high-starch diet. Consequences include retarded brain development, edema, dermatosis, anemia, and depigmentation of hair and skin.

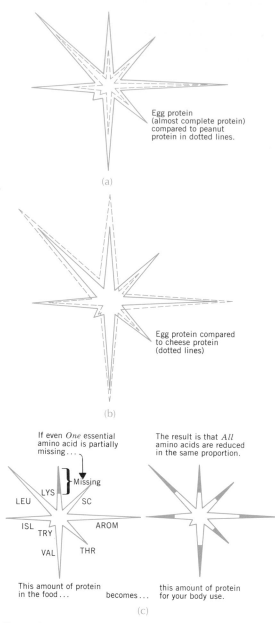

Figure 6.5

Illustration comparing complete and incomplete proteins. (a) With permission from Frances Moore Lappe, *Diet for a Small Planet*, New York: Ballantine, 1975, pp. 67–70; (b) "Amino Acid Content of Foods and Biological Data on Proteins," Food and Agricultural Organizations of the United Nations, Rome, Italy, 1970.

and milk) are complete, while most plant proteins (beans, corn, potatoes) are incomplete. Pure vegetarians have difficulty obtaining all the essential amino acids, which lacto-ovo-vegetarians (eat dairy products and eggs but exclude animal meats) have a much better chance of obtaining the amino acids.

One way to get a balance of amino acids in the diet is to combine protein foods so that they complement

Table 6.4

Essential Amino Acid Requirements (per kg of body weight), mg/day

Amino Acid	Infant (3–6 mo)	Child (10–12 yr)	Adult	Amino Acid Pattern for High-Quality Proteins, (mg/g of protein)
Histidine	33	?	?	17
Isoleucine	80	28	12	42
Leucine	128	42	16	70
Lysine	97	44	12	51
Total S-containing amino acids (includes methionine)	45	22	10	26
Total aromatic amino acids (includes phenylalanine)	132	22	16	73
Threonine	63	28	8	35
Tryptophan	19	4	3	11
Valine	89	25	14	48

Source: U.S. National Academy of Sciences, *Recommended Dietary Allowances,* 1974, p. 44.

each other to create a complete protein meal. Beans and corn complement each other by providing a complete protein that has a balance of the nine essential amino acids (see Figure 6.6). If one of the essential amino acids is missing, even temporarily, protein synthesis in the body will fall to the level of the lowest amino acid (44:36). The lowest amino acid limits the amounts of other amino acids that can be used (see Figure 6.6). For example, if you ingest 100 percent of all the essential amino acids at one meal, except 50 percent of lysine, then only 50 percent of all the es-

sential amino acids are used, the rest is wasted or converted into body fuel (44:37). Sulfur-containing amino acids, methionine and cystine, are the two most limiting amino acids occurring in protein foods, especially in vegetables and fresh fruits (12:100). Once again, the limiting proteins may be balanced out by mixing or combining protein foods so that the limiting amino acids in both foods complement each other and make up a complete protein diet. An example of how this can be done is illustrated in Figure 6.6. For example, the 2.1 percent of protein in a boiled white potato can be

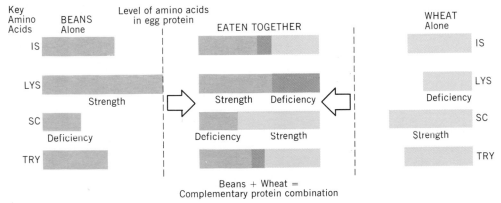

Figure 6.6.

Illustration showing how to combine protein foods in meals so that amino acids complement each other. (From: Amino Acid Content of Foods and Biological Data on Proteins," Food and Agricultural Organization of the United Nations, Rome, Italy, 1970.)

complemented by eating a boiled egg, which provides the necessary amount of sulfur-containing amino acids methionine and cystine. Complementing amino acids in protein foods also reduces the caloric intake, since there is no waste protein to be converted into fat or energy. Since essential amino acids in protein foods are not stored in body cells as such, a person needs a meal's supply of balanced amino acid foods each day. Keep in mind that although foods, such as fruits and vegetables, are low in essential amino acids, they may contain other nutrients, such as vitamins and minerals, that are essential for good health.

How much protein do human bodies need? Although experts on nutrition are unable to agree on the amount (43:41), the amount needed is dependent on the quality of protein eaten. That is, protein foods that contain low amounts of the essential amino acids are low-quality or incomplete protein foods. You need to eat more quantities of these foods to get enough of each amino acid to meet the estimated daily requirements. This would result in overeating and gaining body weight. The National Academy of Science recommended amount of protein needed by a healthy person is 0.40 grams of total protein per pound of body weight per day (43:43), or 0.8 grams of protein per kilogram of ideal body weight per day (69:95). Briggs and Calloway point out that the human body needs a minimum maintenance amount of about 0.5 grams protein per kilogram of body weight and that one needs slightly more than this amount to provide a suitable margin to cover various individual needs, as during periods of stress, tissue building, pregnancy, lactation, or when food is poorly assimilated in the body (12:104). This observation is supported by research done in the 1940s by Dr. Hegsted and his fellow workers at Harvard (32), and Dr. Bricker and his colleagues at the University of Illinois (11). Both of these studies have been substantiated by Swedish, Japanese, and German studies (1); al concluded that about 30 grams of complete protein, or 1 ounce, is sufficient for an adult human. It made no difference whether this protein came from animal or plant sources—both were entirely adequate.

One quick way to assess the protein status of your body—whether or not you are getting enough protein— is by considering the condition of your skin, fingernails, and hair. Because they require newly synthesized protein for growth and health, their condition reflects whether or not you are getting a balance of amino acids in your diet. Are your wounds or abrasions slow to heal? Are your fingernails constantly breaking? Does your hair lack luster? If these conditions prevail, then your diet may be lacking in a balance of amino acids (43:47).

In summary, one needs to pay more attention to the quality and quantity of amino acids in foods. Each meal should be preplanned so that one or more protein foods complement each other in the desirable amounts of essential amino acids.

COMBINING PROTEIN FOODS

You can learn to mix protein foods so that there is a better balance of essential amino acids in each meal. This ensures that the body can maximize the use of all amino acids efficiently and not waste them. Figure 6.4 gives an example of protein complementarity. For more information on this and how to make meals consisting of complete proteins, refer to *Diet for a Small Planet* by Francis Moore.

To find out your individual amino acid requirements, do the following calculation:

Step 1. Convert your body weight in pounds to kilograms, for example,

$$\frac{150 \text{ pounds}}{2.2} = 68 \text{ kilograms}$$

$$\frac{\text{Your body weight in pounds}}{2.2} = \underline{\qquad} \text{ kilograms}$$

Step 2. Multiply this figure times the requirement for each amino acid listed under "adult" (or under child or infant) in Table 6.4. For example, the amount of isoleucine needed each day for a 150-pound person is

68 kilograms × 12 milligrams = 818 milligrams per day

Your own calculation follows:

your body weight in kilograms × _____ milligrams of amino acid = _____ milligrams per day

Calculate your daily amino acid requirements by referring to Table 6.4.

Step 3. Keep a diet diary of the foods you ate for 1 day. Refer to Table A.1 for the value amounts of each of the nine amino acids in the foods eaten. Add the amounts of each amino acid.

Step 4. Compare these totals of daily amino-acid intake to the theoretical requirements. Identify any deficiencies in your daily amino acid intake.

Step 5. Refer to Table A.1 and try to complement the protein foods so as to give you a balance of amino acids in your daily diet.

FATS

Fats are a familiar part of every meal. We often are unaware that many of the foods we eat are rich in fat. Although fats make up 15 to 20 percent of our food on a weight basis, they comprise 40 to 45 percent of the American daily caloric intake. This intake is in excess of what our bodies actually need.

Fats are an essential nutrient to the life of all body cells. But our cells need only minute amounts of fat. All of the body's fat needs can be synthesized from linoleic acid.[1] However, linoleic acid is a fatty acid that cannot be synthesized by the human body and is referred to as an "essential fatty acid." A deficiency of linoleic acid results initially in scaly skin and sore spots. Linoleic acid has many vital cellular functions, so one should not eliminate linoleic acid as a fat completely from the daily diet.

Fats and fat-containing foods are valuable to us in many ways. Fats in food act as carriers of fat-soluble vitamins A, D, E, and K, and also aid in their absorption from the intestine into the bloodstream. Natural oils synthesized from linoleic acid by the body provide the skin and hair with a radiant complexion. Almost half of all the fat in the body is a layer of fat beneath the skin to protect the body from extreme fluctuations in temperature. Fat acts as a protective padding beneath each kidney, as well as the spleen and other organs. The soft fat in the breasts of a woman protects her mammary glands from heat and cold and cushions them against shock. The fat that large muscles contain provides a ready supply of usable energy for their action. Fat is synthesized into cholesterol, which in turn is used in the synthesis of enzymes, hormones, and vitamin D. Fats slow down digestion and the emptying time of the stomach, thereby preventing early recurrence of hunger pangs. Too much fat intake, however, can increase the risks of obesity and heart disease.

Fats, referred to as triglycerides, are mixtures of compounds of the three fatty acids and glycerol. Fats that cannot accept more hydrogen atoms are called saturated fats (Figure 6.7), while those that can accept more hydrogen atoms are referred to as unsaturated or polyunsaturated fats. Most triglycerides are synthesized from fatty acids and glycerol in adipose tissues. The fatty acids, in turn, come either from the diet or from synthesized fatty acids made in tissues from carbohydrates and their metabolites (glucose).

There is a definite relationship between fats and cardiovascular diseases. A dietary deficiency of linoleic acid (an unsaturated fat) may lead to an accumulation of abnormal amounts of cholesterol in the arteries. Similarly, eating an excess of saturated-fat diets, such as beef and pork meats or butter and cheese, may also elevate cholesterol levels in the arteries. Triglyceride levels in the blood may be elevated by ingesting an excess of foods rich in refined sugar (sucrose closely resembles glucose). High blood levels of both cholesterol and triglycerides are found in persons with coronary artery disease. Elevated blood triglyceride levels are associated with abnormally fast clotting of the blood and with "thickness' of the blood, which means that the blood is more likely to form clots within blood vessels.

The kind and amount of fat eaten can affect the levels of various blood fats. Consumption of fats with a low polyunsaturated/saturated (P/S) ratio of 1.1 is effective in reducing the risk of heart disease in persons at risk (overweight, smoking heavily, under work stress, with a history of heart disease, or inactive). Such at risk persons, regardless of age, should cut down their fat intake. Fat foods especially low in linoleic acid (such as beef meats) should be reduced and replaced with foods high in linoleic acid.

The best source of foods high in linoleic acid are vegetable oils; seeds from corn, soybeans, cotton, sunflowers; wheat germ; peanuts and walnuts; vegetables; and poultry fat. Plants store fat in fruits (olives, coconuts, avocados), in seeds (peanuts, soybeans), seed germs (corn germ, cottonseed), or in nuts. Beef meat is mostly fat and not protein. A tender T-bone steak can contain up to 70 to 75 percent fat and only 25 to 20 percent protein (44:215; 47:84). A diet high in beef meat is largely responsible for the large quantity of fat in our diets. The 40 to 45 percent of the caloric intake of an average American should be reduced to about 10 percent, which is much lower than the U.S. recommended dietary goal of 30 percent.

The fat in food gives food its flavor and aroma. For example, skinning chicken meat before cooking the chicken removes the layer of fat in the skin, resulting in a tasteless and odorless meat. In addition, the aromatic nature of many foods, such as french fries, adds to the pleasure of eating. Thus, since fat is also used to cook and flavor other foods, it may be difficult for many to adhere to the prudent 10 percent or less intake of fat in the daily caloric intake of food.

Offsetting the flavoring and tasting advantages of fat is the excess calories contained in fat. A gram of fat supplies about 9 calories of energy, whereas a gram of carbohydrates and protein supply only 4 calories. Thus identifying foods rich in linoleic acid is an excellent way of reducing caloric intake, reducing risk to cancer and heart disease, as well as controlling one's body weight.

There is no set allowance for linoleic acid, but the Food and Nutrition Board (12:73) states that nearly 2 percent of the total calories in the diet should be sufficient for adults, and 3 percent of total calories for infants. Research (18:219) of the diets of people in many

---

[1] Sometimes referred to as Vitamin F.

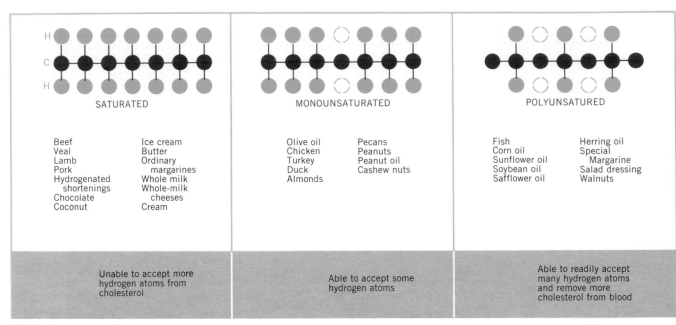

Figure 6.7

Comparison of the three types of fat and the foods containing each. Saturated fats have a long chain of carbon (C) atoms, each of which has two hydrogen (H) atoms. Saturated fats are completely full or saturated with hydrogen atoms and are unable to accept more hydrogen atoms. Monounsaturated fats are similar to saturated fats except that some carbon atoms may be lacking an atom of hydrogen, thereby being unable to accept hydrogen atoms. Polyunsaturated fats may have fewer carbon atoms and fewer hydrogen atoms; these fats are able to readily accept or combine with many hydrogen atoms, thereby removing cholesterol from the blood. (Adapted from George M. Briggs and Doris H. Calloway, *Bogert's Nutrition and Physical Fitness*, Philadelphia: W. B. Saunders, 1979.)

parts of the world suggests that about 10 percent of the daily caloric diet should be adequate in providing all the fat that our bodies need. Although this is in excess of the suggested sufficiency—level of 2 percent, it allows for fat foods that may be low in linoleic acid.

THE CHOLESTEROL CONTROVERSY

A great deal of controversy has existed about cholesterol and its relationship to heart disease. Cholesterol has been portrayed as a kind of coronary time bomb. It was assumed from the results of the Framingham heart study that people with the highest concentration of the fatty molecule in their bloodstreams ran the greatest risk of atherosclerosis and heart disease. Recent research (14; 17; 29:119; 34; 62) points out that not all cholesterol in the blood is bad for us—that one kind may be remarkably protective against heart disease.

Cholesterol is a fatty substance. Eighty percent of it is synthesized mostly by the liver, and to a lesser degree by the small intestine, while about 20 percent comes from food. This balance appears to be regulated by a body thermostat and depends on the amount of cholesterol needed by the body and that which is available in the diet. Cholesterol is one of the raw materials used in the synthesis of stress and sex hormones, vitamin D in the skin, and bile acids for digestion.

Although the body needs a constant supply of cholesterol, excess cholesterol can build up in the body. This happens when our life style becomes sloppy, as when we eat too many fatty, cholesterol-rich foods (e.g., liver, beef meats, hot dogs, and potato chips); are overweight; smoke cigarettes; do not exercise regularly, and do not eat a balanced nutrient diet.

The body uses proteins to remove excess cholesterol from tissues. Since cholesterol is a fatty substance and does not mix with water, the blood cannot carry it in its fat state. Instead, the body attaches it to proteins, forming a fat-protein combination in the blood called lipoproteins. Cholesterol is carried by two major types of lipoproteins: high-density (HDL) and low density

(LDL) lipoproteins, as shown in Figure 6.8. The LDL seem to be involved in transporting cholesterol to, and depositing it in, tissues, including blood vessel walls. On the other hand, the HDL are responsible for removing cholesterol from sites where it is in excess and carrying it back to the liver for disposal.

A diet rich in vegetables, fiber, yogurt, fish, and very little beef meat tends to raise HDL levels (14). The AMA suggests that most Americans lower their cholesterol intake from 600 to 300 milligrams per day. (The average egg yolk contains about 250 milligrams of cholesterol.) Research at Stanford University with marathon runners and at New Orleans with medical students on a vigorous program of physical exercise indicates that increased physical activity greatly increases HDL, thereby lowering and controlling excess cholesterol levels in the body (14;15).

Thus the dietary restriction of cholesterol is no longer necessary for the general population (73:168). The emphasis in coping with cholesterol should be on lowering the intake of animal and dairy fats; lowering the intake of refined sugar; increasing the intake of fresh

vegetables, yogurt, fish, and fiber, which have high-density proteins; and getting more physical activity.

CARBOHYDRATES

Carbohydrate foods are the most abundant and important sources of energy for the majority of people in the world today. We often eat a candy bar in order to get a quick source of energy. Carbohydrates provide economical energy for the body.

Foods high in carbohydrates, such as whole grains, legumes, and potatoes, also supply some proteins and most of the vitamins and minerals. Carbohydrates also supply most of the roughage or fiber that stimulates the digestive system into good working order and prevents constipation. Sugars, in particular, are used to flavor and preserve foods and beverages.

About 46 percent of our total caloric diet is carbohydrate food, of which one-half is refined sugar or sucrose (67). In terms of sugar intake on a weekly basis, the average American eats nothing but sugar every fourth day (see Table 6.5). Many nutritionists and researchers (3;4;15;21;39;44;54;67;73) believe that many health problems, such as depression, diabetes, obesity, dental caries, and heart disease, are aggravated by the high intake of refined sugar.

Although the human body cannot make carbohydrates, plants do build a variety of carbohydrates. The simplest carbohydrate, a monosaccharide, has a single or saccharide unit. Example of monosaccharides include glucose, galactose, and fructose. Glucose, or grape sugar, is found in fruits and honey. Fructose is a fruit sugar that occurs with glucose in fruits and honey. Galactose occurs most often as milk sugar or lactose.

The linkages of these three simple sugars form all complex carbohydrates or starches (see Figure 6.9). Disaccharides, such as honey and refined table sugar or sucrose, are made up of glucose and fructose. Lactose, found in human and cow's milk, is broken down by digestion into glucose and galactose. Babies usually have the enzyme lactase, which digests lactose, but this enzyme often falls to very low levels, or is lacking, in many adults. It is for this reason that many people in the world are unable to tolerate milk in their diet and develop allergic reactions to milk.

Polysaccharides are complex starches that have from 300 to several thousand monosaccharide units jointed together. Plant seeds, tubers, and roots are good examples. It does not matter whether carbohydrates are consumed as simple sugars or starches because digestion breaks them all into glucose (the simplest of all carbohydrates) before they are absorbed into the bloodstream. Simple carbohydrates, such as glucose (candy

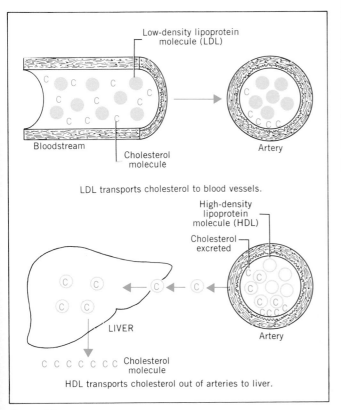

Figure 6.8.
Conceptual illustration of how low-density lipoproteins (LDL) and high-density liproproteins (HDL) function in moving cholesterol.

Table 6.5
Added Sugar in Processed Foods

Food	Serving Size	Weight in Grams	Calories per Serving	Added Grams Sugar	Teaspoons Sugar in Serving	Sugar Weight (%)	Sugar Calories (%)
Beverages							
Frozen concentrate grape juice	6 oz	187	100	4	1	2	15
Coke	12 oz	369	144	36.9	9.2	10	99
Welch's grape juice drink	6 oz	168	110	15.6	3.9	9.3	55
Hi-C orange (Welch's)	6 oz	168	92	19.2	4.8	11.4	81
Kool aid (sugar-sweetened flavors)	6 oz	168	68	17.3	4.3	10	98
Sprite (Coca Cola)	12 oz	369	143	36	9	9.8	100
Bright & Early Frozen Concentrate Imitation OJ	6 oz	168	100	21.6	5.4	13	84
Cereals							
General Mills Cheerios	1¼ cup	28	110	1	0.2	3.6	3.5
GM Wheaties	1 cup	28	110	3	0.7	11	11
GM Total	1 cup	28	110	3	0.7	11	11
GM Kix	1½ cup	28	110	2	0.5	7.1	7
GM Lucky Charms	1 cup	28	110	11	2.7	39.3	39
GM Nature Valley Granola Cin & Raisin	⅓ cup	28	130	7	1.7	25	21
Post Alphabits	1 cup	28	110	11	2.7	39	39
Post Raisin Bran	½ cup	28	90	9	2.2	32	39
Ralston Purina Cookie Crisp (choc chip)	1 cup	28	120	12	3	46	42
Kellogg's Fruit Loops	1 cup	28	110	14	3.5	50	49
Kellogg's Sugar Pops	1 cup	28	100	13	3.2	46	46
Kellogg's Special K	1¼ cup	28	110	2	0.5	7.1	7
Kellogg's Corn Flakes	1 cup	28	110	2	0.5	7	7
Kellogg's Raisin Bran	¾ cup	28	110	3	0.7	10.7	11
Kellogg's All Bran	⅓ cup	28	60	4	1	14.3	26
Kellogg's Apple Jacks'	1 cup	28	110	16	4	57	56
Kellogg's Sugar Frosted Flakes	⅔ cup	28	110	11	2.7	39	39
Kellogg's Country Morning	⅓ cup	28	130	6	1.5	21	18
Kellogg's Rice Krispies	1 cup	28	110	3	0.7	11	17
Kellogg's Sugar Smacks	¾ cup	28	110	16	4.0	57	56
GM Boo-Berry	1 cup	28	110	13	3.2	46	46
GM Cocoa Puffs	1 cup	28	110	11	2.7	39	39
GM Count Chocula	1 cup	28	110	13	3.2	46	46
GM Golden Grahams	1 cup	28	110		2.7	39	39
GM Crazy Cow	1 cup	28	110	12	3.0	43	42
Nabisco 100% bran	½ cup	28	70	6	1.5	21.4	33
Instant Quaker Oatmeal with cin & spice	1⅝ oz	45.5	176	16	4	35.2	35
Quaker Captain Crunch	¾ cup	28	110	12	3	43	42
Quaker Life	⅔ cup	28	105	5	1.2	18	18
Quaker 100% Natural Cereal	¼ cup	28	140	6	1.5	21	17
Shredded Wheat	1 biscuit	25	90	—	—	—	—
Condiments							
Bleu cheese salad dressing	1 tbsp	15	75	1	0.2	6.7	5.0
French salad dressing	1 tbsp	16	65	3	0.7	18.8	18

Food	Serving Size	Weight in Grams	Calories per Serving	Added Grams Sugar	Teaspoons Sugar in Serving	Sugar Weight (%)	Sugar Calories (%)
Hellman's Spin Blend salad dressing	1 tbsp	16	60	3	0.7	18.8	19
Italian dressing	1 tbsp	15	85	1	0.2	6.7	4.5
Cranberry sauce	½ cup	134	203	47	11.7	35	90
Catsup	1 tbsp	15	16	2.5	0.6	17	61
Protein							
Bacon (Oscar Mayer)	2 slices	12	70	0.2	0.0	1.7	1.1
Beef bologna (OM)	2 slices	46	150	1.4	0.3	3	4
Canadian style bacon (OM)	2 slices	56	80	0.2	0.0	0.4	1.0
Canned ham (OM)	3 oz	32	105	0.3	0.1	0.4	1.1
Luncheon meat (OM)	2 slices	54	190	1.4	0.3	3	3
Peanut butter	2 tbsp	32	182	1.3	0.3	4	3
Pork sausage	3 links	54	195	1.2	0.3	2	2
Hard salami	6 slices	54	210	0.6	0.1	1	1
Cotto salami	2 slices	56	110	0.6	0.1	1	2
Spam	3 oz	85	264	3.2	0.8	4	5
Weiners (OM)	one	45	140	1.3	0.3	3	4
Vanilla ice cream, hard	½ cup	67	135	12.6	3.1	19	36
Vanilla ice milk	½ cup	88	112	13.5	3.4	15	47
Yogurt, lowfat flavored	8 oz	227	194	16.3	4.1	7	33
Yogurt, fruit	8 oz	227	231	29.9	7.5	13	50
Snacks							
Applesauce	½ cup	127	116	17.2	4.3	14	57
Columbo frozen yogurt (whole milk)	8½ oz	98	138	21.3	5.3	22	60
Canned pears, heavy syrup	½ cup	128	97	12.5	3.1	10	50
Canned pineapple, heavy syrup	½ cup	128	90	12.2	3.1	10	52
Chocolate pudding	4 oz	130	161	15.6	3.9	12	37
Cool Whip	1 tbsp	4	13	0.9	0.2	23	28
Dannon frozen yogurt (vanilla)	½ cup	105	90	11.2	2.8	11	48
Gino's vanilla milkshake	12.1 oz	338	310	30	7.5	9	37
Graham cracker	2 crackers	14	55	3.5	0.9	25	25
Hershey's milk chocolate	1.2 oz	34	185	17.5	4.4	51	37
Hunt's vanilla Snackpack	5 oz	140	190	17.6	4.4	13	36
Jello, cherry	½ cup	120	80	18	4.5	15	87
Kellogg's brown sugar cinnamon Poptarts	1 tart	49	210	15	3.8	31	28
Vegetables							
Beets, pickled (Delmonte)	½ cup	85	57	8.4	2.1	9.9	57
Sweet peas (canned)	½ cup	85	75	3.8	0.9	4.5	20
Tomato sauce	4 oz	112	30	2.7	0.7	2.4	35
White refined sugar	1 tsp	4	15	—	—	—	—
	1 tbsp	12	46	—	—	—	—

Source: Nutrition Action, August 1979, pp. 10–11.

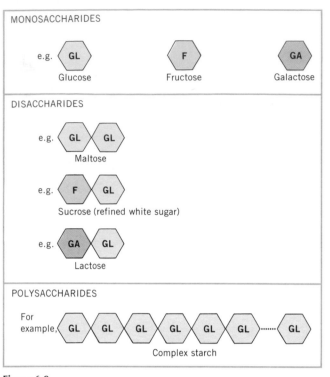

Figure 6.9.

The nature of carbohydrates. Three simple sugars (monosaccharides) whose structures are combined by nature in plants to form more complex carbohydrates: disaccharides and polysaccharides. Sucrose is quickly digested because its structure is relatively small, whereas complex starch takes longer to digest because it has more structures to be broken down through digestion.

and sugar) are easily and quickly digested and absorbed, while complex starches (potato, corn, peas, and bread) obviously take longer to digest.

Once glucose is in the bloodstream, it is circulated to all parts of the body. The brain needs a constant supply of glucose as energy. Glucose is stored in the liver and in body cells as glycogen (as a polysaccharide). Since it has fewer chains of glucose units than starches, glycogen can quickly be converted into glucose for quick energy in the muscle cells and for maintaining a constant blood sugar level.

Foods vary in the amount of sugar and energy they contain, although 1 gram of carbohydrate, regardless of whether it is a monosaccharide or polysaccharide, has 4 calories of energy. Refined carbohydrates, such as white table sugar (sucrose), have had their vitamins and minerals removed. Likewise, the processing and refining of white flour removes all the bran, fiber, and 22 vitamins and minerals (although 6 to 8 of them may be added in the baking process). Thus *processed* cabohydrate foods and their products are very high in calories but usually devoid or very low in the vitamins and minerals necessary to help the body digest and

metabolize them. It is for this reason that refined white sugar and flour products are referred to as "empty calorie" foods.

SUGAR—AN ADDICTION TO SWEETS?

Everyone ingests sugar either directly, as in using it to sweeten coffee and other beverages, or indirectly, when they ingest pastry, desserts, ketchup, soft drinks, and canned fruit and vegetables. Since much of the sugar consumed is hidden, we are often unaware of ingesting it. For example, most persons are unaware that a 6-ounce bottle of Coca-Cola® contains about $4\frac{1}{2}$ teaspoonfuls of sugar and that ketchup contains about 30 percent sugar (3:24). Hence it should not be too surprising that there is considerable controversy about sugar, its use and its effect on the human body and general well-being.

Refined white sugar has been stripped of all of its 10 vitamins and minerals (15:75;74:38). The only part left after the refining and bleaching processes is sucrose—a simple carbohydrate that is basically all empty calories.

Over half of our daily intake of carbohydrates, or 24 percent of our daily caloric intake, comes from sucrose (67). Sugar is used in almost all processed foods and drinks as a preservative and sweetener. When ingested with other foods, or by itself, sugar displaces natural complex starches that have key functions in the body. To make matters worse, the liver drains and leaches the body of precious vitamins and minerals in order to metabolize, detoxify, and eliminate excess sugar from the body (see Figure 6.10).

Although there is very little controversy about sugar's contributing to dental caries (12;15;20;21;44;67;73;74), increasing triglyceride and free fatty acid blood levels in the aorta, and causing the adrenal glands and the liver to overwork (22:20–30;27:58;42:56–59,50–140), there is disagreement among nutritionists, scientists, and medical doctors about the other consequences of using sugar (38:54). Sugar has been implicated in aggravating the condition of diabetes, mental depression, hormonal disorders, overweight, cancer, and heart disease; immobilizing natural body defenses; and causing a general inability to function optimally in life (4:55;18;42:55–59;54:142–145;33:38–144).

A real controversy occurs over the possibility of sugar addiction. Eating a lot of sugar causes insulin to be oversecreted, thereby depleting the liver of glycogen (stored sugar) and flooding the body with too much insulin. This causes large and rapid drops in blood sugar levels and the condition sugar addiction (referred elsewhere as mild hyperglycemia) (23;74:140).

Sugar addiction is the exact opposite of diabetes.

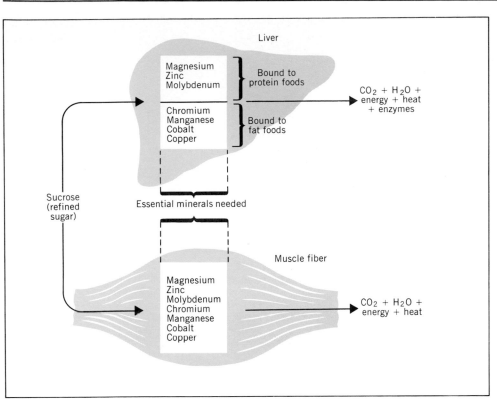

Figure 6.10
Metabolism of sucrose or refined white granular sugar in the body. Since glucose is devoid of the minerals essential for its metabolism, the liver and muscle cells rob stored reservoirs of the essential minerals from other body cells. Unlike sugar, unrefined foods have most of the minerals necessary for their metabolism. Eating refined sugar creates a nutrient deficit.

About 1 in 10 persons inherit a supersensitive pancreas, metabolically incapable of handling large intakes of sugar (15:75). The pancreas in such persons overproduces insulin when the diet is high in sugar. This condition is not the same as the easily medically diagnosed condition of hyperglycemia, where the blood glucose level drops 70 mg% in 4 or more hours after eating. Instead, the blood sugar in a sugar addict may rise in the first hour, only to plummet rapidly 40 to 60 or more mg% about 1 to 3 hours later. Each time the sugar addict gets a sugar fix, the blood sugar goes up, then drops rapidly, profiling a yo-yo effect (see Figure 6.11). It is not how low the blood sugar level drops, but the speed at which it drops, that causes the symptoms of sugar addiction (4:15). The sudden drop in blood sugar level sends the body into a condition of "near-shock." This condition may be further aggravated by caffeine (coffee or Coca-Cola) and intensified by stress. Symptoms of sugar addiction include unprovoked anxiety, insomnia, frigidity in women, and impotence in men, physical fatigue, mental confusion, suicidal depression, and a craving for sweets and alcoholic beverages (18:58). The number of persons suffering from sugar addiction is in the millions (31:128). Children and college students consuming large quantities of soft drinks, chocolate bars, and sweets are probably "sugar addicts."

Sugar addiction is a difficult condition to identify by medical tests, and many physicians are unable to diagnose it. This condition can be readily controlled by eliminating or reducing the intake of refined sugar, nicotine, and alcohol (43:140–145;18:141). Frequent meals should consist of unprocessed complex starches fortified by proteins and some fats. Proteins and fats slow down the digestion and absorption of foods so that carbohydrates trickle gradually into the blood rather than flooding the blood all at once. Pritikin of the Santa Barbara Live Longer Clinic advocates a high (80 percent) complex carbohydrate diet for all persons.

HOW MUCH FAT, PROTEIN, AND CARBOHYDRATES SHOULD YOU EAT?

The minimum and optimal amounts of carbohydrates needed by the body are presently controversial. Research studies of the diets of people in many parts of the world reveal that one can maintain health and live

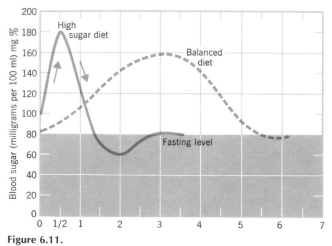

Figure 6.11.

Comparison of the elevation of blood sugar (glucose) in a person eating a high-sugar (sucrose) diet and a person eating a balanced diet of complex starches, fat, and protein (no sugar). The blood sugar of a person on a high-sugar diet rises (arrow) rapidly within the first hour, then drops suddenly (arrow) and rapidly within 2 to 3 hours after eating (referred to by others as hypoglycemia). When this happens the person has a craving to eat something sweet again—hence, a form of sugar addiction. Notice the gradual absorption of sugar into the blood stream and also a more gradual drop in a person eating a balanced or no-sugar diet.

Blood levels in this illustration were adapted from various sources to help conceptualize the idea of sugar addiction.

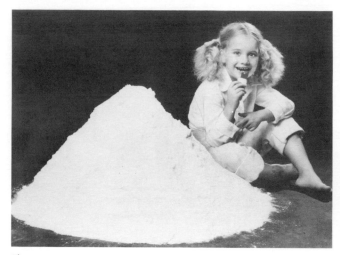

Figure 6.12

The amount of sugar in this picture amounts to 125 pounds. It represents the amount of sugar consumed each year by the average American. We also consume an equal amount of white flour in various forms.

a long time (past age 75) on a high, unrefined, complex carbohydrate diet that is also low in meat and total calories. These studies include people living in Hunzaland in Kashmir (65), Vilcambamba, Ecuador (44), Abkhazia in the USSR (44), the natives of Okinawa during World War II (64), the Otomi Indians of Central Mexico (44), the Sherpas of the Himalayas (49), as well as in Africa and other parts of the world (29;30;32;44). Pritikin and his associates of the Live Longer Center in Santa Barbara (40) have evolved a rehabilitative program for chronically ill and disabled cardiac patients that teaches these patients how to live on an 80 percent complex carbohydrate diet. Their rehabilitation success rate has been remarkable with sick persons. Other studies (1) have compared the effects of three different diets on the performance of a group of athletes and concluded that the human body works best on a diet resembling a high carbohydrate or vegetarian diet (see Figure 6.13).

In the light of such research, a diet made up of 70 to 80 percent complex carbohydrates seems reasonable and safe provided that there is an ample supply of vitamins, minerals, linoleic acid, and essential amino acids and that one does not overeat. In order that fats and proteins not be diverted into energy from their essential

roles, a diet should include a *minimum* of 70 to 100 grams (280 to 400 calories) of complex carbohydrates (12:60). The recommendation (67) of the U.S. Senate Committee on Nutrition and Human Needs in 1977 that Americans in general should decrease by one-half their intake of refined white sugar and double their intake of complex carbohydrates is a step in the right direction. However, it appears to fall drastically short of good, sound nutritional advice and health guidance. Refined sugar is a very poor source of energy; the human body does not need it; and it should be completely replaced by unrefined complex carbohydrates (see Figure 6.3). Also, daily complex carbohydrate intake should have been increased from 22 to 70–80 percent.

The suggested proportions of daily fat, protein, and carbohydrate intake are summarized in Table 6.6.

Vitamins

Vitamins are organic compounds other than fats, carbohydrates, and proteins that are essential to human life. We need to consume minute or trace amounts daily.

Vitamins serve as helpers of enzymes, making possible the processes by which fats, carbohydrates, and proteins are digested, absorbed, and metabolized in the body. They act by helping a biochemical reaction take place but are not changed or incorporated into the products of the reaction. Because of this function, vitamins are called coenzymes. For example, many chemical reactions that take place in the body can be reproduced in a test tube but under different conditions. A

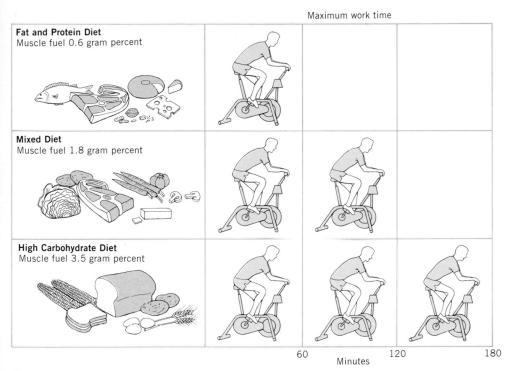

Maximum work time

Fat and Protein Diet
Muscle fuel 0.6 gram percent

Mixed Diet
Muscle fuel 1.8 gram percent

High Carbohydrate Diet
Muscle fuel 3.5 gram percent

60   120   180
Minutes

Figure 6.13

Comparison of the effect of three different diets on the same Swedish athletes using a bicycle endurance test. Athletes were on each of the three diets for 3 days. Endurance was three times greater on a diet resembling a high carbohydrate or vegetarian diet. (Adapted from *A Bircher-Benner Way to Positive Health and Vitality,* Bircher-Benner, Verlag, Zurich, Switzerland: Verlag, Vol. 52, 1975.)

chemical reaction in a test tube may need to be heated to 54 to 60° Celsius (130 to 140°F) before it takes place, whereas a vitamin enzyme inside the liver lowers the need for this high temperature inside the human body to about 37° Celsius (99°F).

Vitamins exist in two forms. Water-soluble forms include the B-complex and C vitamins, while fat-soluble vitamins A, D, E, and K are found in nature associated with fatty foods such as butter, cream, vegetable oils, seeds, and the fats of meats and fish. Water-soluble vitamins are not stored in the body and should be ingested daily. Fat-soluble vitamins are stored within the body tissues (mostly liver). Thus identifying the vitamin as either water- or oil-soluble tells us its source, how it is absorbed into the body, and what happens to it inside the body.

All vitamins are destructible: they can be broken down, oxidized, and altered in shape. Exposure to sunlight, oxygen, or cooking can destroy water-soluble vitamins. Fat-soluble vitamins are more stable to heat than water-soluble vitamins and are less likely to be lost in the cooking and processing of foods. Food processing, storage, and packing can greatly reduce the vitamin content of foods. For example, as much as 80 percent or more of vitamin E may be lost in converting whole wheat to refined white flour (11:154). Green vegetables lose nearly all of their vitamin C in a few days when kept at room temperature (24:22).

The digestive system absorbs these two types of vitamins differently. Water-soluble vitamins cross intestinal and vascular walls directly into the blood, while fat-soluble vitamins are handled laboriously and indirectly. More often than not vitamins are naturally bound to proteins (amino acids), thus facilitating their absorption (72:271). Fat-soluble vitamins must be emulsified and carried across the membranes of intestinal walls with fat. This is usually done through the lymphatic system into the blood system. Anything that interferes with fat absorption also lowers the absorption of fat-soluble vitamins. For example, diarrhea and mineral oil laxatives reduce the absorption rates of such vitamins. Therefore, all human beings need a certain amount of fat in the diet to foster such vitamin absorption.

Water-soluble vitamins are readily transported throughout the body by the blood; they circulate freely among all organs of the body and are used as needed.

Table 6.6

Suggested Minimum Requirements of Protein, Fat, and Carbohydrate and the Percentage of Their Total Daily Caloric Intake

Nutrient	Grams per Day 0.5 Grams Protein per Kilogram of Body Weight		Calorie Intake[a]	Percent of Daily Total Calorie Intake[a]
Protein	35 g	$\left(\begin{array}{c}1\frac{1}{4}\text{ cup}\\ \text{cottage}\\ \text{cheese}\end{array}\right)$	140	10
Fat	6.7–15.6 g	$\left(\begin{array}{c}1\frac{1}{2}\text{–}4\\ \text{tsp}\\ \text{margerine}\end{array}\right)$	60–140	4–10
Carbohydrate	125–268 g	$\left(\begin{array}{c}\frac{1}{3}\text{–}\frac{3}{4}\text{ of}\\ \text{an apple}\\ \text{pie}\\ \text{or}\\ \text{3–7 baked}\\ \text{potatoes}\\ \text{with skin}\end{array}\right)$	500–1070	80
Total	166.7–318.6 g		1350	100

[a] Nutritionists suggest that the average person, weighing 150 lb, should ingest about 2000 calories in order to ensure a proper balance of all nutrients.
Source: George M. Briggs and Doris Howes Calloway, *Bogert's Nutrition and Physical Fitness,* Philadelphia: Saunders, 1979, p. 104.

On the other hand, once fat-soluble vitamins have been transported to the cells of the body, they tend to become sequestered there and associated or stored with body fat.

The kidneys detect and remove excesses of water-soluble vitamins with ease. They do not detect excess fat-soluble vitamins, however, since these vitamins are not soluble in water, are stored in fat tissues, and do not accumulate in the blood. Since water-soluble vitamins are excreted almost as rapidly as they are ingested, toxicity from their overdoses seldom, if ever, happens. However, fat-soluble vitamins (A and D, in particular) can accumulate and reach toxic levels in the body.

The best sources of most vitamins are fresh, leafy, green vegetables because, to begin with, it is plants that synthesize vitamins. Seeds such as legumes, nuts, and whole-grain cereals are also good sources of vitamins. Root vegetables and fruits usually have lesser amounts of vitamins although there are notable exceptions. Lean meats are good sources of the B-complex vitamins. A few vitamins are synthesized in the body—vitamin D is synthesized by the skin with the help of ultraviolet rays, while several B-complex vitamins and vitamin K are synthesized by bacteria in the large intestine. To some extent the microbes in the large intestine are suspected of also synthesizing vitamin B_{12} from cobalt (12:297). This probably explains why true vegetarians can live many years without meat (vitamin B_{12}) in their diet. When vitamins are consumed in ordinary foods, they are readily absorbed into the body and are seldom ingested in toxic levels (12:123). See Table 6.7 for more specific information about vitamin sources and their functions.

Eating a variety of foods and a balanced diet regularly is the best way to provide the body with the vitamins it needs. Much controversy exists about the function of vitamins. Research points out that although vitamins may perform specific functions in specific parts of the body or body processes, vitamins work together as a team. For example, it is erroneous to assume that good eye health is the result of only vitamin A. Indeed, vitamins, A, B_2, C, D, E, P, and minerals calcium, copper, iodine, and iron are all implicated in maintaining eye health. All need to be present in adequate balanced amounts. Vitamins, minerals, and amino acids work collectively with each other on a "shotgun" approach and together exert a "whole" effect on the entire body. Vitamins need each other to be utilized in the body (15:22;33:228). When there is an insufficient intake of one or more vitamins, the entire body—and indeed the person—functions at a lower level of vitality even though signs of deficiency will not be observable or medically evident.

Table 6.7

Vitamins the Body Needs, Their Function, Best Sources, Deficiency Symptoms and Those Most Susceptible to Deficiencies

Vitamin	Those Probably Most Susceptible to Deficiency	Deficiency Symptoms	Function	Best Sources
A	1. College students 2. Cigarette smokers 3. Those who smoke pot 4. Those who take drugs 5. Alcoholics 6. Newborn babies 7. Nursing mothers 8. Chronic respiratory infections 9. Those not eating enough fat 10. Living in polluted areas 11. Excess eye strain	1. Eyes become dry and irritated 2. Dry skin 3. Sties in eyes 4. Glare blindness 5. Inability to see at night 6. Eruptions around hairs 7. Respiratory infections	1. Protects membranes from infections (lungs) 2. Keeps skin healthy 3. Keeps eyes healthy 4. Keeps hair healthy 5. Maintains urinary tract 6. Increases longevity 7. Is essential for protein	1. Fish-liver oil 2. Parsley 3. Dandelion leaves 4. Yellow-green vegetables 5. Kale 6. Spinach 7. Mustard greens 8. Beet greens 9. Apricots 10. Cooked carrots 11. Butter 12. Egg yolk
B₁ (Thiamine)	1. College students 2. Smokers 3. Alcoholics 4. Heavy social drinkers 5. Pregnant women 6. Doing heavy work 7. Stressful conditions 8. Not eating regularly 9. Eating in restaurants 10. Arthritics 11. Eating white bread and refined white flour pastries 12. With infections 13. Irritable, emotional, and high-strung	1. Fatigue 2. Irritability (mental confusion) 3. Depression 4. Headache 5. Flatulence (intestinal gas) 6. Emotional instability 7. Loss of mental alertness	1. Metabolizes CHO 2. Stimulates good feelings and morale (emotional stability) 3. Prevents fatigue 4. Promotes digestion 5. Prevents fat deposits in arteries 6. Promotes child growth 7. Prevents beriberi 8. Keeps heart muscle strong	1. Whole-grain bread 2. Whole-grain cereal 3. Brewer's yeast 4. Liver 5. Milk
B₂ (Riboflavin)	1. College students 2. Irregular eating habits 3. Tense and anxious 4. With infection 5. Depressed 6. Older persons 7. Using oral contraceptives	1. Itchy skin 2. Bloodshot eyes 3. Cracks in corner of mouth 4. Sensitivity to light	1. Aids releasing energy to body cells 2. Enables utilization of fats, proteins, CHO 3. Relieves depression	1. Whole-grain bread and cereals 2. Yellow-green vegetables 3. Brewer's yeast 4. Liver and lean meats 5. eggs
B₃ (Niacin)	1. College students 2. Those not eating fresh green vegetables 3. Under lots of stress 4. Heavy users of sugar 5. Hypoglycemics 6. Users of antibiotics 7. With infection 8. Eating lots of pastry and starches 9. High blood cholesterol	1. General fatigue 2. Bad breath 3. Insomnia 4. Irritability 5. Headaches 6. Skin rashes 7. Depression 8. Inability to concentrate 9. Moodiness	1. Keeps nerves healthy 2. Aids breakdown & utilization of fats, proteins and CHO 3. Reduces blood cholesterol 4. Improves circulation 5. Maintains healthy skin and tongue 6. Synthesizes sex hormones 7. Prevents pellagra	1. Fresh, green leafy vegetables 2. Fish 3. Lean meats 4. Milk 5. Brewer's yeast 6. Peanuts

Vitamin	Those Probably Most Susceptible to Deficiency	Deficiency Symptoms	Function	Best Sources
B₅ (Pantothenic acid)	1. College students 2. Sugar users 3. Hypoglycemia 4. Taking antibiotics 5. Eating refined flour products (white bread) 6. Under emotional-physical stress 7. Work in cold climate 8. Arthritics 9. Eat lots of cooked meat	1. Fatigue 2. Restlessness 3. Anxiety 4. Skin/hair disorders 5. Upper respiratory infections—colds 6. Low blood sugar 7. Hypoglycemia 8. Duodenal ulcers 9. Susceptibility to infections	1. Keeps skin healthy 2. Prevents skin wrinkles 3. Prevents stress 4. Stimulates adrenal glands 5. Forms nerve-regulating substances 6. Aids in metabolism of fats, CHO, and proteins 7. Maintains proper level of sugar 8. Prevents fatigue 9. Helps resist cold temperatures 10. Aids in resisting infection 11. Prevents arthritis 12. Prevents premature aging	1. Organ meats (liver) 2. Brewer's yeast 3. Green leafy vegetables 4. Whole-grain cereals 5. Egg yolk 6. Nuts
B₆ (Pyridoxine)	1. College students 2. On fasting or reducing diets 3. Personal stress 4. Lacking reality of life 5. Heavy meat eaters (high protein diet) 6. Pregnant women 7. Lactating women 8. With infections 9. Heart disease 10. Elderly 11. Alcoholics	1. Emotional instability (irritability) 2. Lack cheerfulness (gloominess) 3. Unrealistic 4. Edema—swelling of feet, hands, and stomach 5. Loss of hair	1. Maintains chemical balance between blood and tissue 2. Influences body metabolism 3. Aids in utilizing fats 4. Aids function of CNS 5. Controls cholesterol level 6. Prevents water buildup and retention in tissues	1. Green leafy vegetables 2. Lean meats 3. Whole-grain cereals 4. Soybeans
B₁₂ (Cyanocobalamin)	1. Vegetarians (nonmeat eaters) 2. Irregular menstruation 3. Taking laxatives 4. Older persons 5. With infections	1. Fatigue 2. Soreness and weakness in arms and legs 3. Mood disorders 4. Mental slowness 5. Anemia (body unable to absorb B₁₂) 6. Growth stunted	1. Promotes growth 2. Prevents pernicious anemia 3. Aids utilization of fats, proteins, and CHO 4. Builds nucleic acid	1. Beef 2. Liver 3. Salt fish 4. Oysters 5. Milk 6. Eggs 7. Synthesized by bacteria in large intestine
B₁₅ (Pangamic acid)				
Biotin (Vit. H)	1. Persons with infections 2. Eating raw egg whites (avidin prevents absorption)	1. Skin rash and scaliness 2. Loss of hair 3. Feeling depressed 4. Insomnia 5. Headache 6. Red skin 7. Muscular pain 8. Poor appetite	1. Aids Utilization of B-complex vitamins 2. Metabolizes fats and CHO 3. Synthesizes lipids in liver 4. Neutralizes allergy to egg whites	1. Green leafy vegetables 2. Eggs 3. Liver 4. Meats 5. Brewer's yeast 6. Synthesized by bacteria in large intestine

Vitamin	Those Probably Most Susceptible to Deficiency	Deficiency Symptoms	Function	Best Sources
Choline	1. College students 2. Smokers 3. Hypoglycemics 4. Overweight 5. Fat and CHO eaters 6. High blood cholesterol 7. Heart disease	1. High blood cholesterol 2. High blood pressure 3. Hypoglycemia 4. Weight control problems	1. Reduces high blood pressure 2. Reduces triglycerides 3. Aids in use of fats and cholesterol 4. Aids in use of amino acids 5. Essential for healthy liver 6. Makes lecithin in body 7. Aids in fat movement 8. Dissolves fats and cholesterol in body	1. Lecithin (soya beans) 2. Brewer's yeast 3. Liver 4. Egg yolk 5. Peanuts (peanut butter) 6. Seeds (wheat germ)
Folic acid (Folacin)	1. Under Stress 2. Alcoholics 3. Diabetics 4. Taking (sulfa) drugs 5. With infections (disease) 6. Pregnancy 7. Excess menstruation 8. Older persons	1. Poor appetite 2. Graying hair 3. Gastrointestinal disturbances 4. Premature birth	1. Essential for function of A, D, E, K vitamins 2. Forms red blood cells 3. Forms nucleic acid 4. Improves circulation 5. Forms body proteins 6. Aids digestion of proteins	1. Green leafy vegetables 2. Liver 3. Brewer's yeast 4. Milk 5. Meat 6. Synthesized by bacteria in the body
Inositol	1. Obese persons 2. Coffee drinkers 3. Cigarette smokers 4. Living in air pollution 5. Cardiovascular proneness 6. Older persons 7. With infections	1. Hair loss 2. Elevated blood cholesterol 3. Constipation 4. Eczema	1. Aids hair growth 2. Interacts with vitamin E 3. Reduces cholesterol in body 4. Helps body synthesize lecithin 5. Prevents arteriosclerosis 6. Resists cirrhosis	1. Same as choline 2. Citrus fruits 3. Synthesized by the body from glucose
PABA	1. With infections 2. Taking sulfa and other drugs	1. Fatigue 2. Skin pigmentation 3. Irritability 4. Depression 5. Constipation	1. Aids skin health 2. Prevents sunburn and other burns 3. Aids intestinal health 4. Helps synthesize red blood cells 5. Aids breakdown and utilization of proteins 6. Fosters intestinal bacteria that manufacture vitamins	1. Liver 2. Brewer's yeast 3. Wheat germ 4. Molasses 5. Synthesized by bacteria in intestine
B-Complex (summary)	1. College students 2. Sugar users 3. Cola drinkers 4. Taking sleeping pills and other drugs 5. Poor diet or eating habits 6. Under stress 7. Alcoholics 8. Cigarette smokers 9. Coffee drinkers 10. Eating processed foods 11. Pregnant women 12. Exposure to insecticides	1. Feeling tired—fatigue 2. Irritability 3. Nervousness 4. Depression 5. Suicidal tendencies 6. Acne 7. Insomnia 8. Anemia 9. High blood cholesterol 10. Falling hair	1. Convert CHO—glucose 2. Healthy skin, hair, eyes, mouth, and liver 3. Muscle tone in digestive tract 4. Normal functioning of nervous system 5. Metabolism of fats and proteins	1. Brewer's yeast 2. Liver 3. Whole-grain cereals 4. Bacteria in large intestine

Vitamin	Those Probably Most Susceptible to Deficiency	Deficiency Symptoms	Function	Best Sources
C	1. College students 2. Not eating fresh fruit and vegetables 3. Alcoholics 4. Cigarette smokers 5. Taking aspirins 6. Taking medication and drugs (antibiotics) 7. With colds, flu 8. With infections (fever) 9. Heroin addicts 10. Excess eye strain 11. Older persons 12. Deficient in vitamin A	1. Tendency to bruise easily (blue marks) 2. Fatigue 3. Painful joints 4. Soreness after exercise 5. Nosebleeds 6. Shortness of breath 7. Bleeding gums 8. Frequent colds and respiratory infections 9. Slow wound healing 10. Skin disorders—e.g., acne, psoriasis, black and blue marks	1. Has all-around function 2. Prevents colds 3. Prevents infections 4. Holds body cells together 5. Reduces allergies 6. Promotes stamina 7. Prevents fatigue and stress 8. Heals wounds and burns 9. Maintains hard bones and teeth 10. Strengthen's blood vessels 11. Stops internal bleeding 12. Aids in metabolism of amino acids and calcium 13. Prevents oxidation of other vitamins 14. Aids absorption of iron	1. Citrus fruits 2. Leafy vegetables 3. Cauliflower 4. Green peppers 5. Cantaloupe 6. Strawberries 7. Tomatoes 8. Raw potatoes
D (D₂ and D₃) D₂-ergocalciferol (synthetic) D₃-cholecalciferol (sunlight and in animal tissues)	1. Lots of reading 2. Using mineral oil 3. With colds, flu 4. Pregnant women 5. Heart disease patients	1. General body flabbiness 2. Dental caries 3. Having colds or flu 4. Eye strain 5. Weak teeth 6. Stomach ulcer	1. Aids use of calcium and phosphorus 2. Builds bones and teeth 3. Promotes normal growth 4. Maintains nervous system 5. Maintains heart action 6. Prevents rickets (soft bones)	1. Fish and liver oil 2. Enriched milk 3. Enriched cereals 4. Egg yolk 5. Liver 6. 15–30 min of sunshine on face each day
E	1. Exposure to air pollution 2. Eating refined white flour bread and pastry 3. Taking mineral oil 4. Taking unsaturated oils 5. Drinking high chlorine water 6. Taking large amounts of iron 7. Exposure to stress 8. Premature babies 9. Diabetics 10. Pregnant women 11. Lactating women 12. Old age 13. Infants 14. Taking birth control pills 15. Heart disease	1. Headaches 2. Rupture of red blood cells 3. Faulty absorption of fats and vitamins 4. High blood cholesterol	1. Aids beauty of skin 2. Postpones aging 3. Protects lungs against air pollution 4. Strengthens capillary walls 5. Regulates menstrual rhythm 6. Prevents loss of other vitamins 7. Prevents scarring 8. Aids in proper focusing of eyes 9. Maintains blood flow to heart (reduces oxygen requirements with diminished blood supply caused by narrowing of blood vessels) 10. Prevents miscarriage 11. Lowers blood cholesterol and fatty acids 12. Prevents infections 13. Prevents muscular dystrophy 14. Vital to cell health 15. Prevents cystic fibrosis 16. Prevents blood clotting and heart disease (thrombosis) 17. Regulates protein and calcium metabolism 18. Improves collateral circulation	1. Vegetable oils 2. Wheat germ 3. Raw peanuts and seeds 4. Cottonseed oils 5. Whole-grain cereals

Vitamin	Those Probably Most Susceptible to Deficiency	Deficiency Symptoms	Function	Best Sources
K (K$_1$, K$_2$, K$_3$)	1. Taking aspirin 2. Bleeders 3. Taking antibiotics 4. Taking anticoagulant drugs (dicumarol) 5. Breathing polluted air 6. Eating lots of frozen foods and fats 7. Poor bile secretion 8. Ingesting mineral oils 9. Recovering from surgery 10. Celiac disease 11. Older persons	1. Excessive bleeding	1. Enhances vitality 2. Extends longevity 3. Vital for normal liver function 4. Helps cells convert glucose into glycogen 5. Helps liver form prothrombin 6. Aids clotting blood 7. Stops fermentation of food 8. Painkiller	1. Kelp 2. Alfalfa 3. Root vegetables 4. Cauliflower 5. Fruits 6. Milk 7. Yogurt 8. Synthesized by bacteria in the body
P (Bioflavenoids)	1. Under stress 2. With constant colds and respiratory infections 3. Overweight obese 4. Diabetics 5. X-ray workers 6. High blood pressure 7. Heart disease 8. Hypertension	1. Similar to vitamin C 2. Tendency to bruise easily 3. Tendency to bleed 4. With vitamin D, contributes to joint pains, rheumatism, and rheumatic fever	1. Essential for absorption of vitamin C and its function 2. Aids Vitamin C with collagen 3. Increases strength of capillaries 4. Protects against infections 5. Prevents colds and influenza 6. Protects against X rays 7. Lowers high blood pressure 8. Prevents arteriosclerosis	1. Same as vitamin C 2. Citrus fruits (white part of orange and lemon skin) 3. Apricots 4. Cherries 5. Blackberries 6. Grapes 7. Cabbage 8. Parsley

Note: This table compiled from many sources (see references in the appendixes).

MINERALS

Minerals in minute or trace amounts are also essential for optimal well-being. They cannot be destroyed during cooking, processing, storage, or freezing. However, cooking often soaks much of the minerals out of the food, thereby decreasing the mineral content of edible foods.

The amounts of minerals needed in the daily diet vary greatly from a few micrograms for the trace minerals (iron, zinc, selenium, manganese, copper, molybdenum, cobalt, chromium, and fluorine) to a million times as much, a gram or more, for the major minerals (calcium, phosphorus, potassium, sulfur, silicon, and magnesium). The best sources and functions of minerals are summarized in Table 6.8; the recommended daily allowances are listed in Table 6-11.

Because they are water-soluble, some minerals, such as sodium and potassium, are readily absorbed into the bloodstream and transported freely; excesses are readily excreted by the kidneys. On the other hand, minerals such as calcium, magnesium, and most trace minerals need to be bound to oxalates or amino acids (chelated as calcium, phosphate, or zinc gluconate) before they can be absorbed from the small intestine. It is also true that trace minerals ingested in pure elemental form can become bound or chelated to nonabsorptive substances in the small intestine, thereby become unavailable, and be poorly absorbed into the bloodstream. For example, only 3 to 10 percent of the amount of iron in food is absorbed, while only about 30 percent of magnesium is normally absorbed. Nature appears to have designed a protective system that prevents the body from absorbing too much of some minerals under normal nonstress conditions.

Diet surveys point out that many Americans are deficient in many trace minerals. Children, girls who begin to menstruate, and women of child-bearing age experience the greatest iron deficiencies. Many persons, ingesting white table sugar and refined white flour products, become deficient in selenium and chromium, since these minerals are removed from sugar cane and whole grains during the milling and refining processes.

Salt, sodium in particular, has been implicated for many years as an important contributing factor to high blood pressure, overweight, and heart disease (71). Nu-

Table 6.8

Minerals the Body Needs, Their Function, Best Sources, Deficiency Symptoms, Those Probably Most Susceptible to Deficiencies

Mineral	Those Probably Most Susceptible to Deficiency	Deficiency Symptoms	Function	Best Sources
Calcium	1. *Taking vitamins A, C, and D* in excess 2. Heavy chocolate eaters 3. Inactive and sedentary 4. Excess stress 5. Over 50 years of age 6. Arthritis 7. Taking laxatives 8. Heavy water drinkers 9. Dysmenorrhea	1. Calcium deposits in joints and tissues 2. Muscle cramps 3. Joint pains 4. Insomnia 5. Acne 6. High pulse rate	1. Maintain healthy skin 2. Build and maintain healthy teeth and bones 3. Maintain healthy blood 4. Eases insomnia 5. Promotes a healthy heart 6. Assists in blood clotting 7. Aids muscle contraction 8. Aids nerve transmission 9. Aids in iron utilization 10. Regulates the passage of nutrients in and out of cells 11. Relieves pain and cramps	1. Milk 2. Dairy products 3. Bone meal 4. Dolomite
Chlorine	1. Working in the hot sun or a hot climate 2. Sweating a lot 3. Excessive vomiting 4. Diuretic intake	1. Loss of hair 2. Impaired digestion 3. Poor muscular contraction 4. Loss of teeth	1. Regulates acid-base balance in blood 2. Aids cell osmosis 3. Stimulates production of hydrochloric acid (HCL) in the stomach 4. Conserves potassium	1. Kelp 2. Table salt 3. Rye flour 4. Ripe olives
Chromium	1. *Eating lots of sugar* refined cereals, and white flour products 2. Diabetics 3. Hypoglycemics 4. Over 50 years of age	1. Inability to deal with starches and sugars 2. Feeling bloated 3. High blood cholesterol levels 4. Retarded growth	1. Regulates blood sugar levels 2. Metabolizes glucose and fatty acids and cholesterol 3. Transports glucose and proteins 4. Forms RNA 5. Forms enzymes 6. Aids insulin	1. Brewer's yeast 2. Bran 3. Whole-grain cereals 4. Meats 5. Clams 6. Corn oil 7. Nuts
Cobalt	1. Vegetarians 2. Anemics	1. Slow growth 2. Fatigue 3. Anemia	1. Prevents pernicious anemia 2. Forms B_{12} 3. Builds red blood cells	1. Liver 2. Oysters and clams 3. Milk 4. Fresh, green leafy vegetables 5. Meats
Copper	1. Excess bleeding 2. Anemics 3. Low red blood cell count	1. Impaired respiration 2. Weakness and fatigue 3. Skin sores 4. Anemia 5. Inability to suntan 6. White spots on fingernails	1. Forms hair color 2. Aids healing 3. Forms hemoglobin 4. Forms red blood cells 5. Facilitates iron absorption 6. Synthesizes enzymes 7. Synthesizes skin pigments 8. Promotes protein metabolism 9. Aids vitamin C oxidation 10. Produces RNA	1. Liver 2. Whole-grain products 3. Almonds 4. Green, leafy vegetables 5. Seafoods
Fluorine	1. Dental caries 2. Older persons 3. Pregnant women	1. Dental caries 2. Poor tooth development 3. Osteoporosis	1. Strengthens bones and teeth 2. Decreases acid in mouth 3. Prevents osteoporosis	1. Fluorinated water 2. Seafoods 3. Gelatin (nonsugar)

Mineral	Those Probably Most Susceptible to Deficiency	Deficiency Symptoms	Function	Best Sources
Iodine	1. Living in an area that has depleted soil 2. Perspiring a lot 3. Excess raw cabbage or cauliflower eaters	1. Dry hair 2. Nervousness 3. Laziness 4. Sluggishness 5. Slow metabolism 6. Goiter 7. Irritability 8. Hardening of arteries 9. Loss of physical vigor	1. Helps maintain beautiful hair, nails, skin, and teeth 2. Aids the thyroid gland and prevents goiter 3. Prevents mental retardation 4. Helps the body burn fat 5. Converts carotene into vitamin A 6. Aids absorption of CHO from the intestine 7. Prevents polio 8. Promotes growth 9. Regulates energy production	1. Kelp 2. Seafood 3. Iodized salt 4. Mushrooms
Iron	1. Women during menstruation 2. Low intake of vitamin C 3. Pregnant women 4. With infections 5. Loss of blood 6. Rapid growth 7. Peptic ulcers	1. Pale skin 2. Fatigue 3. Brittle nails 4. Difficult breathing 5. Constipation 6. Anemia	1. Protein, and copper hemoglobin	1. Liver 2. Oysters 3. Lean meat 4. Leafy green vegetables
Lithium	1. Depressed 2. Alcoholics	1. Depression 2. Up-down moods 3. Contemplating suicide 4. Excessive talking and telephoning 5. Hyperactivity 6. Decreased need for sleep 7. Flamboyant and erratic behavior (e.g., shopping sprees)	1. Acts as mood normalizer 2. Prevents mental illness 3. Reduces tension and anxiety 4. Balances out and decreases high sodium levels	1. Medical prescription 2. Trace amounts present in most foods
Magnesium	1. Eating unbalanced diet 2. Eating lots of meat 3. Diabetics 4. High CHO diet 5. Exposure to lots of noise (working in airport or shipyard) 6. High sugar diet 7. Reducing pills 8. Alcoholics 9. Pregnant women 10. Lactating women 11. High blood cholesterol level 12. Using diuretics 13. Heart disease 14. Low in fresh vegetables 15. Eating white flour bread and pastry	1. Feeling cold 2. Depression 3. Confusion 4. Disorientation 5. Apprehensiveness 6. Muscle spasms and twitching	1. Prevents depression 2. Prevents heart attacks 3. Prevents polio 4. Prevents calcium deposits in bladder 5. Reduces blood cholesterol 6. Fights tooth decay 7. Forms hard tooth enamel 8. Aids in converting blood sugar to energy 9. Helps regulate body temperature 10. Aids nerve function 11. Aids bone growth 12. Helps utilize vitamins B, C, and E 13. Promotes absorption and metabolism of other minerals (Ca, P, Na, and K) 14. Regulates acid-bone balance 15. Activates enzymes for metabolism of CHO and amino acids	1. Fresh, green vegetables 2. Soybeans 3. Wheat germ 4. Figs 5. Apples 6. Seeds, nuts

Mineral	Those Probably Most Susceptible to Deficiency	Deficiency Symptoms	Function	Best Sources
Manganese	1. Eating lots of sugar and sugar products (ice cream and soft-drinks) 2. Eating refined flour products and refined cereals 3. Eating very few, fresh green vegetables 4. Diabetics 5. Older persons 6. Lactating women	1. Diabetes 2. High blood sugar 3. Loss of hearing 4. Ear noises 5. Dizziness	1. Regulates blood sugar and use of sugar in body 2. Aids in removing excess sugar from blood 3. Activates enzymes to utilize vitamins C, biotin, and thiamine 4. Acts as catalyst in synthesis of fatty acids and body cholesterol 5. Activates protein, CHO, and fat metabolism 6. Helps form human milk 7. Nourishes the brain and nerves 8. Aids hearing	1. Unrefined Whole-wheat cereals 2. Egg yolks 3. Leafy green vegetables 4. Tea leaves 5. Nuts
Phosphorus	1. Mental stress 2. Pregnant women 3. Growing children and adolescents 4. Cancer patients 5. Tooth decay 6. Arthritis 7. Taking antacid 8. Taking laxatives	1. Mental-physical fatigue 2. Loss of appetite	1. Essential for all body functions 2. Essential for mental efficiency 3. Aids breakdown of fats 4. Aids breakdown of CHO 5. Stimulates muscle contraction 6. Essential for tooth and skeletal growth 7. Speeds up bone healing 8. Aids B-complex vitamins	1. Meat, fish, poultry 2. Eggs 3. Whole grains 4. Seeds and nuts
Potassium	1. Coffee drinkers 2. Migraine headaches 3. Excessive salt users 4. Alcoholics 5. Extreme stress 6. High blood pressure 7. Older persons 8. Use of diuretics/laxative 9. Cortisone medication 10. Low intake of fruits and vegetables 11. Excessive sweating 12. Hypoglycemics 13. Diarrhea	1. Insomnia 2. Fatigue 3. Headaches 4. Poor reflexes 5. Muscle weakness 6. Constipation 7. Irregular heartbeat 8. Possible acne	1. Keeps skin healthy 2. Aids normal growth 3. Regulates water balance in body cells 4. Converts glucose into glycogen 5. Synthesizes mucle protein from amino acids 6. Stimulates kidneys to eliminate poisons and body wastes 7. Normalizes heartbeat 8. Aids in supply of O_2 to the brain	1. Green leafy vegetables 2. Oranges/bananas 3. Whole grains 4. Sunflower seeds 5. Mint leaves 6. Potato skins 7. Meats
Selenium	1. Living in air pollution 2. Cigarette smokers	1. Loss of skin elasticity 2. Premature aging 3. Fatigue	1. Preserves tissue elasticity 2. Destroys fats in capillaries 3. Aids vitamin E function 4. Prevents cancers of the digestive tract	1. Bran 2. Whole-grain cereals 3. Broccoli 4. Onions 5. Tomatoes 6. Tuna 7. Nuts
Sodium	1. Working in heat and sun 2. Cross-country runners and skiers 3. Diarrhea 4. Excessive sweating 5. Taking diuretics 6. Drinking softened water	1. Fatigue 2. Weakness 3. Nausea 4. Cramps	1. Regulates water balance in cells 2. Regulates blood pressure 3. Aids acid-base balance in blood 4. Aids muscle contraction 5. Purges carbon monoxide from body 6. Maintains blood-lymph health	1. Kelp 2. Table salt 3. Present in all foods 4. Seafoods 5. Beets 6. All meats 7. Cheese

Mineral	Those Probably Most Susceptible to Deficiency	Deficiency Symptoms	Function	Best Sources
Sulfur	1. Vegetarians 2. Inadequate protein intake 3. Psoriasis 4. Eczema	1. Poor skin complexion 2. Dull hair	1. Keeps hair glossy and smooth 2. Keeps skin complexion clear and youthful 3. Keeps nails hard 4. Aids in collagen synthesis 5. Aids manufactured insulin 6. Aids liver to secrete bile 7. Works with vitamin B-complex	1. Meats 2. Fish 3. Legumes 4. Nuts 5. Eggs 6. Cabbage 7. Dried beans
Vanadium			1. May inhibit cholesterol formation in blood vessels 2. May promote blood circulation 3. May prevent tooth decay 4. Aids use of amino acids 5. Regulates fat use in body	1. Kelp 2. Seafood 3. Gelatin (plain and nonsugar)
Zinc	1. Unbalanced diet 2. Alcoholics 3. Men with prostate problems 4. Women taking oral contraceptives 5. Pregnant women (and fetus) 6. Emotional disorders 7. Heart disease 8. Most cancers 9. Eating refined foods 10. Diabetics 11. Injuries and surgery 12. Infertility	1. Fatigue 2. Unalertness 3. Susceptibility to infections 4. Loss of appetite 5. Loss of taste 6. Poor complexion 7. Dull hair 8. Slows healing 9. Hypogonadism	1. Keeps hair glossy and smooth 2. Eliminates cholesterol deposits 3. Aids in absorption of B vitamins 4. Aids manufactured enzymes 5. Aids manufactured insulin 6. Aids CHO metabolism 7. Essential for growth 8. Aids healing 9. Essential for proper functioning of prostate gland 10. Prevents prostate cancer 11. Prevents sterility	1. Brewer's yeast 2. Wheat germ 3. Bran 4. Pumpkin seeds

This table was compiled from many resources (see references in the appendixes).

tritional surveys continuously find Americans eating high-sodium, low-potassium diets (see Table 6.9). More recent research not only finds most Americans deficient in body potassium, but also that it is not so much the excess salt intake but the disruption of the desirable sodium to potassium (Na–K) ratio of 1–20 that may be contributing to high blood pressure, and water retention in adipose tissue. Since Americans ingest 10 to 20 times more than the amount of sodium that the human body needs (½ gram per day), the sodium to potassium ratio varies from 1.5–1 to 6–1.

An excess of sodium causes potassium to be excreted in the urine. The reverse is also true: an excess of potassium increases salt excretion and acts as a natural diuretic by assisting the kidney in flushing excess salt from the body. Just cutting down on salt intake is not enough to restore the sodium to potassium ratio, lose body weight, or lower the risk of high blood pressure. One needs to eat more potassium-rich foods, such as whole-grain cereals, fruits, and fresh, green, leafy vegetables; and less sodium-rich foods, such as meats, dairy products, and salted junk foods (e.g., French fries, pretzels, and popcorn). More dietary suggestions are given in Table 6.10. People with low blood pressure tend to eat more potassium-rich and less sodium-rich foods (71). Those with high blood pressure consume, on the average, four times more salt than those with normal blood pressure (2:139). Research also points out that feeding babies a high-salt diet early in life may result in permanent hypertension in childhood and adulthood.

Table 6.9

Sodium and Potassium (mg/100 g) in Some Unprocessed and Processed Foods

Unprocessed			Processed		
Food	Sodium	Potassium	Food	Sodium	Potassium
Flour, wholemeal	3	360	White bread	540	100
Rice, polished	6	110	Rice, boiled	2	38
Pork, uncooked	65	270	Bacon, uncooked	1400	250
Beef, uncooked	55	280	Beef, corned	950	140
Haddock, uncooked	120	300	Haddock, smoked	790	190
Cabbage, uncooked	7	390	Cabbage, boiled	4	160
Peas, uncooked	1	340	Peas, canned	230	130
Pears, uncooked	2	130	Pears, canned	1	90

Source: McCance and Widdowson, *The Composition of Foods,* H. M. Stationery Office, London, 1978.

Minerals complement vitamins and amino acids in their work. Minerals are used by the body (liver) to synthesize enzymes and to give enzymes their ability to act as catalysts. A few examples follow: along with water, they regulate the acid base and electrolyte balances in the body. They also regulate the functions of the brain, heart, glands, and other organs. Copper, iron, and cobalt combine with amino acids and vitamin C to form hemoglobin and red blood cells, thereby enhancing the oxygen-carrying capacity of the body. Many minerals are also used to synthesize hormones. Iodine, for example, is essential to the synthesis of the hormone thyroxine. The trace mineral, selenium, complements vitamins C and E as a powerful antioxidant and protects cellular membranes. Chromium stimulates the enzymes in body cells to metabolize glucose (carbohydrates) and fats.

Recent research (2), although controversial, points out that minerals work best together in the body only when they are in proper ratio amounts. The ratio of sodium to potassium has already been discussed. The ratio of calcium to magnesium in the body is suspected[2] of probably being about 8–1. If this ratio in the body is exceeded, then the use of magnesium may be inhibited. Many Americans suffer from a potassium deficiency because they ingest too much calcium, which inhibits potassium absorption. Likewise, high dietary sulfate (cabbage) inhibits absorption and increases excretion of molybdenum (12:298). Toxic levels of metal elements, such as lead (from air pollution), mercury, cadmium, and arsenic may build up in the body (from exposure to these metals), thereby inhibiting the functions of trace and major minerals. More research is needed on mineral ratios to resolve the controversy in this nutritional area.

[2] Direct communication with Mineral Laboratory.

FIBER

Fiber or roughage is mostly plant cell wall that cannot be digested because the human digestive system lacks the enzymes to do so. Plant cell wall, such as bran, is made up of cellulose, hemicellulose, lignin, pentosans, and other substances. Although indigestible, fiber is most important to optimal well-being. Besides preventing constipation by promoting mobility of the digestive tract, and regular bowel elimination, it stimulates the workings of the digestive system. Medical evidence (23) suggests that fiber plays a role in preventing atherosclerosis, diverticular disease, and cancer of the breasts and large intestine. Fiber appears to isolate bile acids and steriods in the digestive tract, thereby preventing cholesterol and fat absorption. Since fiber also increases bile-acid excretion, fiber helps regulate and lower cholesterol in the body. By promoting bowel movement several times a day, there is less chance of a buildup of carcinogenic chemicals in the large intestine to irritate the lower colon and cause possible cancer.

Surveys point out that Americans do not ingest enough fiber. Our eating habits have changed since 1900, and we now eat less fresh fruit, fresh vegetables, and whole cereal grains than we should. Refined foods, such as white flour and commercial cereals, lack fiber. The average daily Western diet contains 6.4 grams of crude fiber compared to 24.8 grams for the traditional diet of the Bantu tribesmen (32:235). Consumption has dropped to about a third of its former level, and the fiber that is eaten tends to come from fruits and vegetables rather than from starchy staples (13). We need to eat foods with more fiber in our daily diets (see Table 6.10). Prune and lemon juices and whole-grain brans stimulate intestinal mobility in the same way laxative drugs do (12:56). For example, 5 to 6 tablespoons of wheat bran each day will keep one's digestive system healthy. One

Table 6.10

Fiber in Foods

	Fiber (in grams)
Apple, 1 small	1.0
Banana, 1 medium	0.5
Beans, lima, 1/4 cup	1.8
Beets, diced, 1/2 cup	0.8
Beet greens, cooked, 1/2 cup	1.3
String beans, cooked, 3/4 cup	1.0
Carrots, cubed, 3/4 cup	1.0
Peas, green, fresh, 3/4 cup	2.0
Bread, whole wheat, 3 slices	1.0
Bread, white, 4 slices	0.2
Shredded wheat biscuit, 1	0.7
Oatmeal, cooked, 3/4 cup	0.2
Cream of Wheat, cooked, 1/2 cup	trace
Raspberries, red 3/4 cup	3.0
Prunes, 6 medium + 2 tbsp juice	0.8
Strawberries, fresh, 2/3 cup	1.4

Source: Calculated from figures in *Composition of Foods,* Agriculture Handbook No. 8, Agriculture Research Service, U.S. Department of Agriculture, 1963.

should also eat the skins of baked potatoes, apples, dried beans and peas, and other raw fruits and vegetables instead of discarding plant skins. One should avoid ingesting refined flour products and commercial cereals that are very low in bran. Meats and poultry do not provide fiber.

RECOMMENDED DAILY ALLOWANCES

Just how much of vitamins, minerals, and amino acids we need beyond preventing disease is uncertain. There is no unanimous agreement among nutritionists on the amount needed for average and optimal well-being. Indeed, there is considerable controversy on this matter. For example, how much — if any — vitamin C does a person need to avoid or fight colds? At one extreme are the food enthusiasts, including faddists, while at the other are the majority of practicing physicians who, through the fault of their medical school training, tend to ignore all but the elementary aspects of nutrition. As a result, the amount of nutrients needed for good health is uncertain and controversial. We lack a sophisticated nutrition science in this country.

The National Academy of Science has appointed a Committee on Dietary Allowances to draft a Recom-

mended Daily Allowance (RDA or RMDA) as a nutrient guide for nutritionists (see Table 6.11). Revised every 4 years, the RDA is "intended to provide" acceptable levels of nutrient intake for groups of average people who were healthy to begin with and were without stresses of living. The recommendation (refer to Table 6.13) is not based on minimum requirements but instead represents values in excess of those needed for signs of deficiencies or diseases to appear (42:205;28;54:132–144). Roger Williams, a biochemist, nutritionist, and the discoverer of vitamin B_{15}, points out that RDA is good enough to prevent well-recognized deficiency diseases, but it is not good enough to promote optimal well-being. Those following RDA may not be able to function at their highest level (73:11). This concept may be readily observable from Table 6.12.

Recommended daily allowances may not be realistic guides for many reasons. One is that human beings are distinctive and differ in many ways from each other. Each individual's need for specific nutrients is genetically and biologically programmed; for example, it is estimated that over 1000 different functioning metabolic enzymes are produced in the liver (42:41). If some of these enzymes are absent in a person, he or she cannot digest certain foods (e.g., milk, fish, or fruit). Hence "biochemical individuality" is more the rule than is "the average" in determining a daily nutrient allowance (73:11). But individuals with perfect digestive and metabolic systems are so rare that we cannot assume that one is able to attain well-being on an average nutrient allowance. This rationale sets the stage for the second reason: the concept of supernutrition.

The idea of supernutrition is to provide quality nutrition to all body cells so that the whole body can attain optimal well-being. Supernutrition is based on two biological observations (74). First, living cells, in our bodies and elsewhere, practically never encounter perfect optimal environmental (nutrient) conditions; second, living cells when furnished with wholly satisfactory environments, including the absence of pathogenic organisms, will respond with health and vigor. This means that quality nutrition includes a teamwork balance of all nutrients in a diet for each individual body cell. Although no nutrient by itself is an effective remedy for any common disease, the nutrients acting as a team are probably effective in the prevention of a host of diseases, as well as maintaining resistance to infection. Adequate nutrition must involve the complete chain of nutrients. If a diet is missing one link in the nutrition chain, it may be just as worthless for supporting life as if it were missing 10 links (review the section on amino acids under "Proteins"). One nutrient — mineral, vitamin, or amino acid — added as a supplement to a food can bring very little,

Table 6.11

Recommended Daily Allowances. Revised 1980

	Age (years)	Weight (kg)	Weight (lb)	Height (cm)	Height (in.)	Protein (g)	Fat-Soluble Vitamins Vitamin A (μg RE)[b]	Vitamin A (IU)	Vitamin D (μg)[c]	Vitamin D (IU)	Vitamin E (mg αTE)[d]	Vitamin E (IU)
Infants	0.0–0.5	6	13	60	24	kg × 2.2	420	2100	10	400	3	4.5
	0.5–1.0	9	20	71	28	kg × 2.0	400	2000	10	400	4	6
Children	1–3	13	29	90	35	23	400	2000	10	400	5	7
	4–6	20	44	112	44	30	500	2500	10	400	6	9
	7–10	28	62	132	52	34	700	3500	10	400	7	10
Males	11–14	45	99	157	62	45	1000	5000	10	400	8	12
	15–18	66	145	176	69	56	1000	5000	10	400	10	15
	19–22	70	154	177	70	56	1000	5000	7.5	300	10	15
	23–50	70	154	178	70	56	1000	5000	5	200	10	15
	51+	70	154	178	70	56	1000	5000	5	200	10	15
Females	11–14	46	101	157	62	46	800	4000	10	400	8	12
	15–18	55	120	163	64	46	800	4000	10	400	8	12
	19–22	55	120	163	64	44	800	4000	7.5	300	8	12
	23–50	55	120	163	64	44	800	4000	5	200	8	12
	51+	55	120	163	64	44	800	4000	5	200	8	12
Pregnant						+30	+200	1000	+5	200	+2	3
Lactating						+20	+400	2000	+5	200	+3	4.5

[a] The allowances are intended to provide for individual variations among most normal persons as they live in the United States under usual environmental stresses. Diets should be based on a variety of common foods in order to provide other nutrients for which human requirements have been less defined. See text for detailed discussion of allowances and of nutrients not tabulated. See Table 1 (p. 20) for weights and heights by individual year of age. See Table 3 (p. 23) for suggested average energy intakes.

[b] Retinol equivalents. 1 retinol equivalent = 1 μg retinol or 6 μg β carotene. See text for calculation of vitamin A activity of diets as retinol equivalents.

[c] As cholecalciferol 10 μg cholecalciferol = 400 IU of vitamin D.

[d] α-tocopherol equivalents. 1 mg d-α tocopherol = 1 α-TE. See text for variation in allowances and calculation of vitamin E activity of the diet as α-tocopherol equivalents.

if any, favorable effect, unless the food contains some of all the other nutrients, or unless these are available from the reserves of the person being nourished (74:7). The Recommended Daily Allowances disregard this concept of supernutrition.

The RDA is also based on the assumption that all foods will retain the nutrient values until ingested. In other words, the RDA assumes that the quantity of vitamins and minerals in foods will not be destroyed or depleted during the processing, packaging, transportation, storage, and cooking of foods. The food industry uses preservatives, such as refined sugars, salt, and over 2000 chemical additives to prevent foods from spoiling on the shelves of supermarkets, to improve taste, and to give food aesthetic "sales" appeal (6:185;8:166) Consequently, milling whole-grain wheat into white flour removes the most nutritious part of the wheat. Enriched or fortified white flour usually contains between 4 and 8 of the original 22 nutrients found in whole-grain wheat

(54:22). Fruits and green vegetables begin to lose their vitamin C as soon as they are harvested. Lettuce loses most of its vitamin C in a few days when kept at room temperature (54:22). Over half the foods Americans buy in supermarkets are convenience foods, such as cookies, breakfast cereals, potato chips, and TV dinners (40:142), that are often "empty calorie" foods rich in refined sugar. Such processed foods have lost many nutrients that should be there in the same proportion as the caloric content. The RDA and nutrient values tables overlook such depletions and deficiencies in the real world of people.

Finally, our life styles are stressful, and we often eat in "fast-food restaurants and cafeterias." Food additives and exposure to a life style that includes smog, and cigarette smoke, various drugs, alcoholic beverages, stress on the job and in college, stress in personal life, stress from a fast-pace life style, and junk foods—all collectively accelerate the depletion of vitamins, min-

Table 6.11
Recommended Daily Allowances. Revised 1980 (continued)

Water-Soluble Vitamins								Minerals					
Vitamin C (mg)	Thiamin (mg)	Riboflavin (mg)	Niacin (mg NE)[e]	Vitamin B-6 (mg)	Folacin[f] (μg)	Vitamin B-12 (μg)	Calcium (mg)	Phosphorus (mg)	Magnesium (mg)	Iron (mg)	Zinc (mg)	Iodine (μg)
35	0.3	0.4	6	0.3	30	0.5[g]	360	240	50	10	3	40
35	0.5	0.6	8	0.6	45	1.5	540	360	70	15	5	50
45	0.7	0.8	9	0.9	100	2.0	800	800	150	15	10	70
45	0.9	1.0	11	1.3	200	2.5	800	800	200	10	10	90
45	1.2	1.4	16	1.6	300	3.0	800	800	250	10	10	120
50	1.4	1.6	18	1.8	400	3.0	1200	1200	350	18	15	150
60	1.4	1.7	18	2.0	400	3.0	1200	1200	400	18	15	150
60	1.5	1.7	19	2.2	400	3.0	800	800	350	10	15	150
60	1.4	1.6	18	2.2	400	3.0	800	800	350	10	15	150
60	1.2	1.4	16	2.2	400	3.0	800	800	350	10	15	150
50	1.1	1.3	15	1.8	400	3.0	1200	1200	300	18	15	150
60	1.1	1.3	14	2.0	400	3.0	1200	1200	300	18	15	150
60	1.1	1.3	14	2.0	400	3.0	800	800	300	18	15	150
60	1.0	1.2	13	2.0	400	3.0	800	800	300	18	15	150
60	1.0	1.2	13	2.0	400	3.0	800	800	300	10	15	150
+20	+0.4	+0.3	+2	+0.6	+400	+1.0	+400	+400	+150	h	+5	+25
+40	+0.5	+0.5	+5	+0.5	+100	+1.0	+400	+400	+150	h	+10	+50

[e] 1 NE (niacin equivalent) is equal to 1 mg of niacin or 60 mg of dietary tryptophan.

[f] The folacin allowances refer to dietary sources as determined by *Lactobacillus casei* assay after treatment with enzymes (conjugases) to make polyglutamyl forms of the vitamin available to the test organism.

[g] The recommended dietary allowance for vitamin B-12 infants is based on average concentration of the vitamin in human milk. The allowances after weaning are based on energy intake (as recommended by the American Academy of Pediatrics) and consideration of other factors, such as intestinal absorption; see text.

[h] The increased requirement during pregnancy cannot be met by the iron content of habitual American diets nor by the existing iron stores of many women; therefore the use of 30 to 60 mg of supplemental iron is recommended. Iron needs during lactation are not substantially different from those of nonpregnant women, but continued supplementation of the mother for 2 to 3 months after parturition is advisable in order to replenish stores depleted by pregnancy.

[i] Vitamin A values are expressed as μg RE and IU, Vitamin D as μg and IU, and Vitamin E as mg and IU. IU units of measure as provided since many tables containing nutritive values of foods may not have 1980 recommended units of values [food portions may be expressed as IU (1974 standard)].

Source: Recommended Daily Allowances, Food and Nutrition Board, National Academy of Science National Research Council.

erals, and essential amino acids within the body (38:205;58;60:132–144). Modern habits create a great body demand for vitamins and minerals. For example, long exposure to harsh and glaring lights is common among office workers. This exposure uses up vitamins A and C at an accelerated rate, with consequences of increased susceptibility to colds and minor infections. These and other stressful habits deplete nutrients in the body. Table 6.13 summarizes the nutrients depleted by numerous health habits and disorders. The livers of such persons need more nutrients to continuously synthesize the metabolic enzymes which, in turn, detoxify the many chemicals that find their way into the body. The body also needs more nutrients to synthesize numerous hormones to cope with stress and maintain cellular metabolic integrity. When adequate amounts of nutrients are quickly depleted or are lacking in a diet, one feels fatigued, and becomes sluggish and less active — one runs out of energy much as a car engine stops running when it runs out of gasoline. These are the early signs of poor or inadequate nutrition. The Recommended Daily Allowances fail to give adequate consideration of the American eating habits, life style, and the lack of ample quantities of nutrients in foods.

Thus you should be aware of the shortcomings of RDA. The RDA may or may not apply to you because you may or may not be average. You may need much less than the RDA, or you may need more.

Table 6.12

Relationship of Levels of Wellness to Supernutrition (Nutritional levels), and Ability to Function in Life

Levels of Functioning	Projected Percent Body Efficiency	Levels of Wellness	Probable Levels of Nutrition
Superb functioning; e.g., superman or $6 million man. Olympic champion	95–100	Optimal	Supernutrition
Good functioning in society; e.g., college athlete. Exercises regularly	75–94	Above average	Better than average or RMDA
Average "so-so" functioning; e.g., nonathlete (intramurals). Gets by with moderate exercise or activity	55–74	Average, ordinary health	Meet minimum requirements and some nutrient deficiencies
Difficulty functioning in society; e.g., loser in life. Sedentary	40–54	Below average, poor health	Many nutrient deficiencies—uses RMDA as a guideline
Inability to function in society; e.g., social ineptitude and rejection (lack popularity). Sedentary	25–39	Minor illness infectious state: overweight, depressed, H.B.P., allergies, colds, flus, headaches, or diabetes	Many nutrient deficiencies and serious depletion of nutrients
Inability to care for self. Bedridden	1–24	Major illness disease state: arthritis or heart disease or obesity	Grave deficiencies
	0%	Death	

SHOULD YOU TAKE VITAMIN PILLS?

1. Analyze your daily diet for vitamin-mineral-amino-acid intake. Compare these nutrients to the RMDA:
   (a) Which of these nutrients are you deficient in?
   (b) Which of these nutrients are you getting an overdose of?
2. React to the Nutrient Deficiency Inventory, if you have not already done so.
3. Compare your reaction to Nutrient Deficiency Inventory to your daily diet analysis. If you conclude from this comparison that you need to take nutrient supplements, then follow the suggested guidelines for doing so.

WAYS TO TAKE NUTRIENT SUPPLEMENTS SAFELY AND CORRECTLY

1. The best way to get essential nutrients is from the food you eat each day. Nutrients in nature do not occur alone—they are accompanied by other vitamins and minerals, which help their assimilation for body health.
2. If you take multipe supplements, take a balance of all nutrients as a supplement. The supplement should provide all the essential vitamins, minerals, amino acids, as well as many of the so-called nonessential nutrients. Since vitamins work as a team with other vitamins—and with proteins, minerals, fatty acids, and other nutrients—taking them all at one time ensures having all the essential nutrients present at the same time in the digestive

Table 6.13

Stresses of Living That Cause Depletion of Body nutrients by Most Common Health Habits, Problems, and Disorders (and nutrients needed to counteract or lower the risk to health problem)

Health Problem or Disorder or Health Practice Causing Nutrient Depletion in Body	Nutrients Probably Needed Beyond RMDA to Prevent Depletion or Lower Risk of Disease	
	Vitamins	Minerals
1. Living in air pollution	A, C, E, K, P, inositol	Se, Cu, I, Fe
2. Drinking alcoholic beverages (alcoholism)	Folic acid, inositol, C, K, P	Li, Cu, Fe
3. Anemia	Folic acid, PABA	Cu, Co, Fe
4. Allergies	C, P, A	I, Cu, Fe
5. Appetite (poor)	Biotin, folic acid, P, B-complex	Cu
6. Arteriosclerosis (hardening of arteries)	B_1, inositol, linoleic acid	Ca, I, K
7. Arthritis or rheumatism	B_5, C, P	Ca, P, Cu, Fe
8. Using birth control pills	B_3, C, E, K, P	Fe
9. Cancer	C, P, A	P, Zn, Cu, I, Fe
10. Coffee drinking	Inositol, K	K
11. Digestive disorders— gas, upset stomach	B_1, folic acid, inositol, PABA, C	Chlorine, iron, Cu
12. Drugs (aspirins, sleeping pills, prescriptions, laxatives)	Folic acid, PABA, K, C, P	K, Ca, Cu, Fe
13. Diabetes and hypoglycemia	B_5, B_{12}, biotin, choline, folic acid, C, E, P	Cr, I, K, Zn, Li, Ca, Cu
14. Depression (suicide tendencies/moodiness)	B_1, B_2, B_3, B_6, B_{12} biotin, PABA	Li, P
15. Edema (water buildup in tissues) in women	B_6	—
16. Eyestrain/infection (reading stress, sensitivity to light)	A, B_2, C, D, E, K, P	Ca, Cu, I, Fe
17. Fat metabolism (high-fat diet)	B_3, B_5, B_6, B_{12}, choline, E, K	Cr, I, P, Zn, Vanadium
18. Hair	B_6, biotin, inositol, linoleic acid	Cl_2, Cu, I, Zn, S
19. Fatigue (chronic)	B_1, B_3, B_5, B_{12}, PABA, C, E, P	Ca, Cu, I, Fe, K, Se
20. Headache	B_1, B_3, Biotin, E, K, B_6	—
21. Heart disease	B_1, choline, inositol, D, B_6, E, C, P	Ca, P, K, Mg, Cu
22. High blood pressure	C, P, folic acid, E	Se, Na V, Cu, I
23. Illness, infections, colds, flus, surgery (healing)	A, B_5, B_{12}, C, D, E, biotin, folic acid, inositol, PABA, linoleic acid, P, K	Fe, Zn, P, Cu, Ca, Co, I, Fe
24. Inactivity (sedentary life style)		Ca, I
25. Insomnia	B_3, biotin	Ca, K
26. Irritability	B_3, B_5, B_6, B_{12}, PABA, E, C, P	I, Li, Cu
27. Lactation	E	

Table 6.13 continued

Health Problem or Disorder or Health Practice Causing Nutrient Depletion in Body	Nutrients Probably Needed Beyond RMDA to Prevent Depletion or Lower Risk of Disease	
	Vitamins	Minerals
28. Longevity (delaying aging process)	A, B_5, B_{12}, B_{13}, folic acid, inositol, C, E, K	Ca, Cr, Fe, Li, K, P, Se, Cu, I
29. Meat ingestion	A, B_3, B_5, C, linoleic acid	K, Zn, Cu, I
30. Menstruation	B_{12}, C, folic acid, E	Ca, Fe, Cu
31. Obesity (overweight)	B_6 — Persons gaining weight may be deficient in numerous nutrients.	—
32. Pesticides exposure	C, P	Cu
33. Pregnancy	C, D, E, folic acid	Ca, K, P, F, Fe, Cu (All nutrients essential)
34. Skin disorders or infection (acne, poor complexion)	A, B_2, B_3, B_5, C, E, biotin, inositol, PABA, linoleic acid	Ca, Cu, I, K
35. Smoking tobacco or pot	C, K, P, A (protects mucous membrane), choline, inositol	Se, Cu, I, Fe
36. Soft drinks (coca-cola, etc.)	Inositol, K	K
37. Stress (emotional, physical, etc.)	B_1, B_5, folic acid, P, C, B_6, E	P, K, Ca, Cu, Fe
38. Eating sugar (refined) (sucrose)	See Diabetics	—
39. Vegetarian diet	B_{12}	Co, Zn
40. White flour (refined breads, pastry, etc.)	B_3, B_5, B_{12}, choline, E, K	Cr, I, Zn
41. Weight reduction loss	B_6, choline inositol, C, P	I, Cu, Fe
42. Wound healing and burns, bruising	See Illness	—
43. X-ray or radiation	C, P, linoleic acid	Cu, Fe
44. Dental caries	C, P, D, K	Ca, F, P, K, Cu, I, Fe

tract, a condition essential for optimal absorption into the bloodstream, and for optimal growth, maintenance, and repair of the entire body. Vitamins are absorbed best when taken with other foods and minerals. There are a few exceptions to this practice (discussed later).

Check your supplement by reading the label. The label should list most of the nutrients, including trace minerals, as listed in Table 6.1. Most supplements currently available are unsuitable because they are deficient in providing all the links in the nutritional chain of life. Supplements may also be purchased for a specific vitamin, mineral, or amino acids, and taken separately, although this is not recommended.

3. The amount of supplements to take depends on several factors. Multinutrient preparations fall into three general categories, those that supply:

1. About half the RMDA.
2. One to one and one-half times the RMDA.
3. Three to five times the RMDA.

Good supplements list, in one tablet or capsule, the amount of each nutrient in either I.U. milligrams or grams and/or the percent of the RMDA of each nutrient in each tablet or capsule. In general, the label of a multiple supplement will specify one, two, three, or even eight tablets a day.

Keep in mind that RMDAs serve as a reference point against which the consumer can compare the amount of a nutrient he or she is buying. Since the potency of a vitamin tends to dwindle with the age of the supplement, and some of the vitamin and mineral may not be completely absorbed or metabolized, manufacturers usually put more than the advertized amount of each vitamin.

4. The supplement should be taken before or during each meal to assure your having all the essential nutrients present at the same time in the digestive tract.

5. Minerals need to be in chelated or bound form. Usually, the label informs you how it is bound: for example, as a phosphate, gluconate, or sulfate. Most minerals cannot be absorbed or transported in their elemental state in the human body. Absorption is facilitated by minerals combining with other minerals or with amino acids.

6. Keep the supplements refrigerated to maintain potency.

7. Spread your intake of supplemental nutrients evenly throughout the day. Your body cells need nutrients 24 hours a day; therefore, spreading your intake throughout the day ensures an even concentration of nutrients throughout the day.

8. Take vitamin E and iron separately. Take iron with breakfast, and vitamin E with the evening meal. These two nutrients affect each other adversely in the intestinal tract.

9. Take iron and vitamin C together, as vitamin C aids in the absorption of iron. Likewise, calcium aids the absorption of vitamin D and zinc that of vitamin A.

10. It may also be to your advantage to purchase vitamins C and E separately. These two nutrients are likely to be on the low side in many supplements, and many men and women have life-stye stresses and biochemical needs that far exceed RMDA (see Table 6.13). Just how much of these and other nutrients you need or should take can only be decided by you — often by trial and error. Unfortunately, inexpensive tests to determine the amounts of nutrients one's body needs are not yet available.

11. Supernutrition is a nutrition plan that allows one to attain optimal well-being within 2 or 3 months by supplementing the daily food diet with megadoses of nutrients. It is based on the concepts of orthomolecular medicine that one's body needs the proper amounts of nutrients at the right time, and that the amounts of each nutrient are biochemically and genetically predetermined for each individual. The living cells in our bodies seldom receive perfect optimal nutrition or other environmental conditions. When furnished with wholly satisfactory environments, the cells — and indeed the entire body — respond with optimal health, vigor, and vitality (73:11). Proponents of supernutrition claim that it allows

a person to function optimally instead of vegetating or functioning at half-speed.

Supernutrition, like nutrition, is not very well understood by most scientists and medical doctors — hence it is controversial. You should read more about it in the appropriate references (14;53;73) at the end of this chapter and decide about supernutrition yourself.

BEHAVIOR MODIFICATION TECHNIQUES: ASSESSING YOUR DIET AND EATING HABITS

PURPOSE:
To help you to:
1. Find out why you eat.
2. Find out how you eat.
3. Find out what you eat.
4. Assess your caloric energy requirements.
5. Assess your mineral-vitamin intake (see the earlier section on amino acid analysis).
6. Modify your eating habits (if needed).

This self-contained module is organized into three phases. Each phase allows you to progress slowly, at your own pace, so that you have a chance to change or to modify your eating habits. A slow change helps your body to adjust physiologically, and it also helps to stabilize your body weight.

Each of the three phases are organized in steplike progression so that you will deal with one item or change at a time. All phases focus on analyzing the food you eat and not how you cook or prepare food.

Students using this module should consult with their instructor on classroom procedures for handling in the Daily Food Analyzers, the graphs, and so on. It is important to have periodic checks on whether you are assessing your diet correctly during the first and third week of each phase. You may change the sequence of this module and adjust it to best meet your personal needs.

You should be aware that you should have a medical checkup (health appraisal) prior to changing or modifying your diet, eating habits, or weight. This module is not recommended for pregnant women or persons under medical care (unless approved by their physician). The value portions of foods are for adults; therefore, growing children and teenagers may find these values misleading and incorrect for their ages.

It is hoped that you will find emotional and social reinforcements for such a change during these phases. Discuss reinforcements as aids for this program with your friends, classmates, instructor, and physician. Suggestions for maintaining good eating habits are discussed in the next chapter.

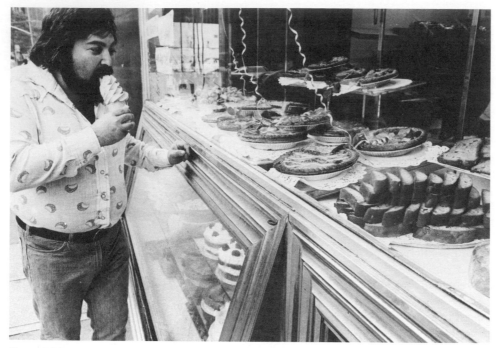

Figure 6.14
Sugar is hidden in many foods. Eating excess amounts of sugar contributes to overweight and poor health.

Suggested Behavioral Modification of Your Eating Habits

Phase	Time Span (weeks)	What To Do
	2	Analysis of present eating habits:
		Step 1. Respond to the Body Statistics Recorder. You should check your body weight each week and your fat measurements every 2–3 weeks as a motivation to continue this modification program.
		Step 2. Respond to the Eating Habits Recorder. This helps you analyze your present eating habits.
		Step 3. Respond to the Daily Food Analyzer and Daily Vitamin-Mineral Analyzer. Keep an honest record of all the foods you eat for 2–3 typical days of a week. This helps you become aware of what you eat. It provides a reference point for future analysis and is vital in making you aware of how successful you are in changing your eating habits.
		By referring to Table 1.2 in the appendices, you will learn the caloric and nutrient values of different foods. You learn by doing!

Phase	Time Span (weeks)		What To Do
		Step 4.	Estimate your Caloric Balance by comparing the total daily caloric food intake with your daily caloric energy expenditures. This gives you an immediate daily picture of whether you gained or lost weight, and whether you are overeating.
		Step 5.	Graph 6.1—Plot your daily or weekly average food intake data in Graph 6.1. This graph gives a picture profile of your eating habits. A graph helps to interpret information and illustrates your eating and food intake trends.
		Step 6.	Graph 6.2—Plot weekly.
		Step 7.	Graph 6.3—Plot weekly.
		Step 8.	Analyze your vitamin-mineral intake. This is similar to the analysis of fats, CHO, and proteins.
II	4		Eliminating junk foods—cutting down fats and refined sugar and starch, and adjusting your intake of vitamins and minerals.
		Step 1.	Continue with Phase I food data recording and analysis.
		Step 2.	Identify junk foods (e.g., circle with red pen all junk foods in previous days). Refer to Table 6.15.
		Step 3.	Identify salt (sodium)-rich foods and cut down on these foods.
		Step 4.	Analyze your daily diet for fiber and check Table 6.10 for best food sources.
		Step 5.	Substitute good nutritious foods (refer to Table 6.16) for junk foods.
		Step 6.	Continue plotting the graphs.
		Step 7.	*Analyze the graphs for trends.* (Look for high-low peaks. Be aware that fat intake usually increases when you increase protein intake, and vice versa. Weight loss of 5–10 pounds will usually occur in 3–5 weeks when you eliminate junk-fat foods, replace these with more nutrient foods, and begin exercising.)
		Step 8.	*Start exercising regularly.* Exercise helps reset and regulate your appestat center in the hypothalmus, which controls the appetite, hunger, thirst, and emotions. Refer to Chapter 5 for infor-

Phase	Time Span (weeks)	What To Do
		mation on this. Exercise will aid you in losing body weight, stabilize your weight, and help you to eat less and not overeat.
		Step 9. *See Chapter 3 — Emotional and Spiritual Well-Being.* Eating habits and weight control are closely related to our emotions and how we feel. Reviewing Chapter 3 will help you to manage and control your eating habits.
		Step 10. *See Chapter 7 — Weight Control.* It has information and suggestions on how to lose weight safely, as well as reinforcements for such a change.
III	4–8	Adjustment and stabilization of eating habits, body weight, and developing new attitudes toward food, eating, health, and life.
		Step 1. Continue with Phases I and II. Adjust your intake of proteins, fats, carbohydrates, vitamins, and minerals. Continuing to analyze your food intake 2–3 times a week will help you do this. Be more conscious of, and give greater emphasis to, eating foods rich in vitamins and minerals instead of counting calories. Getting a daily balance of vitamins and minerals will help squelch your appetite for junk foods and overeating.
		Make sure that your intake of vitamins and minerals does not exceed the RMDA by more than three times. Refer to Table 6.11 for guidance.
		It takes time, will power, and patience to stabilize new eating habits.

BODY STATISTIC RECORDER

Name _____   Date _____

Sex _____ M _____ F

                                                 Beginning   *After*

1. Age: _____ years

2. Weight (with shoes with 1-inch heel and lightweight clothes)   _____   _____

3. Height (with shoes with 1-inch heel)   _____   _____

4. Fat storage site test (pinch of skinfold test)

   (Estimate, using pinch technique, how many inches (meters) of fat there are in various areas of your body.)

	Beginning	*After*
(a) Side of waist	_____ inches	_____ inches
(b) Stomach (navel)	_____ inches	_____ inches
(c) Upper thighs (front)	_____ inches	_____ inches
(d) Triceps muscle	_____ inches	_____ inches

5. Resting pulse rate (beats per minutes)   _____   _____

6. Cholesterol (blood) count   _____   _____

7. Blood glucose count   _____   _____

8. Triglycerides (blood count)   _____   _____

Eating Habits Recorder

1. Check the number of meals you eat per day
   _____ Breakfast
   _____ Lunch
   _____ Dinner
   _____ Snacks

2. Check your salt intake
   _____ Do not use at all
   _____ Salt food on plate once a day (light)
   _____ Salt food on plate (moderately)
   _____ Salt food on plate with every meal
   _____ Only salt food as it is cooked

3. Check foods you eat a lot of
   _____ French fries
   _____ Potato chips
   _____ Hamburgers
   _____ Cookies
   _____ Pies
   _____ Chocolate bars and candy

4. Check beverages you drink each day
   _____ Soft drinks
   _____ Fruit juice
   _____ Beer/wine
   _____ Water
   _____ Other alcoholic beverages

5. Check foods you eat once a day or more
   _____ Lettuce salad
   _____ Cole slaw
   _____ Carrot salad
   _____ Tossed vegetable salad

6. Check which meals you eat in a restaurant
   _____ Breakfast
   _____ Lunch
   _____ Dinner
   _____ Snacks

7. Check which meals you cook each day
   _____ Breakfast
   _____ Lunch
   _____ Dinner
   _____ Snacks

Daily Food Analyzer

NAME _____ DATE _____

ACTIVITY LEVEL _____

DIRECTIONS   List all foods and all drinks for 1 day in the following table. See Table 1.2 in the appendices for caloric values of various foods. Refer to Table 18 to classify your physical activity for the day. Record this estimated activity level in the space above. (Xerox extra copies.)

Food Item (plus drinks)	Approximate Measure of Serving	(1) Protein (grams)	(2) Fats (grams)	(3) CHO (grams)

(Add each column to get grams).   (1)_____ (2)_____ (3)_____

Caloric % of proteins in diet = _____ [a]   (To convert grams to calories)   x4 cal   x9 cal   x4 cal

Caloric % of fats in diet = _____   Total calories eaten[b] =   (4)_____ +(5)_____ +(6)_____

Caloric % of CHO in diet = _____   =   _____ calories (intake for day)

Activity level
(Energy expended same day) =   _____ .

[a] For example, caloric percent of proteins in daily diet $= \frac{\text{cal protein}}{\text{total cal}} \times \frac{100}{1}$.

Conclusion: Calories lost or gained   =   _____ .

[b] See Table 6.6 for the ideal balance of fat, CHO, protein in diet.

Daily Vitamin-Mineral Analyzer

Name _____   Date _____

Food Item	Approx. Measure of Serving	Minerals									Vitamins								
		Cal-cium (mg)	Phos-phorus (mg)	Magne-sium (mg)	Sod-ium (mg)	Potas-sium (mg)	Zinc (mg)	Copper (mg)	Iron (mg)	Vit. A (I/U)	Thia-min (mg)	Ribo-flavin (mg)	Niacin (mg)	Vit. B-6 (mg)	Panto thenic (mg)	Fola-cin (mg)	Vit. B-12 (mg)	Vit. C (mg)
1.																		
2.																		
3.																		
4.																		
5.																		
6.																		
7.																		
8.																		
9.																		
10.																		
11.																		
12.																		
13.																		
14.																		
15.																		
16.																		
Total																		
RMDA																		
Surplus (+) or Deficiency (−)																		

Predicting Your Energy Requirements

There are many ways to determine the amount of energy you expend in a day's activities. Precise laboratory techniques are detailed, complicated, time-consuming, expensive, and usually impractical. An alternative nonlaboratory method is suggested for estimating your total energy needs for a day. It is based on physiological principles of body energy needs and expenditures. You should be aware that, since it is an estimate, it is inaccurate and subject to a small prediction error.

The advantages in using this estimation method over more precise measurements are that you do not need any expensive equipment; it is a quick estimate, easy to calculate; and it is inexpensive.

Method 1—Physical Activity Level

This method predicts your physical activity level. By classifying yourself into one of the five activity levels for a given day in Table 6.14, you use the corresponding body weight factor on the right side of the table. Multiply this factor value by your present body weight. This gives you a theoretical estimate of how many calories of energy your body burns in 24 hours. This theoretical estimate includes the basal metabolic calories needed to sustain or keep you alive, as well as the calories you burn up participating in all daily activities.

CALCULATIONS:
Your daily total:

Energy requirements = body weight (lb.) × body weight factor

For example, a man weighing 150 lb and moderately active, would require:

$$\text{Man} = 150 \text{ lb.} \times 14$$

$$= 2100 \text{ calories}$$

$$\text{You} = \underline{\hspace{2cm}} \times \underline{\hspace{2cm}}$$
$$\phantom{\text{You} =} \text{lb} \qquad\quad \text{factor}$$

$$= \underline{\hspace{2cm}} \text{ calories}$$

Table 6.14

Predicting Your Physical Activity Level

Level	Activity	Body Weight Factor
0	Sedentary, inactive most of the day (e.g., some housewives, some office workers)	13.0
1	Light (seated as student, housewife, or office worker)	13.5
2	Moderate (teacher, housewife)	14.0
3	Vigorous (walking 8 hours a day, factory or construction workers)	14.5
4	Severe (athletes-in-training, lumberjack, heavy labor)	15.0

Source: Adapted from *The Computer Diet* by Vincent W. Antonetti, Copyright © 1973 by Vincent W. Antonetti. Reprinted by permission of the publisher, M. Evans and Co., Inc., New York, p. 14; and Justus J. Schifferes and Louis J. Peterson, *Healthier Living Highlights,* New York: Wiley, 1975, p. 110.

Method 2 — Nomogram

Another way of predicting your caloric body needs and
physical activity is to use the nomogram.

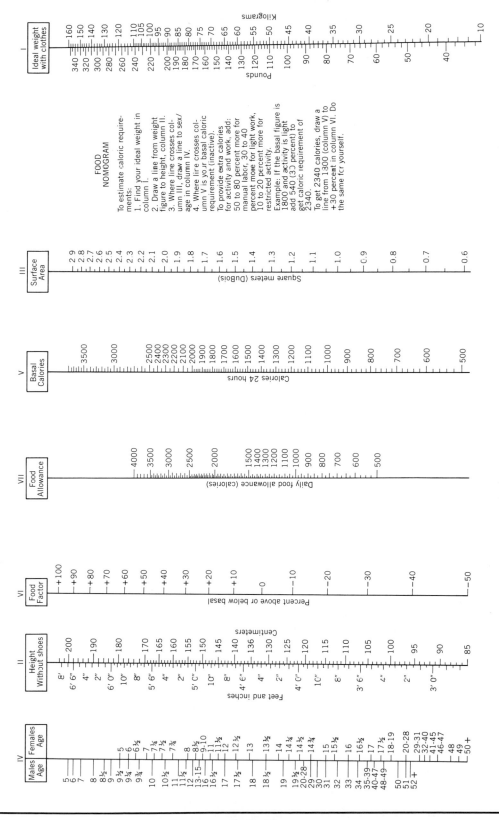

FOOD NOMOGRAM

To estimate caloric requirements:

1. Find your ideal weight in column I.
2. Draw a line from weight figure to height, column II.
3. Where line crosses column III, draw a line to sex/age in column IV.
4. Where line crosses column V is your basal caloric requirement (inactive).

To provide extra calories for activity and work, add:
50 to 80 percent more for manual labor, 30 to 40 percent more for light work, 10 to 20 percent more for restricted activity.

Example: If the basal figure is 1800 and activity is light add 540 (30 percent) to get caloric requirement of 2340.

To get 2340 calories, draw a line from 1800 (column V) to +30 percent in column VI. Do the same for yourself.

Name _____

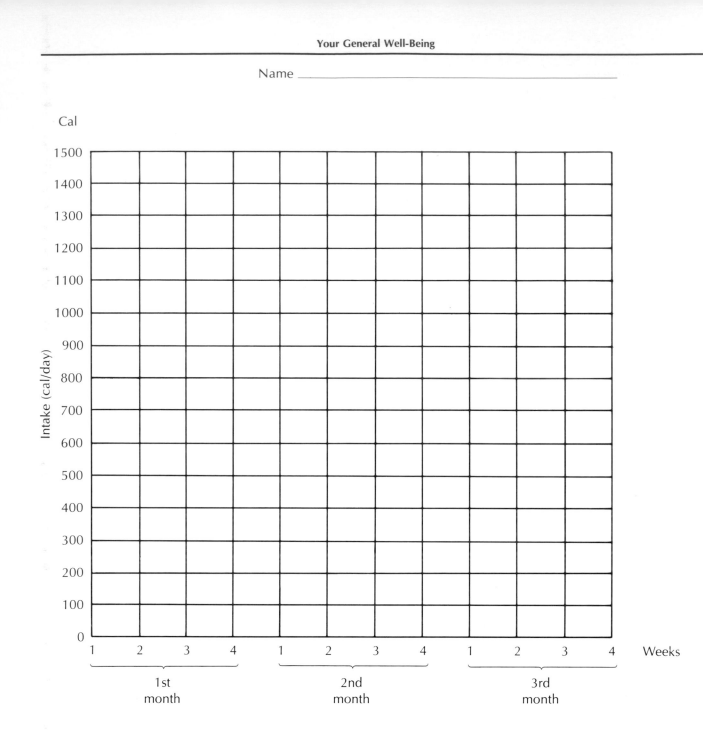

Graph 6.1

A comparison of intake and average weekly caloric intake of protein, fat, and CHO over a 3-month period. Legend: Protein . . . . , fat ---, and CHO ____ (use different colors).

Name _____

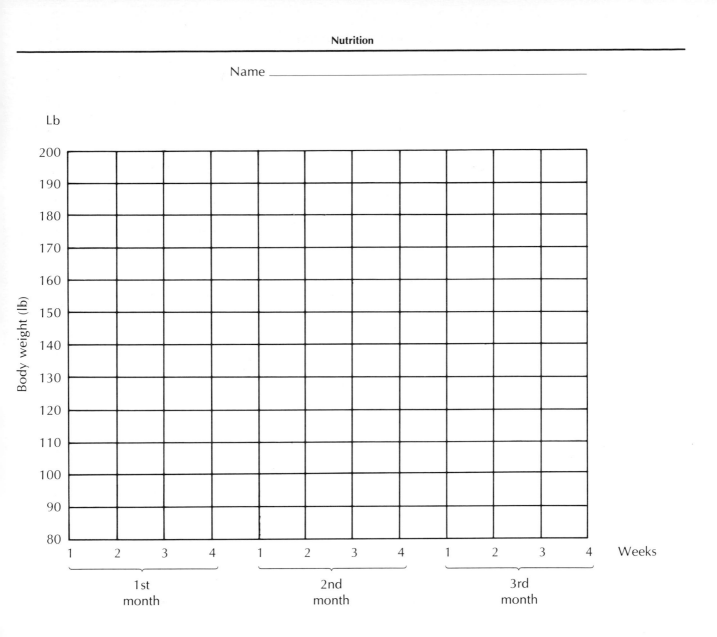

Lb

Body weight (lb)

200
190
180
170
160
150
140
130
120
110
100
90
80

1   2   3   4   1   2   3   4   1   2   3   4   Weeks

1st
month

2nd
month

3rd
month

Graph 6.2
Comparison of actual weekly and desirable body weight (lb) over a 3-month period. Legend: Actual
body weight – – –, desirable body weight ____ (use different colors).

Name _____

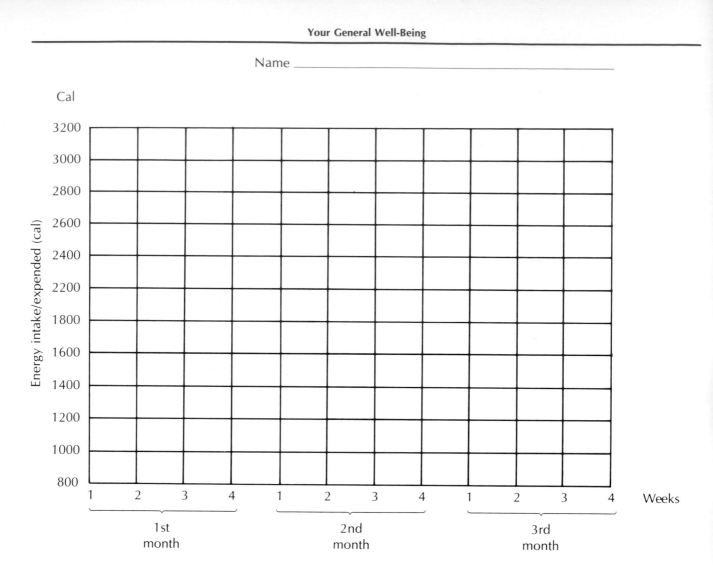

Graph 6.3

Comparison of average weekly caloric intake (food) and caloric expenditure (basal metabolism + activities) over a 3-month period. Legend: Caloric intake –––, caloric expenditure ___ (use different colors).

Table 6.15

Food Values of Junk and Snack Foods[a]

				Portion in Measure		
Food or Drink	Approximate Measure	Weight (grams)	Calories	Protein (gram)	CHO (gram)	Fats (gram)
Bacon, Canadian, fried crisp	1 strip (1 oz)	21	65	6.2	3.0	4.2
Beer	8 oz	240	114	1.4	10.6	8.9
Butter	1 pat		50			5.7
Cake (devil's food chocolate), no icing	2 × 3 × 2	45	165	2.2	23.4	7.7
Candy (milk chocolate bar)	15-cent bar	57	302	4.7	32.4	19.4
Cheese, cheddar (American)	1 oz	28	112	7.0	0.6	9.1
Cookies (1 oatmeal with raisins)	3 in. diameter	14	63	0.9	10.3	2.2
Crackers, cheese Tidbits	15 each	5	8	0.8	3.0	0.8

Food or Drink	Approximate Measure	Weight (grams)	Calories	Portion in Measure		
				Protein (gram)	CHO (gram)	Fats (gram)
Crackers, Ritz	1 each	3.3	17	0.24	2.0	0.87
Crackers, Saltine	1 each	3.2	14	0.29	2.32	0.38
French fries (potato)	10 pieces ½ × ½ × 2 in	50	137	2.1	18.0	6.6
Hot dog (frankfurter), 1 cooked	5½ × ¾ in.	50	124	7.0	1.0	10.0
Ham, fresh, cooked	3½ oz	100	306	32.9	0	18.3
Hamburger, 1 patty, medium cooked	3 × 1	85	224	21.8	0	14.5
Gravy (meat, brown)	1 tbl	18	41	0.3	2.0	3.5
Ice cream	⅙ qt	90	137	4.3	20.2	4.6
Jello (plain), 1 serving	5 per package	65	65	1.6	15.1	0
Lobster (boiled, broiled with 2 tbl butter)	¾ lb	334	308	20.0	0.8	24.9
Olives (green)	2 medium	10	13	0.2	0.4	1.4
Onion dip (with sour cream)	3 tsp	15	31	0.7	1.5	2.5
Oysters, cooked, fried, 1 serving	5–8 each	100	239	8.6	18.6	13.9
Pancakes (waffles), 1	4-in. diameter	45	104	3.2	15.3	3.2
Peanut butter	1 tbl (rounded)	20	115	5.2	4.2	9.6
Peanuts, roasted with skin	1 tbl	15	86	4.0	3.3	7.0
Pie, apple (9-in. pie)	⅙ pie	160	410	3.4	61.0	17.8
Pizza, baked, cheese		100	234	7.8	29.6	9.3
Popcorn, oil and salt	1 cup	18	82	1.8	10.7	3.9
Pork sausage (1 link)	3 × ½ in.	20	94	3.5	0	8.8
Potato chips, crisp (10 each)	2-in. diameter	20	113	1.1	10.0	8.0
Potato salad, parsley	½ cup	100	99	2.7	16.3	2.8
Pretzels, 3-ring	1 each	3.1	12	0.31	2.4	0.12
Pretzels, Veri-thin sticks	10 each	2.8	10	0.28	2.21	0.07
Puddings: Bread with raisins (1 serving)	¾ cup	165	314	8.9	47.8	10.0
Salad dressing, French	1 tbl	14	57	0.08	2.4	5.4
Sausage, bologna (1 slice)	4½ × ⅛ in.	30	66	4.4	1.1	4.8
Soft drinks, carbonated	6 oz	170	78	—	20.4	—
Sour cream	1 cup	240	454	6.7	7.7	43.2
Spaghetti, cooked, enriched	1 cup	146	216	7.3	44.0	0.7
Sugar, white, granular	1 tsp	8	32	0	8.0	0
Wine, port	3½ oz	100	158	0.2	14.0	—
Yogurt (whole milk)	1 cup	244	151	7.3	12.0	8.3

Source: Adapted with permission from C. F. Bowes and H. N. Church, *Food Values of Portions Commonly Used* New York: Lippincott, 1970.

[a] These are foods that have a high proportion of fats or are ''empty'' calorie foods low in vitamins and minerals but rich in CHO and fat calories.

Table 6.16
Foods to Avoid and Foods to Substitute

Avoid or Limit	Substitute — Eat More
Bacon, pork sausages	Lean meats
Beef hamburger	Lean meats (chicken, turkey, and fish)
Beef steaks	Lean meats, mushrooms
Beer, wine, alcohol	Water (8 glasses a day)
Bread	Soybean bread
Butter, margarine	Nonfat dry milk butter
Cakes, cookies, doughnuts, pies, pastries	More protein foods or fresh, green leafy vegetables
Candy bars, chocolate	Celery, fruit
Cheddar cheese	Lowfat cheese, nonfat cottage cheese
Coffee, tea	Decaffeinated coffee, 1–2 cups a day
Cream	Nonfat dry milk
Eggs, omelets	Limit to 1–2 eggs a week
Fish (batter and fried in oil)	Fish with no batter or oil
French fries, potato chips	Fresh, green leafy vegetables (lettuce, celery, cucumbers, onions, tomatoes, green peppers, cabbage, carrots, turnips)
Gelatin desserts	Fresh, green leafy vegetables
Gravies, sauces	
Ham, hot dogs	Lean meats or soybeans (flour)
Ice cream	Fresh fruit (oranges, apples, apricots, peaches, pears, bananas, grapefruit)
Lobster, crab	Fish low in cholesterol
Milk (whole)	Nonfat dry milk
Oils, lard (saturated)	Unsaturated vegetable oils
Olives	Fresh, green leafy vegetables
Pancakes, waffles	Substitute soybean flour
Peanuts	
Pizza	Soybean flour or beans, lean meat
Popcorn	Fresh, green leafy vegetables, or fresh fruit
Pretzels	Fresh fruit
Puddings (custards)	Fresh fruits
Salt	Cut down salting food on plate
Salad dressings	Use diet salad dressings
Sherberts	Fresh fruit
Soft drinks (sweetened)	Water, fresh fruits
Spaghetti and meat balls	Lean meats, soybeans
Syrups	
Yogurt (fruit flavored)	Nonfat cottage cheese

Note: Junk foods—Substitute with more tender loving care (TLC).
Nonfat salad dressing—5 calories per tablespoon: Combine 1/2 cup tomato juice, 2 tb lemon juice or vinegar, 1 tb finely chopped parsley, 1 tb chopped onion, salt, and pepper.

Where to Go for More Help

1. College student health services or center.
2. Local public health department.
3. Dietician at local hospital.
4. Reducing and weight-reduction clubs.

Diet Analysis

For a personalized computer–nutrient analysis of your diet, contact:

Dicalator
P.O. Box 3217
Olympic Station
Beverly Hills, Calif. 90212

Dietronics
c/o Hanson Research Corporation
P.O. Box 35
19727 Bahama Street
Northridge, Calif. 91324

Dietronics
P.O. Box 44244
Dallas, Tex. 75234

Pacific Research Systems
2222 Corinth Avenue
Los Angeles, Calif. 90064

Doctor's Data Inc. (hair and diet analysis)
P.O. Box 111
245 Roosevelt Road West Chicago, Ill. 60185

Mineral Lab Inc.
22455 Maple Court, Suite 301,
Hayward, Calif. 94541

To locate nutrition-oriented doctors in your state or area, write to one of these organizations:

Linus Pauling Institute of Science and Medicine
2700 Sand Hill Road
Menlo Park, Calif. 94025

International Academy of Preventive Medicine
Town and Country Professional Bldg.
Suite 200
10405 Town and Country Way
Houston, Tex. 77024

Rodale Press Incorporated
Emmaus, Penna. 18049

Further Readings

Burkitt, Denis P., "The link between low-fat diets and disease," *Human Nature,* December 1978, pp. 34–41.

Cheraskin, Emanuel, and William Ringsdorf, *Psychodietetics,* New York: Bantam Books, 1976.

Duffy, William, *Sugar Blues,* New York: Warner Books, 1976.

Eckholm, Erik, and Frank Record, "The Affluent Diet: A Worldwide Health Hazard," *The Futurist,* February 1977, pp. 32–42.

Lappe, Frances Moore, *Diet for a Small Planet,* New York: Ballantine Books, 1971.

Leonard, Jon N., J. L. Hofer, and N. Pritikin, *Live Longer Now,* New York: Grosset, 1977.

Passwater, Richard A., *Supernutrition,* New York: Pocket Books, 1976.

Williams, Roger J., *Nutrition Against Disease,* New York: Bantam Books, 1973.

PART C

Potential Behavior Problems

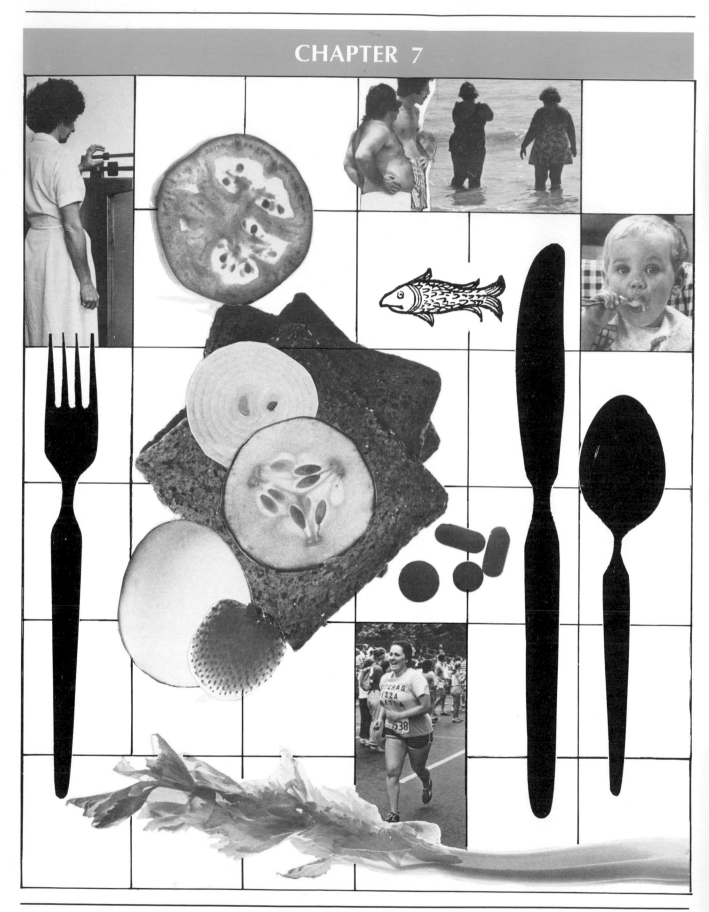

CHAPTER 7

WEIGHT CONTROL AND DIETING

Obesity and overweight have become the number one nutrition problem in the United States. It is estimated that 80 million American adults (about half the adult population) are overweight, with 10 million actually on weight-reducing diets (2). Obesity and overweight are found at all age levels although the proportion of obese adults increases with age. This statistic suggests that physical activity is an important factor in weight gain; as a person grows older, his or her activity level usually declines, and without a corresponding decrease in caloric intake, the person gains weight.

American women tend to add extra pounds at two periods of life: when they are pregnant and after menopause. Men gain extra weight between ages 25 and 40, and they gain weight faster after 40. Many of today's overweight adults were overweight children—close to a fifth of American children are overweight by the time they graduate from high school.

Obviously, being overweight is a major concern of a large proportion of Americans. They are pouring millions of dollars into diet clinics, fat farms, health spas, psychotherapy, exercise equipment, and diet foods in an effort to shed unwanted pounds. What caused them to get fat in the first place? Also, what's so bad about being overweight, anyway? Are fad methods of weight reduction of any value? What is the best way to lose weight and keep it off? These are the questions we will try to answer in this chapter.

☞ WHY DO I EAT? INVENTORY[1]

DIRECTIONS   Here are some statements made by people to describe what they get out of eating. How *often* do you feel this way about eating? Circle one number for each statement. *Important: answer every question.*

	Always	Frequently	Occa-sionally	Seldom	Never
A. I eat to keep myself from slowing down	5	4	3	2	1
B. Handling food is part of the enjoyment of eating	5	4	3	2	1
C. Eating is pleasant and relaxing	5	4	3	2	1
D. When I feel angry about something, I eat	5	4	3	2	1

	Always	Frequently	Occa-sionally	Seldom	Never
E. When I run out of my favorite foods I find it almost unbearable until I can get more	5	4	3	2	1
F. I eat automatically without even being aware of it	5	4	3	2	1
G. I eat to stimulate me, perk myself up	5	4	3	2	1
H. Part of the enjoyment of eating comes from the steps I take to prepare it	5	4	3	2	1
I. I find eating pleasurable	5	4	3	2	1
J. When I feel uncomfortable or upset about something, I eat	5	4	3	2	1
K. I am very much aware of the fact when I am not eating	5	4	3	2	1
L. I eat without realizing what I am doing	5	4	3	2	1
M. I eat to give me a "lift"	5	4	3	2	1
N. When I eat, part of the enjoyment is seeing, smelling, and tasting food	5	4	3	2	1
O. I want food most when I am comfortable and relaxed	5	4	3	2	1
P. When I feel "blue" or want to take my mind off cares and worries, I eat	5	4	3	2	1
Q. I get a real gnawing hunger for food when I haven't eaten for a while	5	4	3	2	1
R. I've found food in my mouth and didn't remember putting it there	5	4	3	2	1

[1] This inventory and interpretation is adapted from *Smoker's Self-testing Kit,* PHS Publication No. 1904, 1969, developed by Daniel Horn, Director of the National Clearinghouse for Smoking and Health of the Public Health Service and members of the Clearinghouse staff.

SCORING

1. Enter the numbers you have circled to the test questions in the following spaces, putting the number you circled to question A over line A, to question B over line B, and so on.

2. Total the three scores on each line to get your totals. For example, the sum of your scores over lines A, G, and M gives you your score on "Stimulation" — lines B, H, and N give you the score on "Handling," and so on.

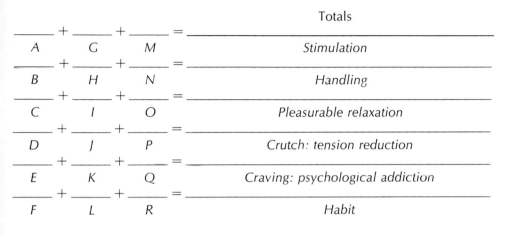

			Totals
_____ + _____ + _____ =			_____
A	G	M	*Stimulation*
_____ + _____ + _____ =			_____
B	H	N	*Handling*
_____ + _____ + _____ =			_____
C	I	O	*Pleasurable relaxation*
_____ + _____ + _____ =			_____
D	J	P	*Crutch: tension reduction*
_____ + _____ + _____ =			_____
E	K	Q	*Craving: psychological addiction*
_____ + _____ + _____ =			_____
F	L	R	*Habit*

Scores can vary from 3 to 15. Any score 11 and above is high; any score 7 and below is low.

INTERPRETATION

What kind of eater are you? What do you get out of eating? What does it do for you? This instrument is designed to provide you with a score on each of six factors that describe many people's eating patterns. Your eating may be well characterized by only one, or by a combination of factors. In any event, this inventory will help you identify why you eat other than to satisfy your hunger, and what kind of satisfaction you think you get from eating.

The six factors measured by this instrument describe one or another way of experiencing or managing certain kinds of feelings. Three of these feeling states represent the positive feelings people get from eating: (1) a sense of increased energy or stimulation; (2) the satisfaction of handling or manipulating things; and (3) the enhancing of pleasurable feelings by reducing the state of tension or feelings of anxiety, anger, and shame, for example. The fifth is a complex pattern of increasing and decreasing "craving" for eating that represents a psychological addiction to food. The sixth, habit, is eating that occurs in an absence of feeling — purely automatic eating.

A score of 11 or above on any factor indicates that this factor is an important source of satisfaction for you. The higher your score (15 is the highest), the more important a particular factor is in your eating and the more useful the discussion of that factor can be in your attempt to cut down on eating.

A few words of warning: If you cut down on eating, you may have to learn to get along without the extra satisfactions that food gives you. Either that, or you will have to find other acceptable ways of getting these satisfactions. In either case, you need to know just what you get out of eating before you can decide whether to forego the satisfactions or find another way to achieve them.

1. Stimulation. *If you score high or fairly high on this factor, it means that you are stimulated by food—you feel that it helps wake you up, organize your energies, and keep you going. If you try to give up eating, you may want a safe substitute: a brisk walk or modest exercise, for example, whenever you feel the urge to eat. Try chewing gum or eating celery or carrot sticks.*

2. Handling. *Handling things can be satisfying, but there are many ways to keep your hands busy without placing food into your mouth. Why not toy with a pen or pencil? Or try doodling. Or play with a coin, a piece of jewelry, or some activity other than eating like knitting, crocheting, painting, or working with handicrafts.*

3. Accentuation of Pleasure—Pleasurable Relaxation. *It is not always easy to find out whether you use food to feel good, that is, get honest pleasure out of eating (factor 3) or to keep from feeling bad (factor 4). Those who get pleasure out of eating often find that an honest consideration of the harmful effects of their habit is enough to help them quit. They substitute chewing gum, drinking fluids, or participating in social and physical activities. With these methods, they find they do not miss the excess food they are not eating.*

4. Reduction of Negative Feelings or "Crutch." *You may be using eating as a kind of crutch in moments of stress or discomfort, and on occasion it may work; food sometimes is used as a tranquilizer. But if you are an excessive eater who tries to handle severe personal problems by snacking many times a day, sooner or later you will discover that foods do not help you deal with these problems effectively.*

When it comes to cutting down, you may find it easy to do so when everything is going well, but you may be tempted to start excessive eating again in a time of crisis. Again, physical exertion, chewing gum, drinking fluids, or engaging in social activity may serve as useful substitutes for eating, even in times of tension. Your choice of a substitute depends on whether the activity will achieve the same effect without having any appreciable risk.

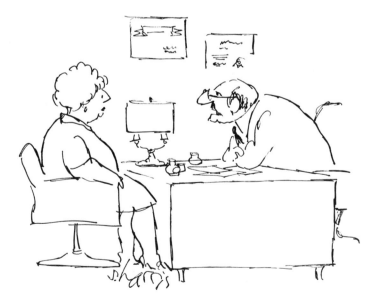

"IT'S PARTLY GLANDULAR AND PARTLY 8,500 CALORIES PER DAY."

5. "Craving" or Psychological Addiction. *Stopping excessive eating will be difficult for you if you score high on the "Psychological Addiction" factor. Probably, for you, the craving for food will continue to build up as your plate begins to empty. To be successful in changing your desire for excess food, you must go "cold turkey"— that is, cut off extra helpings completely.*

You will have to isolate yourself from your favorite rich foods, second helpings, and snacks until the craving is gone. Giving up excess food intake may be so difficult and cause such discomfort that once you do cut down, you will find it easy to resist the temptation to go back to excessive eating.

6. Habit. *If you are a habit eater, you probably are not getting much satisfaction from your food. You probably just eat without realizing you are doing so. You may find it easy to control caloric intake if you can break the habit patterns you have built up. Cutting down gradually may be quite effective if there is a change in the way the food is served and the conditions under which you eat. An example of this might be serving the food from the pots on the stove rather than from bowls on the table. This will make piling on "seconds" a conscious effort. The key to success is becoming aware of all the calories you eat. This can be done by asking yourself, "Do I really want this food?" You may be surprised at how often you do not really want the extra calories.*

SUMMARY

If you do not score high on any of the six factors, chances are that you are not an excessive eater. If so, cutting down calories should be easy.

If you score high on several categories, you apparently get several kinds of satisfaction from eating and will have to find several solutions. Certain combinations of score may indicate that reducing food intake will be especially difficult. Those who score high on both factor 4 and factor 5, "Reduction of Negative Feelings and Craving," may have a hard time cutting down caloric intake. However, there are ways to do it; many excessive eaters represented by this combination have been able to cut down on caloric intake.

Others who score high on factors 4 and 5 may find it useful to change their patterns of eating and cut down at the same time. They can try to eat foods that are lower in calories, such as carrots, fresh fruits, Ry-Crisp, or to substitute exercise and other physical activities for eating. After several months of trying this solution, they may find it easier to develop a habit pattern of low-calorie intake.

You must make a decision to cut down caloric intake either by (1) substituting appropriate volumes of less fattening foods for the high-calorie foods currently in your diet, or (2) reducing or eliminating excess calorie food (like junk foods) from your diet without the substitution of low-calorie foods.

HOW DO YOU KNOW IF YOU'RE FAT?

The standard practice for finding your ideal weight is to refer to a height-weight chart. The basic assumption is that this ideal weight, as related to height, is a good index of both body fat and health. In general, this assumption is useful, which is why we have included such height-weight tables here (Table 7.1). However, there are some definite problems involved in relying on these tables. The height-weight tables in general use today were developed by life-insurance companies and were based on the heights and weights of long-lived policyholders. Weight was measured with clothes on, and height with shoes on (6). Thus the tables were based on a nonrepresentative sample of the population, and they involved nonrepresentative conditions (most people

Table 7.1

Desirable Weights for Men and Women: Weight in Pounds According to Frame (Indoor Clothing)

Men of Ages 25 and Over (with shoes on: 1-inch heels)

Height			Small Frame		Medium Frame		Large Frame	
ft	in	cm	lb	kg	lb	kg	lb	kg
5	2	157.5	112–120	50.8–54.4	118–129	53.5–58.8	126–141	57.2–64.0
5	3	160.0	115–123	52.2–55.8	121–133	54.9–60.3	129–144	58.5–65.3
5	4	162.6	118–126	53.5–57.2	124–136	56.2–61.7	132–148	59.9–67.1
5	5	165.1	121–129	54.9–58.5	127–139	57.6–63.1	135–152	61.2–69.0
5	6	167.6	124–133	56.2–60.3	130–143	59.0–64.9	138–156	62.6–70.8
5	7	170.2	128–137	58.1–62.1	134–147	60.8–66.7	142–161	64.4–73.0
5	8	172.7	132–141	59.9–64.0	138–152	62.6–69.0	147–166	66.7–75.3
5	9	175.3	136–145	61.7–65.8	142–156	64.4–70.3	151–170	68.5–77.1
5	10	177.8	140–150	63.5–68.1	146–160	66.2–72.6	155–174	70.3–78.9
5	11	180.3	144–154	65.3–69.9	150–165	68.1–74.9	159–179	72.1–81.2
6	0	182.9	148–158	67.1–71.7	154–170	69.9–77.1	164–184	74.4–83.5
6	1	185.4	152–162	69.0–73.5	158–175	71.7–79.4	168–189	76.2–85.8
6	2	188.0	156–167	70.8–75.8	162–180	73.5–81.7	173–194	78.5–88.0
6	3	190.5	160–171	72.6–77.6	167–185	75.3–83.9	178–199	80.8–90.3
6	4	193.0	164–175	74.4–79.4	172–190	78.0–86.2	182–204	82.6–92.6

Women of Ages 25 and Over (with shoes on: 2-inch heels)[a]

Height			Small Frame		Medium Frame		Large Frame	
ft	in	cm	lb	kg	lb	kg	lb	kg
4	10	147.3	92–98	41.7–44.4	96–107	43.5–48.5	104–119	47.2–54.0
4	11	149.8	94–101	42.6–45.8	98–101	44.4–49.9	106–122	48.1–55.3
5	0	152.4	96–104	45.3–47.2	101–113	45.8–51.3	109–125	49.4–56.7
5	1	154.9	99–107	44.9–48.5	104–116	47.2–52.6	112–128	50.8–58.1
5	2	157.5	102–110	46.3–49.9	107–119	48.5–54.0	115–131	52.2–59.4
5	3	160.0	105–113	47.6–51.3	110–122	49.9–55.3	118–134	53.5–60.8
5	4	162.6	108–116	49.0–52.6	113–126	51.3–57.2	121–138	54.9–62.6
5	5	165.1	111–119	50.3–54.0	116–130	52.6–59.0	125–142	56.7–64.4
5	6	167.6	114–123	51.7–55.8	120–135	54.4–61.2	129–146	58.5–66.2
5	7	170.2	118–127	53.5–57.6	124–139	56.2–63.1	133–150	60.3–68.1
5	8	172.7	122–131	54.9–59.4	128–143	58.1–64.9	137–154	62.1–69.9
5	9	175.3	126–135	57.2–61.2	132–147	59.9–66.7	141–158	64.0–71.7
5	10	177.8	130–140	59.0–63.3	136–151	61.7–68.5	145–163	65.8–74.0
5	11	180.3	134–144	60.8–65.3	140–155	63.5–70.3	149–168	67.6–76.2
6	0	182.9	138–148	62.6–67.1	144–159	65.3–72.1	153–173	69.4–78.5

[a] For women between 18 and 25, subtract 1 pound for each year under 25.
Source: Prepared from the Metropolitan Life Insurance Company data, derived primarily from data of the Build and Blood Pressure Study, 1959, Society of Actuaries.

weigh themselves nude). According to these tables, a muscular, well-built athlete is overweight, while a chubby, sedentary secretary may be "just right."

Another way to find out whether your present body weight is ideal or desirable is to use the nomogram in Figure 7.1. It classifies you as being either overweight,

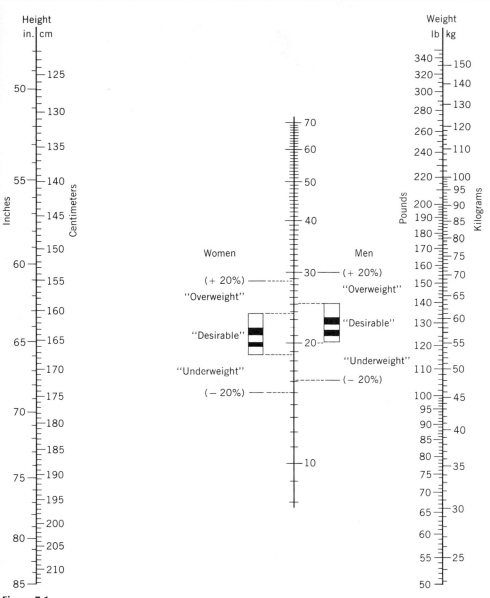

Figure 7.1

Nomograph to classify your body weight as desirable, overweight or underweight from your height and present weight. Nomograph for body mass index (kg/m²). The ratio weight/height² is read from the central scale. The ranges suggested as "desirable" are from life insurance data. (With permission from A. E. Thomas, D. A. McKay, and M. B. Cutlip *American Journal of Clinical Nutrition,* 29:302, 304, 1976.)

underweight, or of desirable body weight. The most accurate method of determining healthy weight is to carefully assess body fat. The oldest and easiest method of assessing body fat is to look at your nude body in the mirror. Since about half of your body fat is stored near the skin surface, it should be noticeable if you have too much of it.

There are a number of more scientific methods used to measure body fatness than by just looking at yourself in the mirror. The simplest and most useful is the *skinfold test.* This test can be done at any site on the body where subcutaneous fat tends to collect: upper arm at the triceps area, middle of the back of the shoulder blade, midchest, waistline, or back of the calf.

Skinfold calipers should be used for accurate measurement (see Figure 7.2). When calipers are not avail-

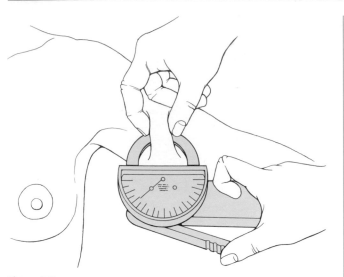

Figure 7.2
The use of fat calipers for skinfold measures.

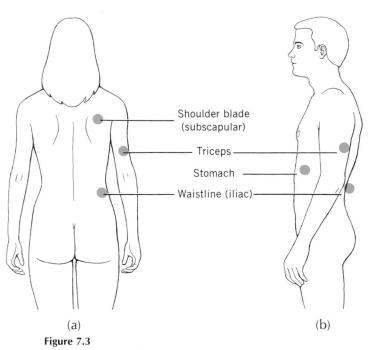

Shoulder blade (subscapular)

Triceps

Stomach

Waistline (iliac)

(a)

(b)

Figure 7.3
Locations of standard sites to measure body fat. (a) Back view of body sites where fat (dotted areas) is stored and location of shoulder blade, triceps, and waistline sites for the pinch test; (b) Side view of body sites for the pinch test.

Table 7.2
Body Fat Norms.[a] This chart classified college-aged men and women

Classification	Women (Fat%)	Men (Fat%)
Very low fat: skinny	14.0–16.9	7.0–9.9
Low fat: trim	17.0–19.9	10.0–12.9
Average fat: normal[b]	20.0–23.9	13.0–16.9
Above normal fat: plump	24.0–26.9	17.0–19.9
Very high fat: fat	27.0–29.9	20.0–24.9
Obese: overfat	30.0 and higher	25.0 and higher

[a] Based on the Sloan formulas for young adult women and men.
[b] Refers to the average for the group that was measured.
Source: With permission from A. W. Sloan, *Journal of Applied Physiology* 23:311–315, 1967.

the shoulder blade (subscapula) and thigh in men, and the triceps (back of arm) and suprailiac (waistline) in women into percent of body fat and body density.

In general, if the measurement of skinfold on any part of the body is greater than 1 inch, you are probably overweight and fat. Table 7.2 classifies college-aged men and women according to body fat.

WHAT IS WRONG WITH BEING FAT?

Fat people are often characterized as jolly, easy-going individuals who get a lot of enjoyment out of life. If they are happy, why should they have to lose weight? Well, the sad fact of it is that most obese people are high health risks. Obesity is a real health hazard. Fat people are greater insurance risks than people of normal weight because they simply do not live as long. Overweight people have a high risk of death from cardiovascular diseases and from ailments of the kidneys, liver, and gall bladder (see Figure 7.5). Fat people are more likely to get cancer, to have diabetes, and to be involved in accidents (6). Furthermore, overweight pregnant women have more complications during delivery and are more likely to deliver a stillborn baby.

Obesity damages more than physical health. The negative self-image generated by fatness can cause numerous psychological problems. Fat children are ridiculed by their playmates, and fat girls have lower chances of getting married. Fat people tend to be discriminated against in employment and in other social situations.

The extra burden of fat on the body also hampers the individual's general feeling of well-being. People who have lost excess weight often describe their fat life as one of lethargy and fatigue; without that weight they find themselves with energy to spare.

able, you can measure the thickness of your skin by the *pinch test.* Locate the triceps muscle by referring to Figure 7.3. Pinch the skin gently between thumb and forefinger and measure the skin thickness. Take the average of three measurements. You can use the nomogram to predict the amount of fat in your body by referring to Figure 7.4. The nomogram converts skinfold thickness of

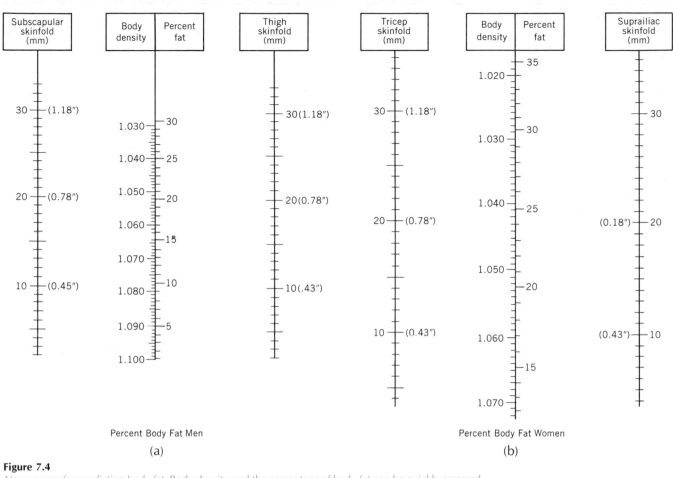

Figure 7.4

Nomograms for predicting body fat. Body density and the percentage of body fat can be quickly assessed for men and women from the graphs. A straight line joining your skinfold values will intersect the corresponding values for body density and the percentage of fat. The nomogram converts skinfold to percent body fat and body density. With permission from (a) A. W. Sloan, *Journal of Applied Physiology,* 23: 311–315, 1967, and J. F. Brozek, et al., *Annals of New York Academy of Science,* 101:113–140, 1963. Permission granted by the New York Academy of Sciences. (b) A. W. Sloan, et al. *Journal of Applied Physiology* 17:967, 1962, and J. F. Brozek, et al., *Annals of the New York Academy of Science* 101:113, 1963.

Thus there are lots of reasons why being overweight is harmful—physically, psychologically, and socially. But how do people get to be overweight in the first place? Is overweight unavoidable for most people or can it be prevented?

WHAT CAUSES OBESITY?

Basically, obesity is caused by taking in too many calories. It does not take much to become obese over a period of time. For example, eating a piece of pie every day (300 calories) above normal caloric needs of the body will put on 30 pounds in 1 year, or 90 pounds in 3 years. Other 300-calorie foods that can do the same are a chocolate brownie, 2 slices of pizza, 2 cinnamon rolls, or 15 pretzels. Even one extra Coke a day (100 calories) will add 10 pounds in a year.

Of course, the reason for obesity is much more complex than just "too many calories." Some people seem to eat all the time and never gain weight, while others are constantly dieting but continue to stay fat. It turns out that there are a number of causes of obesity, and they all interact. For example, some types of obesity are genetic or are caused by disorders in the nervous system or endocrine system. However, it turns out that these physiological problems are the source of only a very small percentage of obesity cases.

Some physical factors do seem to *predispose* one to obesity (see Figure 7.6). According to one theory, fat people have more fat cells in their body than nonobese people. Although one is born with a specific number of

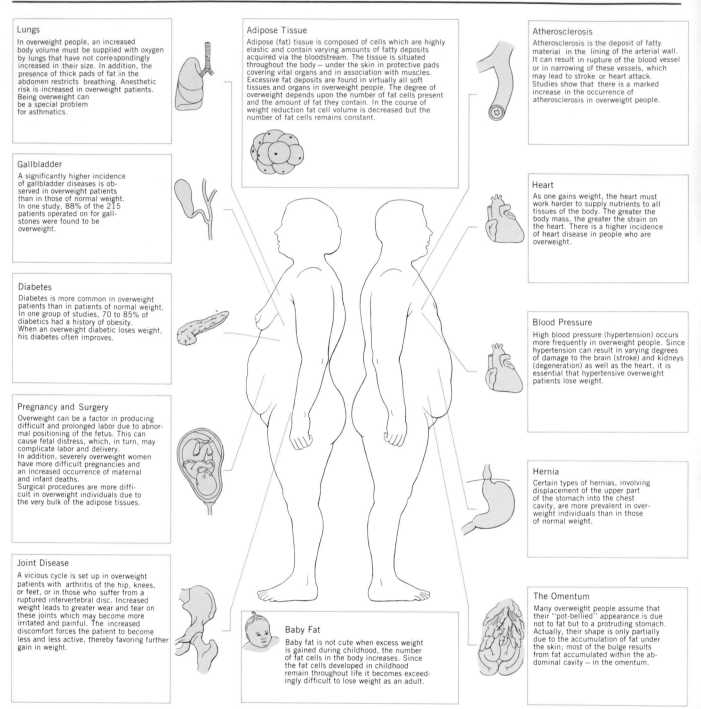

Lungs

In overweight people, an increased body volume must be supplied with oxygen by lungs that have not correspondingly increased in their size. In addition, the presence of thick pads of fat in the abdomen restricts breathing. Anesthetic risk is increased in overweight patients. Being overweight can be a special problem for asthmatics.

Gallbladder

A significantly higher incidence of gallbladder diseases is observed in overweight patients than in those of normal weight. In one study, 88% of the 215 patients operated on for gallstones were found to be overweight.

Diabetes

Diabetes is more common in overweight patients than in patients of normal weight. In one group of studies, 70 to 85% of diabetics had a history of obesity. When an overweight diabetic loses weight, his diabetes often improves.

Pregnancy and Surgery

Overweight can be a factor in producing difficult and prolonged labor due to abnormal positioning of the fetus. This can cause fetal distress, which, in turn, may complicate labor and delivery. In addition, severely overweight women have more difficult pregnancies and an increased occurrence of maternal and infant deaths. Surgical procedures are more difficult in overweight individuals due to the very bulk of the adipose tissues.

Joint Disease

A vicious cycle is set up in overweight patients with arthritis of the hip, knees, or feet, or in those who suffer from a ruptured intervertebral disc. Increased weight leads to greater wear and tear on these joints which may become more irritated and painful. The increased discomfort forces the patient to become less and less active, thereby favoring further gain in weight.

Adipose Tissue

Adipose (fat) tissue is composed of cells which are highly elastic and contain varying amounts of fatty deposits acquired via the bloodstream. The tissue is situated throughout the body — under the skin in protective pads covering vital organs and in association with muscles. Excessive fat deposits are found in virtually all soft tissues and organs in overweight people. The degree of overweight depends upon the number of fat cells present and the amount of fat they contain. In the course of weight reduction fat cell volume is decreased but the number of fat cells remains constant.

Baby Fat

Baby fat is not cute when excess weight is gained during childhood, the number of fat cells in the body increases. Since the fat cells developed in childhood remain throughout life it becomes exceedingly difficult to lose weight as an adult.

Atherosclerosis

Atherosclerosis is the deposit of fatty material in the lining of the arterial wall. It can result in rupture of the blood vessel or in narrowing of these vessels, which may lead to stroke or heart attack. Studies show that there is a marked increase in the occurrence of atherosclerosis in overweight people.

Heart

As one gains weight, the heart must work harder to supply nutrients to all tissues of the body. The greater the body mass, the greater the strain on the heart. There is a higher incidence of heart disease in people who are overweight.

Blood Pressure

High blood pressure (hypertension) occurs more frequently in overweight people. Since hypertension can result in varying degrees of damage to the brain (stroke) and kidneys (degeneration) as well as the heart, it is essential that hypertensive overweight patients lose weight.

Hernia

Certain types of hernias, involving displacement of the upper part of the stomach into the chest cavity, are more prevalent in overweight individuals than in those of normal weight.

The Omentum

Many overweight people assume that their "pot-bellied" appearance is due not to fat but to a protruding stomach. Actually, their shape is only partially due to the accumulation of fat under the skin; most of the bulge results from fat accumulated within the abdominal cavity — in the omentum.

Figure 7.5

Fat sites in the body and health risks.

fat cells, the infant body is very sensitive to overfeeding and eating the wrong kinds of foods. Babies who are overfed up to 6 months of age tend to develop more fat cells. Once somatic cells become fat cells, they remain as fat cells for life (see Figure 7.7). A person gains weight by increasing the size of his fat cells and lose weight by shrinking the size of his fat cells. This is one explanation of why fat babies usually grow up to be fat adults.

Another theory is that obese people have a malfunctioning "appestat," the control center in the hypothalamus of the brain that regulates food intake (see Figure 7.8). This center is responsible for letting you know when you need food and for turning off your desire to eat once you have taken in sufficient fuel for the body's needs. If the appestate is "set too high," the body takes in more fuel than it needs, and the excess is stored in fat.

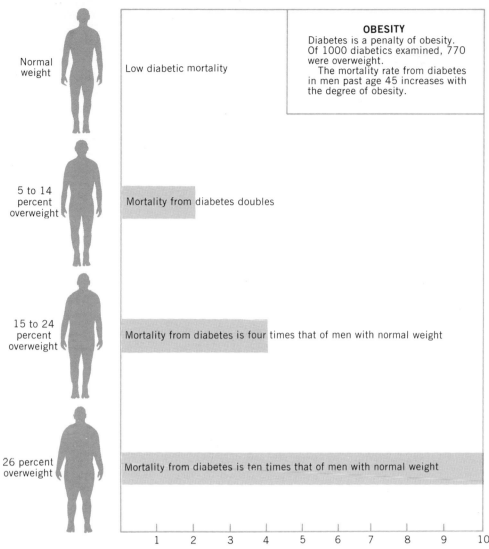

Normal weight — Low diabetic mortality

OBESITY
Diabetes is a penalty of obesity.
Of 1000 diabetics examined, 770
were overweight.
The mortality rate from diabetes
in men past age 45 increases with
the degree of obesity.

5 to 14 percent overweight — Mortality from diabetes doubles

15 to 24 percent overweight — Mortality from diabetes is four times that of men with normal weight

26 percent overweight — Mortality from diabetes is ten times that of men with normal weight

1 2 3 4 5 6 7 8 9 10

Figure 7.6
There is a distinct relationship between obesity and death from diabetes. Obese persons have a high predisposition to diabetes. (Courtesy of the Eli Lilly and Co.)

Sugar, soft drinks, alcohol, nicotine, and other chemicals are suspected of disrupting a normal functioning appestat—sending it out of control. When this happens, the affected person usually is unable to control his or her weight.

Another approach to the causes of obesity is based on the observation that obese people eat in response to food cues—to seeing, smelling, or thinking about food—whereas, nonobese people eat in response to internal cues of hunger. Fat people eat until the food supply is gone, whereas normal-weight people eat until their hunger is satisfied. It has, therefore, been suggested that there is a fundamental psychophysiological difference between obese and nonobese people.

Many psychologists have suggested that obesity is often the result of emotional problems. For some people,

food is a substitute for love or a reward for being good. Many react to stress by eating or nibbling. Some people hide behind fatness saying that they could accomplish great things in their lives if they were not fat; staying fat protects them from having to attempt those accomplishments. People who overeat often use food as a way to reduce tension when angry or as a means of comfort when depressed. There are probably as many emotional problems related to overeating as there are overweight people (see Figure 7.9).

There are essentially three approaches to weight loss. First, you can increase energy expenditure (exercising) and enjoy eating. Second, you can cut down food intake (calories) and be miserable because you cannot eat. Third, you can combine both. If you can get your exercise level up to a minimum of 40 to 50 minutes a day,

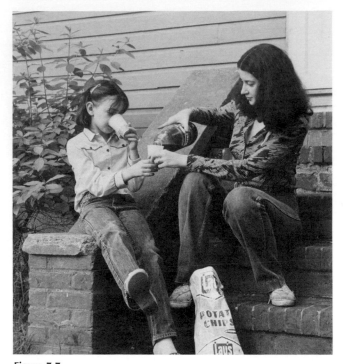

Figure 7.7
Eating habits begun in childhood are partially responsible for weight problems in adult years.

four times a week, then you can ease up on counting calories and dieting. Research (5) suggests that inactivity is of greater importance than excessive food intake in the development of obesity in adolescents. Studies of obese children and adults have revealed that most of them ate about as much as individuals of normal weight but that they were much less active physically (3:562). Thus they were overeating only in terms of their needs. Those who were more active had their appetites suppressed.

THE AMERICAN WAY OF DIETING

Millions of Americans want to lose weight, but they want to do it without sacrificing their favorite fattening foods, without major effort, and as painlessly as possible (see Figure 7.10). The plain fact of it is, it is fun to eat and easy to gain weight but difficult to lose it and keep it off. Less than 20 percent of those trying to lose weight have any long-term success with dieting (5).

Fat people have tried just about everything to shed those unsightly and unhealthy pounds and inches: diet pills, hormone shots, fat farms, hypnosis, group therapy, acupuncture, health clubs, and even having their jaws wired shut (see Figure 7.11). Some of these approaches

are plain quackery (such as those belts that are supposed to take off inches quickly); some are dangerous; and some are useful if followed carefully and correctly.

By far, the most popular approach to weight loss is to follow a diet plan, usually one proposed by a doctor in a best-selling paperback book. These diets range from "eat all you want and still lose weight" approaches to total fasting. How useful are these diets? Are any of them dangerous? Here is a brief rundown on the most popular diets, discussing their advantages and disadvantages (2).

Low-Calorie Diets

Almost all self-styled diet experts will admit that the key to losing weight is to eat less, cut down on calories, and exercise more. *Calories* are the units of energy burned by the body. Proteins and carbohydrates contain 120 calories per ounce; fats contain 270 calories per ounce. When the calories in food are not burned, they are stored as fat. One pound of fat is equal to 3500 calories. That means that you have to eat 3500 calories less than you body normally needs in order to lose 1 pound of fat. So, for example, if your body needs 2000 calories a day, you can lose a pound in 1 week by eating only 1500 calories a day (500 less a day times 7 equals 3500 calories).

The number of calories needed each day varies from person to person, depending on one's body weight, metabolism, and activity level. In general, a person with a moderately active life needs 16 calories per pound per day. Thus a moderately active 125-pound woman would need about 2000 calories a day, while a similarly active 150-pound man would need about 2400. Eating more than that amount of calories will produce weight gain; eating fewer will bring weight loss.

Most diets are designed to lower the total calorie intake in some way. Here we are focusing on those diets in which calories are specifically counted. The goal of the basic low-calorie diet is to keep a balance of nutrients and a varied diet while reducing the overall caloric intake. Commercially available low-calorie diets include the Prudent Diet, the New York Health Department Diet, the American Diabetic Association Diet, a number of computer diets, and the Astronaut's Diet (many go by this name, but only one was actually developed for the U.S. astronauts).

The advantages of the low-calorie diet are that it is based on sound nutritional principles, it is healthy, it is tailored to the individual, and it encourages the dieter to become aware of the caloric content of foods. The main disadvantage is that it depends totally on will power—there are no gimmicks to inspire or motivate the dieter.

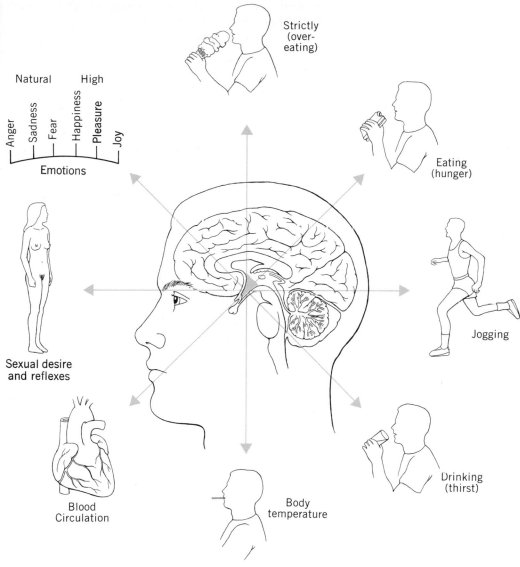

Strictly
(over-
eating)

Eating
(hunger)

Natural   High

Anger Sadness Fear Happiness Pleasure Joy

Emotions

Jogging

Sexual desire
and reflexes

Drinking
(thirst)

Blood
Circulation

Body
temperature

Figure 7.8
Location of the hypothalamus, which contains the "appestat," or control center for the many body functions.

Low-Carbohydrate Diets

People on low-carbohydrate diets count carbohydrate grams instead of calories. They eat as much of other foods as they normally would, but they cut down on sugars and starches. Carbohydrate counters limit themselves to 50 to 60 carbohydrate grams a day. Many gram-counter books are available to help the dieter determine the carbohydrate content of various foods.

The main advantage of this diet is that it is easy to handle. The dieter ends up eating primarily protein foods, which leave him or her with a full feeling. Weight loss is rapid at first and inspires the person to stay on the diet. Unfortunately, most of the initial weight loss is water weight (carbohydrates retain salt and water in the body). After a low-carbohydrate diet, people tend to jump back up to their previous weight level.

High-Protein Diets

The best-known, high-protein diet is the Stillman Quick Weight Loss Diet (2) and most other high-protein diets are patterned after it. This diet is based on the idea that the body spends more energy metabolizing proteins than it does on the other food elements. Dr. Stillman says you can eat all you want of meats, poultry, fish,

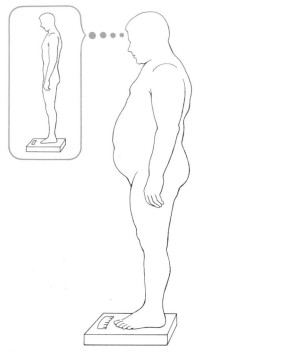

Figure 7.9
Think less. Losing weight requires a good attitude toward food, eating, exercise, and yourself.

seafoods, and eggs, but you must severely limit your fats and carbohydrates. This diet is also called the water diet, since it calls for eight glasses of water a day. All protein-high diets, including nonweight reduction, necessitate a large amount of water.

There are several criticisms of this diet. First of all, the theory it is based on may not be valid—it has not been proved. Second, the diet is lacking in many important nutrients. Third, high-protein consumption coupled with a lack of carbohydrates produces major metabolic changes in the body, including a condition called *ketosis*. This condition is characterized by the presence of *ketones,* by-products of fat metabolism, in the urine. Ketosis produces bad breath, frequent urination, and can be harmful to the liver and kidneys (the eight glasses of water are included to help minimize these effects). It has also been shown that this diet increases the blood cholesterol level and that it produces fatigue in the dieter. Dieters have also criticized it for being monotonous.

The main advantage of a high-protein diet is that it does provide rapid weight loss, although it, too, is subject to the bounce-back effect when the dieter returns to regular eating habits.

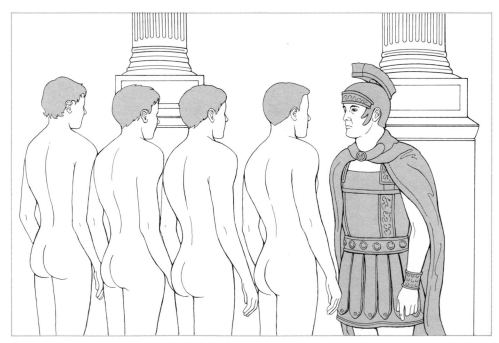

Figure 7.10
Social pressure is usually needed to motivate people to stay trim. As an example, Spartan young men lined up naked every month for inspection to detect corpulency. The Spartans were so concerned with good physique that fat citizens were assigned special exercises.

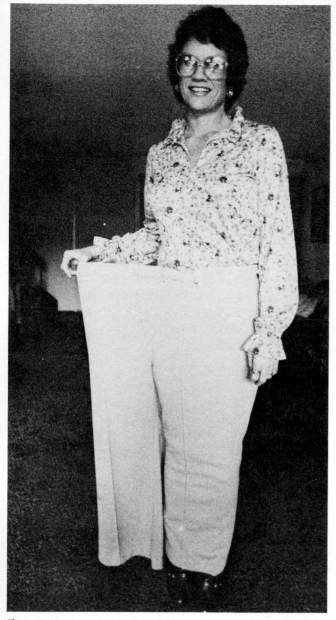

Figure 7.11
Solving obesity by an intestinal bypass operation. This patient lost 200 pounds—from 350 to 150 pounds.

High-Fat Diets

The most famous high-fat diet was popularized in *Dr. Atkins' Diet Revolution* (1). It is based on the idea that high-fat intake stimulates fat metabolism so greatly that both stored fat and dietary fat are burned. Atkins believes that fat people are victims of "carbohydrate poisoning," so his diet excludes all carbohydrates. Like the high-protein diet, this diet produces ketosis. But, Dr. Atkins considers ketosis to be a positive condition because it shows that fats are being burned.

The Atkins high-fat diet has been severely criticized by doctors, nutritionists, and other diet experts. They say that the diet (1) is highly unscientific, (2) is nutritionally deficient, (3) promotes heart disease, (4) produces fatigue and low blood pressure, and (5) is harmful to the kidneys. They definitely dispute the idea that ketosis is a beneficial condition. All in all, the high-fat diet can be very dangerous and should be tried only for short periods and only by people who have received their doctor's approval.

One-Food Diets

Many fad diets are centered around one food. There is the rice diet, the banana and milk diet, the grapefruit diet, the seafood diet, the yogurt diet, and many others. These diets can be valuable if they get the dieter to make important changes in his or her eating habits, and if the individual actually does lose weight. However, they are lopsided nutritionally and should be followed for only short periods of time.

Fasting

In recent years fasting has become a popular method for quick weight loss. Fasting involves total abstinence from food, existing primarily on clear liquids. Ex-Harvard nutritionist, Jean Mayer, (6), has pointed out that there are a number of dangers in this practice. Not only is the body being deprived of its necessary fuel, but fasting actually causes the body to be depleted of essential minerals. According to Mayer, the body does not immediately draw on stored fats, but instead turns first to the protein in muscle tissue to satisfy energy needs. Fasting also produces ketosis, fluid loss, light-headedness, and general weakness. Long periods of fasting are definitely dangerous to health. Short fasts should be done only under a doctor's supervision.

Other Diets

One commercially available approach to dieting is formula diets, such as Metrecal and Sego. These formulas contain essential nutrients for a balanced diet. Used in combination with a low-calorie diet, such formulas can be quite helpful to the dieter.

Many overweight persons turned to liquid protein diets in the 70s. Most of these diets attempt to provide a nutrient balance.

Not so helpful is the so-called Zen macrobiotic diet. Not actually related to Zen Buddhism, this diet proceeds in a series of six stages, with the diet at the final stage consisting of only brown rice and tea. This diet is actually a form of starvation, and in fact, several people have reportedly died from it.

In summary, all diets have similar drawbacks. They can be lacking in essential nutrients, so the dieter should be sure to take supplements. Many diets reduce fiber intake, which can result in intestinal upsets. Any major change in diet can upset the body's metabolism and digestive system; the dieter should be prepared to abandon a diet that creates major physical discomfort or that the body does not seem willing to adapt to. Some diets can be expensive—a factor most of us have to consider. Only nutritionally balanced diets should be followed for more than a 2-week period. Finally, any diet can be effective if it is followed carefully, and if it produces long-term positive changes in one's eating habits. Most weight-reducing programs fail because they neglect or overlook to change eating habits, to stabilize the new dietary habits, and to help the overweight person to fulfill his or her emotional needs. Most weight-reducing programs are initiated at the wrong time in a person's life—when the person is under considerable emotional stress. Such poor timing makes it more difficult to stabilize new eating habits and to keep weight off permanently.

BEHAVIOR MODIFICATION TECHNIQUES: DESIGN YOUR OWN WEIGHT LOSS PROGRAM

You are the best person to decide how you should go about losing weight. You have to assess your own attitudes toward food, your eating habits, your likes and dislikes, and other factors that will influence your success at undertaking a weight loss program. But, before starting any program, you should get a thorough medical examination. There are many conditions that can be aggravated by a major change in your diet, and you may find out that you are allergic to certain foods. Your doctor can tell you whether you have any physical conditions that will affect your diet plans.

In order to design your weight reduction program you will first need to decide how much weight you want to lose. Next determine how long you want to take to shed those pounds (it is healthiest to lose about 1 to 2 pounds a week—and you are then more likely to keep them off). You can now calculate how many calories you must cut from your diet in order to reach this goal.

Say, for example, that you weigh 145 and your ideal weight is 125. You decide you want to lose those 20 pounds in 10 weeks. To lose 2 pounds a week, you will have to cut 1000 calories from your diet each day. Thus, if the normal number of calories burned by a 125-pound person is 2000, you will have to go on a 1000-calorie diet.

Now, 1000 calories is a very limited diet. But you can increase your daily intake of calories and still lose weight if you add one more component to your weight-reduction program: exercise. For example, 30 minutes of jogging, bicycling, or swimming each day will burn up 400 calories a day. Exercise does more than burn calories: it reduces your appetite and improves your emotional outlook by reducing stress and tension. Furthermore, exercise causes the body to mobilize its stored fat. (Exercise programs were described in more detail in Chapter 5.)

Last, but not least, respond to the "Why Do I Eat? Inventory." It will help you gain an insight into the psychological satisfactions you receive from eating. These insights could help you change your eating patterns, thereby reducing your caloric intake.

Guidelines for Dieting and Weight Loss

Here are some helpful hints for dieting, losing weight, and stabilizing your body weight:

1. *Get a thorough medical examination* (this should include biochemical tests and physical examination).
2. *Get a nutritional food-eating habits analysis.*
3. *Stop smoking*—smoking impairs the satiety (braking) mechanism in the hypothalamus (12:105).
4. *Avoid alcoholic beverages.*
5. *Eliminate all or most sugars* from the diet (empty calories) (11:106). Eliminate refined granular table sugar (brown and white), honey, molasses, syrups, pies, cokes, donuts and pastries, ice cream. Avoid canned, preserved, and frozen foods that contain sugar. Avoid flavoring oils: e.g., sugar salad dressings, ketchup. For amount of sugar in various food substances, see Reference 9.
6. *Cut down or stop eating empty-calorie junk foods:* e.g., potato chips, popcorn, and crackers.
7. *Cut down or eliminate table salt and salty foods* (most cooked foods contain adequate amounts of salt). Salt holds back cell water. Before losing fat, the fat cells must first become partially dehydrated. You and your doctor should also check your sodium/potassium ratio.
8. *Eliminate coffee and tea.* Caffeine disrupts the appetite control center.
9. *Do not overeat.* Overeating impairs the satiety (braking) mechanism in the brain (12:106).
10. *Cut down your intake of high-fat foods* such as beefsteak, pork, bacon, and luncheon meats, such as hot dogs, bologna, salami, and sausages.
11. *Avoid refined foods (empty calories):* e.g., cere-

als, white flour, pasta products, instant white rice, etc.

12. *Exercise regularly* (see Chapter 5).

13. *Eat balanced vitamin-mineral meals,* as well as CHO-protein-fat calorie meals (see Chapter 6).

14. *Eat 4–6 small meals* instead of one or two big ones.

15. *Eat slowly,* with pleasant company, in pleasant surroundings; be in a happy mood. It takes about 20 minutes for the food in the stomach to signal the brain that you have had enough food (satiated). By eating rapidly, you never give this communication a chance to work. Take several breaks (2–3 minutes) in the middle of a meal to chat.

16. *Drink 8 glasses of fluids daily.* Water flushes wastes out of kidneys and body.

17. *Fulfill your other human health needs,* such as emotional and social needs.

18. *Get reinforcements for losing weight* and maintaining desirable body weight from your family, friends, and modifications in your life style.

19. *Change your cooking habits* — preparation of foods (6:238–241):

  (a) *Peeling or trimming foods* diminishes vitamins and minerals — avoid it if possible.

    (1) There is more vitamin C in the peel and just under the skin on oranges and tomatoes, and niacin in the skin of carrots, than in the inside. Cooking and frying destroys most vitamin C.

    (2) Inner leaves of cabbage, lettuce, and similar vegetables are practically devoid of carotene (vitamin A), but the outer green leaves are loaded with it.

  (b) *Boiling vegetables* — water-soluble vitamins, especially B complex, leak out from vegetables into the cooking water. Riboflavin and niacin are heat-resistant but do dissolve in water.

  (c) *Avoid frying foods* — but if you do, use a non-stick finish pan (no fat added to the food).

  (d) Trim off all fat before cooking meat.

  (e) Drain fat from food before serving it.

  (f) Drain oil from canned food, like tuna.

  (g) Use as little water as possible.

  (h) Use a steam-cooker to steam.

  (i) Cook food for the shortest possible time — *do not overcook!*

  (j) Conserve vitamins in foods. Never fry foods, as frying doubles calories.

20. *Improve your protein-eating efficiency.* Balance out the protein (essential amino acids) intake for each meal so as to obtain the best possible protein from foods and to encourage maximum protein use and synthesis in your body. Balancing out the proteins in your diet means

that smaller quantities of food can be consumed, the body's nutritional needs will be taken care of, and you can cut down on the caloric or energy intake (see Chapter 6).

21. *Include fiber in your diet.* Fiber helps regulate your daily bowel movement, aids in digestion, and the assimilation of nutrients.

22. *Snack, if you must,* on low-calorie vegetables (celery, carrots), on fruit, or on high-protein nuts and soybeans.

23. *Plan your meals* ahead of time so that you can control what you eat; shop for food with a ready-made list, and buy only a one-or-two-day supply of food. Shop only when you are not hungry.

24. *Keep your cupboards and refrigerator empty of snack foods.*

25. *Take nutrient supplements* as needed and medically recommended.

26. Continue to take body measurements. Although your weight may not change for several weeks, your body measurements (e.g., thigh, girth, and waistline) may change indicating that adipose tissue is probably reduced in size and muscle tissue is becoming firmer and therefore heavier. This is a positive unnoticed change. Reassess your body-fat composition by referring to Figure 7.4. Has your total body fat dropped?

Eating Habits

To get thin, you have to assess how you got fat in the first place. Why are you overweight? Does your overeating stem from a lack of will power? Emotional insecurity? A poor self-image? Sloppy eating habits? The "Why Do I Eat?" Inventory at the beginning of this chapter should help you to identify some of the reasons why you overeat. Only you can do something to change your attitudes about yourself and about food. If your social and emotional needs are not being met elsewhere, you may be trying to meet them with food.

Perhaps you have unconscious eating habits that are slowly adding pounds. Once you have identified such habits, you can change them. To analyze your eating habits, you should keep a food log for 1 week, indicating not only what you eat but when you eat, the amount of time you take to eat, your physical position while eating (sitting or standing), associated activities (talking, watching television, or reading), your mood, and how hungry you are. You may find, for example, that you eat a lot quick snacks while standing up. If you make a rule for yourself that you will eat all meals and snacks sitting at a table, you may be able to break this habit. Look for patterns in your eating that you can do something about. Do you tend to eat when you feel tense? Find an alternative response, such as exercise or some other physical activity. Do you often eat lunch at a high-calorie fast-food place? Try a new lunch spot or make your own lunches.

You can change your eating habits by removing temptations to eat. Keep food out of sight. Avoid stocking up on goodies—buy only those foods that require preparation before they can be eaten. You cannot eat it if it is not in your house or room.

Another way to change your habits is to make the eating of "forbidden" foods unpleasant. Do you like to eat chocolate cupcakes? Deliberately eat so many cupcakes that you get sick. Or chew on your favorite food and spit it out on an empty plate. Does it appeal to you? Do you have a craving for a dish of ice cream? Try to imagine it covered with bugs—not so tempting any more, right?

Try to take your thoughts off food. Become involved with other people and their projects. Take an interest in what they do and participate. Join a group whose goals appeal to you. Develop a new interest or hobby that will not only take your mind off food but will enrich your life and improve your self-image.

Motivation to Control Your Weight

Weight control is a personal problem that can only be managed by you. To be successful in your weight-loss program, you must be highly motivated. Sometimes all you need to do is to look in the mirror. Not only can the sight of your pudgy body motivate you to want to lose weight, a mirror allows you to see progress in a more telling way than a scale does. A mirror reflects how you feel about yourself. You can use clothes as motivation, too. Bring out an outfit that has become too small. Try it on every week—are you making progress? Being able to fit comfortably into clothes that were too small for you is a satisfying reward for reducing and a motivator for continued weight control.

Think thin! Think of wearing a bathing suit, of suntanning and playing on the beach. Think of feeling good with that heavy weight gone and of being successful in life and love.

If you need some outside help in keeping motivated, join a diet group. There are several self-help organizations made up of people with the same problems as yours. You can provide each other with willpower and motivation. Popular weight-control clubs include TOPS, Overeaters Anonymous, Weight Watchers, Diet Workshop, and Diet Watchers. Such groups can be found in the telephone book under "Reducing and Weight Reduction Services." In selecting a diet group, one should remember that gadgets and gimmicks don't work, there are no shortcuts, and one does need to cut down caloric intake and increase exercise.

Going on a diet is often not enough. Most of us need the support of people other than family members and fellow students or co-workers. It has been found that overweight and obese persons do better losing weight with other people than by themselves. These diet organizations offer rewards of various types for those who are successful, and some even have penalties for those who gain weight. Perhaps they have a program that will be helpful to you.

Keeping Weight Off

One of the worst consequences of dieting is the "yo-yo" effect. Many dieters lose weight fast, then gain it back just as rapidly. Not only is this problem psychologically depressing, it is dangerous to the body. The brain cells are unable to rely on a stable supply of nutrients to maintain their equilibrium, so they function in an unstable manner. Thus "yo-yo" dieters often experience emotional instability, irritability, anxiety, hypersensitivity, and the inability to concentrate and think rationally (4). College students cannot afford to diet this way and be academically successful, much less get along with their friends.

The "yo-yo" effect usually occurs because once the dieter reaches his or her desirable weight, he or she goes back to the old eating habits that caused the weight gain in the first place. Thus the only way to keep the weight off once it is lost is to break those old eating habits. A number of popular diets are designed in stages: an initial "crash diet" stage of low calories, followed by later stages of higher calories at "maintenance" levels.

As with losing weight, it is important in keeping weight off to be motivated to do so, to change eating habits, and to avoid "no-no" foods. One way to keep motivated is to dress attractively and to go places where people will notice you and comment on your weight loss. Maintaining an exercise program will help keep your weight where you want it, and it will also help to keep your appestat set at the right level.

Where to go for More Information

For detailed information on popular diets, read Consumer Guide's *Rating the Diets* (2).

For more information on nutrition and dieting, see your college health services or center, your local health department, or a dietician at a local hospital.

For help in weight reduction, see your local weight-reduction clubs.

Further Readings

Berland, Theodore, and Editors, "Rating the Diets," Skokie, Ill, *Consumer Guide,* 1974.

Williams, Roger J., *Nutrition Against Disease,* New York: Bantam Books, 1973.

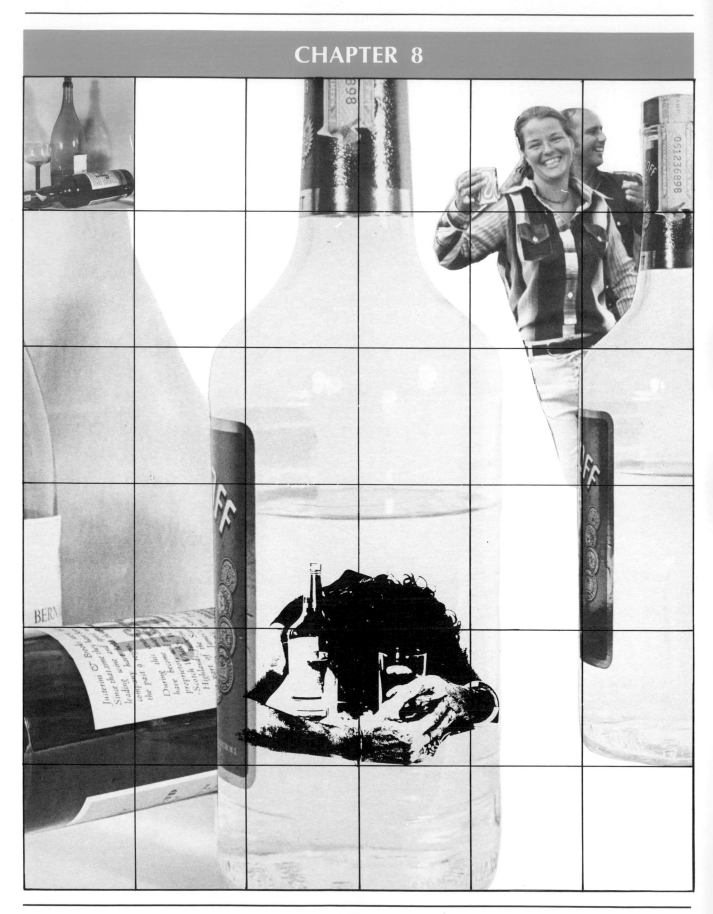

CHAPTER 8

ALCOHOLISM AND SOCIAL DRINKING

The abuse of alcohol is the number one drug problem in the United States today. Not only do more people abuse it than any other drug, alcohol abuse also has far-reaching consequences for the abuser's health, for the economy, and for American society as a whole.

Approximately 100 million Americans, or 68 percent of the population 18 years and older, are social drinkers (16). Of this number, about 10 million either have a serious drinking problem or are chronic alcoholics. Each chronic alcoholic in turn affects the lives of several family members and close friends, thereby imposing the problem of alcoholism on others. Alcohol contributes to more than 50 percent of all traffic accidents and causes more than 28,000 fatalities, countless injuries, and immeasurable property damage each year (7). There is no way to estimate the costs and damages involved in decisions made by alcoholic executives or shoddy work done by drunk or hungover workers. The economic cost associated with the misuse of alcohol is estimated at $25 billion a year.

In addition to the social and economic consequences of alcohol abuse, this drug affects the user in a number of harmful ways. Long-term drinking may eventuate in cirrhosis, a disease of the liver that is usually fatal. Alcohol is implicated with tobacco smoke in the development of certain cancers and heart disease. Long-term alcohol abuse eventually damages the brain. Furthermore, the woman who drinks heavily during pregnancy can severely harm her developing fetus. Over 1500 American babies are born each year with a set of birth defects and physical malformations referred to as fetal alcohol syndrome (13). Babies who have the syndrome are born with serious health problems, including mental retardation, small heads, narrow eyes, joint deformities, and heart defects.

Spontaneous abortions are more frequent in alcoholic mothers, suggesting that the alcoholic state is lethal to many developing embryos (5). Two drinks taken by a mother are suspected of raising the child's blood alcohol level 10 times that of the mother. Some researchers have suggested that millions of today's children and teenagers may be suffering from mental and emotional disorders because their mothers drank alcohol during pregnancy.

Why is alcohol such a menace? What are its effects on the mind and body of the user? What causes people to develop drinking problems or to become alcoholics? What can people do to avoid problems with drinking or to overcome alcoholism? What does our society offer as alternatives to alcohol? These and other questions will be explored in this chapter.

But first, classify your drinking habit as one of the six categories in the table that follows and interpret your category.

☞ WHERE ARE YOU IN YOUR DRINKING?

Using the following table, classify your drinking habits into one of the six categories.

Category	Drinking Frequency	Number of Drinks per Day—Month (e.g., beer, cocktails)	Examples of Drinking Occasions
1. Abstainer	Do not drink	none	—
2. Infrequent drinker	Once a month or less	1–2	Party
3. Light or occasional drinker	1–4 times per month	1–4	Party, dance, bar
4. Moderate-to-heavy drinker	1–4 times per week regularly	1–3	Parties, bars, before/after meals, during ballgames
5. Heavy, problem drinker	Once a day	2+	Any or all occasions
6. Alcoholic	Two or more times a day	2+	Any or all occasions, including mornings

INTERPRETATION

Categories 1 to 3

If you fall into Category 1 or 2, alcohol is not a problem for you. If you fall into Category 3, you should examine your drinking habits. When you drink, is it to excess? Are there specific situations in which you are more likely to drink? Do you drink before driving or engaging in other activities in which your impaired judgment could have adverse effects on yourself or others? If so, be sure to read the section on being a responsible drinker in the following chapter. Your drinking habits may not qualify as problem drinking or alcoholism, but you should be aware of how drinking affects your behavior and your interactions with others.

Category 4: Moderate to Heavy Drinking

If you fall into this category, you may be on your way to becoming a problem drinker. Do you have any of the symptoms of the early stages of problem drinking? Answer these questions:

	Yes	No
1. Are you beginning to lie about your drinking?	_____	_____
2. Do you ever feel guilty about your drinking?	_____	_____

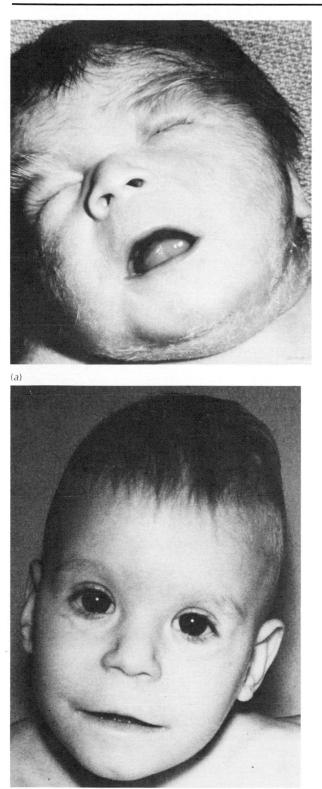
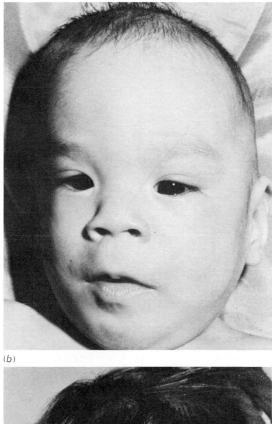
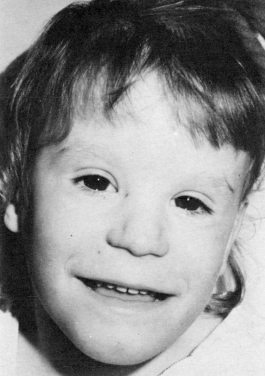

(a)

(b)

(c)

(d)

Figure 8.1

Facial features of two children with fetal alcohol syndrome. (a) Newborn American Indian boy. (b) Same infant at 6 months of age. (c) Sixteen-month-old white girl. (d) Same child at 4 years. Note short palpebral fissures, low nasal bridge with short nose, midface hypoplasia, and long convex upper lip with narrow vermillion border. Other not uncommon features are ocular ptasis, strabismus, wide mouth, and prominent ears.

	Yes	No
3. Do you gulp your drinks?	_____	_____
4. Do you try to have a few extra drinks before joining others in drinking?	_____	_____
5. Must you drink at certain times—e.g., before lunch or a special event, or after a disappointment or quarrel?	_____	_____
6. Do you drink because you feel tired, depressed, or worried?	_____	_____
7. Are you annoyed when family or friends talk about your drinking?	_____	_____
8. Are you beginning to have occasional blackouts or to pass out from drinking?	_____	_____
9. Do you drink more than your friends?	_____	_____
10. Do you sneak drinks on occasion?	_____	_____

If you answered yes to more than one of these questions, you show signs of becoming a problem drinker. You should examine your drinking habits now and try to change them. Read the sections in the chapter on responsible drinking and alternatives to drinking, and try to follow the suggestions that are presented.

Category 5: Problem Drinker

If you fall into this category, alcohol plays a major role in your life and interferes with your work, your interpersonal relations, and your emotional well-being. You are definitely a problem drinker if you answer yes to one or more of the following questions:

	Yes	No
1. Are you making promises and telling lies to cover up or explain your drinking?	_____	_____
2. Are there many times and situations when you find you must have a drink?	_____	_____
3. When sober, do you regret what you have said or done while drinking?	_____	_____
4. Are you drinking alone more often, avoiding family or friends?	_____	_____
5. Do you have weekend drinking bouts and Monday hangovers?	_____	_____
6. Have you lost your job because of drinking?	_____	_____
7. Have you been "going on the wagon" to try to control your drinking?	_____	_____

	Yes	No

8. Do you have numerous arguments and disagreements with others? _____ _____

9. Are memory blackouts and passouts becoming more frequent? _____ _____

10. Do you have trouble paying your bills? _____ _____

11. Do you have trouble with the law? _____ _____

If you answered yes to any of these questions, you must face up to the fact that you are a problem drinker. You need to realize that alcohol has begun to control your life. It is not too late to regain control. Read the section in the chapter on problem drinking and follow the suggestions offered for problem drinking and alcoholics.

Category 6: Alcoholic

If you fall into this category, you are one of an estimated 10 million Americans who are psychologically and physically dependent on alcohol. You are an addict, and withdrawal of your drug will cause you to experience withdrawal symptoms: delirium tremens (DTs). You are an alcoholic if you answer yes to one or more of these questions:

	Yes	No

1. Do you drink to live and live to drink? _____ _____

2. Do you drink alone? _____ _____

3. Are you openly drunk on important occasions at which drinking is inappropriate? _____ _____

4. Do your drinking bouts last for several days at a time? _____ _____

5. Do you sometimes get the "shakes" in the morning and think it helps to take a "quick one"? _____ _____

6. Do blackouts and passouts now occur more often? _____ _____

7. Have you lost concern for your family and others around you? _____ _____

8. Has drinking endangered your health? _____ _____

9. Would you rather drink than eat? _____ _____

If you are an alcoholic, you first need to recognize your condition and admit to it. Thousands of alcoholics have faced their drinking problem and overcome it. You can, too. Read the section on alcoholism in the chapter, and follow the suggestions provided for problem drinkers and alcoholics. If you need help with your problem, look into the resources listed at the end of the chapter.

ALCOHOL IS A DRUG

Alcohol is the most commonly used and misused drug in the United States. Many Americans do not realize that alcohol is a drug, because it is such a normal part of their lives. They do not see drinking as a means to an altered state of consciousness, but rather as a means to some other end, such as promoting conviviality or stimulating conversation. They see alcohol primarily as a social lubricant. Other people consider alcohol to be a normal part of their diet—wine with meals, beer and chips during the ball game, and so on. Unlike other drugs, alcohol is also a possible food; that is, it provides calories (although no other food nutrients). Furthermore, rituals involving alcohol have reached us through many cultures and religious ceremonies, further ingraining this substance into our daily lives (see Figure 8.2).

Nevertheless, alcohol *is* basically a drug, and it has definite short-term and long-term effects (see Figure 8.3).

SHORT-TERM EFFECTS

Alcohol is often thought of as a stimulant because it appears to make people more lively and uninhibited. Indeed, in moderate quantities alcoholic beverages do slightly increase the heart rate, dilate blood vessels in the extremities, and stimulate appetite. However, alcohol is basically a depressant, since it primarily depresses functions of the central nervous system. Alcohol anesthetizes the brain.

The reactions caused by alcohol are related not so much to the amount of alcohol consumed as to its concentration in the blood. Unlike most other foods, alcohol does not have to be digested slowly before reaching the bloodstream. Instead, it is immediately absorbed into the blood, passing through the walls of the stomach and the small intestine. The blood rapidly carries it to the brain.

When blood-alcohol levels are low, the effect is usually mild sedation, relaxation, or tranquility. Slightly higher levels may produce behavioral changes that seem to suggest stimulation of the brain: the individual may become talkative, aggressive, and excessively active. However, these changes are thought to result from depression of the most highly developed brain centers that normally inhibit or restrain such behavior. At still higher levels, great depression of lower parts of the brain occurs, producing incoordination, confusion, disorientation, stupor, anaesthesia, coma, or even death (see Figure 8.4).

Blood-alcohol levels have important legal applications. In most parts of the United States, and in some countries of Europe, an individual with a blood-alcohol level of 0.05 percent or less is legally presumed to be sober and in condition to operate a motor vehicle. A person with a level of 0.15 percent or more is legally intoxicated or "under the influence" in some states, while in others the 0.10 level constitutes legal intoxication.

It is still uncertain whether there is a threshold below which alcohol has no detectable influence on reflex responses, reaction time, and various complex skills. However, when the blood-alcohol level reaches 0.03 or 0.05 percent, it is generally agreed that changes are evident. At very low blood-alcohol levels, such simple reflex responses as the knee-jerk seem to be more rapid. At levels about 0.03, or 0.04, reflex responses, reaction

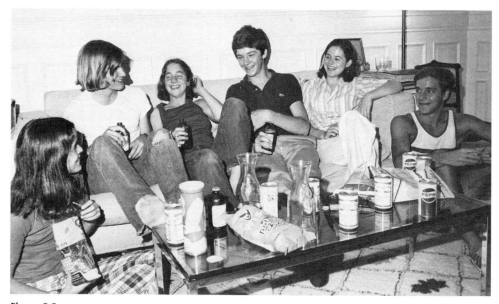

Figure 8.2
Alcoholic beverages being used as a social lubricant.

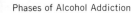

Phases of Alcohol Addiction

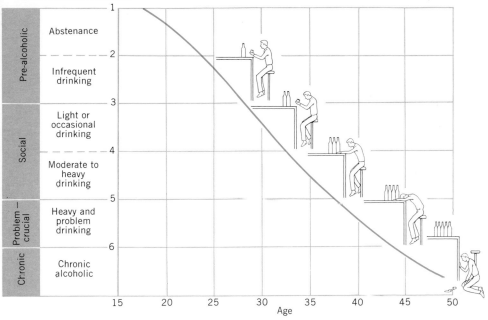

Figure 8.3

Progressive phases of alcohol addiction. Studies of alcoholism show that, on an average, the classical signs of alcoholism occur after a decade of social drinking (ages 20–30), then progressing to another decade or more of heavy-problem drinking (ages 30–40). Contrasting phases of addiction to age are deceiving, for one may progress very rapidly into chronic alcoholism or become arrested as a social drinker. (Adapted from U.S. Department of Transport, "First Aid for the Drunken Driver Begins in Your Office" (pamphlet for physicians, GPO-717-793), Washington, D.C. U.S. Government Printing Office, June 1973, p. 7.)

time, and performance in such activities as automobile driving and many kinds of athletics generally change for the worse. Significantly, as a driver's performance is impaired, his or her judgment often deteriorates and the person believes he or she is driving better (see Figure 8.5).

FACTORS AFFECTING ALCOHOL ABSORPTION

The rate at which alcohol is absorbed into the bloodstream and its behavioral effects are influenced by a number of interacting factors. On the physical side, how fast a person drinks, his or her weight, whether the person has eaten, his or her drinking history and body chemistry, the type of beverage used, and the interaction with other drugs are all major factors. On the psychological side, the drinking situation, the drinker's mood, his or her attitudes, and the person's previous experience with alcohol, all contribute to his or her reactions to drinking.

1. *Speed of drinking.* The more rapidly an alcoholic beverage is ingested, the higher will be the peak blood-alcohol concentrations. Thus, these levels are lower when the beverage is "nursed" or taken in divided amounts than when it is gulped or taken in a single dose.

2. *Body weight.* The greater the weight of the body muscle (but not body fat) of an individual, the lower will be his blood-alcohol concentration resulting from a given amount of alcohol. For example, the blood-alcohol level produced in a 180-pound man drinking 4 ounces of distilled spirits will be substantially lower than that of a 130-pound man drinking the same amount in the same length of time—and the larger man will show fewer effects. The large person has a larger amount of body fluid to dilute the alcohol ingested (see Figure 8.6).

3. *Presence of food in the stomach.* Eating while drinking notably retards the absorption of alcohol, especially when alcohol is consumed in the form of distilled spirits or wine. When alcoholic beverages are taken with a substantial meal, peak blood-alcohol concentrations may be reduced as much as 50 percent.

4. *Drinking history and body chemistry.* Each person has an individual pattern of physiological functioning that may affect his or her reactions to alcohol. For example, in a number of physical conditions, such as that

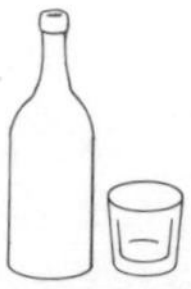

Whisky
100 proof
(50% alcohol)
AVERAGE DRINK
1 ounce
(.5 oz. alcohol)

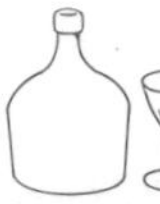

Wine
(15% alcohol)
AVERAGE DRINK
3½ ounces
(.525 oz. alcohol)

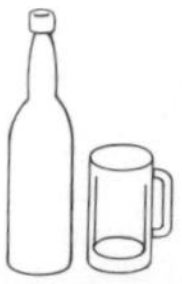

Beer
(4½% alcohol)
AVERAGE DRINK
12 ounces
(.54 oz. alcohol)

Alcohol Concentration in Blood Stream (percent)	Number of drinks per Hour	Part of Brain Affected	Area of Brain Affected	Behavior Affected
0.03	1 bottle of beer (12 oz) 1 cocktail (whiskey) (90 percent proof)	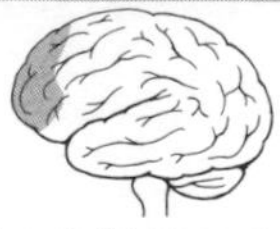	1. Reason/judgment (minor)	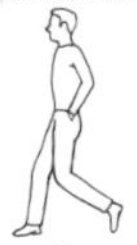
0.05	2 bottles of beer 2 cocktails	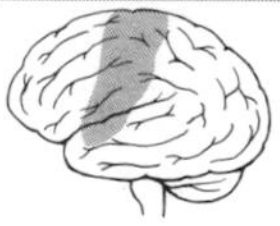	2. Coordination 3. Self-control	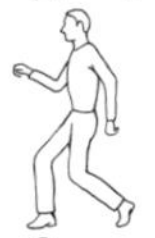
0.10	4 bottles of beer 4 cocktails	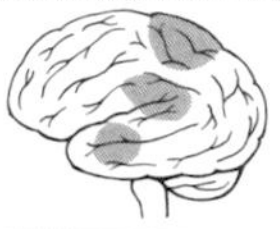	4. Vision 5. Speech 6. Hearing 7. Reaction time	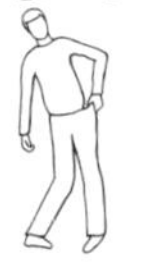
0.15	6 bottles of beer 6 cocktails	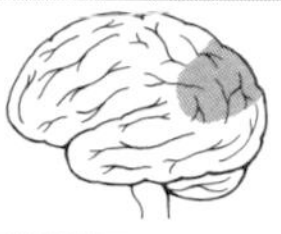	8. Balance 9. Coordination 10. Judgment	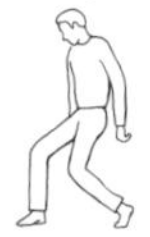
0.30	12 bottles of beer 12 cocktails	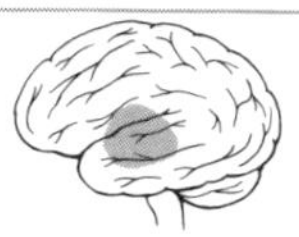	11. Memory 12. Unconsciousness	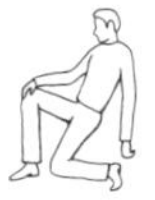
0.60	24 + bottles of beer 24 + cocktails 4 percent alcohol in beer; 90 percent proof distilled beverages	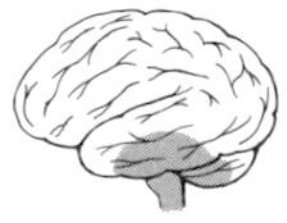	13. Respiratory center inhibited 14. DEATH possible	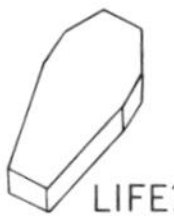 LIFE?

Figure 8.4.
Six stages of intoxication showing the brain areas and behavior affected by the increasing concentration of alcohol in the blood for a 155-pound moderate drinker. The best measurement of drunkenness is the alcohol content of the blood (left column). The blood-alcohol level is the ratio of alcohol present in the blood to the total volume of blood.

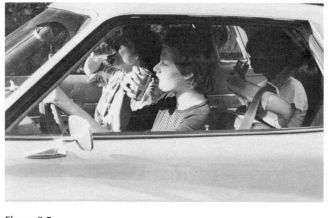

Figure 8.5
Drinking and driving do not mix.

marked by the "dumping syndrome," the stomach empties more rapidly than normal, and alcohol seems to be absorbed more quickly. Emptying time may be either slowed or speeded up by anger, fear, stress, nausea, and the condition of the stomach tissues. In individuals with a long history of drinking, tolerance to alcohol develops so that an increased dosage must be used to give effects similar to those obtained with the original dose. Thus, a person with extensive drinking problems is likely to require far more alcohol to get "high" than an inexperienced drinker.

5. *Type of beverage.* In all the major alcoholic beverages—beer, table wines, cocktail or dessert wines, liqueurs or cordials, and distilled spirits—the chief ingredient is identical: ethyl alcohol, known also as ethanol

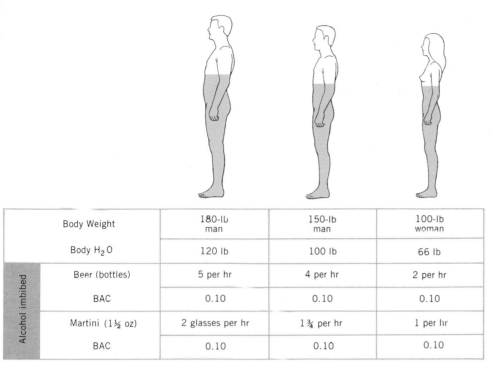

	Body Weight	180-lb man	150-lb man	100-lb woman
	Body H$_2$O	120 lb	100 lb	66 lb
Alcohol imbibed	Beer (bottles)	5 per hr	4 per hr	2 per hr
	BAC	0.10	0.10	0.10
	Martini (1½ oz)	2 glasses per hr	1 ¾ per hr	1 per hr
	BAC	0.10	0.10	0.10

Figure 8.6
Concentration of blood alcohol (BAC) and its effects depend on the size of the person. It is based on the general concept that your body is two-thirds water. The 180-pound man needs to drink five cans of beer, while the 150-pound man four drinks and the 100-pound man two drinks per hour to have a blood alcohol concentration of 0.10.

or simply as alcohol (see Figure 8.7). It is a natural substance formed by the reaction of fermenting sugar with yeast spores. The concentration of alcohol is usually about 4 percent by volume in American beers, 10 to 12 percent in table wines, between 17 and 20 percent in cocktail or dessert wines such as sherries, 22 to 50 percent in liqueurs, and 40 to 50 percent (80 to 100 proof) in distilled spirits. In addition, these beverages contain a variety of other chemical constituents. Some come from the original grains, grapes, and other fruits. Others are produced during the chemical process of fermentation or during distillation or storage. Still others may be added as flavoring or coloring. These nonalcoholic "congeners"* contribute in their own right to the effects of certain beverages, either directly affecting the body or affecting the rates at which alcohol is absorbed into the blood and metabolized in the tissues.

A number of studies in the United States and abroad have demonstrated that beers, wines, and distilled spirits

*Congeners are substances other than water and alcohol in beer and wine (e.g., dextrins, maltose, vitamins, organic acids, and salts).

may vary markedly in the rate at which the alcohol they contain is absorbed into the blood (16). In general, the higher the concentration of congeners, the slower the effects of the same amount of alcohol consumed in the form of liquor. However, any two drinks that contain the same amount of alcohol will eventually have the same effects. Diluting an alcoholic beverage with another liquid, such as water, also helps to slow down absorption, but mixing with carbonated beverages can increase the absorption rate.

6. *Other drugs.* When alcohol is ingested with other drugs or when other drugs are already present in the body, the second drug may intensify and change the effects of alcohol. For example, the use of both alcohol and tranquilizers may increase the effects of both drugs tenfold, resulting in bizarre, unpredictable effects and possible death. Especially deadly is the combination of alcohol with barbiturates, since they synergistically interact to depress all body functioning. Anyone under medication, especially with sleeping pills, antihistamines, or other depressants, should avoid drinking alcoholic beverages.

7. *Psychological factors.* The effects of alcohol are

ALCOHOLIC CONTENT OF SOME COMMON ALCOHOLIC BEVERAGES

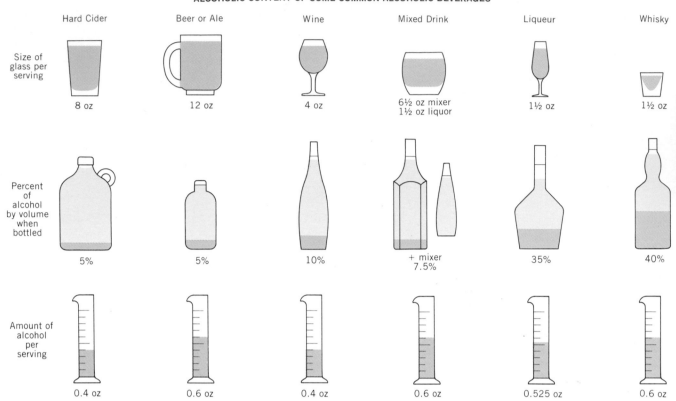

	Hard Cider	Beer or Ale	Wine	Mixed Drink	Liqueur	Whisky
Size of glass per serving	8 oz	12 oz	4 oz	6½ oz mixer 1½ oz liquor	1½ oz	1½ oz
Percent of alcohol by volume when bottled	5%	5%	10%	+ mixer 7.5%	35%	40%
Amount of alcohol per serving	0.4 oz	0.6 oz	0.4 oz	0.6 oz	0.525 oz	0.6 oz

Figure 8.7.
Although the percent of alcohol varies from drink to drink, the actual amount of alcohol remains about the same, as the bottom row shows.

often influenced by the drinker's mood, expectations, and previous experience with alcohol. Some people can get very intoxicated on small amounts of alcohol because they expect alcohol to have that effect. Some individuals who have a great deal of experience with alcohol may be able to control themselves to an extent that belies the amount of alcohol they have ingested.

Step 1.　ethyl alcohol + enzyme alcohol → acetaldehyde.
　　　　　　　　dehydrogenase
Step 2.　acetaldehyde + 　enzyme → acetic acid.
　　　　　　　　aldehydeoxidose
Step 3.　acetic acid ⟶ $CO_2 + O_2$ + heat + energy.
　　　　　　　coenzyme A

THE METABOLISM OF ALCOHOL IN THE LIVER

Alcohol is changed first to acetaldehyde, a highly irritating toxic chemical. Acetaldehyde rarely accumulates, since it is oxidized quickly into acetate by another enzyme aldehydeoxidase.

Acetate is transformed into a variety of other compounds that are eventually oxidized completely into carbon dioxide and water. The drug Antabuse or Disulfiram is sometimes used to treat alcoholism. It inhibits the action of the enzyme dehydrogenase and causes the accumulation of toxic acetaldehyde. The immediate effects are nausea, vomiting, flushing, tachycardia collapse in shock, and potentially death.

Antabuse should be used only by the skilled physician who can continuously monitor the biochemical changes taking place in the body of an alcoholic.

FACTORS AFFECTING ALCOHOL METABOLISM

The speed of alcohol *absorption* generally affects the rate at which one becomes intoxicated; conversely, the speed of alcohol *metabolism* (oxidation by the liver), affects the rate at which one becomes sober again. Research has demonstrated that the rate of alcohol metabolism, like that of absorption, may be influenced by a number of factors. A Massachusetts General Hospital study has shown that both alcoholic and nonalcoholic subjects maintained on good diets can moderately increase their rate of alcohol metabolism if they consume substantial amounts over a long period of time. As a general rule, it will take as many hours as the number of drinks consumed to sober up completely (see Figure 8.8). Old wives tales notwithstanding, drinking black coffee, taking a cold shower, or breathing pure oxygen will not hasten the process. All one can do is wait and let the liver do its work.

A familiar aftereffect of overindulgence is the *hangover*—the morning-after misery of extreme fatigue combined with nausea, upset stomach, anxiety, and headache. The hangover is common and unpleasant, but rarely dangerous. It affects the moderate drinker who occasionally drinks too much (especially if tired or under stress), as well as the excessive drinker after a prolonged drinking bout. The exact mechanism is unknown, but physiologists theorize that a hang-up is probably due to alcohol dehydrating the brain tissues (since alcohol is an unstable chemical and has a high affinity for water). The symptoms are usually most severe many hours after the peak of the drinking bout, when little or no alcohol can be detected in the body. Although the hangover has been blamed on mixing drinks, it can be produced by any alcoholic beverage alone or by pure alcohol. There is inadequate evidence to support beliefs that it is caused by vitamin deficiencies, dehydration, fusel oils (nonalcoholic components of alcoholic beverages that are relatively toxic but present in clinically insignificant amounts), or any other nonalcoholic components.

No satisfactory treatment for hangover is known. There is no scientific evidence to support the curative claims of popular remedies, such as coffee; raw egg; oysters; chili peppers; steak sauce; "alkalizers"; vitamin preparations; "the hair of the dog"; or such drugs as barbiturates, amphetamines, or insulin. The hang-up usually dissipates when the water balance in the brain tissue is restored. One can help restore this balance by drinking water during and after drinking alcohol. Hangovers can be prevented by drinking slowly, with food in the stomach, under relaxed social circumstances, and with sufficient self-discipline to avoid intoxication. A hangover is your body's way of telling you that you have given it an overdose of a poisonous substance.

LONG-TERM EFFECTS

Drinking alcohol in moderation apparently does the body little permanent harm. Drinking does deplete vitamins—folic acid, inositol, C, K, P and minerals—lithium, copper, and iron. But when taken in large doses over a long period of time, alcohol can prove disastrous, impairing both the quality and length of life. Structural damage to several major organs, such as the liver, heart, and brain, may result.

Prolonged heavy drinking has long been known to be associated with various types of muscle disease and tremors. Alcohol, in high concentrations, is suspected of slowly killing brain cells by forming wads or blood clots that plug up capillaries in the brain. When enough cells in that part of the brain dealing with neuromuscular coordination are destroyed, as in many chronic alcoholics, the chronic alcoholic exhibits nervous twitches, tremors, and partial loss of coherent speech. One essential muscle affected by alcohol is the myocardium, the chief muscle of the heart. Although chronic alcoholism and heart disease have often been observed together, until recently liver disease was thought to be the cause of the heart damage. Investigators at several large hospitals have now found that alcohol can produce heart disease without the presence of liver impairment. These scientists have also established that heart disease is commonly found among alcoholics (16).

When large quantities of alcohol are consumed, especially "straight," the gastrointestinal system can become irritated. The body metabolism of protein and amino acids is disrupted. Nausea, vomiting, and/or diarrhea are mild indications of trouble. The more frequently such ingestion takes place, the greater the irritation. Gastritis, ulcers, and pancreatitis commonly occur among alcoholics.

Cirrhosis of the liver occurs about six times as frequently among alcoholics as among nonalcoholics. Yet, it also occurs among nondrinkers, and its cause is the subject of continuing investigation. Many scientists seem convinced that adequate nutrition provides an effective protection against cirrhosis. Some investigators, however, have shown that large amounts of alcohol may cause liver damage even in properly fed subjects (16).

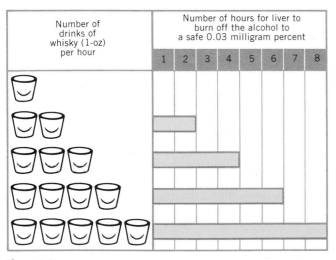

Figure 8.8.
Burn-off time is the amount of time needed for the liver to metabolize alcohol to a safe driving 0.03 mg %.

Very heavy drinkers also have lowered resistance to pneumonia and other infectious diseases.

Heavy drinking over may years may result in serious mental disorders or permanent, irreversible damage to the brain or peripheral nervous system. Critical mental functions, such as memory, judgment, and learning ability can deteriorate severely, and an individual's personality structure and reality orientation may disintegrate as well.

With serious brain damage in alcoholics, Korsakoff's syndrome may result. In this psychotic condition, patients cannot remember recent events and compensate for their memory loss with confabulation; that is, the making up of fictitious events. In addition, these individuals often suffer from polyneuritis, an inflammation of the nerves that causes burning and prickly sensations in the hands and feet. Vitamin deficiency caused by excessive drinking and inadequate intakes of nutritious foods appears to be the primary cause of this condition. Vitamin therapy is often used to treat the polyneuritis and memory deficit although the effects are not always reversible.

Thus we see that in moderate doses alcohol has few long-term effects on the body, whereas the frequent use of large doses of alcohol can have major irreversible effects on the liver, brain, and heart, often directly leading to the death of the drinker. The life span of the chronic alcoholic is shortened by 10 to 12 years.

YOU AND ALCOHOL

The use of alcohol is a pervasive part of American society. Alcoholic beverages are served before, during, and after meals; at parties and dances; on special occasions; and with leisure events, especially at spectator sports.

Studies have shown that alcohol use and abuse is particularly high among college students, although college men tend to drink three times as much as college women (16). Most college students have reached a point in their lives at which they feel a need to emancipate themselves from home and parents, to discover or reaffirm their identities, to refine social skills, to stand up on their own and assume personal and financial responsibilities, and to try to establish commitments—to an education, to society, to a profession or job, and to intimate relationships. Drinking plays a major role in this transitional period for many persons. For some, it is an escape from the pressures of coping with all these new-found needs and responsibilities. For others, drinking is a symbol of having made the transition—it is an "adult" behavior. Still others use alcohol as a form of rebellion against parents and other authorities who disapprove of drinking.

People of all ages use alcohol for a wide variety of reasons. Some are born into cultures or families that encourage or discourage particular drinking practices. For example, "hard drinking" is considered a sign of manhood among many societies. Most drinkers consume alcohol only in specific social situations in order to be "sociable" or just out of habit. Some individuals, especially young people, are pressured into drinking by their peers. Finally, many people use alcohol for the "high" it provides or as an escape from tensions, worries, and psychological problems.

WAYS TO MAINTAIN A NONDRINKING LIFE STYLE

What most people do not realize is that drinking alcoholic beverages is a negative approach to psychological and social well-being. One does not need alcohol to feel better, to make or meet with friends, to be entertained, or for any other reason. Perhaps one of the greatest skills to be mastered early in life is being able to experience a "natural high" from life itself. Being able to control your destiny and behavior requires an inner spiritual strength that must be learned and practiced. Drinking involves giving up some of that control over your life and your well-being.

If you would like to eliminate alcohol from your life, there are a number of things you can do to accomplish this goal. First, you should examine the situations and circumstances under which you are most likely to drink (see Table 8.1). Do you drink to release tension? Do you drink to be sociable? Do you drink to get high? Do you drink only when you are with a certain crowd? Do you drink because there is not much else to do in particular situations?

Analyze your drinking habits, then read through the following suggestions. Many of them will not apply to you, but some may be helpful to you in your desire to reduce or eliminate the role of alcohol in your life.

1. Get a thorough medical checkup if you have not had one in the past 3 years. Make sure that your body is in good health.

2. Assess your eating habits and nutrition (see Chapter 6). Your diet may be missing essential nutrients, causing you to function at less than optimal levels.

3. Get regular exercise (see Chapter 5). Exercise alleviates tensions and anxieties.

4. Start a self-improvement program aimed at improving your physical appearance. Take care of your skin, hair, and nails, and fix up your wardrobe. You will feel better about yourself and will improve your self-image.

5. If you tend to combine drinking and smoking, cut down on or eliminate cigarettes (see Chapter 9).

Table 8.1

Theories Surrounding the Causes of Alcoholism

Name	Physiological Theories
Genetic	It is suggested that an alcohol-prone individual may have inherited the susceptibility to be influenced adversely by alcohol.
Genetotropic	It is postulated that an inherited effect of metabolism in some people causes them to require unusual amounts of some of the essential vitamins. Because they do not get these large amounts that are needed in their normal diet, they have a genetically caused nutritional deficiency. Those who have this deficiency develop an abnormal craving, in this case, for alcohol.
Endocrine	This theory suggests that alcoholism is a result of a dysfunction of the endocrine system. Similar symptoms found in alcoholics and patients with endocrine disorders suggest that some failure of the endocrines might be casually related to the onset of alcoholism.
	Psychological Theories
Psychoanalytic	This theory is based on the idea that alcoholism develops as a response to inner conflict between dependency drives and aggressive impulses.
Learning	This theory suggests that alcohol ingestion is a reflex response to some stimulus as a way to reduce an inner-drive state, such as fear or anxiety.
Personality trait	It is postulated that in the prealcoholic stage, a personality pattern or constellation of characteristics is discernable.
	Sociological Theories
Cultural	The degree to which the culture operates to bring about inner tensions or acute needs for adjustment in its members may influence the use of alcohol as an adjustment behavior.
Deviant behavior	The alcoholic represents someone who, through a set of circumstances, becomes publicly labeled as a deviant and is forced by society's reactions into playing a deviant role.

6. Attend parties and social functions that emphasize recreational activities, such as games and dancing, rather than conversation and drinking. Do not plan social functions around alcohol consumption.

7. Associate more with nondrinking friends and friends who have given up alcohol.

8. Try to identify a personal, family, job, or other problem that may be causing anxiety, making you feel uncomfortable, inadequate, and discontent with yourself. Tackle the problem yourself or seek help from a counselor or other professional.

9. Explore ways to experience "natural highs" (see Chapter 3 and refer to alternatives to drugs in Table 10.6 of Chapter 10).

10. When you are offered a beverage, choose something nonalcoholic, such as juice, milk, or water.

11. Resist social pressures to drink. If you decide to abstain from alcohol for moral, medical, economic, or other reasons, you should not be placed under pressure to drink by other members of society. If someone pressures you to drink, explain your decision tactfully and stand your ground.

12. Develop new interests and hobbies—you may find that you have hidden talents or abilities. Join a club or organization where you can share your ideas and interests with others.

13. Try to get a job that you are best suited for and that you are well prepared for. Doing so will help you to have a more positive attitude about your work and about life.

14. Redefine or clarify your values. Make a list of your immediate and long-range goals, and put them in order of priority. Keep the list and review your attainment of these goals from time to time.

15. Reassess your life style. How are your work, family, friends, home, and community contributing to making you a better and happier person? What changes could you make that would improve your life situation? For example, you might decide to move to a new environment, fix up your room or home, change your major, or cut off relations with someone who angers or upsets you.

16. Examine your daily habits and develop a new sense of responsibility. For example, you could get up earlier in the morning to accomplish more before class or work; you could eat a regular breakfast; and you could plan each day ahead of time to make sure that you will accomplish everything you want to do.

17. See a counselor or psychologist to help you with any personal problems or stresses that are causing you discomfort and that you have difficulty resolving.

18. Seek out friends who fulfill your social needs for companionship and sharing.

19. Form a union of nondrinkers to lobby for reduced auto insurance rates, legislation, etc.

Many of these suggestions may seem rather unrelated to drinking. They are designed to help you (a) improve your physical well-being and self-esteem, (b) deal with problems and stresses that could eventually drive you to alcohol for relief or escape, and (c) finding things to do that will give you a sense of enjoyment and satisfaction and add meaning to your life.

WAYS OF BEING A RESPONSIBLE DRINKER

More than half the adults in the United States are social drinkers. Most of these people drink only occasionally (categories 2 and 3). Undoubtedly, you will encounter social situations in which you choose to have a drink or two: weddings, graduations and other special events. Or you may feel that drinking poses no problems for you and that you enjoy alcoholic beverages from time to time at parties or in other social situations (see Figure 8.9).

If you do drink, you should realize that you have a responsibility to yourself and others to avoid intoxication and the loss of self-control. Being drunk is not funny. Even though drinking is socially sanctioned, public drunkenness is not. If you wish to drink socially in a responsible manner, without becoming inebriated, here are a few suggestions:

1. Do not mix alcohol with driving. Do not drive while under the influence of alcohol. Wait for your liver to detoxify the alcohol. Refer to the dry-out chart. Arrange with someone else for

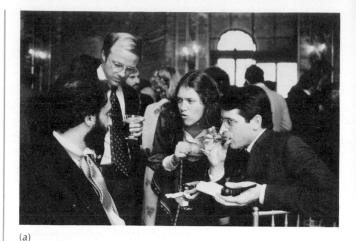

(a)

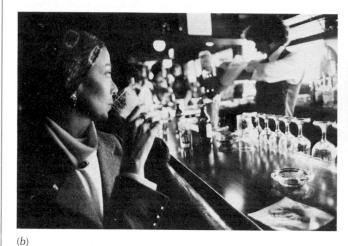

(b)

Figure 8.9
(a) Alcoholic beverages are used as a social lubricant at parties and social functions, as well as to symbolize and celebrate birthdays, weddings, and religious holidays. (b) Drinking alone is not much fun.

safe transportation home or wait until you are sober (see Figures 8.5, 8.8, and 8.11).
2. Never drink when you have a problem to solve.
3. Do not drink on an empty stomach—serve and eat food with drinks.
4. Do not drink on the job or when going to classes.
5. The safe way to drink is one drink per hour.
6. Make provisions, as the host of a party, to provide alternative nonalcoholic refreshments for those who do not care to drink. (Better yet, do not serve alcoholic drinks.)
7. Plan to get natural and social highs without alcohol highs.
8. Do not impose your drinking habits on others as contingencies for socializing, doing business, studying, etc.

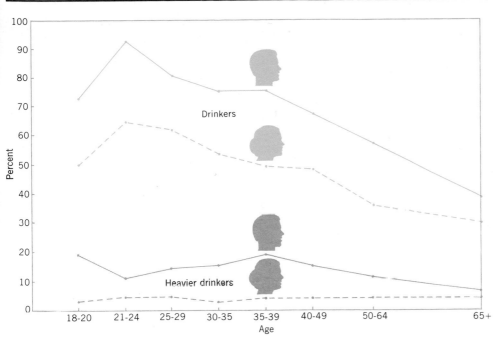

Figure 8.10.
Percent of social drinkers and heavy drinkers among adults, by sex and age, in the United States in the fall of 1972. There are more social drinkers of college age than in any other age group. Although there are more young social drinkers, the heavy drinkers are those around age 40.

Figure 8.11.
Nomogram to predict your blood alcohol concentration (BAC). Equate the amount of alcohol imbibed to 80 percent proof liquor. The example illustrates the proper use of this nomogram. The weight has been identified as 150 pounds in the left column. The number of drinks consumed in 1 hour was either 3, 5, or 8. An arrow was drawn through the body weight and the liquor consumed per hour. The column on the right gives you your BAC. (Reprinted with permission from *Current Health 1:* Vol. 2, No. 4, December, 1978, p. 4, Curriculum Innovations, Inc.) (Teacher's ed. Dawn Graff, ed.)

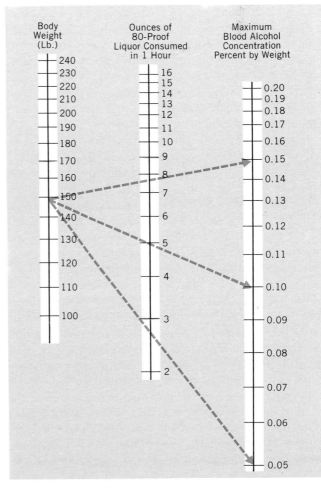

9. Do not use alcohol as a social lubricant — do not plan social functions around alcohol.
10. Do not integrate drinking with other life-style routines such as leisure activities, eating, and social functions.
11. Do not drink when conducting business or studying.
12. When at a party (or as a host), stop drinking alcohol for an hour before the scheduled end of the party.
13. Do not allow intoxicated guests or others to drive.
14. Stop serving drunk guests.

BEHAVIOR MODIFICATION TECHNIQUES FOR PROBLEM DRINKING AND ALCOHOLISM

It has been estimated that 10 million American adults are *problem drinkers* (Category 5). According to alcohol expert, Robert Straus (14), problem drinkers are "individuals who *repeatedly* use alcoholic beverages in ways which, for *them*, lead to problems of health or interpersonal relationships, destroying their sense of self-worth, or interfering with their abilities to carry out their basic responsibilities to family, job, and community in accordance with prevailing social expectations." Straus emphasizes "repeatedly" because this category does not include those social drinkers who may, on isolated occasions, become intoxicated.

About half (10 million) of all problem drinkers are full-fledged *alcoholics* (Category 6). That is, they are unable to stop drinking once they have started and they cannot refrain from drinking in inappropriate situations. The major distinction between problem drinkers and alcoholics appears to be that problem drinkers are capable of controlling their drinking and becoming purely social drinkers, whereas alcoholics have a compulsive need to use alcohol in self-destructive ways and are unable to return to controlled forms of drinking (14).

Contrary to popular belief, less than 5 percent of the nation's alcoholics are found on Skid Row. The average alcoholic is a man or woman with a good job, a home, and a family (see Table 8.2). This is a person who has an uncertain life style, has people who care about him or her, and has valuable possessions that may have taken a lifetime of hard work to accumulate.

However, the very nature of this drinking addiction will find alcoholics suffering from a noticeable inability to manage their lives properly. The obvious result of this difficulty is an enormous strain on personal relationships, with family and friends inevitably sharing the pain and suffering the alcoholic experiences. Often, alcohol acts as a demon in the mind of an otherwise rational and responsible individual, converting him into a tool of destruction to himself and to others. The debilitation continues until the alcoholic sinks to the "bottom of the pit of life." Only when he becomes aware of this, admits that he has a drinking problem, and seeks help, can he be helped by others. The best insurance against becoming an alcoholic is not to drink in the first place, and instead, gradually as a young adult, assume responsibilities for an orthobiotic life style (see Figure 8.12).

If you have taken the test at the beginning of the chapter and find yourself in Category 5 or 6, you need to make some major changes in your life. Or perhaps you have a friend or relative who qualifies as a problem drinker or alcoholic. Here are a few suggestions to help

Table 8.2

The Most Common On-the-Job Drinking Signs
1. Hangovers on the job
2. Morning drinking before going to work
3. Absenteeism, half-day or day
4. Increased nervousness, jitteriness
5. Drinking at lunchtime
6. Hand tremors
7. Drinking during working hours
8. Late to work
9. More unusual excuses for absences
10. Leaving work early
11. Leaving one's post temporarily
12. Avoiding the boss or associates
13. More edgy and irritable
14. Using 'breath purifiers'
15. Longer lunch periods

Source: Kenneth A, Rouse, "Detour—Alcoholism Ahead," Kemper Insurance Company booklet, 1964, p. 2.

you, or your friend, overcome dependence on alcohol and regain control over life.

1. Face the fact that you have a problem and that you will be hurting yourself and others if you do not try to do something about it.

2. Read as much as you can about alcohol and alcoholism to better understand the nature of your problem.

3. Realize the health benefits of stopping drinking: add 10 to 12 years to your life; reduce the risk of heart disease and certain cancers; avoid cirrhosis of the liver and nervous system disorders; and reduce the risk of serious auto accidents.

4. Realize the psychological benefits of not drinking: regain control over your life; increase your self-esteem; get greater pleasure from what life has to offer; accomplish more; and have a greater chance of achieving self-actualization.

5. Realize the social benefits of not drinking: better chance of being a successful marriage partner and parent; greater acceptance by friends and members of your community; and less chance of committing a crime or being arrested.

6. Realize the economic benefits of not drinking: more income as a result of efficient work; fewer expenses from medical bills; and money saved from not purchasing alcohol.

7. Read the suggestions provided earlier in the

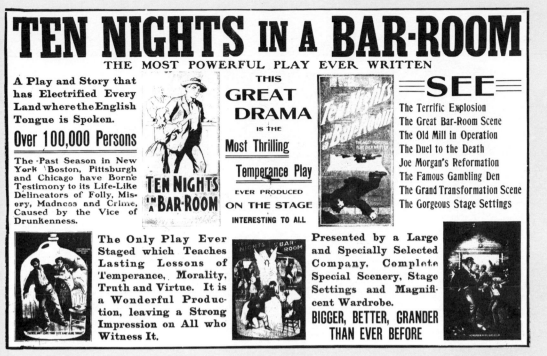

Figure 8.12
A poster depicting a popular temperance movement play about the evils of alcohol.

chapter in the section on alternatives to alcohol. Follow these suggestions that will help you to improve your physical and psychological well-being and reduce your need for alcohol.

8. Work on developing greater self-control and self-discipline. Avoid arguing and quarrelling with others.

9. Avoid situations in which you would normally be offered drinks—do not go to cocktail parties or bars. Avoid "drinking buddies."

10. Get rid of all alcohol and drinking paraphernalia in your home.

11. Join Alcoholics Anonymous.

12. Enroll in a behavioral change class or seminar designed to help problem drinkers and alcoholics.

13. See a psychologist or other professional who specializes in helping people with drinking problems.

14. Enlist friends and relatives in helping you to abstain from alcohol.

15. If all else fails, ask your doctor to put you on Antabuse, a chemical that will make you feel ill when you ingest any alcohol.

16. Review the previous section on ways of maintaining a nondrinking life style.

Kicking the drinking habit is not easy because it involves both physical and psychological dependence and because so many factors are involved. We hope that by following the previous suggestions you will be able to identify the major factors that have contributed to your dependence on alcohol and will do something about them.

Where to Go for More Information and Help

1. Campus counselor.
2. Your health instructor.
3. Your county or city Public Health Department.
4. Your community mental health clinic or state Mental Health Department.
5. Your local alcohol center.
6. Your local drug abuse center.
7. The National Counsel on Alcoholism, 2 Park Avenue, New York, N.Y. 10016.
8. The National Clearing House for Alcohol Information, Box 23115, Rockville, Md. 20852.
9. Alcoholics Anonymous (main office: 468 Park Lane South, New York, N.Y. 10016).
10. Al-Anon Family Groups Council (main office: 115 East 23rd Street, New York, N.Y. 10010).
11. NCALI, P.O. Box 2345, Rockville, Md. 20852.
12. DISCUS, Suite 1300, 425 13th Street N.W., Washington, D.C. 20004.

Suggested Reading

Hafen, Brent, Q., *ALCOHOL: THE CRUTCH THAT CRIPPLES*, Minneapolis, Minn.: West Publishing Co., 1977.

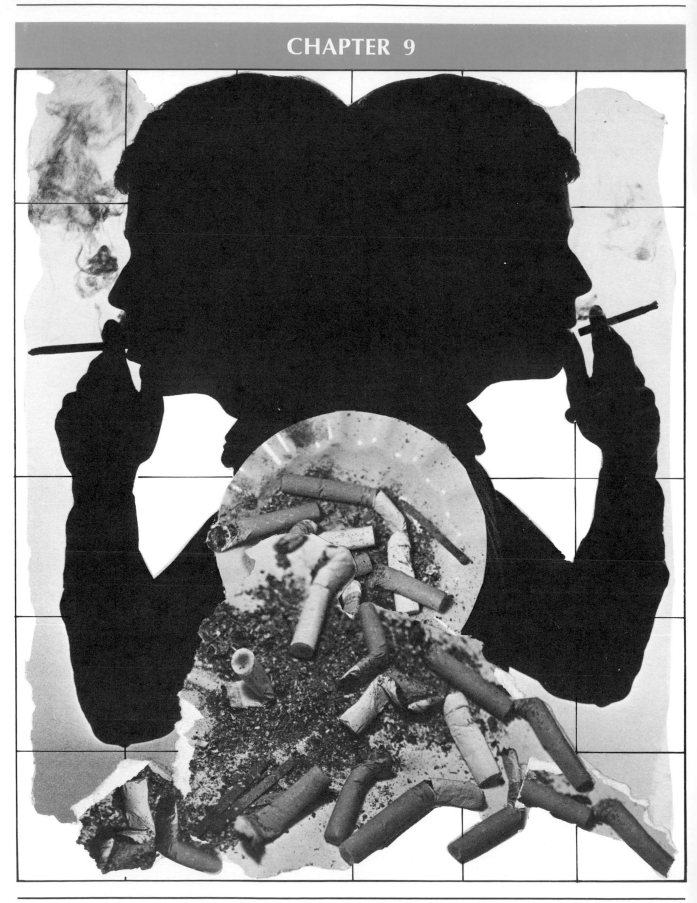

"Cigarette smoking is dangerous to your health." This familiar warning, found on all cigarette packages and in all cigarette advertising, has proved to be an enormous understatement. The fact is, cigarette smoking *is* hazardous to your health—so hazardous that it has killed millions of people. Smoking contributes to more than 320,000 deaths each year in the United States, including 75 percent of all preventable cancer deaths. Smoking plays a major role in heart disease, emphysema, bronchitis, cancer, liver disorders, birth defects, and numerous other life-threatening diseases. In this chapter we will see how smoking contributes to these illnesses and how people hooked on cigarettes can free themselves of this deadly habit.

☞ SMOKER'S SELF-TESTING KIT (ADULTS)[1]

There are four short tests in this kit to help you find out what you *know* about cigarette smoking and how you *feel* about it. These tests can tell you:

1. Whether you really want to quit smoking.
2. What you know about the effects of smoking on health.
3. What kind of smoker you are (why you smoke).
4. Whether the world you live in will help or hinder you if you do try to stop.

We believe that if you take a good, hard look at the facts and if you analyze your real feelings, you may decide to quit smoking. Tests 1 and 2 are designed to help you take this look at yourself.

Tests 3 and 4 will give you some insight into what kind of smoker you are and will reveal some of the problems you may run into when you try to quit.

The purpose of these tests is to develop your insight, to help you understand your smoking habit and to decide what you want to do about it.

An explanation of what the scores mean follows the tests. Make sure, before reading this explanation, that you have answered each question and totaled your scores on all four tests. Then go on to the interpretation of your scores.

---

[1] *Permission to reprint this instrument was granted by the National Clearinghouse for Smoking and Health (USPHS), Bethesda, Md., 1974.*

☞ TEST 1. DO YOU WANT TO CHANGE YOUR SMOKING HABITS?

For each statement, circle the number that most accurately indicates how you feel. For example, if you completely agree with the statement, circle 4, if you agree somewhat, circle 3, and so on.

Important: Answer every question.

	Completely Agree	Somewhat Agree	Somewhat Disagree	Completely Disagree
A. Cigarette smoking might give me a serious illness	4	3	2	1
B. My cigarette smoking sets a bad example for others	4	3	2	1
C. I find cigarette smoking to be a messy kind of habit	4	3	2	1
D. Controlling my cigarette smoking is a challenge to me	4	3	2	1
E. Smoking causes shortness of breath	4	3	2	1
F. If I quit smoking cigarettes, it might influence others to stop	4	3	2	1
G. Cigarettes cause damage to clothing and other personal property	4	3	2	1
H. Quitting smoking would show that I have willpower	4	3	2	1
I. My cigarette smoking will have a harmful effect on my health	4	3	2	1
J. My cigarette smoking influences others close to me to take up or continue smoking	4	3	2	1
K. If I quit smoking, my sense of taste or smell would improve	4	3	2	1
L. I do not like the idea of feeling dependent on smoking	4	3	2	1

HOW TO SCORE

1. *Enter the numbers you have circled to the Test 1 questions in the spaces below, putting the number you have circled to question A over line A, to question B over line B, and so on.*
2. *Total the 3 scores across on each line to get your totals. For example, the sum of your scores over lines A, E, and I gives you your score on* Health — *lines, B, F, and J give the score on* Example, *and so on.*

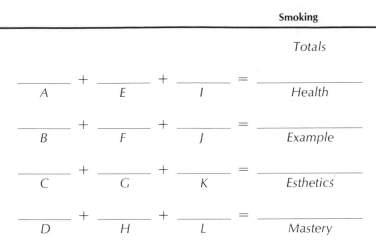

Totals

_____ + _____ + _____ = _____
A   E   I   Health

_____ + _____ + _____ = _____
B   F   J   Example

_____ + _____ + _____ = _____
C   G   K   Esthetics

_____ + _____ + _____ = _____
D   H   L   Mastery

Scores can vary from 3 to 12. Any score 9 and above is high; *any score 6 and below is* low. *Learn from Part 2 what your scores mean.*

☞ TEST 2. WHAT DO YOU THINK THE EFFECTS OF SMOKING ARE?

For each statement, circle the number that shows how you feel about it. Do you strongly agree, mildly agree, mildly disagree, or strongly disagree?

Important: Answer every question.

	Strongly Agree	Mildly Agree	Mildly Disagree	Strongly Disagree
A. Cigarette smoking is not nearly as dangerous as many other health hazards	1	2	3	4
B. I do not smoke enough to get any of the diseases that cigarette smoking is supposed to cause	1	2	3	4
C. If a person has already smoked for many years, it probably will not do him much good to stop	1	2	3	4
D. It would be hard for me to give up smoking cigarettes	1	2	3	4
E. Cigarette smoking is enough of a health hazard for something to be done about it	4	3	2	1
F. The kind of cigarette I smoke is much less likely than other kinds to give me any of the diseases that smoking is supposed to cause	1	2	3	4
G. As soon as a person quits smoking cigarettes, he begins to recover from much of the damage that smoking has caused	4	3	2	1
H. It would be hard for me to cut down to half the number of cigarettes I now smoke	1	2	3	4

	Strongly Agree	Mildly Agree	Mildy Disagree	Strongly Disagree
I. The whole problem of cigarette smoking and health is a very minor one	1	2	3	4
J. I have not smoked long enough to worry about the diseases that cigarette smoking is supposed to cause	1	2	3	4
K. Quitting smoking helps a person to live longer	4	3	2	1
L. It would be difficult for me to make any substantial change in my smoking habits	1	2	3	4

HOW TO SCORE

1. *Enter the numbers you have circled to the Test 2 questions in the spaces below, putting the number you have circled to question A over line A, to question B over line B, and so on.*
2. *Total the 3 scores across on each line to get your totals. For example, the sum of your scores over line A, E, and I gives you your score on* Importance *— lines B, F, and J give the score on* Personal Relevance, *and so on.*

Totals

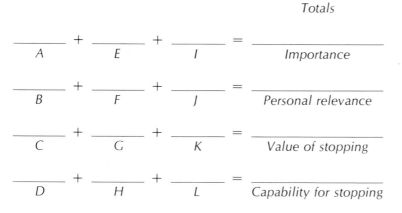

_____ + _____ + _____ = _____			
A E I Importance			
_____ + _____ + _____ = _____			
B F J Personal relevance			
_____ + _____ + _____ = _____			
C G K Value of stopping			
_____ + _____ + _____ = _____			
D H L Capability for stopping			

Scores can vary from 3 to 12. Any score 9 and above is high; *any score 6 and below is* low. *Learn from Part 2 what your scores mean.*

☞ TEST 3. WHY DO YOU SMOKE?

Here are some statements made by people to describe what they get out of smoking cigarettes. How *often* do you feel this way when smoking them? Circle one number for each statement.

Important: Answer every question.

	Always	Frequently	Occasionally	Seldom	Never
A. I smoke cigarettes in order to keep myself from slowing down	5	4	3	2	1
B. Handling a cigarette is part of the enjoyment of smoking it	5	4	3	2	1
C. Smoking cigarettes is pleasant and relaxing	5	4	3	2	1
D. I light up a cigarette when I feel angry about something	5	4	3	2	1
E. When I have run out of cigarettes I find it almost unbearable until I can get them	5	4	3	2	1
F. I smoke cigarettes automatically without even being aware of it	5	4	3	2	1
G. I smoke cigarettes to stimulate me, to perk myself up	5	4	3	2	1
H. Part of the enjoyment of smoking a cigarette comes from the steps I take to light up	5	4	3	2	1
I. I find cigarettes pleasurable	5	4	3	2	1
J. When I feel uncomfortable or upset about something, I light up a cigarette	5	4	3	2	1
K. I am very much aware of the fact when I am not smoking a cigarette	5	4	3	2	1
L. I light up a cigarette without realizing I still have one burning in the ashtray	5	4	3	2	1
M. I smoke cigarettes to give me a "lift"	5	4	3	2	1
N. When I smoke a cigarette, part of the enjoyment is watching the smoke as I exhale it	5	4	3	2	1
O. I want a cigarette most when I am comfortable and relaxed	5	4	3	2	1
P. When I feel "blue" or want to take my mind off cares and worries, I smoke cigarettes	5	4	3	2	1

	Always	Frequently	Occasionally	Seldom	Never
Q. I get a real gnawing hunger for a cigarette when I haven't smoked for a while	5	4	3	2	1
R. I have found a cigarette in my mouth and did not remember putting it there	5	4	3	2	1

HOW TO SCORE

1. Enter the numbers you have circled to the Test 3 question in the spaces below, putting the number you have circled to question A over line A, to question B over line B, and so on.

2. Total the 3 scores on each line to get your totals. For example, the sum of your scores over lines A, G, and M gives you your score on Stimulation—lines B, H, and N give the score on Handling, etc.

Totals

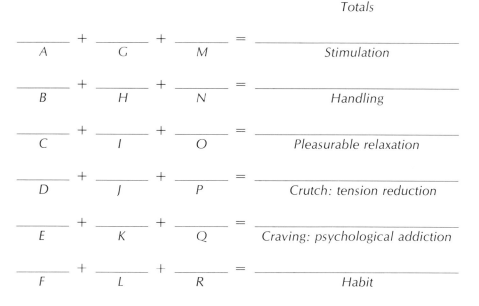

```
_____  +  _____  +  _____  =  _____
   A          G           M             Stimulation

_____  +  _____  +  _____  =  _____
   B          H           N             Handling

_____  +  _____  +  _____  =  _____
   C          I           O             Pleasurable relaxation

_____  +  _____  +  _____  =  _____
   D          J           P             Crutch: tension reduction

_____  +  _____  +  _____  =  _____
   E          K           Q             Craving: psychological addiction

_____  +  _____  +  _____  =  _____
   F          L           R             Habit
```

Scores can vary from 3 to 15. Any score 11 and above is high; *any score 7 and below is* low. *Learn from Part 2 what your scores mean.*

☞ TEST 4. DOES THE WORLD AROUND YOU MAKE IT EASIER OR HARDER TO CHANGE YOUR SMOKING HABITS?

Indicate by circling the appropriate numbers whether you feel the following statements are true or false.

Important: Answer every question.

	True or Mostly True	False or Mostly False
A. Doctors have decreased or stopped their smoking of cigarettes in the past 10 years	2	1
B. In recent years there seem to be more rules about where you are allowed to smoke	2	1
C. Cigarette advertising makes smoking appear attractive to me	1	2
D. Schools are trying to discourage children from smoking	2	1
E. Doctors are trying to get their patients to stop smoking	2	1
F. Someone has recently tried to persuade me to cut down or quit smoking cigarettes	2	1
G. The constant repetition of cigarette advertising makes it hard for me to quit smoking	1	2
H. Both government and private health organizations are actively trying to discourage people from smoking	2	1
I. A doctor has, at least once, talked to me about my smoking	2	1
J. It seems as though an increasing number of people object to having someone smoke near them	2	1
K. Some cigarette commercials on TV make me feel like smoking	1	2
L. Congressmen and other legislators are showing concern with smoking and health	2	1

M. The people around you, particularly those who are close to you (e.g., relatives, friends, and office associates), may make it easier or more difficult for you to give up smoking by what they say or do. What about these people? Would you say that they make giving up smoking or staying off cigarettes more difficult for you than it would be otherwise? (Circle the number to the left of the statement that best describes your situation.)

3   They make it much more difficult than it would be otherwise.
4   They make it somewhat more difficult than it would be otherwise.
5   They make it somewhat easier than it would be otherwise.
6   They make it much easier than it would be otherwise.

HOW TO SCORE

1. *Enter the numbers you have circled on the Test 4 questions in the spaces below, putting the number you have circled to question A over line A, to question B over line B, and so on.*

2. *Total the 3 scores across on each line to get your totals. For example, the sum of your scores over lines A, E, and I gives you your score on Doctors—lines B, F, and J give the score on General Climate, and so on.*

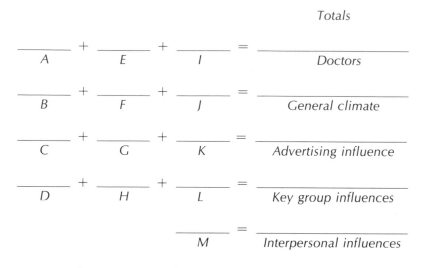

Totals

			Totals
A	+ E	+ I	= Doctors
B	+ F	+ J	= General climate
C	+ G	+ K	= Advertising influence
D	+ H	+ L	= Key group influences
		M	= Interpersonal influences

Scores can vary from 3 to 6; 6 is high; *5,* middle; *4, low middle; 3,* low. *Learn from Part 2 what your scores mean.*

You have now taken the four tests and are ready to read the explanation of what your scores mean.

TEST 1. DO YOU WANT TO CHANGE YOUR SMOKING HABITS?

Why do you want to quit smoking? Are your reasons strong enough for you to make the effort to quit? Do you have enough reasons? This is something only you can decide.

Four common reasons for wanting to quit smoking cigarettes are: Concern over the effects on *health;* desire to set an *example* for others; recognition of the unpleasant aspects (the *esthetics*) of smoking; and desire to exercise *self-control.*

Test 1 of the Smoker's Self-Testing Kit was designed to measure the importance of each of these reasons to you. The higher you score on any category, say *health,* the more important that reason is to you. A score of 9 or above in one of these categories indicates that this is one of the most important reasons why you may want to quit.

1. Health. Research during the past 10 or 15 years has shown that cigarette smoking can be harmful to health. Knowing this, many people have recently stopped smoking and many others are considering it. If your score on the *health* factor is 9 or above, the health hazards of smoking may be enough to make you want to quit now.

If your score on this factor is low (6 or less), look at your scores on Test 2. They tell how much you know about the health hazard. You may be lacking important information or may even have incorrect information. If so, health considerations are not playing the important role they should in your decision to keep on smoking or to quit.

2. Example. Some people stop smoking because they want to set a good example for others. Parents do it to make it easier for their children to resist starting to smoke; doctors do it to influence their patients; teachers want to help their students; sports stars want to set an example for their young fans; husbands want to influence their wives, and vice versa.

Such examples are an important influence on our behavior. Research shows that almost twice as many high school students smoke if both parents are smokers compared to those whose parents are nonsmokers or former smokers.

If your score is low (6 or less), it may mean that you are not interested in giving up smoking in order to set an example for others. Perhaps you do not appreciate how important your example could be.

3. Aesthetics (The Unpleasant Aspects). People who score high, that is, 9 or above, in this category, recognize and are disturbed by some of the unpleasant aspects of smoking. The smell of stale smoke on their clothing, bad breath, and stains on their fingers and teeth might be reason enough to consider breaking the habit.

4. Mastery (Self-Control). If you score 9 or above on this factor, you are bothered by the knowledge that you cannot control your desire to smoke. You are not your own master. Awareness of this challenge to your self-control may make you want to quit.

Summary of Test 1

Test 1 has measured your attitude toward four of the most common reasons why people want to quit smoking. Consider those that are important to you. Even if none are important, you still may have a highly personal reason for wanting to change your habit. All in all, you may now see that you have reasons enough to want to quit smoking.

If you are still not sure, study the interpretation of your scores on Test 2 (the next test) to determine what you know about the effects of smoking on your health and what part that knowledge may play in your decision.

TEST 2. WHAT DO YOU THINK THE EFFECTS OF SMOKING ARE?

To attempt to give up smoking you must do more than simply acknowledge that "cigarette smoking may be harmful to your health." You must be aware that smoking is an *important* problem, that it has *personal* meaning for you, that there is *value* to be gained from stopping, and that people are *capable* of stopping. Test 2 measures the strength of your recognition of each of these factors.

If your score is 9 or above on any factor, that factor supports your desire to try to stop smoking. If your score is 6 or below, that factor will not help you, but note that you may have scored low, because you lack correct information. For every factor for which you *do* have a low score, read the accompanying explanatory material with special care.

1. Importance. Cancer, heart disease, respiratory disease—all related to smoking —are among the most serious to which man is exposed. You should not shrug off the growing evidence that they cause death and severe disability. Yet you may be doing this if your score is 6 or lower on the first part of Test 2.

Research has shown that one death in every three is an "extra" death among men who die between the ages of 35 and 60, because cigarette smokers have higher death rates than nonsmokers. One day of every five lost from work because of illness, 1 day in every 10 spent in bed because of illness, 1 day of every 8 days of restricted activity —are all "extra," because cigarette smokers suffer more disability than nonsmokers.

2. Personal Relevance. Some smokers kid themselves into thinking: "It can't happen to me—only to the other guy." If you score 6 or below, you may be one of these people.

Your reasoning may go something like this: "I don't really smoke enough to be hurt by it. It takes two packs a day over a period of many years before harmful effects show up."

Unfortunately, this is not true. Even people who smoke less than half a pack a day show significantly higher death rates than nonsmokers. Breathing capacity can diminish after only a very few years of regular smoking. Even what used to be considered light smoking, such as half a pack a day, can be harmful.

3. Value of Stopping. Evidence shows that there are benefits to health when you give up smoking—even if you have smoked for many years. A score of 6 or lower indicates that you do not realize this.

There are real advantages in giving up smoking even for long-term smokers; people who quit before any symptoms of illness or impairment occur suffer lower death rates than those who continue to smoke, and reduce the likelihood of serious illness.

People who have had heart attacks and those with stomach ulcers and chronic respiratory diseases should definitely give up smoking. It is difficult if not impossible to control such illnesses if they do not.

4. Capability for Stopping. If your score is 6 or lower on this part of the test, you believe that it will be hard for you to quit. But you may find encouragement in the fact that over 20 million adults are now successful exsmokers. Of these, over 100,000 doctors, well over half of those who were ever cigarette smokers, have successfully quit.

In the following Test, No. 3, you will gain some insight into the reasons why you smoke. With this new knowledge, it may be easier for you to give up smoking than you thought it would be. At any rate, you must develop confidence that it is possible for you to control your smoking; if you do not, you are less likely to succeed in your attempt to quit.

Summary of Test 2

Review your scores on the four factors that this test measures. For those on which you scored in the *middle* or *low* brackets, study the explanatory material. If this pamphlet does not answer all your questions, you may get additional material from the Public Health Service, your local health department, and such agencies as the National Tuberculosis and Respiratory Disease Association, American Cancer Society, American Heart Association, or your public library.

Now, you should be ready to decide whether or not you are going to try to give up smoking. If you have strong enough reasons to do so, if you know enough about the real effects of smoking, if you have not been led astray by misinformation, and if you will not try to fool yourself, you are ready.

TEST 3. WHY DO YOU SMOKE?

What kind of smoker are you? What do you get out of smoking? What does it do for you? This test is designed to provide you with a score on each of 6 factors which describe many people's smoking. Your smoking may be well characterized by only one of these factors, or by a combination of factors. In any event, this test will help you identify what you use smoking for and what kind of satisfaction you think you get from smoking.

The six factors measured by this test describe one way or another of experiencing or managing certain kinds of feelings. Three of these feeling-states represent the *posi-*

tive feelings people get from smoking: (1) a sense of increased energy or *stimulation,* (2) the satisfaction of *handling* or manipulating things, and (3) the enhancing of *pleasurable feelings* accompanying a state of well-being. The fourth is the *decreasing of negative feelings* by reducing a state of tension or feelings of anxiety, anger, shame, and so on. The fifth is a complex pattern of increasing and decreasing "craving" for a cigarette representing a psychological *addiction* to cigarettes. The sixth is *habit* smoking, which takes place in an absence of feeling—purely automatic smoking.

A score of 11 or above on any factor indicates that this factor is an important source of satisfaction for you. The higher your score (15 is the highest), the more important a particular factor is in your smoking and the more useful the discussion of that factor can be in your attempt to quit.

A few words of warning: If you give up smoking, you may have to learn to get along without the satisfactions that smoking gives you. Either that, or you will have to find some more acceptable way of getting this satisfaction. In either case, you need to know just what it is you get out of smoking before you can decide whether to forego the satisfactions it gives you or to find another way to achieve them.

1. Stimulation. If you score high or fairly high on this factor, it means that you are one of those smokers who is stimulated by the cigarette—you feel that it helps wake you up, organize your energies, and keep you going. If you try to give up smoking, you may want a safe substitute, a brisk walk or moderate exercise, for example, whenever you feel the urge to smoke.

2. Handling. Handling things can be satisfying, but there are many ways to keep your hands busy without lighting up or playing with a cigarette. Why not toy with a pen or pencil? Or try doodling. Or play with a coin, a piece of jewelry, or some other harmless object.

There are plastic cigarettes to play with, or you might even use a real cigarette if you can trust yourself not to light it.

3. Accentuation of Pleasure—Pleasurable Relaxation. It is not always easy to find out whether you use the cigarette to feel *good,* that is, get real, honest pleasure out of smoking (Factor 3) or to keep from feeling so *bad* (Factor 4). About two-thirds of smokers score high or fairly high on *accentuation of pleasure,* and about half of those also score as high or higher on *reduction of negative feelings.*

Those who do get real pleasure out of smoking often find that an honest consideration of the harmful effects of their habit is enough to help them quit. They substitute eating, drinking, social activities, and physical activities—within reasonable bounds—and find they do not seriously miss their cigarettes.

4. Reduction of Negative Feelings, or "Crutch. Many smokers use the cigarette as a kind of crutch in moments of stress or discomfort, and on occasion it may work; the cigarette is sometimes used as a tranquilizer. But the heavy smoker, the person who tries to handle severe personal problems by smoking many times a day, is apt to discover that cigarettes do not help him deal with his problems effectively.

When it comes to quitting, this kind of smoker may find it easy to stop when everything is going well, but may be tempted to start again in a time of crisis. Again, physical exertion, eating, drinking, or social activity—in moderation—may serve as useful substitutes for cigarettes, even in times of tension. The choice of a substitute depends on what will achieve the same effect without having any appreciable risk.

5. "Craving" or Psychological Addiction. Quitting smoking is difficult for the person who scores high on this factor, that of *psychological addiction.* For him, the craving for the next cigarette begins to build up the moment he puts one out, so tapering off is not likely to work. He must go "cold turkey."

It may be helpful for him to smoke more than usual for a day or two, so that the taste for cigarettes is spoiled, and then isolate himself completely from cigarettes until the craving is gone. Giving up cigarettes may be so difficult and cause so much discomfort that once he does quit, he will find it easy to resist the temptation to go back to smoking because he knows that some day he will have to go through the same agony again.

6. Habit. This kind of smoker is no longer getting much satisfaction from his cigarettes. He just lights them frequently without even realizing he is doing so. He may find it easy to quit and stay off if he can break the habit patterns he has built up. Cutting down gradually may be quite effective if there is a change in the way the cigarettes are smoked and the conditions under which they are smoked. The key to success is becoming *aware* of each cigarette you smoke. This can be done by asking yourself, "Do I really want this cigarette?" You may be surprised at how many you do not want.

Summary of Test 3

If you do not score high on any of the six factors, chances are that you do not smoke very much or have not been smoking for very many years. If so, giving up smoking—and staying off—should be easy.

If you score high on several categories, you apparently get several kinds of satisfaction from smoking and will have to find several solutions. Certain combinations of scores may indicate that giving up smoking will be especially difficult. Those who score high on both Factor 4 and Factor 5, *reduction of negative feelings* and *craving,* may have a particularly hard time in going off smoking and in staying off. However, there are ways to do it; many smokers represented by this combination have not been able to quit.

Others who score high on Factors 4 and 5 may find it useful to change their patterns of smoking and cut down at the same time. They can try to smoke fewer cigarettes, smoke them only halfway down, use low-tar-and-nicotine cigarettes, and inhale less often and less deeply. After several months of this temporary solution, they may find it easier to stop completely.

You must make two important decisions: (1) whether to try to do without the satisfactions you get from smoking or find an appropriate, less hazardous substitute, and (2) whether to try to cut out cigarettes all at once, or taper off.

Your scores should guide you in making both of these decisions.

TEST 4. DOES THE WORLD AROUND YOU MAKE IT EASIER OR HARDER TO CHANGE YOUR SMOKING HABIT?

What will happen when you try to quit smoking? Aside from the problems that may arise within yourself because of the strength of the smoking habit and what you get out of it, to what extent will you get help from what is happening around you?

This test will help you identify which of 5 factors may be of particular importance to you in providing support to your efforts to quit smoking. A factor on which your score is 5 or 6 represents a part of your environment that can be a help to you. A factor on which your score is 3 or 4 indicates a situation that may hurt your chances of staying off cigarettes.

1. Doctors. Many people are influenced by what their physicians do and say about the smoking problem. We know that the overwhelming majority of doctors accept cigarette smoking as a serious health hazard and that well over half of the doctors who used to smoke have given it up. If you score 5 or 6 on this factor, talk to your doctor about smoking and get his support.

2. General Climate. A score of 3 or 4 on this factor indicates that the environment in which you live and work will not be very helpful in your effort to quit smoking. You may need to seek a more congenial environment. If so, make a point of talking to, or associating with, people who are trying to stop smoking or who have suceeded in doing so. Also, avoid places where smoking is permitted in favor of places where smoking is prohibited.

3. Advertising Influence. A score of 3 or 4 on this factor indicates that you are strongly influenced by cigarette advertising. You may have to avoid exposing yourself to these influences until you can withstand them. Reducing your television viewing or watching educational television may help.

4. Key Group Influences. Knowing the position taken by certain "key groups" can be very important for some people, and a score of 5 or 6 on this factor indicates that you are aware of the influence of such groups. Some people are strongly influenced by the actions of the federal government, some by public and private health agencies, others by schools. All these are on public record that smoking is harmful and all are engaged in programs to reduce cigarette smoking.

5. Interpersonal Influences. For most of us there are certain people who are particularly important to us. What these people think, do, and say can make a big difference in the way we behave. For some it is a husband or a wife. For others it is their children or their parents. For still others it is the people at work. Because there are so many possible influences, it is difficult to determine which ones are important to you through a simple set of questions. Your answer to Question M should serve as a guide in this area. If your score is 5 or 6, the people who are important to you are likely to be helpful in your effort to quit smoking. If, however, your score is 3 or 4, these important people may not be helpful unless you actively seek their support.

Summary of Test 4

Your chances of staying off cigarettes permanently depend to a large extent on the support you get from the world around you. Your scores on this test identify the "helps" and "hindrances" in your own environment. With this knowledge, you may be able to find ways to improve your chances.

ENCOURAGING TRENDS

The percentage of adult smokers in this country is shrinking fast. In 1965, 52 percent of men and 32 percent of women smoked. By 1975, only 39 percent of men and 29 percent of women smoked (14), while in 1978, only 37.5% of the men smoked (2). Overall, smokers dropped from 42 percent to 34 percent of all adults. The greatest decline in smokers has occurred in males aged 21 to 24. In 11 years the percentage of smokers in this age group dropped from 67 to 41. Smoking among young people is down. Only 12 percent of these teenagers in the 12 to 18 group now smoke (2). There has been a sharp drop in smoking among 17 to 18-year-old boys but a disturbing rise among girls of the same age (2). There has been a significant drop in total U.S. cigarette consumption for the first time in 10 years. Cigarette consumption per person is at its lowest level in 20 years (2).

There are other signs that smoking is on the decline. About 95 percent of smokers in the United States have indicated that they would like to kick the habit. Of the 54 million smokers in this country, 17 million, or 31 percent, tried to quit in 1978, and 3.5 million were successful (2). In 1975, about 84 percent of smokers were able to stop smoking for at least 30 days (18). Today smoking is a little easier to give up than it was in the past because the nicotine content in American cigarettes has been decreased by more than 50 percent in the last 20 years. The tar content, which contributes greatly to a cigarette's taste and feel and which also contains cancer-causing ingredients, has been cut by two-thirds. There has been a major shift away from cigarettes with high tar and nicotine to low tar and nicotine brands (2).

The decline in cigarette consumption has been a sign for U.S. cigarette companies to manufacture new low-poison brands that reduce—but do not eliminate—the risk of disease and death from smoking. Seeing the handwriting on the wall, cigarette companies have begun to diversify their investments in enterprises unrelated to smoking: dog food, container shipping, industrial solvents, beer, and so on.

The decline in smoking is an encouraging sign that Americans have realized that smoking is a dangerous habit, as illustrated in Figure 9.1, and have decided either to quit or not to smoke in the first place. Despite these hazards, however, millions of Americans still smoke, and even though they would like to quit, many have not succeeded. Later in the chapter we will offer some programs to help smokers break this habit. But, first, let us examine what smoking actually does to the body.

DEATHS FROM SMOKING

... 300,000 Annual
... 800 Per Day
... 34 Per Hour

Smoking Kills

27 times more than *murders*
20 times more than *Vietnam*
15 times more than *suicides*
 9 times more than *diabetes*
 6 times more than *auto accidents*
2.4 times more than *all infectious diseases*

Figure 9.1

The mortality hazards of smoking. *Source:* U.S. Surgeon Generals Luther Terry and William Stewart, World Conference on Smoking and Health.

SMOKING AND HEALTH

Cigarette smoke contains 1200 different chemicals, many of which are poisonous or cancer-producing (carcinogenic), as shown in Figure 9.2. Among the major diseases attributed to inhalation of these chemicals are lung cancer; heart disease; emphysema; bronchitis; and cancers of the bladder, esophagus, pancreas, and oral cavity (lips, mouth, tongue, and pharynx) (see Figure 9.3).

Nicotine is one of the most poisonous chemicals in tobacco smoke. Trace amounts of nicotine, when injected into the bloodstream, cause vomiting, weak and rapid pulse, and may even cause death. In the respiratory system, the nicotine from cigarettes paralyzes the cilia (the tiny hairs that normally sweep things out of the system); constricts passageways; and disrupts phlegm clearance in the bronchial tree, thereby predisposing the smoker to frequent respiratory infections, especially chronic bronchitis, influenza, and colds.

Nicotine also affects the cardiovascular system. It increases the heartbeat and constricts the blood vessels in the extremities. It is also known to cause the adrenal glands to release adrenalin (epinephrine), which in turn causes fat cells in the body to release fatty acids into the bloodstream. Thus nicotine increases fat levels in the blood, a condition related to atherosclerosis and heart disease.

In addition, the nicotine in cigarettes raises the blood sugar level. Although this phenomenon is not clearly un-

New
Compounds

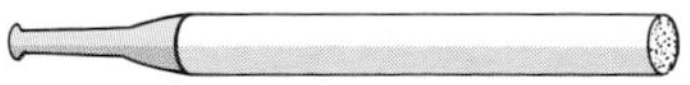

Main
Stream
Smoke

Chemical Compounds

Particulate Phase
1. Water
2. Irritants
   (a) Acids
   (b) Alcohols
   (c) Many other irritating chemicals
3. Carcinogens (cancer causers)
   (a) Many hydrocarbons
4. Co-Carcinogens (speed up cancer process)
   (a) Phenols

Volatized Compounds (uncondensed vapors)
1. Nicotine
   (a) Speeds up the heart rate
   (b) Makes the heart wasteful of energy
   (c) Increases blood pressure
   (d) Increases blood sugar
   (e) Increases blood fat
   (f) Accelerates the clotting time of blood
   (g) Produces a carcinogen when burned

Heterogeneous Mixture of Gases
1. Carbon dioxide
2. Carbon monoxide
   (a) Reduces oxygen transport
3. Hydrogen cyanide, formaldehyde, ammonia, and acetaldehyde
   (a) Inhibits ciliary movement and increases the probability of respiratory infection

Tar

Note: Tar includes all of the particulate phase plus the condensable components of the gas phase. Cigarettes generally contain between 2 and 31 milligrams of tar. Nicotine makes up approximately 7 to 8 percent of the tar and ranges between 0.1 and 2.2 milligrams per cigarette.

Figure 9.2

Composition of inhaled tobacco smoke. (From: Smoking Research/San Diego, 1968. Health, Education, and Welfare Department.)

derstood, nicotine is suspected of stimulating the adrenal glands to secrete hormones that cause the body to burn more of the sugar stored in the liver. Nicotine's combined action of increasing the heartbeat, increasing blood pressure (because of restricted blood vessels), and increasing blood sugar act as a strong stimulant and produce a lift that many smokers find necessary and enjoyable.

Of the many noxious gases in cigarette smoke, the most debilitating is *carbon monoxide* (CO), which interferes with the oxygen-carrying capacity of the blood. Carbon monoxide has 200 times the affinity for red

blood cells that life-giving oxygen does. Thus carbon monoxide prevents red blood cells from picking up enough oxygen to distribute to the tissues. Furthermore, carbon monoxide inhibits the blood cells from releasing oxygen to tissues that need it. For this reason, a pack-a-day smoker who lives at sea level gets only as much oxygen as a nonsmoker 8000 feet above sea level (16). This explains why cigarette smokers often experience shortness of breath and physiological "lows." If you are a smoker, you should be aware that you inhale only 25 percent of the 120 milligrams of carbon monoxide emitted per cigarette smoked; the remaining 75 percent is

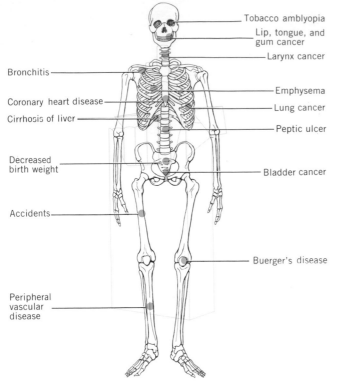

Figure 9.3.
Many diseases and conditions can be considered to be associated with smoking. Not all are casually related, but they should not be overlooked. For instance, accident rates are higher for smokers than nonsmokers. This includes fires in the home caused by the smoker who dozes off with a lighted cigarette in hand. The blood level of carbon monoxide is higher in smokers during the time they are smoking. Increasing attention is being given to the question of whether this carbon monoxide in the blood may be dulling the alertness of drivers to the point where this is a contributory factor in auto accidents. (From National Clearinghouse for Smoking and Health, United States Public Health Service.)

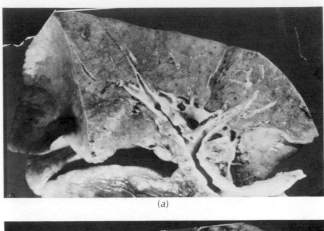

(a)

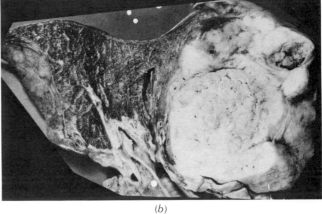

(b)

Figure 9.4
(a) A biopsy longitudinal section of a normal human lung. (b) A biopsy longitudinal section of a cancerous lung.

Table 9.1

Life Expectancy (years) at Various Ages Estimated for United States Males Who Smoke

Age	Never smoked regularly	Number of cigarettes smoked per day			
		1–9	10–19	20–39	40+
25	48.6	44.0	43.1	42.4	40.3
30	43.9	39.3	38.4	37.8	35.8
35	39.2	34.7	33.8	33.2	31.3
40	34.5	30.2	29.3	28.7	26.9
45	30.0	25.9	25.0	24.4	23.0
50	25.6	21.8	21.0	20.5	19.3
55	21.4	17.9	17.4	17.0	16.0
60	17.6	14.5	14.1	13.7	13.2
65	14.1	11.3	11.2	11.0	10.7

Note: A 25-year-old male, who never smoked, can expect to live 6.2 years longer than a male of the same age who smokes 2–3 packs of cigarettes a day.
Source: Chartbook on Smoking, Tobacco, and Health, Department of Health, Education, and Welfare, Washington, D.C.,.

released as sidestream smoke (17). Thus your cigarette smoking is just as hazardous to the nonsmoker as it is to you. The smoker's right to risk his or her own health by smoking does not include the right to jeopardize the health of others.

The *tars* and particulate matter in cigarette smoke are among the chemicals implicated in cancer, emphysema, and heart disease in smokers (see Figure 9.4).

The younger one is when smoking is started, the greater the chances are of dying prematurely (see Table 9.1). For example, a boy who begins smoking before age 15 and continues to smoke is only half as likely to live to age 75 as a boy who never smokes (2). Smokers have six times the risk of dying of lung cancer as nonsmokers, and the risk for someone who smokes two or more packs a day increases to 19 times that of a nonsmoker (4). Lung cancer has a very low cure rate—only 10 percent who get it live more than five years. This smoking-caused disease accounts for 22 percent of all cancer deaths.

Cigarette smoking, in general, has been implicated in disrupting the "appestat" in the hypothalamus of the brain. The appestat is the control center for emotions, thirst, hunger, and appetite (see Chapter 7). Smoking aggravates the hypothalamus, disrupting its ability to function normally. Since the hypothalamus is sensitive to both nicotine and hunger, nicotine probably blocks off the ability of the hypothalamus to tell the brain that the body is no longer hungry. The person overeats. When the appestat malfunctions, people have difficulty controlling their appetite; thus smoking aggravates weight problems and obesity.

Another destructive impact of the numerous chemicals in cigarette smoke is on the liver. It is the liver's job to detoxify the body of noxious chemicals. Smoking places an extra burden on the liver, forcing it to use up extra quantities of vitamins A, C, B₆, and E in order to detoxify cigarette chemicals. In 1952 W. J. McCormick (8) claimed that smoking one cigarette destroyed about 25 milligrams of vitamin C in the body. Thus two cigarettes would just about wipe out the recommended daily allowance (60 mg) of vitamin C for a male. Although McCormick's study has been challenged by Omer Pelletier's 1968 study (13), there is ample evidence that smokers excrete only about half the vitamin C excreted in urine by nonsmokers. Thus smoking depletes the body of at least one essential nutrient.

Chemicals in cigarette smoke affect more than just the smoker. A pregnant woman who smokes can create trouble for her unborn baby (11). Smoking increases the likelihood of miscarriage, fetal distress, premature babies, and stunted fetal growth. A Cleveland study found that mothers who smoke have increased levels of lead in their blood and so do their babies. This form of lead poisoning can cause unusual irritability, drowsiness, and mental retardation. According to Professor Stanley Garn of the University of Michigan, about half of all American babies are spending their prenatal months in smoke-filled wombs (18). New studies indicate that a pregnant woman who smokes is smoking for two persons; nicotine not only affects her own body but constricts the blood vessels in her unborn child, cutting down on fetal blood flow. Furthermore, carbon monoxide cuts down the amount of oxygen in the already reduced blood supply. The fetus just cannot get enough oxygen (see Figure 9.6). Thus the smoking mother indirectly "suffocates" her baby. In addition, the babies of mothers who smoke during pregnancy weigh an average of 6 ounces less at birth than the babies of nonsmoking mothers.

Smoking parents affect the well-being of their chil-

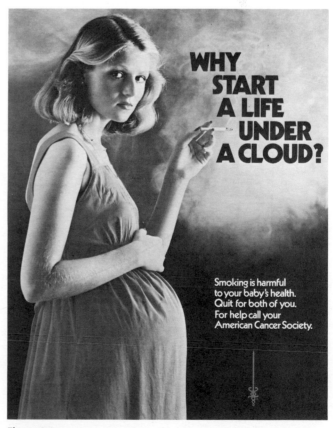

Figure 9.6
The chemicals of cigarette smoke pass through the umbilical cord and into the baby's bloodstream. Smoking restricts a baby's normal growth, causes underdevelopment, and makes a baby more susceptible to illness in the first delicate weeks of life. Why handicap your child at birth? The baby suffocates from smoke.

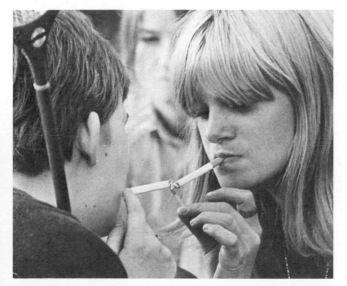

Figure 9.5
Smoking as a habit is started early in life.

dren. Children of smokers have an increased incidence of respiratory ailments.

Recent research indicates that women have a lot more at stake in smoking than the health of their future children. Lung cancer, usually considered a major killer of men smokers, is taking a greater and greater toll among women. For the first time, more women than men in the 35 to 44 age bracket have developed cases of lung cancer. It appears that women may be more susceptible to the cancer effects of smoking; the lung cancer for smoking women is 16 times the risk for nonsmokers, whereas the risk for smoking men is 10 times that of nonsmokers.

Women who smoke also run the risk of heart disease (see Figure 9.7). There is a synergistic effect that seems to drastically increase the chances of myocardial infarction. With more younger women smoking and the earlier use of birth control pills, it is possible that the risk of heart disease in middle-aged women may increase dramatically in the near future.

In assessing the health consequences of smoking, one must also keep in mind the interaction of cigarette chemicals with other chemicals that are taken into the body. For example, those who smoke have 3 to 10 times the chance of getting oral cancer, and those who are heavy alcohol drinkers have twice the chance of getting oral cancer as nondrinkers. But those who both smoke and drink have 15 times the chance of getting oral cancer compared to those who neither smoke nor drink (4). Cigarette smoke also interacts synergistically with a number of air pollutants, increasing the negative effects of both (see Chapter 15).

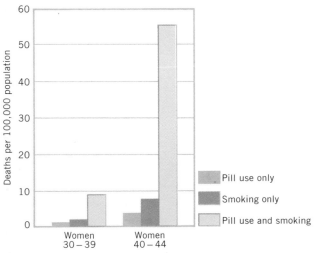

Figure 9.7

Comparisons of risks of death from heart disease in women who smoke and use birth control pills. Of the approximately 10 million women who take the pill 30 to 40 percent also smoke cigarettes. If you take the pill, do not smoke! Source: USHEW.

There are many other deleterious consequences of smoking, and most smokers have heard the evidence many, many times. When all the health consequences of smoking are added together, the unemotional and realistic conclusion is that cigarette smoking is not only bad for one's health, it is a stupid, expensive, and unnecessary habit. Furthermore, quitting smoking immediately reduces all the health risks involved—the body is able to recover its normal functioning and to again seek optimal health. As Table 9.1 shows, the incidence of lung cancer, heart disease, and emphysema drops significantly when one stops smoking and even when one decreases the number of cigarettes smoked per day. It is estimated that the average young man who smokes heavily shortens his life by about 8 years. It is obvious, then, that thousands of lives could be saved and many more thousands enriched if people would take one simple action: stop smoking.

We realize that this is easier said than done. So, the rest of the chapter will be devoted to ideas, suggestions, and programs for helping the smoker join the growing ranks of ex-smokers and nonsmokers.

WAYS TO MAINTAIN YOUR NONSMOKING LIFE STYLE (FOR THOSE WHO DO NOT SMOKE)

If you do not smoke, you may think that this chapter has little relevance for you. However, knowing about smoking—its effects and how smoking can be mastered—can be useful to you in a number of ways. First of all, you may have loved ones who smoke: parents, grandparents, a brother or sister, or a friend. You can help them to get rid of this health-destroying habit and to live longer, fuller lives (see Figure 9.8). Give them the smoker's self-test and discuss with them the reasons they smoke and the dangers of smoking. Tell them you will help to reinforce their effort not to smoke if they try to quit. If you are successful, you will not only have helped someone you love, but you will have enriched your own life.

Second, the smoking of others can be harmful to your health. Studies have shown that in closed rooms or small spaces (such as in cars and elevators) cigarette smoke enters the lungs of nonsmokers and has noticeable effects on their well-being. Smoking is a type of air pollution. In many smoke-filled rooms, cigarette smoke chemicals, such as carbon monoxide and nitrogen oxide, far exceed the National Industrial Hygiene standards for health and safety. Cigarette smoke irritates the nonsomoker's eyes and produces headaches, sneezing, coughing, wheezing, and increased heart rate and blood pressure (20). Many people are allergic to cigarette smoke and suffer from irritation of the eyes, nose, and

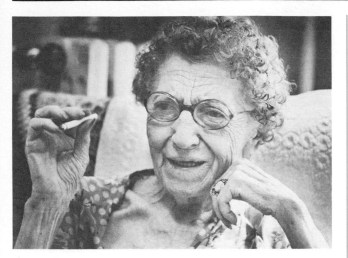

Figure 9.8
How much effect did smoking tobacco have in causing wrinkles on this elderly woman's skin?

throat. The National Occupational Safety and Health Act encourages people to work in clean air (smoke-free) environments. You should tactfully refuse to work in a cigarette-filled environment.

What can you do to keep smokers from endangering your health and reducing your enjoyment of life? If you are in a closed room or a car with smokers, be sure to open windows or to have adequate ventilation so that the smoke will be less likely to affect you. Do not allow smoking in your car or home. If nearby smokers in a res-

taurant, at a concert, or in a theater annoy you so that you cannot enjoy your meal or the program, politely ask them to put out their cigarettes. Compliment smokers for not smoking in your presence. In many cities and states there are now laws against smoking in public places, elevators, supermarkets, and other such locations. Become aware of the laws in your community and do not be afraid to point them out to those violating the laws. If restaurants, buses, airlines, and other places have No Smoking sections, be sure to take advantage of them. If you patronize an eating place or other establishment that does not have No Smoking areas, suggest to the management that such areas be established. Point out that smokers are now a minority of adults: 34 percent and dropping.

It is essential that you continue to fulfill your basic human needs. These include the need to get plenty of physical exercise; eat balanced nutritious diets; and become emotionally, spiritually, and socially fulfilled.

Choose nonsmoking friends. Go to parties and social functions where there is no cigarette smoking or cigarette smoking is discouraged.

Finally, if you feel that smokers are infringing on your rights, you may want to join an active organization such as ASH (Action on Smoking and Health), GASP (Group Against Smoking Pollution), or FANS (Fresh Air for Non-Smokers). Your local Lung Association can provide information on what groups are available in your community. Some groups may also be listed under "Smokers Information" in the Yellow Pages of your phone directory.

BEHAVIOR MODIFICATION TECHNIQUES

The longer one smokes and the older one gets, the more difficult it is to break away from the addiction to smoking. This means that it will be easier for you to stop smoking now than next month or next year. Time is on your side! Research also suggests that once you have stopped smoking, there is a very good chance that former smokers can reduce the lung damage substantially even reducing the risk to that of a lifelong nonsmoker (see Figure 9.9) (2). Research also suggests that the longer you smoke, the more permanent the damage can become. If you smoke, you can do what over 21 million Americans have successfully done before you, they gave up their craving for nicotine and they did it without major trauma. Most exsmokers followed one of three major approaches in achieving their goal.

1. *Cold turkey.* They stopped suddenly, with no tapering off. This approach is difficult at the

beginning, but it becomes easier; it is the best approach if you are psychologically prepared for it and can handle withdrawal.

2. *Tapering off alone.* Many people wean themselves from cigarettes over a period of 5 days to a month or two. You can do so on your own if you have the inner strength, willpower, and self-control. If you do not, the third approach might be best for you.

3. *Tapering off with help.* Smokers often call on others to help them kick the habit. Others can give you emotional support and reinforcements to help you quit. There are a number of different ways to get help. One is to join a smoking clinic, class, or group on your campus or in your community. Or you could take a special behavior modification class that will help put you in control of your habit. Several stop-smoking clinics

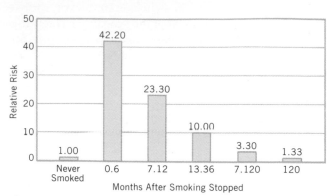

Figure 9.9

The risk of lung cancer drops after a smoker stops smoking tobacco. (With permission from Vickery, *Life Plan for Your Health*, Reading, Mass.: Addison-Wesley, 1978, p. 140.)

are likely to be available to your community. Some are expensive (such as the Schick Center), while others have a nominal fee (such as the 5-day stop-smoking clinics offered at Seventh Day Adventist hospitals and centers). Finally, you could join an antismoking organization (such as GASP or ASH, Smokenders, Smoke Watchers International, and others) in your community; such groups usually have excellent cessation programs.

The key to your successfully becoming an ex-smoker is *you*—you and the desire to quit smoking. Perhaps you are not quite convinced that smoking could really harm you. Or perhaps you have resigned yourself to the fact that you are hooked. Maybe it is time to rethink these issues and to tackle the problem head on. Often smoking is a reflection of a person's overall life style. There are probably many other habits and behaviors in your life that tend to reinforce your smoking habit. In order for you to successfully give up smoking, you will need to modify your life style a bit. Otherwise, you will probably end up going back to old patterns and resume the smoking habit. The suggestions that follow are organized with this fact in mind—you need to change patterns of thinking, behaving, and living in order to get rid of your habit.

The following program is designed to provide the smoker with as much latitude and flexibility as possible and allow for individuality and personal needs. The program is organized in six steps, although they are not meant to be followed in any particular order. Steps 1 and 2 are fundamental to the program, but the rest of the steps consist of strategies to complement steps 1 and 2 and should be used concurrently with the first steps.

Step 1. Be Motivated to Quit

The first step on the road to being an exsmoker is admitting that you have a problem—that you *are* hooked on cigarettes. You can become aware of this problem more fully if you take the four-part smoker's self-test at the beginning of this chapter. Reading the interpretations of your responses should give you major insights into the extent and nature of your problem.

Once you admit that smoking is a problem for you, you must convince yourself that you want to quit. One way to do so is to make two lists: one giving reasons why you should not smoke, and the second giving reasons why you should continue to smoke. Table 9.2 provides a wide variety of reasons for giving up smoking; perhaps it contains some points that will hit home with you.

Table 9.2

Reasons for Quitting Smoking

1. You will have improved personal appearance—cleaner teeth and a better complexion.
2. Your breath will be more pleasant (no tobacco breath).
3. Your hair will smell cleaner (no tobacco odor).
4. You will be free of smoker's cough.
5. Your popularity with the opposite sex will increase.
6. Your eyes will no longer be constantly irritated.
7. Your senses of smell and taste will be improved.
8. You will experience fewer colds, flu, and respiratory illnesses.
9. You will be able to accomplish more.
10. You will no longer have tar stains on your fingers.
11. Your clothing will smell fresh (no tobacco smell).
12. You will have control over your mind and body (you will have proved you can overcome your dependence on tobacco).
13. You will not be exposing others to the irritations of cigarette smoke.
14. You will have greater social acceptance—your habit will no longer be irritating others.
15. Your self-image will improve.
16. You will not have cigarette butts and ashes to clean up anymore.
17. You will save money.
18. You will cut down on the risk of having lung cancer and heart disease.
19. You will pay less for health insurance.
20. You will pay less for home and personal property insurance.
21. You can switch to "natural highs" and experience the joys of taste and smell, deep breathing, and optimal physical well-being.
22. You will feel more in control of your health and your fate.

If you are skeptical about the effect smoking is having on your health, you might ask your doctor or campus health service to give you a special lung test (7) that can show smoking damage to lungs long before visible symptoms appear. Developed at Hines Veterans Administration Hospital in Chicago, the test measures lung function and uses the gas krypton, which you are asked to inhale. The gas is unable to penetrate lung tissue that has been damaged by smoking, and those tissues appear blank on film exposed in a special camera. You may find the results of this test to be startling.

Step 2. Change Other Physical Habits

The object of step 2 is to alter your internal body environment so that you will feel good without cigarettes. Instead of polluting your body with all sorts of chemical substances (in addition to tobacco smoke) and neglecting your physical well-being, you should focus on changing your overall physical habits in a healthful direction. This means not only quitting smoking but:

1. Reassessing your eating habits so that you begin to eat nutritiously balanced meals (see Chapter 6).
2. Exercising regularly (see Chapter 5). Most smokers do not exercise regularly. Exercise appears to act as a catalyst not to smoke.
3. Getting regular rest and sleep (fatigue is an enemy of will-power; jangled nerves scream for a cigarette).
4. Cutting down on drinking coffee, cola drinks, and alcoholic beverages (all reinforce the craving for nicotine).

In addition, you should drink plenty of orange juice during the first few days after quitting, take a shower or bath every day (to wash off the nicotine), brush your teeth three to five times a day, and practice deep breathing to clear the lungs.

Your program of quitting smoking thus becomes part of an overall self-improvement program aimed at making you feel better, look better, and live longer. Furthermore, it is designed to make you become aware of your whole pattern of living and to change it so that is is more conducive to optimal well-being.

Step 3. Find Substitutes for Smoking

When you get the urge to smoke a cigarette, try one of the following instead:

1. Be physically active (running is best).
2. Relax or rest for 15–30 minutes.
3. Chew a stick of gum.

4. Eat an apple, a celery stick, a carrot, or an orange, but be careful not to substitute eating for smoking.
5. Telephone a sympathetic friend and share your feelings.
6. Take a warm bath or shower.
7. Go for a walk.
8. Drink a glass of water (try to drink 6–8 glasses per day, between meals).
9. Calculate the cost of your smoking habit for 1 year (see Table 9-3). Make a reservation for a holiday that will be paid for with money saved by not smoking.
10. Work out any problems that may be bothering you and inciting you to light up. Most smokers have certain times when they especially crave a cigarette, such as right after meals. Try to schedule activities (such as a long walk) for after meals; do not sit around. Go outside and inhale deeply of the fresh air.
11. Do something with your hands (doodle, hold your napkin, or drive with both hands on the steering wheel).

Step 4. Build Social Reinforcers

Try to get cigarettes totally out of your life and add things to your life that will reinforce your nonsmoking. Keep all

Table 9.3
The Cost of Smoking Tobacco Cigarettes

Cigarettes Smoked per Day (Packs)	Cost (based on 1980 dollar value)		
	Day	Month	Year
½	$0.35	$ 10.50	$ 126.00
1	0.70	21.00	252.00
1½	1.05	31.50	378.00
2	1.40	42.00	504.00
2½	1.75	52.50	630.00
3	2.10	63.00	756.00
3½	2.45	73.50	882.00
4	2.80	84.00	1008.00
4½	3.15	94.50	1134.00
5	3.50	105.00	1260.00
5½	3.85	115.50	1386.00
6	4.20	126.00	1512.00
6½	4.55	136.50	1638.00
7	4.90	147.00	1764.00
8	5.60	168.00	2016.00
9	6.30	189.00	2268.00
10	7.00	210.00	2520.00

cigarettes, matches, and ashtrays out of sight. Do not offer cigarettes to others or light their cigarettes for them. If someone offers you a cigarette, turn them down. Do not allow others to smoke in your room or home—put up a "No Smoking" sign for others to see. Try to stay away from people who smoke, and instead, surround yourself with nonsmoking friends. Nonsmokers, and those who are trying to stop smoking, should avoid smoke-filled places and occasions. This is especially important for those allergic to cigarette smoke.

When you go out to restaurants, ride on buses, and so on, insist on sitting in the nonsmoking section. Perhaps you could get together with some friends who also want to stop smoking and view one or more of the following films: "The Embattled Cell," "Times Pulls the Trigger," "I Am Joe's Heart," and "I'm Sorry, Baby" (effects of smoking on the fetus). These films are available from your local Cancer Association. You could also join an antismoking group, such as ASH or GASP. Use biofeedback machines to provide motivation-reinforcement not to smoke. For example, the ecolyzer monitors and shows on a meter the amount of carbon mondioxide in your blood. Perform a handsteadiness test before and after smoking a cigarette by trying to keep a metal probe centered in a small hole. Monitor your heart rate (pulse) before and after smoking a cigarette. Use a krypton gas test to photograph the impact that cigarette smoking has on your lungs. According to the New Hampshire Lung Association, these and other biofeedback demonstrations have a dramatic impact on both smokers and nonsmokers.

Step 5. Taper Off

There are a number of ways to cut down on smoking or on the amount of chemicals that actually make their way into your system. You can, for example, smoke low-tar, low-nicotine cigarettes. Or you can smoke one-third of each cigarette and then stop (most tar and nicotine are concentrated near the butt or filter tip). Perhaps you could try not to inhale the smoke or you could inhale every second or third time and taper down to not inhaling. It might be helpful to keep track of the number of cigarettes you inhale each day.

One way to taper off is to cut down on the number of times you light up in various situations when you normally smoke a lot: after meals, driving to and from work or school, in tense situations, while studying, and so on. Finally, you could cut down one to two cigarettes per day and gradually taper off.

Step 6. Learn to Live Without Smoking

Find things in your life that you enjoy doing and concentrate on them. Set attainable goals, and enjoy your successes and accomplishments. Throw yourself into attending to your basic human health needs, especially your emotional, social, ego, intellectual, and self-actualization needs (see Chapter 1). Learn to plan ahead in order to avoid stress, and work purposefully toward your goals. When you *are* tense and under stress, learn to work out your tensions in socially and physiologically sound ways (such as by playing tennis).

Need things to keep you going? Take up a cause or a hobby that fulfills you. Do something you always wanted to do but somehow never got around to. Identify your undeveloped abilities and improve yourself by developing some of them. Get involved in social activities; join groups that share an interest or hobby of yours. Above all, start exercising regularly. Doing things to add meaning and enrichment to your life will help to free you from your dependence on smoking.

When All Else Has Failed

What should you do if you just cannot seem to kick the habit no matter how hard you try? One drastic measure is to try products such as lobeline sulfate tablets, Bantron, or Nicoban, which are designed to make you ill if you try to smoke.

If You Choose to Smoke

If you are dead set on smoking, get a good health insurance policy. Set money aside for a future chronic disease —cancer, emphysema, and/or heart disease. Unless you have adequate coverage and savings, your hospital and medical bills in 10 to 30 years may bankrupt you.

If you must continue to smoke:

1. Do not smoke all the way.
2. Take fewer drags on each cigarette.
3. Reduce inhaling.
4. Smoke fewer cigarettes per day.
5. Smoke only the mildest cigarettes.
6. Do not be in a rush to buy another pack.
7. Walk through an intensive care unit of a hospital and observe emphysema victims struggling for breath. Could you be one of these patients in 10 years' time?
8. Begin a regular exercise program.

Further Readings

Surgeon General's Report, *The Health Consequences of Smoking*, Washington, D.C.: U.S. Government Printing Office, 1972.

Ochsner, Alton, *Smoking: Your Choice Between Life and Death*, New York: Simon and Schuster, 1970.

Olshavsky, Richard W., *No More Butts*, Bloomington, Ind.: University Press, 1978.

Geisinger, David L., *Kicking it: the New Way to Stop Smoking Permanently*, New York: Grove Press, 1979.

The Smoke Watcher's How-to-Quite Book, New York: Bernard Geis Associates, 1970.

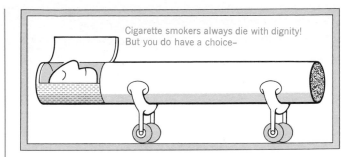

Cigarette smokers always die with dignity! But you do have a choice–

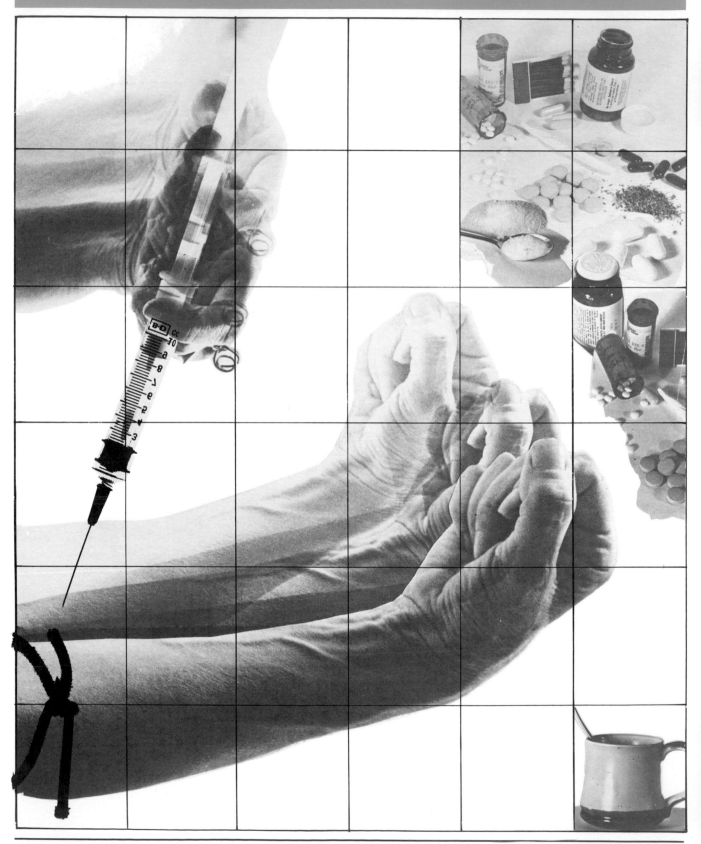

CHAPTER 10

THE WAY OF TRUTH

Wake up with caffeine,
Keep going on nicotine,
Move bowels on serutan,
Kill pain with aspirin,
Stay alive with geritol,
Grow slender with alba,
Walk on arches of steel,
Drown worries in alcohol,
Adjust stomach on tums,
Write examinations on benzedrine,
Relax with tranquilizers,
Stop backaches with kidney pills,
Sleep on barbiturates,
Start the new day with bubbling alkalizers
     to get rid of yesterday's brown taste,
To make room for today's.

Author Unknown

It is no secret that the use of drugs of every type—from aspirin to alcohol—is at an all-time high in the United States. We have already seen that about 70 percent of all American adults imbibe alcohol from time to time. Another three-quarters of a million people are regular users of amphetamines, while the nonmedical use of sedatives and tranquilizers is prevalent among millions of adults. It is estimated that 3 to 4 million young adults alone are nonmedical users of sedatives. Millions drink coffee, tea, and a variety of soft drinks. Furthermore, government surveys indicate that 25 to 40 million Americans have tried marijuana at least once. Pot smoking is particularly popular among young people; 50 percent of high school seniors, and more than half of college students report having used the drug (50).

It appears that a great percentage of American teenagers and adults are swallowing, inhaling, and injecting a wide variety of substances with the intent of altering their moods, thoughts, sensations, and perceptions. Most of the current drug experimentation is among those in the 10 to 25 age group, few people being regular drug users after age 30 (47). With the increased drug use among young people and with the changing availability of various drugs, American attitudes toward drug use and abuse are changing as well. Marijauna, for example, has achieved such widespread use that legal constraints against its sale and possession have been relaxed in many states. Other drugs become fads for short periods when they are particularly available or when they are considered "in."

What are the major substances that Americans most often turn to for relaxation, kicks, or alteration of thoughts and perceptions? In this chapter we will be examining the nature and effects of several of these substances, as well as their drawbacks. We will also be looking at America's overreliance on over-the-counter drugs, and we will offer some suggestions for dealing with drug dependence and for finding alternatives to drug use. But, first, evaluate the role drugs play in your life.

☞ WHAT ROLE DO DRUGS PLAY IN YOUR LIFE?

1. Identify the psychoactive substances that are a regular part of your life. Indicate how much of the substance you use and how often. Calculate the expense of your drug use both in the cost of the drug and in the time involved obtaining and/or preparing it. (Alcohol and nicotine are not included.)

Drug	How much?	How often?	Expense (money)	Expense (time)
Coffee/tea				
Cola Drinks				
Bariburates				
Heroin/PCP				
Cocaine/or tranquilizers				
Marijuana				
Sleeping Pills				
Over-the-counter medicines				

2. Try to identify the motivation for taking the drugs you take. Choose one or more from the following list (answer separately for each drug you use):
relaxation_____ stimulation_____ sensory alteration_____ to get high_____ as a social lubricant_____ for the interesting experience_____ for fun_____ nothing better to do_____ to enhance other experiences_____ for insight_____ for self-examination_____ out of sheer habit_____ other_____.

3. List five "benefits" of each drug that you use regularly. After each benefit, give another source (nondrug) from which you could be getting the same or similar benefits.

4. List several drawbacks for each drug that you use regularly. In what ways might your life be improved if you reduced or eliminated your drug use?

5. Reassess and clarify your goals in life (see Chapter 3). How does your use of drugs fit in with these goals and values?

6. Assess your physical fitness and diet (see Chapters 5 and 6). How does your drug use relate to these aspects of your life? Would improvement of your diet and increased exercise affect your drug use? How?

7. How much do you really know about the drugs you use—their psychological, physiological, and long-term effects? From what source has most of your drug information come? If you were to research the effects of your drugs, would it affect your drug use?

If you would like to change the role that drugs play in your life, turn to the end of this chapter for suggested alternatives to drug use.

DRUGS: SOME BASIC CONCEPTS

A *drug* is any chemical substance that, when taken into the body, produces physiological, emotional, or behavioral changes. This definition thus includes the entire spectrum of substances used in the treatment of illness, for recreation or pleasure; from aspirin, antibiotics, and antacids to marijuana, cough syrups, morphine, soft drinks, coffee, chocolate bars, mescaline, and methamphetamine.

Drugs that are taken for the sole purpose of altering consciousness in some way are usually referred to as *psychoactive drugs*. There are many types of psychoactive drugs with a wide variety of psychological effects. *Depressants,* for example, slow down body functioning by depressing the central nervous system; they thus have a relaxing effect. Depressants include alcohol, barbiturates, tranquilizers, and the opiates. At the other end of the spectrum are the *stimulants,* which speed up body functioning. They include the amphetamines, caffeine, and cocaine (see Table 10.1). Other drugs work primarily on sensation and perception — for example, marijuana and psychedelics (LSD and mescaline). In addition, people have used such wide-ranging substances as gasoline fumes, nutmeg, glue, and nitrous oxide to alter consciousness. Many people use a variety of nonprescription or over-the-counter drugs when feeling discomfort, nausea, and pain.

Each psychoactive drug has different properties, effects, and side effects. The experience produced by a particular drug depends on the dose, the method of ingestion (swallowing, inhaling, or injecting), the purity of the drug, and the user's biochemistry, mood, and expectations (see Tables 10.2 and 10.3). Thus any description of a particular drug's effects is very general and subject to numerous individual variations.

Table 10.1

Drug Use Among Young Adults (percent)

	Ever Used			Used in Past Year (1976)		
	12–17	18–25	26+	12–17	18–25	26+
Marihuana	22.4	52.9	12.9	18.4	35.0	5.4
Amphetamines	4.4	16.6	5.6	2.2	8.8	0.5
Barbiturates	2.8	11.9	2.4	1.1	5.7	0.5
Tranquilizers	3.3	9.1	2.7	1.8	6.2	0.8
Cocaine	3.4	13.4	1.6	2.3	7.0	*a*
Heroin	0.5	3.9	0.5	*a*	0.6	*a*

a Less than 0.5%.
Source: Federal Strategy, *Drug Abuse Prevention,* 1976, p. 16.

One thing we can say for sure about many drugs is that they are addictive. More properly speaking, certain drugs produce *physical dependence* in the user. Physical dependence on a drug means that the body actually adapts to the drug and makes it a part of the body's chemistry. When the user stops taking the drug, the body must adjust to the new chemical situation. This readjustment — called the *withdrawal syndrome* — can involve convulsions, hallucinations, nausea, sweating, muscular pain, and a number of other symptoms, depending on the drug being withdrawn.

Physical dependence occurs only with the depressant drugs: alcohol, sedatives, and the opiates. Such dependence is characterized not only by the withdrawal illness [called delirium tremens (DTs) in alcoholics], but by drug *tolerance*. Tolerance refers to the body's gradual adaptation to a drug over prolonged use so that more and more of the drug is required to obtain the desired effect. Amounts of the drug that might have killed the individual when trying it for the first time come to be "normal" doses for that person.

Psychoactive drugs that do not produce physical dependence often have a potential for producing psychological dependence, or *habituation;* that is, use of the drug becomes a habit that is hard to break, even though the drug is not physically addicting. When the drug is withdrawn — whether caffeine, nicotine, or amphetamines — the person becomes restless, irritable, and nervous (11). Psychological dependence is a phenomenon that can be seen not only with drugs but with a number of other habits, ranging from TV watching to sexual activity.

Another problem that has become increasingly important in recent years is *polydrug use:* using more than one psychoactive drug at a time. Looking for extra kicks or a new experience, many young people take two or more drugs at the same time. They smoke pot and drink beer, mix barbiturates with alcohol, drop acid while on uppers, and so on.

Many drug combinations produce a *synergistic effect;* that is, their combined effect is much greater than that of the two drugs taken at separate times. Drugs are most likely to interact synergistically if they are similar chemically. For example, when alcohol and barbiturates, both depressants, are taken together, body functions can become so depressed that coma and even death may result. In fact, thousands of deaths a year are attributed to this deadly combination. Many persons self-medicate with nonprescription drugs and drink alcoholic beverages, thereby creating potential synergistic drug effects.

Most persons are unaware that drug use or abuse places additional stress on the liver to metabolize the

Table 10.2

Motives for Drug Abuse

Motivation	Purpose
Well-being	Seeking a drug-induced nebulous state of optimal physical or mental well-being
Rebellion	Using drugs as an agent to defy societal or parental authority; a rejection of parental values or an attempt to gain recognition
Mystical-religious	An urge to transcend the self through a drug-induced self-consciousness, the desire to obtain an intense religious experience, or an intense need for deep, meaningful personal experience
Insight-Identity	A desire to know the self and to gain insight into who "I" am as a person, "What is life and its purpose?" a quest for personal engagement, or an attempt to change one's personality and life style
Peer pressure	Attraction to a deviant subculture; a desire to maintain, gain, or elevate one's status within a group by adopting drug-use behavior patterns
Imitation	A conformity, being like others, imitating adult behavior; attempting to treat symptoms without examining the underlying real problems; sidestepping feelings, avoiding emotions, and evading difficult situations.
Aesthetic	An attempt to increase creativity, expand one's mind and increase one's ability to appreciate the arts and "beauty."
Curiosity	A desire to see what it is like; to be able to say "I did thus and so"; demonstrating a willingness to take a risk.
Recreation	An attempt to re-energize body and soul, to obtain social companionship and facilitate social interaction, to experience pleasure, and to avoid boredom.
Relaxation	To help unwind from mental or physical activity; dealing with increasing amounts of free time; a way of life.
Aphrodisiac	An attempt to heighten one's sexual desire.

Source: Adapted from Alton V Dohner, "Motives for Drug Use: Adult and Adolescent," *Psychosomatics,* Vol. 13, No. 5, September-October, 1972.

drugs and detoxify them. To do this, the liver requires extra amounts of vitamins and minerals to synthesize many hormones to metabolize the drugs. As a consequence, drug users may often become deficient in the vitamins folic acid, PABA, K, C, P and the minerals calcium, copper, iron, and potassium.

There is no such thing as a safe chemical or drug. At least 5 percent of patients in hospitals in the United States and the United Kingdom are admitted because of side effects of the drugs they are taking (6). Of the patients already hospitalized, as many as 18 percent may suffer from adverse reactions to drugs (6). Since biochemical individuality varies from person to person, this also reinforces the idea that there is no safe drug. Any-

thing ingested or inhaled to an excess can cause a metabolic adverse reaction in the body.

Now that we have covered some very basic concepts, let us examine each of the major drugs to see their specific effects and potentials for physical and psychological dependence.

DEPRESSANTS

Depressants are drugs that slow down or reduce the activity of the central nervous system. These drugs decrease brain activity, thereby causing a reduction in behavioral output and in the level of awareness. The most widely abused depressant drug is alcohol (see Chapter 8). Other major depressants include barbiturates, other sedative-hypnotics, tranquilizers, and the opiates.

BARBITURATES

Barbiturates, often referred to as "downers," are drugs most often medically prescribed as sleeping pills and as anxiety reducers. Barbiturates are classified as *sedative-hypnotics* because they have both relaxing (sedative) and sleep-inducing (hypnotic) effects. They are often used nonmedically to achieve behavioral effects similar to those of alcohol—relaxation, reduced inhibition, and a pleasant tipsiness. In fact, one can get "drunk" on downers (3). The barbiturates most often abused include secorbarbital (Seconal), pentobarbital (Nembutal), and phenobarbital.

Barbiturates are very commonly abused, and physiological dependence can develop with regular heavy use of about a month. With this dependence comes the need for larger and larger doses (tolerance), and withdrawal produces an illness that is worse than the DTs of alcoholics, or the withdrawal syndrome of heroin addicts (see Fig. 10.1). In fact, the withdrawal illness for sedative-hypnotics is known to be fatal in some cases.

Although barbiturates may be prescribed by physicians to cure insomnia, it has been found that these drugs can actually cause sleep problems. It seems that sedatives suppress the dreaming stage of sleep (REM sleep), the part of sleep that makes a person feel refreshed and recharged. Thus a person who takes sleeping pills may feel tired and exhausted after a drug-induced sleep. Sleeping pills are usually effective for a few nights but become ineffective after a week or two of regular use. At this point, the drug can begin to cause disorders that create insomnia or anxiety. If the person stops taking the pills, anxiety increases; the resulting insomnia and restlessness lead to represcriptions, and drug dependence is established.

Barbiturates carry with them a number of other potential dangers. For one thing, they can impair mental and motor functioning the day after they are used as sleeping pills, thus increasing the chance of work errors and accidents. More important, they can interact in the body with other drugs. As we saw earlier, polydrug use, such as combining barbiturates with alcohol, can be fatal. Finally, barbiturates are the drugs most often used in suicide attempts and in successful suicides (48).

Although nonmedical abuse of barbiturates continues, physicians who are concerned with the negative effects of these drugs have begun to turn to short-term sedatives and other alternatives to replace the dangerous barbiturates.

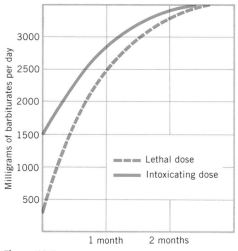

Figure 10.1

Tolerance and Toxicity in barbiturate use. With the daily use of barbiturates, tolerance develops and larger and larger doses are needed to achieve an effect. The lethal dose (the dose that can be fatal) rises more slowly. Thus, during the second or third month of use the two doses become dangerously close. (Adapted from the Department of Health, Education, and Welfare.)

OTHER SEDATIVE-HYPNOTICS

There are several nonbarbiturate sedative-hypnotics that have effects similar to those of the barbiturates and have found their way into nonmedical use. These drugs include methaqualone (Quaalude, Sopor), meprobamate (Miltown, Equanil), and glutethimide (Doriden). Like barbiturates, they have a sedative effect in small doses, and a hypnotic effect in higher doses. They also have the same potential for physical addiction as the barbiturates.

Overdose on downers, such as barbiturates and Quaaludes, has become common among young people in this country. If you suspect that someone you know has taken too many downers, or has mixed them with alcohol, get him or her to a hospital immediately. Signs of overdose include a drunkenlike stupor and passing out. If the person is conscious, try to induce vomiting, and do your best to keep him or her awake so that the physician can induce vomiting and treatment. Do not give the person coffee, uppers, or any other drugs—they will only make the condition worse.

Those who have become physically hooked on downers have found that trying to break the habit can be dangerous. Going "cold turkey" brings on the withdrawal illness, which is very severe with these drugs. Any attempt at withdrawal should therefore be done under medical supervision.

Table 10.3

Controlled Substances: Uses and Effects

Drugs	Schedule[a]	Often Prescribed Brand Names	Medical Uses	Dependence Physical
Opium	II	Dover's Powder, Paregoric	Analgesic, antidiarrheal	High
Morphine	II	Morphine	Analgesic	High
Codeine	II III V	Codeine	Analgesic, antitussive	Moderate
Heroin	I	None	None	High
Meperidine (Pethidine)	II	Demerol Perhadol	Analgesic	High
Methadone	II	Dolophine, Methadone, Methadose	Analgesic, heroin substitute	High
Other narcotics	I II III V	Dilaudid, Leritine, Numorphan, Percodan	Analgesic, antidiarrheal, antitussive	High
Chloral hydrate	IV	Noctec, Somnos	Hypnotic	Moderate
Barbiturates	II III IV	Amytal, Butisol, Nembutal, Phenobarbital, Seconal, Tuinal	Anesthetic, anti-convulsant, sedation, sleep	High
Glutethimide	III	Doriden	Sedation, sleep	High
Methaqualone	II	Optimil, Parest, Quaalude, Somnafac, Sopor	Sedation, sleep	High
Tranquilizers	IV	Equanil, Librium, Miltown Serax, Tranxene, Valium	Anti-anxiety, muscle relaxant, sedation	Moderate
Other depressants	III IV	Clonopin, Dalmane, Dormate, Noludar, Placydil, Valmid	Anti-anxiety, sedation, sleep	Possible
Cocaine[b]	II	Cocaine	Local anesthetic	Possible
Amphetamines	II III	Benzedrine, Biphetamine, Desoxyn, Dexedrine	Hyperkinesis, narcolepsy, weight control	Possible
Phenmetrazine	II	Preludin	Weight control	Possible
Methylphenidate	II	Ritalin	Hyperkinesis	Possible
Other stimulants	III IV	Bacarate, Cylert, Didrex, Ionamin, Plegine, Pondimin, Pre-Sate, Sanorex, Voranil	Weight control	Possible
LSD	I	None	None	None
Mescaline	I	None	None	None
Psilocybin-Psilocyn	I	None	None	None
MDA	I	None	None	None
PCP[c]	III	Sernylan	Veterinary anesthetic	None
Other hallucinogens	I	None	None	None
Marijuana Hashish Hashish Oil	I	None	None	Degree unknown

[a] Scheduling classifications for individual drugs since controlled substances are often marketed in combination with other medicinal ingredients.
[b] Designated a narcotic under the Controlled Substances Act.
[c] Designated a depressant under the Controlled Substances Act.

Potential Psychological	Tolerance	Duration of Effects (in hours)	Usual Methods of Administration	Possible Effects	Effects of Overdose	Withdrawal Syndrome
High	Yes	3 to 6	Oral, smoked	Euphoria, drowsiness, respiratory depression, constricted pupils, nausea	Slow and shallow breathing, clammy skin, convulsions, coma, possible death	Watery eyes, runny nose, yawning, loss of appetite, irritability, tremors, panic, chills and seating, cramps, nausea
High	Yes	3 to 6	Injected, smoked			
Moderate	Yes	3 to 6	Oral, injected			
High	Yes	3 to 6	Injected, sniffed			
High	Yes	3 to 6	Oral, injected			
High	Yes	12 to 24	Oral, injected			
	Yes	3 to 6	Oral, injected			
Moderate	Probable	5 to 8	Oral	Slurred speech, disorientation, drunken behavior without odor of alcohol	Shallow respiration, cold and clammy skin, dilated pupils, weak and rapid pulse, coma, possible death	Anxiety, insomnia, tremors, delirium, convulsions, possible death
	Yes	1 to 16	Oral, injected			
	Yes	4 to 8	Oral			
	Yes	4 to 8	Oral			
Moderate	Yes	4 to 8	Oral			
Possible	Yes	4 to 8	Oral			
	Yes	2	Injected, sniffed	Increased alertness, excitation, euphoria, dilated pupils, increased pulse rate and blood pressure, insomnia, loss of appetite	Agitation, increase in body temperature, hallucinations, convulsions, possible death	Apathy, long periods of sleep, irritability, depression, disorientation
	Yes	2 to 4	Oral, injected			
	Yes	2 to 4	Oral			
	Yes	2 to 4	Oral			
Possible	Yes	2 to 4	Oral			
Degree unknown	Yes	Variable	Oral	Illusions and hallucinations (with exception of MDA); poor perception of time and distance	Longer, more intense "trip" episodes, psychosis, possible death	Withdrawal syndrome not reported
Degree unknown	Yes	Variable	Oral, injected			
Degree unknown	Yes	Variable	Oral			
Degree unknown	Yes	Variable	Oral, injected, sniffed			
Degree unknown	Yes	Variable	Oral, injected, smoked			
Degree unknown	Yes	Variable	Oral, injected, sniffed			
Moderate	Yes	2 to 4	Oral, smoked	Euphoria, relaxed inhibitions, increased appetite, disoriented behavior	Fatigue, paranoia, possible psychosis	Insomnia, hyperactivity, and decreased appetite reported in a limited number of Individuals

TRANQUILIZERS

Tranquilizers are depressants with effects milder than those of the sedative-hypnotics and with less potential for addiction or overdose. The most popular tranquilizers include Librium, Valium, and the phenothiazines (Thorazine, Compazine, and Stellazine).

These drugs are used medically to calm patients with emotional and psychological problems. Used nonmedically, they provide a mild euphoria or high without the side effects and dangers found with other downers. However, they are potentially dangerous when used in combination with other downers or with alcohol.

One tranquilizer that has recently come into vogue is phencyclidine (PCP). Also known as "angel dust," PCP is actually an animal tranquilizer although it is pushed on the streets as a hallucinogen. Because PCP is a depressant, it carries with it the dangers of polydrug use. Furthermore, high doses of PCP are known to have a number of adverse effects, including poor coordination, dulled sensations, feeling of death or doom, paranoia, memory problems, speech problems, and bizarre behavior that can be self-destructive (17).

Phencyclidine is often sold on the street as THC, or as various psychedelics (mescaline, psilocybin), as well as being marketed in pill or powder form. According to *Newsweek* (39), more than 100 deaths and 4000 emergency room cases were attributable to PCP in 1977, a year of peak experimentation with the drug.

OPIATES

The opiates are central nervous system depressants derived from, or chemically similar to, the juice of the unripe seed pods of the opium poppy. Opiates (also called narcotics) include opium, morphine, heroin, codeine, and methadone. Opium is one of the mildest drugs in this class, as morphine is refined from opium, and heroin is refined from morphine. Medically, the milder opiates are used to reduce psychological pain; that is, they reduce tensions and decrease drive.

The potential for physical dependence on the opiates is very high, especially because the method of administration (injection of heroin into a vein) puts the drug directly into the bloodstream (see Figure 10.2). As with other depressants, tolerance develops in time and a withdrawal illness follows withholding of the drug. Side effects of heroin addiction include constipation and constricted pupils. Most of the other physical impairments associated with addiction (malnutrition, sallow skin, etc.) are not a result of the drug itself but of the life style of the typical user. More significant are the disorders that can result from the use of needles, including hepatitis and bacterial endocarditis, which is a fatal disease.

Much has been made in recent years of the dangers of heroin overdose. However, it appears that a large majority of "overdose" deaths have actually had related or several other causes—usually the mixing of heroin with other downers, especially barbiturates and alcohol. Rock star, Janis Joplin, for example, apparently died from taking heroin while intoxicated.

Heroin abuse among young people (ages 15 to 25) appears to be on the upswing in the United States, especially in the middle class. Because marijuana has been lumped with narcotics for so long, and because they have found marijuana to be relatively harmless, many young people have arrived at the conclusion that heroin is likely to be just as harmless. Thus many teenagers are finding themselves mixed up with a drug that is highly addictive, for which tolerance develops quickly, and that becomes an expensive habit. They are also finding

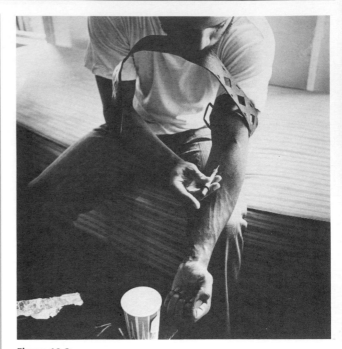

Figure 10.2
A young man shooting heroin (mainlining).

that getting rid of the habit is not as easy as it was to begin it.

Is there a "cure" for heroin addiction? Statistics from various addiction treatment programs give a very bleak answer of those who enter such programs, from Synanon to government plans, a very high percentage return to heroin after having been "cured." Some experts suggest that even after physical dependence has been conquered, there is a "postaddiction syndrome" that produces a craving for the drug in former users (3). One solution to this problem has been the introduction of the methadone maintenance program. Former heroin addicts go to government-sponsored clinics where they are given daily doses of methadone, a synthetic opiate. Although methadone is a narcotic, it appears not to produce the "intoxicating" effects of heroin but rather to simply satisfy the body's craving for the drug. The "success" of such programs is yet to be determined, and they are highly controversial, but they constitute one approach being tried to help the heroin addict become a functioning member of society.

STIMULANTS

Stimulants are drugs that speed up the activity of the central nervous system (brain and spinal cord). They elevate arousal level, mood, and activity. The major stimulants used psychoactively are nicotine, caffeine, amphetamines, and cocaine.

Caffeine

Caffeine is a chemical found in coffee, tea, cola drinks, and chocolate. The stimulating effects of caffeine are mild when compared to those of the amphetamines, but the effect is similar. Caffeine produces slight increases in heart rate and blood pressure, impairs hand-steadiness, reduces drowsiness and fatigue, elevates blood glucose levels, and increases urination (31).

Caffeine has become America's national nonalcoholic drink. We consume half the world's entire coffee supply: 16 pounds per person per year (50). A cup of regular coffee contains 100 to 180 milligrams of caffeine, 6 ounces of a cola drink contains 20 to 36 milligrams of caffeine, and one aspirin tablet contains 15 to 30 milligrams. Without realizing it, a person who drinks three cups of coffee, takes a couple of aspirins, and has a Coke in one day, consumes about 500 milligrams of caffeine. The intake of more than 250 milligrams per day can bring on "coffee nerves"—symptoms such as nervousness, irritability, muscle twitching, diarrhea, sensory disturbances, irregular heartbeat, and decreased blood pressure. Caffeine appears to produce psychological dependence in a number of regular users.

Amphetamines

Amphetamines are synthetic chemicals that are used medically to combat fatigue and depression. They are no longer prescribed to help lose weight. Major amphetamines include Benzedrine, Dexedrine, Dexamyl, methamphetamine (Methedrine), and Desbutol. Other stimulants with similar effects that are not chemically amphetamines include Ritalin and Preludin. The amphetamines "speed" have become a favorite with those who wish to exert themselves beyond their physical limitations: long-haul truck drivers, students cramming for exams, and even athletes. Some people take large amounts of amphetamines (usually in pill form but sometimes by injection) to keep going, to feel high, to counteract depression, and to deal with psychological and emotional problems. Such persons can develop a strong psychological dependence on the drug.

Amphetamines mimic the action of adrenalin in the body. They cause the heart to race at high speed; they increase blood pressure, heart rate, and breathing rate, while decreasing appetite and gastrointestinal activity. A person who is high on "speed" feels mentally and physically charged, and his or her euphoria continues until stored energy reserves are depleted. Then the person becomes restless, irritable, extremely fatigued, and depressed. Headache, dizziness, agitation, apprehension, and confusion replace ecstasy. After having been to the top of the roller coaster, the person has crashed to the bottom.

Many "speed" freaks go on binges that last for days, taking the drug every few hours and avoiding food and sleep. During this period, the user can easily become agitated and paranoid and may begin to hallucinate. Eventually, the trip must end and the person gives in to total exhaustion. The phrase "speed kills" comes from the fact that long-term use of large amounts of amphetamines puts such a strain on all body systems that the heart, liver, kidneys, or brain will eventually suffer major damage.

Cocaine

Cocaine is a drug derived from the leaves of the coca plant. It is used both as a local anesthetic and as a stimulant. When taken internally, many of its effects are similar to those of the amphetamines: arousal of the cardiovascular and respiratory systems, stimulation of the nervous system, and reduced appetite. Cocaine is probably the strongest antifatigue agent available.

On the street, "coke" or "snow" is sold as a white powder that has been cut with other substances, such as caffeine or cheap amphetamines. Cocaine is usually sniffed or snorted, as it is absorbed quickly through the mucous membranes of the nose into the bloodstream. This practice often results in damage to the nasal septum (the tissue between the nostrils), producing a regular "postnasal drip" and periodic nose bleeds.

The cocaine user experiences a high similar to that achieved with speed—a feeling of euphoria, increased energy, and excitability. The drug's powers are intense but short-acting, lasting about half an hour. Coming

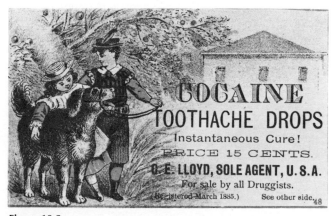

Figure 10.3
An old advertisement encouraging people to use cocaine drops to stop toothache.

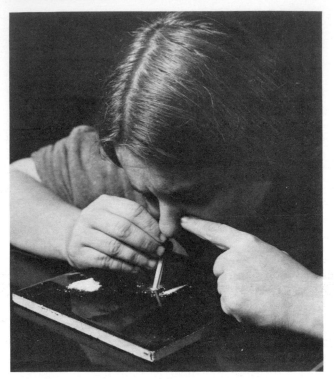

Figure 10.4
What are the long-term consequences of sniffing cocaine?

down produces a depression for which more cocaine seems to be the immediate remedy. Cocaine is an expensive drug and it also produces tolerance, so a cocaine habit can be very rough on the pocketbook. The long-term abuse of cocaine results in loss of appetite, weight loss, malnutrition, insomnia, digestive disorders, paranoia, and hallucinations (see Figure 10.4).

Marijuana

Marijuana ("pot") is a drug in a class by itself, because it is not a stimulant or depressant and is not really a psychedelic. Marijuana ("pot," "grass") is a leafy substance derived from *Cannabis sativa,* or Indian hemp. As a psychoactive drug, it is usually smoked, although occasionally it is ingested (e.g., baked in brownies). Related drugs include hashish (about eight times more potent a drug made from the resin of the hemp plant), and THC (tetrahydrocannabinol), the synthesized psychoactive ingredient of marijuana and hashish.

Marijuana is one of the oldest drugs known to human culture. It was originally used 4000 years ago in China as a medicine, and the poor in India and the Middle East have used cannabis for centuries as an escape from the daily dreariness of a marginal existence. Marijuana has been used in the United States for various medical purposes since the early 1800s and has been used as a psychoactive drug by various cultural groups for dec-

ades. However, it was not until the 1960s that the drug began to achieve widespread recreational popularity. Studies indicate that today marijuana is the third most widely used drug in America, after alcohol and nicotine (see Figure 10.5).

The physiological and psychological effects of marijuana are influenced by a number of factors, including the size of the dose; potency of the drug; environmental setting; interaction with other drugs; and the individual's metabolism, mood, and expectations. Among the psychological effects that most pot smokers experience are changes in vision, hearing, and touch; the subjective slowing of time; floating sensations; a feeling of depersonalization; relaxation; the loss of attention and immediate memory; difficulty of concentration; and a euphoria that often includes giggling and laughter. Common physiological effects include increased heart rate, dryness of the mouth, reddening of the eyes, decreased hand-steadiness, and increased appetite.

What are the long-range effects of the chronic use of pot? Advocates of marijuana claim that it is relatively harmless and cite numerous scientific studies to support this claim. For example, the National Commission on Marijuana and Drug Abuse (Shafer Commission) in its 1972 report to the President and Congress stated, "No conclusive evidence exists of any physical damage, disturbances of body processes, or proven human fatalities attributable solely to even very high doses of marijuana." Recent Department of Health, Education, and Welfare reports continue to support this statement. However, scientists such as Columbia University's Gabriel Nahas (24) contend that there is scientific support for such negative long-term marijuana effects as irreversible brain damage, lowered body resistance to infectious diseases, chronic bronchitis, cancer, and possible sterility or impotence. Further research will give us a better idea of the actual long-term effects of chronic pot smoking.

Regular marijuana use does have one known important negative effect: psychological dependence. Some regular users come to rely on the drug to see them through social situations or to help them cope with daily problems. When they are forced to go without their drug for a while, they become irritable and nervous and tend to become obsessed with obtaining more cannabis. (See any resemblance to the nicotine habit?) Another danger of pot smoking comes from the adulterants that often are smoked with the herb. The most dangerous of these "additives" is paraquat, a herbicide used by the Mexican government to kill marijuana plants. In 1978 about 20 percent of the marijuana crossing the Mexican border into the United States was contaminated with paraquat. Paraquat poisoning may lead to coughing up of blood, difficulty in breathing, and possible permanent lung

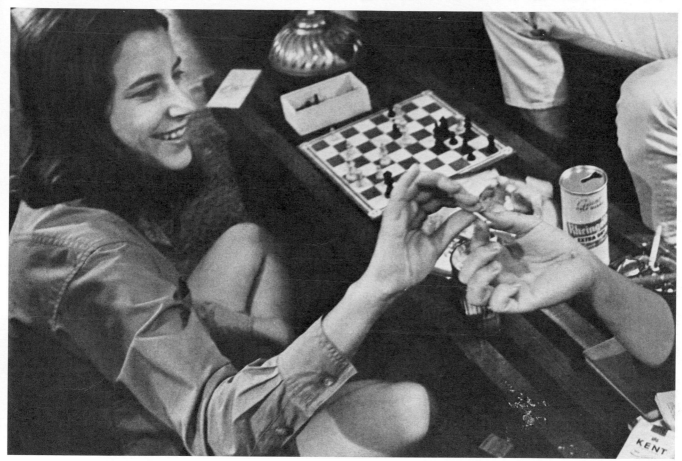

Figure 10.5
A pot party for pot-heads. What is a roach?

damage. The long-term effects of paraquat on the body are not known.

Because marijuana impairs sensory-motor functioning to some extent, those who smoke pot should not drive or take on tasks that require a great deal of coordination. Furthermore, marijuana is likely to interact synergistically with amphetamines, caffeine, and other drugs, with unpredictable results. Nevertheless, the greatest danger of marijuana use continues to be the risk of arrest and penalty involved with possession of an illicit substance.

PSYCHEDELICS

Psychedelics are drugs that produce hallucinations and that alter perception, mood, time sense, and thought processes. The most widely used psychedelics are LSD (lysergic acid diethylamide), peyote, mescaline, psilocybin, DMT, and MDA (see Table 10.4). These drugs are similar in effect but vary in potency and duration of action.

Derived from ergot fungus, LSD ("acid") is a clear, tasteless, and odorless substance. It is available on the street in tablets and capsules or on blotter paper. It is effective in extremely small doses. Medically, it has been used in the treatment of psychosis and schizophrenia, in therapy for sexual disorders, in rehabilitation of criminals, and in easing the final days of terminal patients. Nonmedically, LSD has been used for people who want to expand their consciousness or to experience the alterations in perception known as a "trip." The main hazard of "dropping acid" is a bum trip—a negative experience while on the drug. Such "bummers" can result from a negative setting, the person's mood, an unknown dosage level, or impurities in the drug. A person on a bum trip should be treated gently and should be carefully "talked down." Making the setting as pleasant as possible (soft music and darkened lights) often helps.

The use of LSD and other psychedelic drugs may sometimes result in psychotic reactions and "flashback" phenomena. Flashbacks are the brief, sudden, unexpected perceptual distortions and bizarre thoughts of an LSD trip that occur after the pharmacological effects of

Table 10.4

Comparative Strengths of LSD and Other Hallucinogens (approximate)

Hallucinogen	Comparative Strength[a] (mg)
Marijuana (leaves and tops of *Cannabis sativa,* swallowed)	30,000 (very weak)
Peyote buttons *(Lophophora williamsii)*	30,000
Nutmeg *(Myristica fragrans)*	20,000
Hashish (resin of *Cannabis sativa*)	4,000
Mescaline (3,4,5-trimethoxyphenylethylamine)	400
Psilocybin (4-phosphoryltryptamine)	12
STP (2,5-dimethoxy-4-methyl-amphetamine)	5
LSD (d-lysergic acid diethylamide tartarate)	0.1 (very strong)

[a] That is, each of these dosages has an equivalent effect.

Source: With Permission from Sidney Cohen, "Pot, Acid and Speed," *Medical Science,* Vol. 19, No. 2, February 1968, p. 31.

the drug have worn off (perhaps months or years after the last ingestion). In some individuals, LSD can precipitate serious depressions, paranoid behavior, or chronic psychoses. Fatal accidents and suicide have occasionally occurred with the use of LSD. Whether LSD or other mind-altering drugs, such as mescaline, nutmeg, or jimson weed, is used, the users find such trips unsatisfactory because of such side effects as nausea, vomiting, and diarrhea.

Peyote buttons, derived from the peyote cactus, are hallucinogens that have been used by American Indians in religious ceremonies for many generations. Mescaline is a psychedelic derived from peyote or made synthetically. Like LSD, both peyote and mescaline produce consciousness-altering effects. The main side effect of these drugs is stomach disorders, often leading to vomiting. Another "organic" psychedelic is psilocybin, found in the psilocybe mushroom. The mushrooms themselves are usually eaten to achieve the psychoactive effects.

Among the various synthetic drugs known to have psychedelic properties are DMT (dimethyltryptamine), a drug with effects of very short duration; MDA, a more mellow substance related to nutmeg; and STP, which requires a fairly large dose to achieve psychedelic effects.

OTHER PSYCHOACTIVE SUBSTANCES

In their efforts to achieve drug highs, people have experimented with a wide variety of chemicals. Sniffing of various vaporous substances has become particularly popular. For example, the inhalation of fumes from gasoline and toluene (airplane glue) provides a certain kick. Both these practices can be dangerous: the lead in gasoline is poisonous, while toluene can produce a nausea, impaired coordination, headache, and similar symptoms. Furthermore, many people have died from sniffing

aerosol products because some of these products contain deadly chemicals in addition to the propellants.

IS SUGAR A DRUG?

Refined sugar, or *sucrose,* is usually considered a food. It is, after all, a type of simple carbohydrate, and as such provides energy (calories). However, sucrose provides no other nutrients and is thus referred to as an "empty calorie" food (see Chapter 6). Sugar in various forms is the leading food additive in the United States today. Other aspects of sugar, including its suspected contribution to many diseases and disorders, are discussed in Chapter 6.

Because excessive intake of sugar can alter body metabolism and thereby influence mood (causing both highs and lows), many people consider sugar to have drug properties. Furthermore, sugar produces psychological dependence in many people, who often refer to their sugar habit as "having a sweet tooth." Sucrose is obviously a pervasive part of the American diet and its effects on mood and behavior, as well as on physical health, should not be discounted.

OVER-THE-COUNTER DRUGS

Over-the-counter (OTC) drugs, also referred to as self-medications, are chemicals considered safe for use by the general public when they are taken according to directions on the package. Such drugs can be obtained without a prescription. There are more than 4000 over-the-counter products to choose from, designed to provide relief from such ailments as colds, headaches, constipation, skin disorders such as acne, and obesity (see Figure 10.7). Most people learn about OTC drugs from

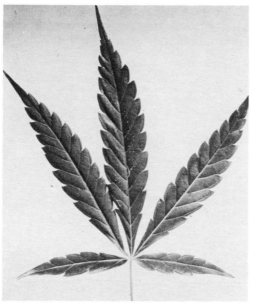

(a)

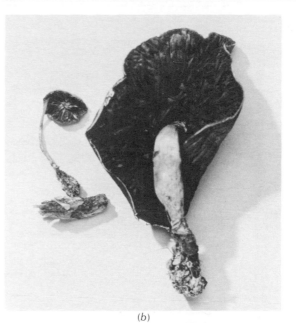

(b)

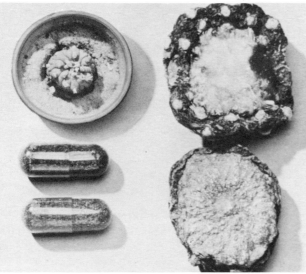

(c)

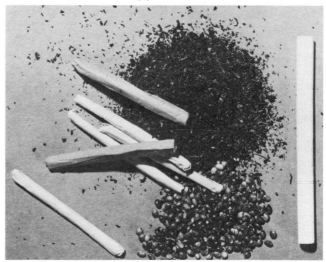

(d)

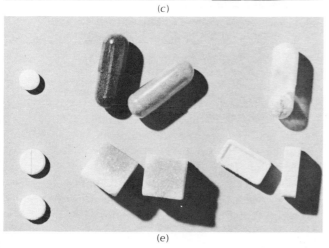

(e)

Figure 10.6

A variety of psychoactive drugs that may be abused. (a) marijuana leaf, (b) psilocybe mushroom, (c) peyote, (d) marijuana, and (e) LSD.

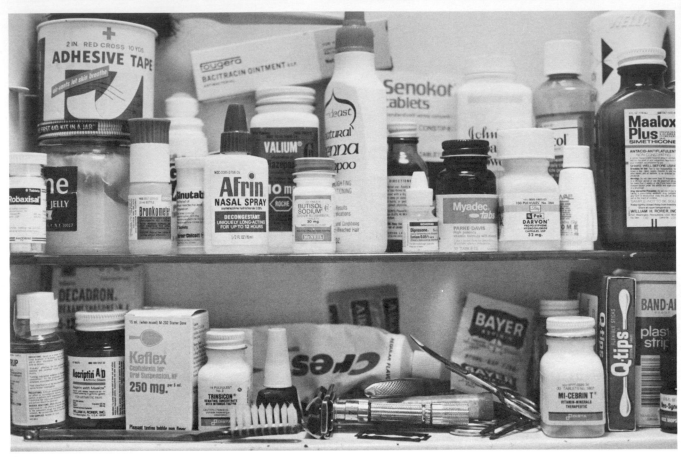

Figure 10.7
A medicine cabinet usually reflects the many drugs that a family may abuse or misuse.

advertising and at home, and on the basis of this information they self-prescribe OTC medication.

There are many problems inherent in the use of OTC drugs. First, most are rather ineffective because they are prohibited from containing the effective doses found in prescription drugs. Thus people tend to take more of the drug than is recommended. For another thing, people may choose the wrong medication for their ailment; taking a laxative when the real problem is appendicitis, for example, can be fatal. Furthermore, people tend to try to put up with or treat daily ailments without really going to the source of the problem. Such ailments are often messages from the body that should be heeded and not covered up. Finally, OTC drugs can be dangerous when taken in conjunction with other substances. Many cold remedies, for example, contain depressants that can interact synergistically with alcohol or barbiturates.

Many minor ailments can be corrected without recourse to OTC drugs. For example, headache and tension can be relieved by regular exercise, and many

disorders disappear with improvements in diet. One common complaint, constipation, can be eliminated through the addition of fiber to the diet and regular exercise.

Some self-medication has a place in our daily lives, but it must be done with discretion. When in doubt, consult a physician or other health professionals about self-medication. Know why you are taking a drug. Participate in deciding on your treatment and ask your physician for alternatives to drugs. In general, take only those drugs prescribed for you or recommended by a doctor. Keep a record of all medications you take. Follow your doctor's instructions exactly, especially regarding the frequency and time of taking the medicine (e.g., meals can alter the effects of a drug). Continue to take a prescribed medicine until it is used up or until your doctor tells you to stop. Never lend prescribed drugs to others or borrow someone else's prescription. Be sure to destroy any "left-over" medications, especially since they deteriorate with age.

WAYS TO MAINTAIN A DRUG-FREE LIFE STYLE

The surest way to maintain a drug-free life style is to fulfill your basic human needs in the following areas:

1. Physical activity (see Chapter 5).
2. Balanced daily nutrient diet (see Chapter 6).
3. Emotional-spiritual satisfactions (see Chapters 3 and 16).
4. Social-cultural satisfactions (see Chapter 4).

In addition to fulfilling your basic human needs, you need to:

1. Socialize with drug-free friends and acquaintances.
2. Cultivate good-quality persons who can help to make you a better person.
3. Patronize drug-free parties, dances, and other social activities.

4. Identify goals and aspirations for yourself and strive to attain some; this will give you direction and purpose in life.
5. Give high priority to experiencing natural highs over chemical highs.
6. Develop your latent talents and aptitudes and strive toward self-development and self-actualization (see Table 10.5).
7. Develop skills for living early in life. These include one basic employment or vocational skill. While working, learn a second alternative job skill as a backup to the first. Other skills of living should include optimal health self maintenance, socialization skills—such as dancing, playing card games, relating to others—and several hobby (cultural) skills—such as playing a musical instrument, painting, acting, flower growing, clothes making, etc.
8. Aspire for optimal well-being and orthobiosis.

Table 10.5
Levels of Experience and Examples of Alternatives to Drugs

A. Physical

1. Relaxation exercises; "hatha" (physical) yoga
2. Dance and movement training
3. Training in preventive medicine; positive health habits
4. Dietary and nutritional training and habits
5. Physical recreation: competitive athletics (especially for *fun*); individual physical conditioning (e.g., jogging or exercises); hiking, nature study, certain outdoor work, etc.
6. Gentle addiction withdrawal
7. Experience and training in the martial arts (e.g., aikido, karate, or judo)

B. Sensory

1. Sensory awareness training (including increased awareness of body position, balance, coordination, small muscle control, and learning to diminish or intensify sensory input)
2. Massage
3. Visual exploration of nature
4. Responsible sexuality

C. Emotional

1. Competent, empathic individual counseling
2. Competent, empathic group psychotherapy
3. Special therapeutic techniques (e.g., psychodrama and role-playing, expertly conducted)
4. Instruction in the psychology of personal development (e.g., in secondary schools)
5. Affective education (including techniques like values clarification, especially in the primary grades)
6. Emotional awareness exercises (e.g., learning body language, honest, open self-awareness; psychological awareness workshops and seminars (especially for adults)

D. Interpersonal

1. Creation of alternate peer groups
2. Competently run, empathic experiences in peer and group process (including group discussion, and sensitivity and encounter groups)
3. Competent, empathic group psychotherapy
4. Various "experiences in being," including interpersonal workshops aimed at development of caring, personal responsibility, confidence, and trust and respect for others
5. Psychodrama, role-playing, and other special techniques (expertly conducted)
6. Competent, empathic individual counseling for interpersonal troubles
7. Goal-directed, positive group activities through organizations such as Scouts, 4-H, F.H.A., school clubs, church organizations, etc.
8. Social confidence training; instruction in social customs, "manners" of human interaction (especially for shy children)
9. Self-examination of relationships
10. Family life education and training
11. Family therapy, family counseling, parent education
12. Premarital and marital counseling and education
13. Temporary alternate families, alternate foster homes
14. Emotional "tutoring" (e.g., big brothers and sisters helping younger people)
15. Creation of community "rap centers"

E. Mental-Intellectual

1. Mental or intellectual hobbies and games (e.g., puzzles, chess, etc.)
2. Intellectual excitement through reading and discussion
3. Intellectual challenge through education: exploring frontiers of knowledge and stimulating curiosity
4. Introspection; analysis of thought
5. Memory training
6. Training in problem-solving and decision-making (e.g., "Synectics" training)
7. Concentration and attention exercises
8. Training in mind control (e.g., "Psychocybernetics," autosuggestion, positive thinking, etc.)

F. Creative-Aesthetic

1. Nongraded instruction or experiential opportunity in appreciation of artistic productions (e.g., music, art, drama, etc.)
2. Opportunities for artistic participation (e.g., nongraded lessons in art, music, drama, etc.)
3. Creative hobbies (e.g., crafts, sewing, cooking, gardening, handiwork, photography, etc.)
4. Experience in communication skills (e.g., writing, public speaking, media, conversation, etc.)
5. Theater games; other procedures encouraging imagination and creative fantasy
6. Creation of community centers for the arts

G. Experiential

1. Self-generated play experience
2. Experiments in sensory deprivation
3. Biofeedback training (e.g., alpha wave training)
4. Sleeplessness and fasting (natural procedures for "intoxicated" states, only with health parameters)
5. "Mind-tripping" (e.g., guided daydreams and fantasy)
6. Hypnosis (expertly conducted)

H. Stylistic

1. Exposure to others deeply and meaningfully involved in nonchemical alternatives
2. Exposure to "hero" figures unfavorable to chemical abuse
3. Enlistment in antidrug or pro-alternative programs
4. Exposure to philosophy of enjoying the *process* of attainment, not just the *product*
5. Parental abstinence and moderation in drug use (parent agreement to cut down to give better example to children)
6. Exposure to philosophy of the "natural," education regarding the artificiality of chemical dependence

I. Social-Political

1. Partisan political action (e.g., helping candidate campaigns)
2. Nonpartisan lobbying (e.g., for ecological projects)
3. Personal political involvement (e.g., running for elective or organizational office)
4. Field work with politicians and public officials
5. Involvement in social service, including:
    (a) Providing voluntary service to the poor (e.g., day care for working mothers, helping to locate housing, assisting access to health services, etc.)
    (b) Providing companionship to the lonely (e.g., companions for the aged, foster children, prison inmates, etc.)
    (c) Work with schools (e.g., student tutoring programs, volunteer teaching assistants and counselors, etc.)
    (d) Work with drug abuse problems (e.g., peer or volunteer counseling, information provision)
    (e) Work in preserving the environment (e.g., recycling, identifying pollution, and preservation of areas of natural beauty)
6. Participation in ACTION (e.g., VISTA and the Peace Corps)
7. Citizen "potency" training (learning effectiveness with government and bureaucracy)
8. Voluntary efforts through organizational sponsorship (e.g., YMCA, Boys Clubs, Big Brothers, etc.
9. Construction of responsible roles in community organization and governance for young people.

J. Philosophical (General and Personal)

1. Seminars and workshops on values and meaning of life (adults)
2. Courses on values, ethics, morality, meaning, etc. (schools)
3. Reading philosophical literature
4. Values clarification procedures; identity clarification procedures
5. Exposure to philosophical (nonviolent) aspects of martial arts (e.g., aikido and karate)
6. Exposure to metaphysical literature and thought
7. Humanistic counseling oriented toward meaning and values clarification
8. Achievement values, for meaningful challenge from career or employment
9. Exposure to individuals committed to varieties of personal philosophies
10. Creation of community "growth centers"
11. Strengthening of ethnic, racial, and minority pride

K. Spiritual-Mystical

1. Study of spiritual literature; increased library holdings relevant to nonchemical spiritual methods
2. Creation of information centers for spiritual alternatives
3. Exposure to holy men of different belief systems; exposure to different techniques of applied spirituality
4. Meditation

5. Yoga (especially nonphysical components)
6. Contemplation and prayer
7. Spiritual dance and song
8. Increased course offerings in intellectual and experiential components of spiritual study (especially college level and secondary level)

L. Miscellaneous

1. Sky-diving, scuba-diving, etc.
2. "Outward Bound" survival training
3. Exploration of new physical environments (e.g., flying, soaring, camping in wilderness areas, etc.)
4. Competence or "self-reliance training" (e.g., vocational and occupational education, instruction in household technology (autos, electronics, plumbing, household appliances, etc.)
5. Family management education (e.g., accident prevention, childcare, money management, first-aid, menu and diet planning, etc.
6. Vocational counseling leading to meaningful employment
7. Accredited work experience through schools (e.g., house-building, merchandising, service station maintenance, restaurant training, etc.)

Source: With permission of Allen Y. Cohen and the National Institute on Drug Abuse; *Alternative Pursuits for America's 3rd Century: A Resource Book on Alternatives to Drugs,* Washington, U.S. Government Printing Office, 1975 pp. 40–43.

BEHAVIOR MODIFICATION TECHNIQUES

What role do drugs play in your life? Answer the questions in the survey provided at the beginning of this chapter. If you feel that you are too dependent on drugs, whether caffeine, grass, or pills, there are a number of things you can do to alter your drug-use patterns. There are innumerable ways of achieving "natural highs" or of finding meaning and satisfaction in life and dealing with life's problems without resorting to chemical assistance. Only you know what activities and interests will help you to fulfill your particular needs and aspirations. Study Table 10.5 and identify the experiences and motivating alternatives that have the greatest possibility of fulfillment for you.

Suggestions for Managing a Drug Problem

1. Find out your motivation for taking drugs.
2. Relate your motivation for drug taking to your human health needs.
3. Assess your human health needs. Which ones are most fulfilled? Least fulfilled?
4. Identify ways *best for you* to fulfill your basic human health needs (see Chapters 3, 4, 5, 6 and 16).
5. Assess your nutrition-eating habits (if you have not done so). Often one's drug problems may have causative roots in one's diet.

6. Assess your living skills. These include skills for a job, socializing, community involvement, and personal growth; development for health, satisfaction, and happiness. What degree of competencies do you have in each area? Relate these to your motivation for taking drugs.
7. Reassess and clarify your goals in life. This should be done each year. Is your present style of life functional, purposeful, and meaningful?
8. Assess your physical fitness and whether you are getting enough exercise regularly (see Chapter 5).
9. *Alternatives to drugs:* You need to discover new and better ways to gain satisfaction and meaning from life. The number of possible alternatives is infinite. The alternatives are readily available in all communities and college campuses. Alternatives to drug approaches and experiences that are relevant to unfulfilled needs and aspirations of the drug abuser or user are listed in Table 10.5. You need to select the alternative(s) that "turn you on" and will help fulfill your needs and aspirations. These alternatives will help you to switch from a chemical high to a natural high.

Developing an interest in more than one alternative is very desirable and practical. Having many such alternative outlets not only fulfills many of your basic health needs, but also makes you more interesting and diversified. It broadens your horizons for living. One philosophical approach to positive living is to maximize your talents and natural abilities along with fulfilling your basic needs. Decide on your immediate priority needs and then map out a long-range plan whereby you can explore and participate in new but appealing alternatives every 3 to 5 years. This way, you will never get bored with life and will always have a fresh outlook on life.

10. Learn to listen to your body and respect its messages (pain, discomfort, nausea, insomnia, etc.). Treat the cause, not the symptoms!

11. Refer to previous chapters (4–9) for alternatives to drugs.

Managing Your Drug Problem

If you are taking a drug now and wish to stop using it, here are a few suggestions to help you:

First 3 days (check immediately to safeguard your health):

1. Take only one drug at a time (avoid polydrug use)
2. Take a dose that causes minimum hassle.
3. Do not drink alcoholic beverages if you are using a drug.

4. Do not drive a car or motorbike if you take drugs.

First week:

5. Eat well-balanced nutrition meals.
6. Get plenty of fresh air and sunshine.
7. Get regular exercise.
8. Ask yourself—do you really need it?
9. Get accurate information about the drug you are using.
10. Contact a drug agency, counseling agency, or your physician for help or more information. You need professional aid to help you kick your drug habit.
11. Make friends with one or more drug-free persons.
12. Assess your life style (see previous chapters).

Where To Go For More Information

1. Authoritative books and journal articles in your campus or community library.
2. Your campus health services center.
3. Your local public health department.
4. Your local substance abuse (drug) agencies.
5. Your health instructor.
6. Your physician.
7. Your local pharmacist.

Further Readings

Fort, Joel, *The Pleasure Seekers,* New York: Bobbs-Merrill, 1969.

Graldon, Joe, *The People's Pharmacy: A Guide to Prescription Drugs, Home Remedies and Over-the-Counter Medications,* New York: Avon Books, 1976.

Ray, Oakley S., *Drugs, Society and Human Behavior,* St. Louis, Mo.: C. V. Mosby, 1978 or current edition.

The Editors of Consumer Reports, *The Medicine Show: Consumers Union's Practical Guide to Some Everyday Health Problems and Health Products,* Mount Vernon, N.Y.: Consumer's Union, 1976.

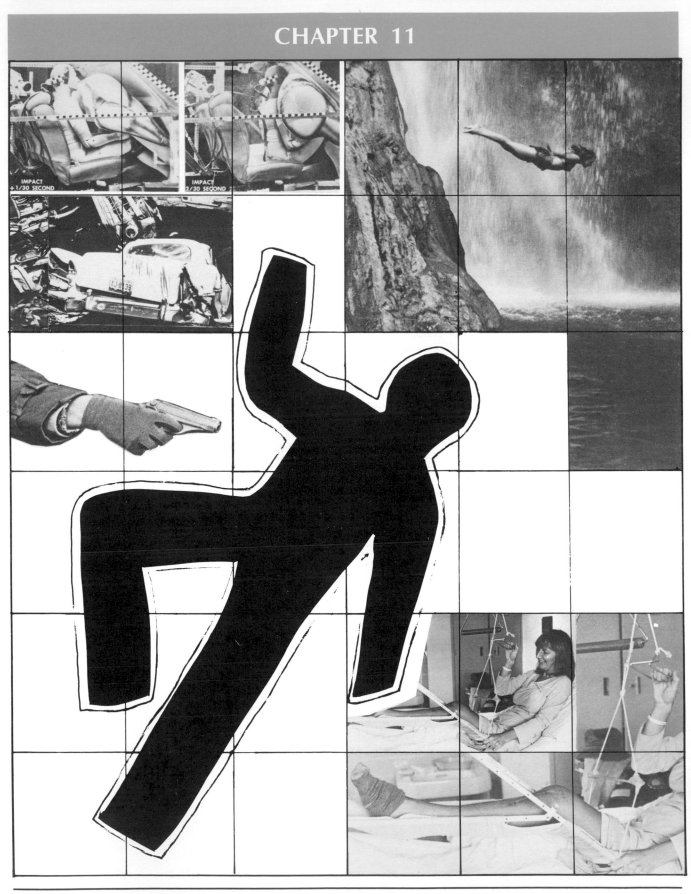

ACCIDENTS, SUICIDE, AND CRIME

The greatest threats to the life of those under age 35 are accidents, homicides, and suicides. These are summarized in Table 11.1. These threats occur while driving on highways and freeways, at home, or in residence halls, at work, in the college environment, and while enjoying recreational activities.

Table 11.1

Causes of Death of College-Aged Persons and the General Population for 1976

Cause	Number of Deaths			Death Rates*		
	Total	Male	Female	Total	Male	Female
All Ages						
All Causes	1,892,879	1,050,819	842,060	888.5	1,013.2	770.3
Heart disease	716,215	399,501	316,714	336.2	385.2	289.7
Cancer	365,693	199,443	166,250	171.7	192.3	152.1
Stroke (cerebrovascular disease)	194,038	84,286	109,752	91.1	81.3	100.4
Accidents	103,030	72,376	30,654	48.4	69.8	28.0
Motor-vehicle	45,853	33,597	12,256	21.5	32.4	11.2
Falls	14,896	7,696	7,200	7.0	7.4	6.6
Drowning	8,000	6,782	1,218	3.8	6.5	1.1
Fires, burns	6,071	3,733	2,338	2.9	3.6	2.1
Poison (solid, liquid)	4,694	3,147	1,547	2.2	3.0	1.4
Pneumonia	51,387	28,514	22,873	24.1	27.5	20.9
Diabetes mellitus	35,230	14,414	20,816	16.5	13.9	19.0
Cirrhosis of liver	31,623	20,830	10,793	14.8	20.1	9.9
Arteriosclerosis	28,887	11,822	17,065	13.6	11.4	15.6
Suicide	27,063	19,622	7,441	12.7	18.9	6.8
Homicide	21,310	16,553	4,757	10.0	16.0	4.4
Emphysema	18,795	14,849	3,946	8.8	14.3	3.6
15 to 24 Years						
All Causes	47,545	35,508	12,037	118.9	176.8	60.5
Accidents	24,121	19,416	4,705	60.3	96.7	23.7
Motor-vehicle	15,672	12,244	3,428	39.2	61.0	17.2
Drowning	2,520†	2,280†	240†	6.3	11.4	1.2
Poison (solid, liquid)	1,332	1,048	284	3.3	5.2	1.4
Firearms	758	681	77	1.9	3.4	0.4
Homicide	5,493	4,258	1,235	13.7	21.2	6.2
Suicide	4,736	3,787	949	11.8	18.9	4.8
Cancer	2,701	1,626	1,075	6.8	8.1	5.4
Heart disease	1,045	631	414	2.6	3.1	2.1

*Death rates per 100,000 population.
Source: Accidents Facts, Chicago: National Safety Council, 1977.

Accidents are related to our fulfillment of the need for adventure. All the things that we accept as being worthwhile in life—love, friendship, loyalty, knowledge, art, music, drama, sports, religion—are adventures in which the human spirit endeavors to experience the unknown or uncommon realities of life. Life is lived to the fullest when we experience the thrill of adventure. But, in the process of experiencing new adventures of living, we often risk life and limb for the cherished benefits of success. Such circumstances are conducive to the occurrence of accidents that often result in injury and death.

The innate need for adventure and something new in life is compounded by tremendous stresses throughout life, thereby creating inner conflicts and frustrations. Most young people bring family-home-emotional problems with them to college. This is a time of life when young men and women are also confronted with facing decisions about their life and work—breaking home ties, confronting new thoughts and values, and clarifying their commitments while searching for a stable self-identity. Academic pressures frequently aggravate these and other problems that young persons have. Collectively, such stresses increase a person's susceptibility to accidents and suicide. Their behaviors often become extensions of their frustrations, anxieties, and stresses. For example, many football players play overly aggressive football that results in unnecessary injuries. Many persons extend their own personalities to their cars, thereby expressing their inner turmoil through their automobiles. Others act out their hostilities and frustrations, while at the same time satisfying the need for adventure by taking unnecessary and unsafe risks while snow skiing, scuba diving, surfing, and so on.

These observations do not imply that one should forego the pleasures of and satisfactions of adventure or driving a car. Instead it is important to recognize the potential hazards of the automobile, sports, and other high-risk adventures, and then take proper steps to reduce the risk of accidents. Related to accidents is crime, in that both are unexpected, unpremeditated, and often result in injury and death; muggings, rape, burglary, and robbery reflect the degree of safety and security we find in everyday life.

Most accidents do not just happen. They are man-caused (see Figure 11.1). They result from violations of rules, regulations, procedures, and courtesies that have evolved over the years as an attempt by man to survive and extend his longevity. More often than not, accidents are symptomatic of disorders and/or the failure to adapt. The occurrence of an accident, or a near-miss accident, no matter how trivial or how serious, is a signal that something—or someone—is not functioning properly. Accidents seem to occur when a number of determining factors come together to set a person up for accidents. The key to escaping accidents is to become aware of these factors. This chapter discusses the leading causes of accidents and suggests ways to cut down your accident risk.

Respond to the Inventory on the next page before reading this chapter. Doing so will help make you aware of behaviors that may increase your chances of having an accident.

15%

Environmentally
caused

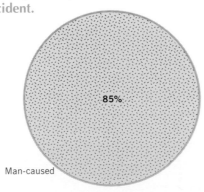

85%

Man-caused

Figure 11.1
Most accidents are caused by man himself.

☞ SUSCEPTIBILITY TO ACCIDENTS INVENTORY[1]

DIRECTIONS   Circle the number in the frequency column opposite the behavioral statement that best describes your behavior or best fits you.

Behaviors	Frequency			
	Usually or Always	Often	Sometimes/ Seldom	Never
A. Recreational Activities				
1. Fly a private plane or glider	5	3	1	0
2. Skydive	5	3	1	0
3. Drive a racing car or dune buggy	5	3	1	0
4. Drive a motorcycle, snowmobile, or power boat	5	3	1	0
5. Skin dive or scuba dive	5	3	1	0
6. Drive on weekends to go skiing or camping	5	3	1	0
7. Board or body surf	5	3	1	0
8. Hunt	5	3	1	0
9. Play body contact sports, like football, hockey etc.	5	3	1	0
10. Snow or water ski	5	3	1	0
11. Mountain climb or spelunk	5	3	1	0
12. Swim alone	5	3	1	0
Total	+	+	+	
B. Vocational				
13. Work with explosives or chemicals	5	3	1	0
14. Work as a lineman	5	3	1	0
15. Work in constructing bridges, high rise buildings, etc.	5	3	1	0
16. Smoke cigarettes in no-smoking areas	5	3	1	0
17. Drive 20,000 miles or more per year	5	3	1	0

[1] The author is grateful to Dr. Bernard Loft, Progessor of Health and Safety, Indiana University, for his reactions and suggestions in the construction of this instrument.

Behaviors	Frequency			
	Usually or Always	Often	Sometimes/ Seldom	Never
18. Work in a noisy environment	5	3	1	0
19. Work with X-ray or ultraviolet equipment	5	3	1	0
20. Work with hot metals	5	3	1	0
21. Work with heavy construction materials or equipment	5	3	1	0
Total	+	+	+	
C. Home				
23. Store cleaning materials, insecticides, etc., in unlabeled or improperly labeled containers	5	3	1	0
24. Store old clothes, papers, paints, or solvents in garage or attic	5	3	1	0
25. Cut lawn when grass is wet	5	3	1	0
26. Inadequate lighting in stairways	5	3	1	0
27. Use long light or TV electric cords	5	3	1	0
28. Smoke cigarettes in bed	5	3	1	0
29. Use underground electrical appliances or extension cords	5	3	1	0
30. Electrical appliances connected when not in use	5	3	1	0
31. Have slippery shower or bathtub floor	5	3	1	0
32. Smoke cigarettes while using aerosol cans (e.g., hairspray)	5	3	1	0
33. Have small rugs that skid on floor	5	3	1	0
34. Do own house repairs	5	3	1	0
35. Store guns and ammunition at home	5	3	1	0
36. Windows nailed shut	5	3	1	0
37. Stairs without adequate handrails	5	3	1	0
38. Use pot holders (towel) to handle hot pots and pans	5	3	1	0

Behaviors	Frequency			
	Usually or Always	Often	Sometimes/ Seldom	Never
39. Forget to replace burned-out lighbulbs	5	3	1	0
40. Wear high heel shoes	5	3	1	0
41. Unable to find shutoff switch for electricity	5	3	1	0
42. Wear pants with wide cuffs	5	3	1	0
43. Unable to find shutoff valve for water	5	3	1	0
44. Unable to find shutoff valve for gas or oil	5	3	1	0
45. Unable to find flashlight or do not have one	5	3	1	0
46. Postpone getting fire extinguisher (or do not have one)	5	3	1	0
Total	+	+	+	

D. Personality

Behaviors	Usually or Always	Often	Sometimes/ Seldom	Never
47. Tend to overlook "doing things"	5	3	1	0
48. Postpone making repairs to car, house, boat etc.	5	3	1	0
49. Postpone paying bills on time	5	3	1	0
50. Get a kick out of taking chances	5	3	1	0
51. Postpone getting sleep	5	3	1	0
52. Feel tired a lot	5	3	1	0
53. Drink beer or alcoholic beverages	5	3	1	0
54. Procrastinate, then rush to meet deadlines	5	3	1	0
55. Difficulty in making decisions	5	3	1	0
56. Trip over obstacles	5	3	1	0
57. Experience failure more often than success	5	3	1	0
58. Worry over your clumsiness and lack of coordination	5	3	1	0
59. Have difficulty seeing faraway objects (without glasses)	5	3	1	0
60. Get mad or lose temper often	5	3	1	0

Behaviors	Frequency			
	Usually or Always	Often	Sometimes/ Seldom	Never
61. Get into trouble with others	5	3	1	0
62. Have difficulty hearing others speak	5	3	1	0
63. Feel you are more important than others	5	3	1	0
64. Driving gives you a sense of power	5	3	1	0
65. Worry over what happened the day before	5	3	1	0
66. Carry a knife with a blade more than 6 ins. long	5	3	1	0
67. Carry a gun or handle one	5	3	1	0
Total	+	+	+	
E. Pedestrian				
68. Wear dark clothes at night	5	3	1	0
69. Cross street wherever it is convenient	5	3	1	0
70. Step off curb when waiting for light to change	5	3	1	0
71. Cross intersection when light is red or amber	5	3	1	0
72. Expect cars to stop for you	5	3	1	0
73. Jaywalk to cross street	5	3	1	0
74. Walk in same direction as traffic	5	3	1	0
75. Walk frequently at night	5	3	1	0
76. Walk after drinking alcoholic beverages	5	3	1	0
Total	+	+	+	
F. Bicycling				
77. Ride with poor or no brakes	5	3	1	0
78. Ride with low or unchecked air pressure in tires	5	3	1	0
79. Ride on sidewalk	5	3	1	0
80. Ride at night without a headlight	5	3	1	0
81. Ride without light reflectors	5	3	1	0
82. Forget to give traffic signals	5	3	1	0

	Usually or Always	Often	Sometimes/ Seldom	Never
83. Ride two abreast on street	5	3	1	0
84. Like to show off	5	3	1	0
85. Ride with handlebars curled low	5	3	1	0
Total	+	+	+	
G. Driving (car/motorcycle)				
86. Park improperly or illegally	5	3	1	0
87. Drive when tired	5	3	1	0
88. Drive at excessive speeds for conditions	5	3	1	0
89. Cut in and out of traffic	5	3	1	0
90. Drive when ill or upset	5	3	1	0
91. Drive when under drug medication	5	3	1	0
92. Drive after having two or more beers or cocktails	5	3	1	0
93. Forget to buckle safety belt or harness	5	3	1	0
94. Drive over 20,000 miles a year	5	3	1	0
95. Carry gasoline in a can in trunk of car	5	3	1	0
96. Drive when signal lights and brakes do not work	5	3	1	0
97. Drive car or motorcycle with engine not tuned up	5	3	1	0
98. Drive with leaky exhaust	5	3	1	0
99. Drive with low air pressure in tires or with worn-out tires	5	3	1	0
100. Drive with mechanical problems	5	3	1	0
101. Drive in rain or icy conditions	5	3	1	0
102. Drive with poor car brakes	5	3	1	0
103. Judgment of distance is poor	5	3	1	0
104. Receive traffic citations or warnings	5	3	1	0
Total	+	+	+	

SCORING   Add all the circled numbers in each section.

Score Range	Degree of Susceptibility
151–520	*Extreme*
70–150	*Average*
0–69	*Low*

It is important to have each person identify those behaviors, habits, attitudes, and environments in his life style that make him susceptible to accidents. This inventory helps you to become aware of your risk of accidents and motivates you to do something about these high risks.

Pay special attention to those behavioral or habit statements in each section that you circled as "always" or "often." These behaviors collectively identify you as having high or above-average proneness to accidents. Keep in mind that scoring "always" or "often" on just a few behavioral statements in a section may provide significant clues in predicting a future accident for you.

It is more important to pay attention to how you score in each section than to interpret your total score for this inventory. A total score for all sections is included although your scores in each separate section are more important.

Confer with your health science and safety instructor about your reactions to this inventory. Select alternative behaviors and habits that will make you less prone to accidents. Another alternative would be to modify some of your habits and behaviors that structure your present life style.

You can avoid accidents and still experience exciting adventures.

Most of the topics covered in the inventory are discussed in this chapter.

ACCIDENTS AND THEIR CAUSES

An accident is that occurrence in a sequence of events which usually produces unintended injury, death, or property damage (1:97). Real accidents are viewed as unpredictable, uncontrollable, and unavoidable circumstances. Although unplanned and unpremeditated, accidents *can* be predicted and controlled. Even natural catastrophies—such as earthquakes, tidal waves, and tornados—may be predicted and planned for.

Accidents should be perceived as an end result of an "accident process" in which there is a causal chain of events, conditions, and behaviors that precede the accident (14:113). A hypothetical example of such a causal chain is contained in Table 11.2. For example, speeding can be regarded as the effect of aggressive driving and as the cause of delayed recognition of a dangerous situation. It is the last combination of efforts, as noted in Table 11.2 by capital E, that directly leads to the accident. It is easiest to identify this last combination of effects, and more difficult to identify the preceding effects as we regress in accident time. That is, one often focuses (as in accident investigations) on the extrinsic environmental causes of an accident and less on such intrinsic human causes as a family fight or quarrel, or other personal distress, such as a divorce or financial, social, or job failures, or a poor attitude toward life (14:32–33).

The leading cause of death for the 15–24 age group is accidents, followed by homicides and suicides. Table 11.1 summarizes how the general population died in 1976. More specifically, Figure 11.2 illustrates that those of age 15–24 have a higher incidence of dying from motor vehicle accidents, drowning, poisonings, and firearms than other age groups.

Since motor vehicle accidents cause five times more accidents in the 15–24 age group than the next two causes of death, the focus is on helping you to become aware of how young persons died in motor vehicle accidents, and the causes contributing to such accidents. Figure 11.3 summarizes how persons of all ages died in motor vehicle accidents. An interpretation of the individual graphs tells us that the 15–24 age group died because of various collisions, overturning, or running off the road. The 15–24 age group died from collisions more often than any other age group. What conditions predispose this age group to die this way?

Table 11.2

Hypothetical Human, Vehicle, and Environmental Causal Chains That Combine in a Traffic Accident

Human Causal Chain

c: Man fights with wife
e: Late departure for work
c: Late departure for work
e: Aggressive driving
c: Aggressive driving
e: Driver speed too fast for conditions
C: Speed too fast for conditions
E: Driver did not immediately comprehend danger of slower vehicle ahead around curve

Vehicle Causal Chain

c: Faulty inspection
e: Worn brakes not detected
C: Worn brakes
E: Increased stopping distance

Environmental Causal Chain

c: It was raining
e: Wet roadway
C: Wet roadway
E: Lower coefficient of friction on roadway
   Human + vehicle + environmental causal chains = CRASH

Source: With permission from David Shinar, *Psychology on the Road,* New York: Wiley, 1978.

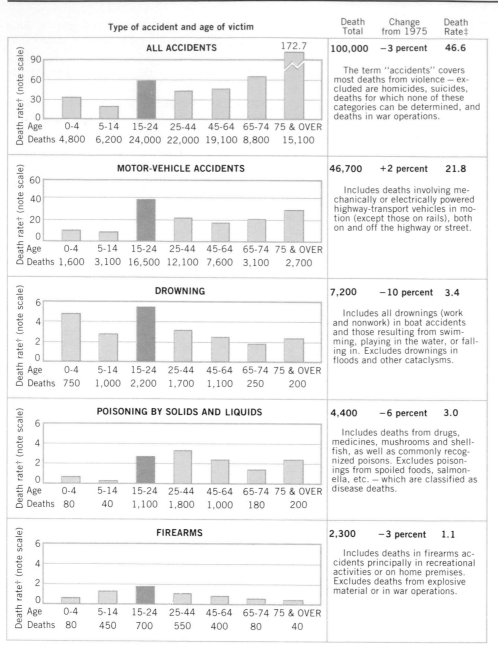

Type of accident and age of victim	Death Total	Change from 1975	Death Rate‡

ALL ACCIDENTS 172.7

Age	0-4	5-14	15-24	25-44	45-64	65-74	75 & OVER
Deaths	4,800	6,200	24,000	22,000	19,100	8,800	15,100

100,000   −3 percent   46.6

The term "accidents" covers most deaths from violence — excluded are homicides, suicides, deaths for which none of these categories can be determined, and deaths in war operations.

MOTOR-VEHICLE ACCIDENTS

Age	0-4	5-14	15-24	25-44	45-64	65-74	75 & OVER
Deaths	1,600	3,100	16,500	12,100	7,600	3,100	2,700

46,700   +2 percent   21.8

Includes deaths involving mechanically or electrically powered highway-transport vehicles in motion (except those on rails), both on and off the highway or street.

DROWNING

Age	0-4	5-14	15-24	25-44	45-64	65-74	75 & OVER
Deaths	750	1,000	2,200	1,700	1,100	250	200

7,200   −10 percent   3.4

Includes all drownings (work and nonwork) in boat accidents and those resulting from swimming, playing in the water, or falling in. Excludes drownings in floods and other cataclysms.

POISONING BY SOLIDS AND LIQUIDS

Age	0-4	5-14	15-24	25-44	45-64	65-74	75 & OVER
Deaths	80	40	1,100	1,800	1,000	180	200

4,400   −6 percent   3.0

Includes deaths from drugs, medicines, mushrooms and shellfish, as well as commonly recognized poisons. Excludes poisonings from spoiled foods, salmonella, etc. — which are classified as disease deaths.

FIREARMS

Age	0-4	5-14	15-24	25-44	45-64	65-74	75 & OVER
Deaths	80	450	700	550	400	80	40

2,300   −3 percent   1.1

Includes deaths in firearms accidents principally in recreational activities or on home premises. Excludes deaths from explosive material or in war operations.

‡ Death per 100,000 population 1976.

Figure 11.2

A graphic summary of how college-age persons and others died accidentally in 1976. (With permission from *Accident Facts*, National Safety Council, Chicago, 1977.)

Traffic Accidents

Approximately 15 percent of all traffic accidents are due to hazardous conditions in the environment. The vast majority of accidents, 85 percent, are man-made. Although it is impossible to precisely pinpoint the reasons for the high rate of traffic deaths and injury cases, we can identify those forces that contribute heavily to traffic accident losses.

Role of Alcohol in Causing Accidents

The drinking driver is the foremost factor in the traffic accident problem. Reports (18:27) coming in from accident-investigating teams, medical examiners, and other sources show that although problem drinkers constitute under 10 percent of the driving population, alcohol is involved in more than 50 percent of traffic fatalities. Hard core drinking drivers are responsible for two-

Type of accident and age of victim

	Death Total	Change from 1975	Death Rate‡

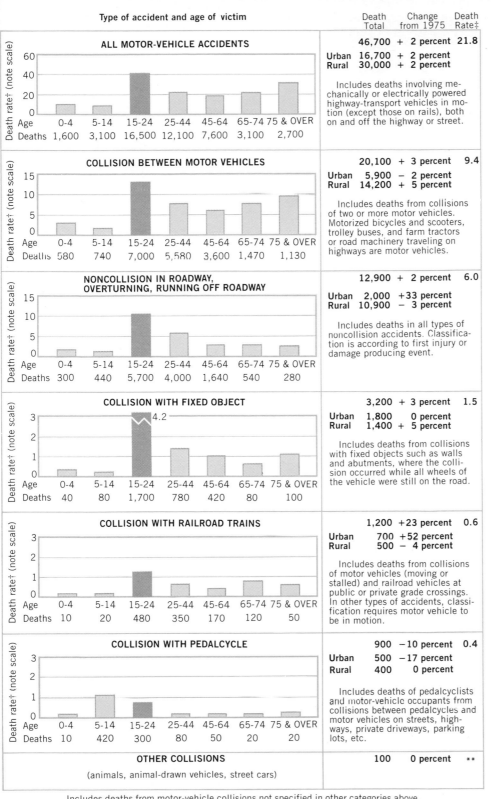

ALL MOTOR-VEHICLE ACCIDENTS

Age	0-4	5-14	15-24	25-44	45-64	65-74	75 & OVER
Deaths	1,600	3,100	16,500	12,100	7,600	3,100	2,700

46,700 + 2 percent 21.8
Urban 16,700 + 2 percent
Rural 30,000 + 2 percent

Includes deaths involving mechanically or electrically powered highway-transport vehicles in motion (except those on rails), both on and off the highway or street.

COLLISION BETWEEN MOTOR VEHICLES

Age	0-4	5-14	15-24	25-44	45-64	65-74	75 & OVER
Deaths	580	740	7,000	5,580	3,600	1,470	1,130

20,100 + 3 percent 9.4
Urban 5,900 − 2 percent
Rural 14,200 + 5 percent

Includes deaths from collisions of two or more motor vehicles. Motorized bicycles and scooters, trolley buses, and farm tractors or road machinery traveling on highways are motor vehicles.

NONCOLLISION IN ROADWAY, OVERTURNING, RUNNING OFF ROADWAY

Age	0-4	5-14	15-24	25-44	45-64	65-74	75 & OVER
Deaths	300	440	5,700	4,000	1,640	540	280

12,900 + 2 percent 6.0
Urban 2,000 +33 percent
Rural 10,900 − 3 percent

Includes deaths in all types of noncollision accidents. Classification is according to first injury or damage producing event.

COLLISION WITH FIXED OBJECT

Age	0-4	5-14	15-24	25-44	45-64	65-74	75 & OVER
Deaths	40	80	1,700	780	420	80	100

3,200 + 3 percent 1.5
Urban 1,800 0 percent
Rural 1,400 + 5 percent

Includes deaths from collisions with fixed objects such as walls and abutments, where the collision occurred while all wheels of the vehicle were still on the road.

COLLISION WITH RAILROAD TRAINS

Age	0-4	5-14	15-24	25-44	45-64	65-74	75 & OVER
Deaths	10	20	480	350	170	120	50

1,200 +23 percent 0.6
Urban 700 +52 percent
Rural 500 − 4 percent

Includes deaths from collisions of motor vehicles (moving or stalled) and railroad vehicles at public or private grade crossings. In other types of accidents, classification requires motor vehicle to be in motion.

COLLISION WITH PEDALCYCLE

Age	0-4	5-14	15-24	25-44	45-64	65-74	75 & OVER
Deaths	10	420	300	80	50	20	20

900 −10 percent 0.4
Urban 500 −17 percent
Rural 400 0 percent

Includes deaths of pedalcyclists and motor-vehicle occupants from collisions between pedalcycles and motor vehicles on streets, highways, private driveways, parking lots, etc.

OTHER COLLISIONS
(animals, animal-drawn vehicles, street cars)

100 0 percent ∗∗

Includes deaths from motor-vehicle collisions not specified in other categories above. Most of the deaths arose out of accidents involving animals or animal-drawn vehicles. Deaths from accidents involving street cars are not yet known for 1976.

†Deaths per 100,000 population in each age group, 1976.

‡Deaths per 100,000 population
∗∗Death rate was less than 0.05.

Figure 11.3

Summary of how college-aged persons and others died in motor-vehicle accidents in 1976. (With permission from *Accident Facts,* National Safety Council, Chicago, 1977.)

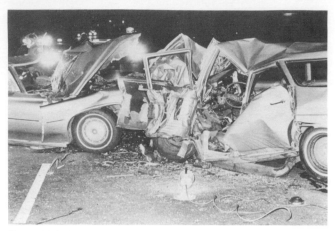

Figure 11.4(a)
Wreckage of cars in a head-on crash. Both drivers dead in this crash.

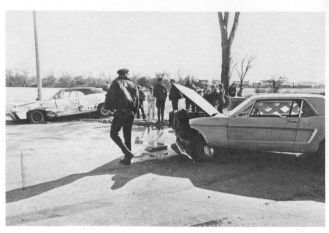

Figure 11.4
A two-car accident that resulted in minor injuries but extensive damage to both cars.

thirds of the traffic fatalities. Surveys conclude that one out of every 25 cars on the highway during late evening hours, when fatal accidents occur most often, is driven by a drunk—not a person who has had a drink or two but by a "drunk" (18:127). The use of alcohol is a major contributing cause of highway crashes. Social drinkers are also involved in auto crashes, but their exact involvement is unknown because of insufficient research. But, social drinkers are not off the hook as far as drinking and driving are concerned. If you drink, don't drive!

The probability of being involved in a crash while drinking alcoholic beverages (18:128) can be estimated from Figures 11.5 and 11.6. The probability of a fatal crash increases appreciably when the concentration reaches about 0.10 percent. For example, the probability of a fatal crash is seven times greater for a driver with

Weight	Drinks During 2-Hour Period 1½ ounces 86° Liquor or 12 ounces Beer											
100	1	2	3	4	5	6	7	8	9	10	11	12
120	1	2	3	4	5	6	7	8	9	10	11	12
140	1	2	3	4	5	6	7	8	9	10	11	12
160	1	2	3	4	5	6	7	8	9	10	11	12
180	1	2	3	4	5	6	7	8	9	10	11	12
200	1	2	3	4	5	6	7	8	9	10	11	12
220	1	2	3	4	5	6	7	8	9	10	11	12
240	1	2	3	4	5	6	7	8	9	10	11	12

Be careful BAC to 0.05   Driving impaired 0.05-0.09   Do not drive 0.10 and up

Figure 11.6
The effect of the number of drinks on responsible driving. The top part of the table, above the shaded area, shows that, depending upon one's weight, one or at the most two drinks, rarely affect responsible driving. Beyond that, the probability of being seriously affected becomes much greater. The odds increase seven times that your guest or you with a 0.10 percent BAC will be involved in an auto accident. (From U.S. Department of Transport., *How to Talk to Your Teenager About Drinking and Driving*, Pamphlet 625-636, Washington, D.C. U.S. Government Printing Office, October 1975.)

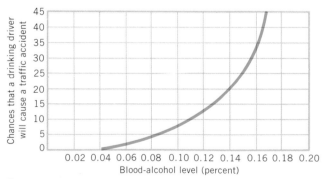

Figure 11.5
Predicting the probability of a drinking driver causing an automobile accident. As the blood level rises (drinks per hour), the chances (risk) of having an accident increase sharply. (With permission from R. F. Borkenstein, et al., "The Role of the Drinking Driver in Traffic Accidents," Department of Forensic Studies, Indiana University, Bloomington, 1964.)

a blood alcohol concentration (BAC) of 0.10 percent than for a driver with no alcohol. The chances of having a fatal auto accident are 25 times greater when the BAC in a driver reaches 0.15 percent. The probability of being involved in a fatal car accident also increases when the drinking driver drives during late night or early morning hours (14:124). Alcohol depresses the brain center, thereby impairing judgment and coordination. This impairment increases the likelihood of being mentally distracted, speeding, and overcompensating to the extent of causing an accident. Alcohol impairs the three main driver functions: perception, decision, and response (14:124). Other drugs, such as marijuana; depressants like Librium, Valium, antihistamines, and even antibiotics, when used alone, may also impair the brain and driving task. An Indiana study (14:125) revealed that in over 90 percent of accidents, the drinking driver committed some error, causing an accident that an alert and defensive driver would not have made.

Other causes, such as falling asleep from fatigue and resultant inattention, lack of experience, lack of familiarity with the condition of the road, being in a hurry, or being emotionally upset, all increase the likelihood of an accident.

The Vehicle — A Lethal Weapon

Although alcohol undoubtedly is the major factor contributing to the cause of crashes, the vehicle itself is the dominant factor determining the severity of bodily injuries once a crash occurs (18:129). Its structural strength, interior padding, seat belts, and shoulder harnesses, and the placement of knobs and projections on the instrument panel undoubtedly determine crash survivorability. The majority of fatal injuries occur when the head or chest hits the steering assembly, the instrument panel, or the windshield. Without the protection of proper "packaging," a rider in a crash continues moving at the precrash speed of the vehicle, and consequently, hits some part of the vehicle at this speed.

Speed. Reducing the speed results in a dramatic reduction of traffic injuries and fatalities. This became most obvious when the energy crises of 1973–1974 mandated reduced speed limits. The higher the speed of a crashing automobile, the greater the number of fatalities. Three out of ten fatalities involve vehicles being driven too fast (18:131). The risk of auto death doubles when the motorist increases the speed from 55 to 65 mph. At high speeds, the car travels a longer distance before it can be stopped or brought under control.

Vehicle Condition. Another major factor contributing to traffic death tolls is the mechanical working condition of the vehicle. About half of the vehicles in use are estimated to be deficient in one or more aspects of safety operation (18:131). These deficiencies are due to normal deterioration with use, improper maintenance, inadequate initial design, or faulty construction. Poor brakes definitely contribute to accidents.

Driver Attitude and Accident Proness. "A man drives as he lives." This idea has been embraced by Shinar (14:32) as depicting perhaps why some drivers are more accident-prone than others. Research (14:32) points out that when one's personal life is marked by caution, tolerance, thrift, loyalty, foresight, and consideration of others, one drives in the same manner and has a safe driving record. On the other hand, an aggressive and emotionally unstable driver, who lacks these desirable personality characteristics, has a much higher accident rate than the emotionally stable driver. Similarly drivers with antisocial behaviors, such as poor citizenship, negative and pessimistic attitudes, have poor driving records (14:32-40). Those with deviant behavior have a high accident-proneness profile (18:133).

Many use driving as a way of coping with, and acting out, their feelings about personal problems. Thus college students and others under personal stress are likely to have dangerous driving habits and, as a result, be involved in more accidents (14:35). For example, during the time of a divorce — from 6 months before to 6 months after filing for divorce — the percentage of drivers involved in accidents was greater than for persons not involved in divorce suits (14:35). The greatest time of accident involvement is in the 3 months following the filing for divorce. This 3-month period following the filing for divorce reflects the high degree of deep emotional turmoil that a person is going through and the likelihood of being involved in an accident.

The notion that life stresses may be reflected in driving behavior has led to the hypothesis that many highway collisions may not be accidents at all, but rather premeditated suicides, or an outcome of behavior patterns reflecting suicidal tendencies. A 1970 study of accident and violation records of persons hospitalized for suicidal gestures revealed that suicidal patients had an 81 percent higher accident rate, and a 146 percent higher violation rate than those of the total population (14:36). Suicidal persons were overinvolved with drunken driving, and reckless and negligent driving, such as speeding and improper turns.

Accident proneness appears to vary according to the length and resolution of personal problems (14:31). Young drivers, in particular, need to change some of their attitude toward life in order to reduce their predisposition to accidents.

Seat Belts. The universal use of seat belts could save about 15,000 lives in this country each year (18:147). Studies show that at least 30 percent of those who died in highway accidents would have been saved if they had been wearing safety belts (18:147). Death in crashes is frequently the result of victims being thrown from the

Table 11.3

Risk of Death and Injury When Not Using Seat Belts

Instant death	30 times as high
At least severe injury	9 times as high
At nontrivial injury	6 times as high
Any injury	4 times as high

Source: U.S. Department of Transportation, *Traffic '72,* A Report on the Activities of the National Highway Traffic Safety Administration and the Federal Highway Administration, 1973.

automobile. Seat belts or lap and shoulder harnesses could have prevented such deaths. Estimates of the chances of survival and avoidance of injury to ejectees (generally unbelted) have been contrasted with the risk of nonejection (generally belted) in Table 11.3. There has been a sharp decrease in traffic deaths and injuries in Australia and New Zealand with the enforcement of mandatory safety belt use (18:147). All drivers and automobile passengers should use seat belts all the time.

Motorcycle Accidents

Driving a motorcycle is a young person's thing. Riding a motorbike provides thrills and a sense of adventure for young people. The majority of motorcycle victims are young people under 25 years of age (18:153). Female drivers have one-half the risk of serious injury of male drivers. The higher incidence of male motorcycle accidents probably reflects a cultural expectation: young men are expected to display daring as a masculine trait and live up to their "macho."

Much of the hazard associated with motorcycles can be attributed to the nature of the vehicle itself. When compared to automobiles, motorcycles are less stable, are less visible to other road users, and offer less protection to the driver in the event of a crash (see Figure 11.7).

The automobile is the motorcyclist's worst enemy. Drivers of larger vehicles do not always see the motorcyclist in time to avoid an accident. Many automobile drivers may be antagonistic toward the motorcyclist. Speed too fast for conditions is a main contributor to motorcycle accidents. The most dangerous driving hours of the day are those between 4:00 and 6:00 P.M. when traffic is heavy and visibility is bad.

The main cause of death is skull-brain injury. Studies show that the risk of serious head injury is 50 percent less for those who wear helmets (18:154).

Mopeds, a bicycle transformed into a minimotorcycle, are as unsafe and dangerous as they are attractive and fun to ride.

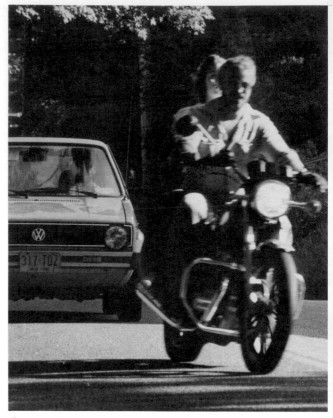

Figure 11.7

The risk of having a traffic accident while riding a motorcycle is greater than driving an automobile. How much greater is this risk?

Bicycles

Bicycles have become a physical fitness status in the United States in the past few years. The dramatic increase in the number of cyclists has brought an equally dramatic increase in the number of bicycle injuries and fatalities (see Figure 11.8). The 15 to 24 age group is heavily involved in bicycle accidents.

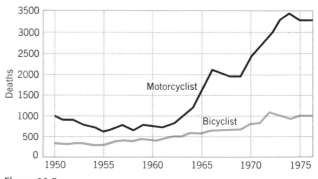

Figure 11.8

Motorcycle and bicycle fatalities, 1950 to 1976. (From Federal Department of Transportation.)

The loss of control is the major problem in bicycle accidents. Other important causal factors are mechanical and structural problems and entanglement of body parts in the bicycle. Bicyclers are most negligent of observing traffic rules and signs, which no doubt, contribute to traffic accidents.

Drowning

The greatest hazard of swimming is drowning. Over 2500 of the 8000 annual drownings, or 31 percent, happened to young people between the ages of 15 and 24. Men outnumber the women 10 to 1. Most drownings are unnecessary. The greatest protection against drowning for both swimmers and nonswimmers is to learn the technique of *drownproofing*. This technique permits a swimmer or nonswimmer to remain afloat for hours without the full use of the limbs, while fully dressed. One learns to control panic and fear and breathing, thereby preventing fatigue and exhaustion. No effort is made to keep the head out of the water, except for the few seconds that a person needs to take a fresh breath of air. One simply thrusts the arms and legs downward to help sustain buoyancy, while raising the head and breathing through the nose and mouth (see Figure 11.9).

Most drownings occur because people do not understand the laws of buoyancy and floating bodies. More than 99 percent of human beings will float when the lungs are full of water. Instead of struggling, all persons should learn the drownproofing technique before participating in water sports or activities.

Homicide

Homicide is the death of a person resulting from violence, such as being knifed, or shot with a gun, or murdered. When a person dies from self-inflicted causes, such as shooting oneself, or from an overdose of a drug, then this death is classified as a suicide.

Homicide is the second leading cause of death among 15 to 24-year-olds (see Table 11.1). Death by firearms most often occurs from handling firearms that are loaded while in storage or while cleaning and showing off with guns. Over three times more males than females die from homicide accidents. Nonwhites have a higher death rate for these accidents than do whites in all age groups (9:94). Most homicides occur in the home. Firearm accidents are related to (1) violence—self-protection, settling of arguments; (2) recreational hunting—nearly all of these victims are males; (3) alcohol—half of

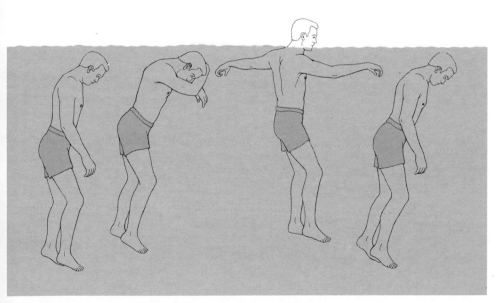

Figure 11.9
Drownproofing technique: 1, Rest just below the surface, letting arms and legs hang limp. 2. Slowly raise arms as if to fend off a blow to forehead. 3. Extend arms and float to surface. 4. After rising for breath, rest by hanging limp under water. (Redrawn after *Today's Health*, June 1969.)

all homicides are alcohol-related; and (4) crime—robbery and arguments over money.

Since about half of all American homes have a firearm, it should be no surprise that next to motor vehicle accidents, homicides are the second leading cause of death for the college-age student (see Table 11.1). Homicide rates are also highest for divorced persons, for widows and widowers, and for all color-sex groups (9:115). Rates in the South are almost twice the rate of the United States as a whole (9:116). Victims are usually known personally to the offender and are frequently a member of the same family (9:117).

The frightening aspect of firearm accidents is that about 50 percent of these accidents occur in situations where there is no intent to do any shooting at all (18:225). Although men are the primary victims in hunting accidents, women are usually the ones shot in the home (18:257). Individuals who purchase guns for self-defense are more likely to accidentally injure a friend or relative than to be called to use the gun against an attacker.

WAYS OF MAINTAINING ACCIDENT-FREE LIFE STYLE

1. Avoid alcohol and drugs that deliberately distort your mental state.
2. Do not drive or partake in hazardous activities when emotionally upset. Anger and lots of distress reduce your ability to protect yourself.
3. Avoid hazardous situations when feeling tired or fatigued.
4. Get ample sleep and rest each day so as to avoid fatigue.
5. Concentrate on one thing at a time.
6. Always plan a new and unfamiliar task.
7. Develop the skills for a new task, sport, or job before going all out.
8. Recognize certain situations and circumstances as being hazardous (e.g., handling guns, playing in street, hunting, or driving fast).
9. Analyze behavior in near-miss accidents, such as almost breaking a glass, almost falling or tripping over an object, or hitting a car.
10. Look for other's errors—anticipate that someone may make a mistake that will require adjustment on your part.
11. Look for changes in routines and in planned situations. We operate on assumptions, which hold up until a routine or situation changes, causing one's behavior to change.
12. Do not gamble against yourself (e.g., jaywalking across a freeway). The odds of a situation should be in favor of keeping you safe and well.
13. Be prepared to unlearn habits (cigarette smoking) that contribute to accidents.
14. Stay physically fit and avoid obesity. Exercise keeps muscles strong, maintains body stamina, sharpens our sense of balance and coordination, and increases mental alertness.

BEHAVIOR-MODIFICATION TECHNIQUES FOR REDUCING ACCIDENT RISK

The information up to now has provided you with cues about ways of reducing accident risks. Keep in mind that most accidents are man-made. This means that you can do something about reducing your own risks.

If you have a high predisposition to accidents (as predicted from your responses to the inventory or you have a history of accident proneness or near misses), then you should try to reduce your high risks. A few ways to reduce your chances of having an accident (automobile and others) follow.

1. *Have accident foresight.* Assess the chances of an accident's occurring before you drive or do something. Are the odds in your favor of being successful and accident-free? Which factors increase the risk?

2. *Take precautions.* Before driving or doing something, make a checklist of what can go wrong to cause an accident (e.g., snow on all car windows blocking your driving vision or a dull kitchen knife causing a cut

on a finger. Doing so will help to make you aware of existing accident hazards.

3. *Assess your personality and attitude.* Do you have an accident-prone personality? Are you emotionally unstable and overaggressive? Do you have a negative attitude toward life? Are you overly cocky? Are you a showoff? Are you inconsiderate of others? Do you have many traffic violations?

4. *Assess your habits and behaviors.* Do you drive while intoxicated from alcohol or drugs? Do you drive while emotionally upset or depressed (as after a family quarrel or divorce)? Do you become easily distracted while driving or doing other things (cannot concentrate on what you are doing)? Do you fail to use seat belts? Do you speed too fast because you fail to budget your time or plan ahead? Do you stop to stretch and exercise after driving for several hours? Do you like to show off while driving, as by drag racing others? Do you smoke in bed?

5. *Control your physical environment.* Are the roads icy or wet? Is vision impaired by fog, ice, rain, or darkness? Is the automobile in good working order? When did you last check the air pressure in the tires? Do you use skid-resistant rugs at home? Are your stairs and hallways well lighted? Do you leave toys and other objects scattered on the floor?

6. *Assess your life style.* Take time out from work, school, or other activities to assess your life style and factors in your life style that may be making you accident-prone. In other words, get "yourself together." The inventory at the beginning of this chapter should have helped you to accomplish this. Ask your friends to help you become less accident-prone.

Identify the contributory causes of accidents and try to change or modify them now. Doing so now may save your life tomorrow!

Where To Go For Help

1. Your friends and relatives.
2. Your instructor.
3. The Local American Red Cross.
4. The local police, traffic, and fire departments.
5. Write to the U.S. Consumer Product Saftey Commission, Washington, D.C. 20207 (concerning product-related injuries).
6. Write to the National Safety Council, 444 North Michigan Avenue, Chicago, Ill. 60611.

SUICIDE

Suicide is taking one's own life. Taking one's life usually means losing the will to live and wanting to die, while the body is still physically able to function. Suicide is the third leading cause of death among college-age students (see Table 11.1). This tragedy afflicts persons of both sexes and every race, color, and creed. Suicides among whites is about three times greater than among non-whites. About three times as many women as men attempt suicide, but nearly three times as many men as women complete the act. About 80,000 young people between 15 and 24 attempt suicide each year, with about 5000 succeeding. It is estimated that about 24,000 persons of all ages committed suicide in 1975. These estimates may only be a small percentage of the actual numbers, since death certificates may not list suicide as the cause of death. These estimates are probably only displaying the tip of the suicide iceberg. Many persons do not die by their own hand but lose the will to live and are listed as dying from natural causes, although their deaths could be considered as suicide or from accidents precipitated by loss of the will to live.

Professional people commit suicide more often than nonprofessionals. Psychiatrists have the highest suicide rate of any occupational specialty in this country, followed by business executives, doctors, lawyers, dentists, and mental health workers. These professionals appear to suffer from the stresses associated with their work and from stresses resulting from great changes in their status.

Among college students, the suicide rate is now two and one-half times that of the general population. Among those who attempt suicide, nearly one-third will try again within the next 6 months.

Male college students most frequently commit suicide by the use of firearms, hanging, and other violent means.

On the other hand, females use poisoning first (overdoses of sleeping pills), then firearms, and then a variety of other means.

The majority of persons attempting suicide do not die from suicide. Some researchers estimate that there are 10 attempts for every completed suicide.

Many would-be suicides give many warnings and clues about their suicidal intent. These warnings and clues are "cries for help." Thus recognizing suicidal tendencies and perceiving impending attempts in yourself or your friends may save a life. Most suicidal persons are a danger to themselves for only a brief period of time (a few critical days). Most successful suicides do not occur in the depth of a depression but rather when the person is improving. This concept is illustrated in Figure 11.10.

Suicidal persons give many clues regarding their suicidal intentions. The first step in preventing suicide is recognition of these warnings (6:185):

1. Depression (this is the key symptomatic behavior).
2. Psychosomatic complaints.
3. Insomnia.
4. Withdrawal or rebellious behavior.
5. Neglect of schoolwork.
6. Inability or unwillingness to communicate.
7. Promiscuity.
8. Use of alcohol or drugs.
9. Truancy or running away.
10. Neglect of personal appearance.
11. Difficulty in concentration.
12. Sudden changes in personality.
13. Sexual anxieties.
14. Deflated self-image.
15. Irritability and hypersensitivity.
16. Temper outbursts.

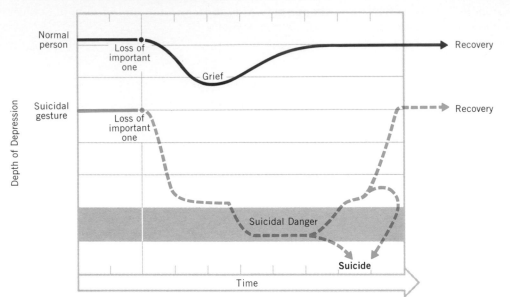

Figure 11.10

Graphic profiles of a normal person and a person with suicidal gestures and how each might react to a life crisis and grief. Note that the vulnerable person regresses into suicidal danger (shaded area). The normal person with good social-emotional fortifications recovers much quicker from grief while the vulnerable person slumps into a more severe depressed state and vegetates for a long time in this prosuicidal state. Recovery is slow and prolonged. Suicide does not occur in the depth of depression, but rather, when the patient is improving. (Adapted from Edgar Draper, ''A Developmental Theory of Suicide,'' *Comprehensive Psychiatry*, January/February, 1976, p. 70.)

17. Hostility.
18. Lack of friends.
19. Extreme parent-child conflicts.
20. Long history of problems.
21. Broken home or disorganized family life.
22. Death or loss of a parent or other important person.
23. Accident proneness.
24. Loss of appetite.
25. Inability to cope with the stresses of life.
26. Sense of hopelessness.
27. Inability to establish close ties with others.
28. Unhappiness—no reason for living.
29. Having a double failure pattern.
30. Having few close friends.
31. Dating opposite sex infrequently.
32. No plans for the future.

Social isolation, withdrawal, and depression appear to be the most important reasons precipitating a suicide. Whether a person with a few or many of the characteristics in the above list attempts a suicide depends on the availability of his or her emotional and social resources.

Meaningful relationships with others act as an essential buttress against suicide and also help to maintain emotional well-being. Persons committing suicide usually have no close friends with whom they can share confidences or receive psychological support. It is suspected that many fatal automobile crashes may be successful suicide attempts (12).

Although the pressures of college alone rarely cause a suicide, they may precipitate it. College students bring with them their parental pressures, their emotional hang-ups, and personal problems. Stresses of college merely aggravate an already existing condition. Consequently, most males attempt suicide during the freshman year (academic pressure), while women attempt suicide most often during the sophomore year (after breaking up with a boyfriend).

Those most vulnerable to suicide (suicide attempters) had unstable home-family backgrounds (6:123):

84 percent of suicide attempters with stepparents felt that they were contending with an unwanted stepparent.
74 percent viewed their family conflict as extreme.

72 percent had one or both natural parents absent from the home (divorced, separated, or deceased).

62 percent had both parents working (or one parent at work when there was only one parent present).

58 percent of all cases had a parent who was married more than once.

40 percent had a parent, relative, or a close friend who attempted suicide.

20 percent of all adolescent suicide attempters had a parent who attempted suicide.

Large numbers lived with persons other than parents (foster homes or relatives).

There was marked residential mobility, an abnormal number of school changes, and siblings leaving home.

16 percent had serious problems with a parent who drank alcohol.

Obviously, the predisposition toward suicidal behavior is laid in early childhood. Poor parental relationships set the stage for later life when socioemotional stresses trigger suicidal gestures and attempts. Family stability is most essential in the development of stable, nonsuicidal persons.

A suicide rarely occurs without warning. Doctors (15) have observed that 70 percent of all people attempting suicide express ideas of self-destruction. They communicate their suicidal ideas to their immediate family members and friends. Such statements as "I'm going to kill myself"; "I wish I were dead"; "I don't care anymore"; "Do whatever you wish, life isn't worth living anymore"; and "I'm no good" should be taken seriously. Such expressions should be considered a "cry for help." Many persons who attempt suicide are not fully intent on dying. They are intent on changing something, to restore a lost relationship, to recover self-esteem, to escape from an intolerable situation, or to activate support and a response from significant other persons. Even at the moment of decision, there is a wish to be rescued, a hope for another way, a counterforce for life.

WAYS OF PREVENTING SUICIDE

You can immunize yourself (and others) against suicide in the following ways.

1. Develop big and small goals—evolve 2- or 5-year plans for attaining these goals. This gives you a sense of direction in life and is a good way to counteract hopelessness, lack of purpose in life, and lack of a will to live. Everyone needs a purpose for living.
2. Learn ways to relieve tension, anxiety, and depression (see Chapter 3).
3. Develop numerous social skills as a way to combat loneliness and withdrawal. We all need to relate to others. A good alternative to suicide is people. "People need people."
4. Develop a close relationship, perhaps even fall in love and fulfill your emotional needs.
5. Become involved in a worthwhile cause, such as working for a political party or an ecology, or health cause.
6. Identify your strengths and weaknesses and learn to live with them. Maximize the positive and deaccentuate the negative.
7. Diversify your interests and activities by participating in various extracurricular activities such as sports, intramurals, dancing, painting, music, hobbies, etc.
8. Begin a self-improvement program. Develop not just your many talents and abilities, but also skills for more effective living.
9. Select a marriage partner with whom you can evolve an emotionally stable home and a loving and caring family. Give your future children an opportunity to become productive, successful, and optimally healthy persons.
10. Evolve and try to live a well-balanced life style that allows time for serious work, as well as play, rest, exercise, and opportunities to recharge your battery.

BEHAVIOR MODIFICATION TECHNIQUES

What can you do if you or your friend have suicidal feelings and gestures (2;3;6:40)?

1. Go to the campus counseling center.
2. Go to the local crisis intervention center (suicidal persons need professional help).
3. Talk to your health instructor or someone you feel comfortable with and in whom you can confide. You need someone other than yourself to use as a sounding board, for determined suicidal persons do not initially go to a suicidal prevention or crisis center. They usually steer clear of preventors (3). A person in the throes of a mental crisis needs someone who will listen and really hear what he or she is saying.
4. Telephone your local Suicide Hot Line or local Crisis Center for help.
5. Socialize and spend time with the potential

suicidal person. Such persons are lonely and need companionship desperately. Do things with him or her regularly, helping to fuse a sense of belonging with others (6:254). This sense of feeling "fused" with a larger entity than ourselves is essential to the maintenance of meaningful living. Also, involve the suicidal person in social, community, and other activities. You may need to initially (figuratively) lead him or her by the hand, for suicidal persons may not be able to muster the energy to become involved. Be definitive by taking the initiative to pick up the person or telephone him or her instead of waiting for him or her to call you.

6. Talk about what you suspect. If you broach the subject, you will not be planting suicide seeds in the person's mind. Chances are good that the response may be positive, and the admission of suicidal thoughts often lessens their impact and opens the door for further discussion. Do not try to talk the person out of suicide; instead just get them to put it off. Talk about a "No Suicide Contract." Express hopefulness and radiate positiveness and cheerfulness but do it sincerely.

7. Get acquainted with, and talk to, the suicidal person's family if possible. Do not confront the family with your suspicions. Merely point out that significant changes in your friend have occurred while in college. This attempt may not work and is of lesser importance than getting the person to communicate with someone who can establish rapport, and gain the person's confidence and trust. Your campus counseling service may include such persons.

8. Write for suicide information to:

> Center for Studies of Suicide Prevention
> Room 12A-01
> 5454 Wisconsin Avenue
> Chevy Chase, Md. 20015

CRIME: PROTECTING YOURSELF AND YOUR PROPERTY

We all need to feel and to be safe from the threat of crime. Violent crimes include murder, forcible rape, robbery, and assault. Property crimes involve break-ins, burglary, larceny, theft, and auto theft.

It is impossible to accurately determine the number of crimes committed in this country. The FBI crime clocks (Figure 11.11) give some insight into the extent of the crime problem. Fewer than half of all crimes actually committed are ever reported.

We live in a violent society and must learn to cope with crime. Feeling unsafe and insecure when walking on the street, or having to lock all the doors and take extra precautions to burglar-proof your home or apartment—all stifle one's potentials for optimal well-being. It is an emotionally stressful way to live. Yet college students must realize that they are easy prey for theft, burglary, and assault.

College students and others should take the following safety precautions, whether living in a dormitory, apartment, or home:

1. Close and lock all windows and doors when leaving or before going to bed, or working in the back of your home.

2. Leave porch lights on after dark. Use a special timing device that turns lights on and off in different rooms at intervals.

3. Report all strangers loitering in your building or strange vehicles parked on the street to the security or police.

4. Do not tack up notes on your door to deliverymen, friends, etc. It advertises your absence.

5. Create an impression of occupancy. Keep a light on or a radio playing where it can be heard.

6. Make a safety check every night before retiring.

7. Ask your friends or driver to wait until you enter your residence safely.

8. Use the chain or bolt on hotel or motel rooms at all times.

9. Women living alone should list only their first initial in the telephone directory, on mail boxes, and apartment house listings.

10. Do not leave shopping bags and attractive goods in the front or rear seat of the car. Lock them in the car trunk so as not to entice break-ins.

11. Tell your next door neighbors when you are going away and when you will be back. Ask your neighbor not to tell others of your plans.

12. Join a Neighborhood Watch program in your community. Such programs are organized to prevent and stop all crime.

13. Walk with a flashlight at night and with another person.

14. Do not hitchhike. Hitchhiking for women is playing rape roulette.

15. Lock all car doors and keep windows rolled up to discourage car thieves.

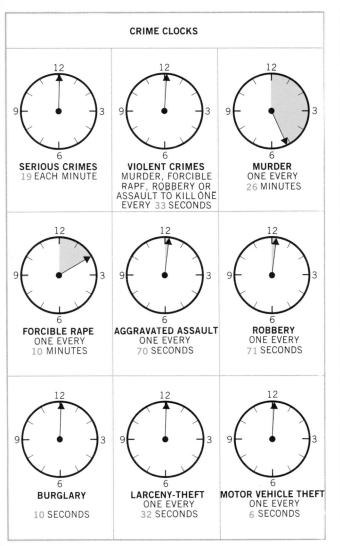

CRIME CLOCKS

SERIOUS CRIMES
19 EACH MINUTE

VIOLENT CRIMES
MURDER, FORCIBLE RAPE, ROBBERY OR ASSAULT TO KILL ONE EVERY 33 SECONDS

MURDER
ONE EVERY 26 MINUTES

FORCIBLE RAPE
ONE EVERY 10 MINUTES

AGGRAVATED ASSAULT
ONE EVERY 70 SECONDS

ROBBERY
ONE EVERY 71 SECONDS

BURGLARY
10 SECONDS

LARCENY-THEFT
ONE EVERY 32 SECONDS

MOTOR VEHICLE THEFT
ONE EVERY 6 SECONDS

Figure 11.11
Crime Clocks depict the variety of crimes and how often they occur. (From the Federal Bureau of Investigation, U.S. Department of Justice, 1975 ed.)

16. Drive to a gas station, fire station, or police station if a car is following you.
17. Do not leave your car parked for long periods at airports or parking lots.
18. Travel with companions when using mass transit.
19. On a public conveyance, sit near the driver or conductor if possible.
20. Give up your valuables without a fight when being robbed—better your purse than your life.
21. Try to escape when assaulted.
22. If being assaulted, strike with a purse, or book, or heavy object at the Adam's apple, eyes, nose, solar plexus, or the crotch (see Figure 11.12).

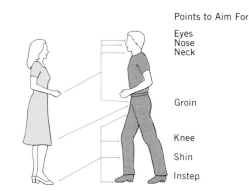

Points to Aim For
Eyes
Nose
Neck
Groin
Knee
Shin
Instep

Defense Tactics if Approached from the Front

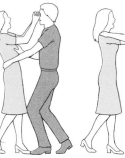
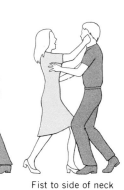

Double fist to bridge of nose   Thumbs into eyes   Fist to side of neck

Figure 11.12
Defense tactics to use when a woman is attacked. These and other tactics may be learned in a self-defense class.

These are all sensitive places. Use the defense arsenal in your purse (nail file, keys, comb, ball point pen) to scratch or rake the assassin's face. Use your heels and shoes as weapons.

Rape

Rape occurs when a man (or men) forces a woman or child to have sexual intercourse without consent or with violent physical assault. Research points out that most rapes are probably planned in advance and premeditated by the attacker. In the light of this observation, it should not be surprising that most rapists strike in the victim's own home, in a college dormitory, or in a nearby street. Almost all rapes involve people of the same race. Women who walk alone on a street between the hours of 8:00 P.M. and 2:00 A.M., on weekends, and especially during warm weather, have the highest risk of rape.

Although rape can happen to any woman, most victims are young—over half are under age 21 (8:18). The so-called date rape, in which a woman is forced to have sexual relations with a man she is out with, is thought to be the most common unreported offense. The majority of all reported rapes involve strangers or a man who has been watching a particular woman and waiting for her to make her next move. There are many reasons why so many rapes are unreported. Fear of family reaction, job security, public trial, and embarrassment are probably the main reasons, although many rapes are also unreported because the rapist is a family member, an estranged husband, an employer, a neighbor, or a former boyfriend.

Most rapists are young men between the ages of 17 and 25 years. The rapist is a person who has difficulty relating to women, as well as other persons.

Although most police departments and Rape Crisis Centers help rape victims and assist with prosecution, there is only a 50-50 chance that the police will arrest an accused rapist (8:23). Furthermore, there is only 1 chance in 100 that the rapist will be tried and convicted (8:23). Reasons for such low prosecutions and convictions are that the information describing the rapist and physical evidence of rape is destroyed, is not available, is out of date, or is incomplete. A woman should be aware that the chances of seeing her attacker brought to justice are very slim indeed. This sense of awkwardness and futility should not discourage a raped woman from seeking arrest of the rapist.

What can a woman do *not* to provoke a sexual assault, a mugging, or avoid rape? Here are a few suggestions (16:1):

1. Mentally prealert yourself to possible causes of action if attacked: scream, yell "fire," tell the rapist you are pregnant or with venereal disease, talk to him, strike a disabling blow or kick, blow a whistle, vomit to turn the rapist off, etc.
2. Heed your survival instincts in dangerous or suspicious situations. Avoid strangers who watch you on various days and occasions.
3. Double-date with friends until you get to know your date.
4. Never allow a man whom you just met drive you home from a singles' bar or party, or from work.
5. Lock the doors in your car when driving alone during the day and night. Check your car before entering it at night.
6. Do not ride in elevators with a stranger.
7. Do not let unscheduled repairmen into your home or apartment.
8. Do not walk alone in the streets, especially after dark.
9. Take a course in self-defense.
10. Contact your local Rape Center or write for information to: The Rape Center P.O. Box 21005

Washington, D.C.; or Women Against Rape P.O. Box 02084 Columbus, Ohio 43202.

11. Help all your male friends to enjoy wholesome, social experiences and establish interpersonal communications. Help mold emotionally stable men.
12. Acquaint yourself with police and court procedures in case of sexual assault.
13. Simulate or role play a rape situation with your friends—so you will be prepared in case you are assaulted.
14. Examine your behavior and habits to determine when and how they might predispose you to be raped.

The following are suggestions of what to do if you are attacked (8:22;16):

1. Drop everything and run—kick off your shoes, blow your whistle, scream "fire" as you run, on the first indication of possible rape. Hopefully, someone will notice your plight and help.
2. If Number 1 doesn't work, confront the rapist verbally, using all the assertiveness and confidence you can muster to counter the image of the stunned, passive victim he needs to maintain to carry out his dehumanizing act. Stare him in the eye and confront him. Tell him to "Get Lost!" Most rapes do not begin with surprise attacks but with periods of conversation, where the man tests his victim (4:26). The proper response can make fighting unnecessary.
3. Begin empathetic communication if the above two approaches do not work or if the rapist has a weapon. "You must have a lot of problems dating if you have to rape women. Maybe I can help you talk easier with women. What do you usually talk about?" Treat him as a human being while, at the same time, regaining your emotional stability. Try to gain his confidence. Try this approach until the threat is over or the man becomes physically aggressive.
4. Put up a fight if he becomes physically aggressive. How much of a fight to put up depends on the woman. Hopefully, putting up a fight will discourage the rapist. Use a foot to scrape down his shin; stomp his instep; punch his eyes, nose, or throat with a fist; punch or kick him in the testicles (groin area). However, you should keep in mind that with certain rapists, any kind of resistance may increase the chances of injury beyond the rape itself.
5. If rape takes place, despite all these efforts, reassure the rapist that you will not tell anyone of

what has happened. As soon as you are safe, phone the police and have your attacker arrested.

There is no unanimous agreement on what a woman should do if assaulted. It is important to remember that a rapist is often a violent person committing a crime. Storaska in his book *How to Say No to a Rapist and Survive* suggests that, in his opinion, survival is the first priority—a dead victim cannot report a rape. Such an outlook does not suggest that a woman give in to rape but instead suggests that a woman should think in terms of saving her life, as well as her honor.

What to do immediately after the rape:

1. Try to regain your emotional stability. Call a friend to accompany you to the police station and hospital.
2. Save all evidences of a rape. Take special care not to contaminate or alter the evidence.
   (a) Do not remove the semen from the vagina or oral areas until you have reported the crime to your doctor or a hospital.
   (b) Save any evidence of the rapist's hair, fingernails, clothes, etc.
3. Immediately call the police and your nearest Rape Crisis Center to have a counselor assist and accompany you.
4. Be prepared to provide information to the police about:
   (a) A description of the rapist—height, age, hair color, eyes, face, other noticeable features, such as his accent, speech, and mannerisms.
   (b) Means of travel.
   (c) How assault took place.
5. Undergo an immediate physical medical examination. If you were raped, a gynecological examination is necessary to confirm penetration. This is essential in proving the crime in court. An examination may be conducted by your personal physician or a physician at the nearest hospital. But it must be performed as soon as possible after the assault. You will be examined not only to confirm vaginal penetration, but also for injuries and additional evidence, such as the rapist's hair. You may request pregnancy and venereal disease tests, while being examined.
6. Submit to a private in-depth interview. The interviewer will help you to recall the incident and detail the assailant's appearance, speech, mannerisms, and visible injuries you may have. These details are essential for identification of the assailant and for the thorough presentation of evidence in court.
7. After the interview, the investigators will review with you possible court proceedings and inform you of assistance available to you at various agencies.
8. Make every effort to communicate with and soften the impact of your misfortune for your husband, boyfriend, father, or brother. You may need the help of your friends and someone from the local Women's Rape or Crisis Center.

Further Readings

Accidents

Accident Facts, Chicago: National Safety Council, latest edition.

Rape

Self-Defense for Women: A Simple Method, Ventura, Calif.: Thor Publishing Co., 1973.

Storaska, Frederic, *How to Say No to a Rapist and Survive,* New York: Random House, 1975.

Tegner, Bruce, and Alice McGrath, *Self-Defense for Girls and Women: A Physical Education Course,* Ventura, Calif.: Thor Publishing Co., 1973.

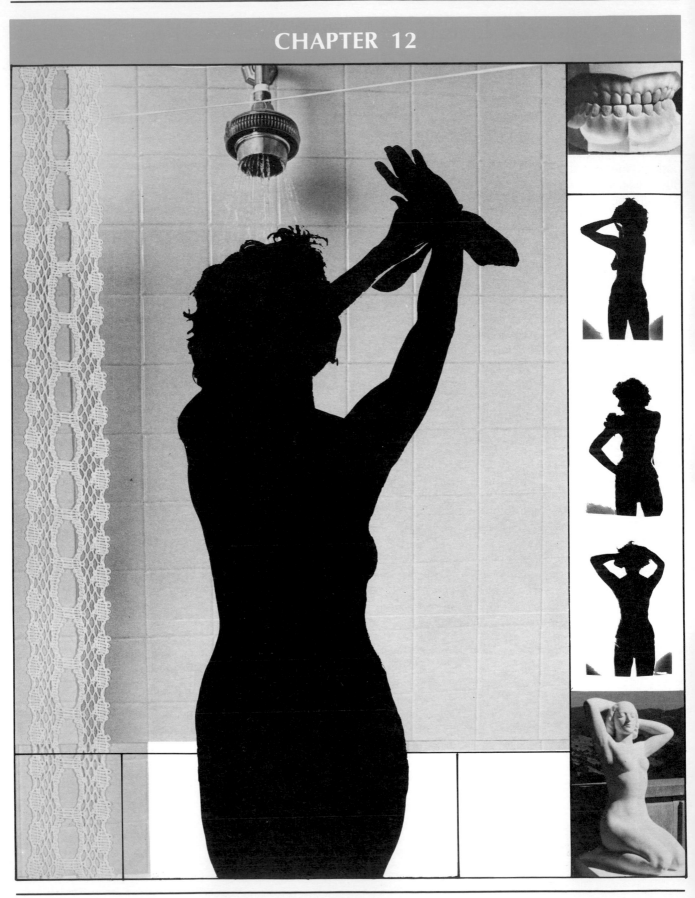

Your job interview is often successful because of your personal appearance and grooming. People notice your outer appearance—they recognize you by the way you look. Your skin, hair, teeth, and clothes make up your appearance. How well you look is a reflection of how well your body is functioning and how well you take care of it. Your skin complexion, for example, is a barometer of your state of well-being.

Because your appearance complements your personality, you need to maintain your body on a daily basis, much like your automobile needs servicing and a tuneup from time to time. A daily hygienic routine not only wards off infection, but is also the first step toward looking good, feeling good, and attaining optimal well-being. Attention to hygiene will make you more attractive and improve your social popularity and self-esteem.

Ever wonder what causes bad breath? Or how you can brush teeth so as to avoid tooth decay? How can you suntan safely and avoid skin cancer? These and other questions will be answered in this chapter.

Respond to the Dental Habits Inventory before reacting to the rest of this chapter.

☞ DENTAL HABITS INVENTORY[1]

NAME _____ DATE _____

DIRECTIONS React to each behavioral statement by circling the number that most accurately indicates how you perform the statement.

Important—React to every statement.

Behavioral Statement	A Always	B Usually	C Sometimes	D Never
1. Brush your teeth at least twice a day	0	5	15	20
2. Use dental floss at least once a day	0	5	15	20
3. Drink fluoridated water daily	0	5	15	20

Behavioral Statement	A Always	B Usually	C Sometimes	D Never
4. Use a red-dye disclosing tablet several times a year	0	5	15	20
5. Visit the dentist every 6 months	0	3	12	15
6. Have your teeth cleaned at the dental office every 6 months	0	3	12	15
7. Brush your tongue when brushing your teeth	0	4	12	15
8. Rinse your teeth and mouth out with water after meals	0	3	7	10
9. Use a soft bristle toothbrush	0	1	3	5
10. Brush your teeth before a meal	0	1	3	5
	Never	Sometimes	Usually	Always
11. Eat sweets and snacks between meals	0	5	10	15
12. Chew gum containing sugar	0	1	3	5
13. Others complain about my breath	0	1	3	5
14. Feel a need to use mouthwash	0	1	3	5
15. Munch food between meals	0	1	3	10
Subtotals				

SCORING:

Total all the numbers you circled in column A and write it at the bottom of the column (subtotals). Do the same for columns B, C, and D. Add the totals for all four columns. This is your dental habits score.

[1] I am grateful to Dr. Robert Prario, D.D.S., to Dr. Ray Stewart, D.D.S., and to dental hygienist Mary Ellen Montgomery, all of San Diego, for their reviews of, and reactions to, this instrument.

INTERPRETATION

Classify your total score into a range below:

Score Ranges	Total Dental Health Practices
136–185	*Very poor dental health habits*
91–135	*Poor dental health habits*
51– 90	*Fair-good dental health habits*
0– 50	*Very good dental health habits*

Those behaviors and habits that contribute most to conserving your teeth have the greatest value weight. For example, brushing your teeth at least twice a day breaks up bacterial plaque and prevents the buildup of calculus. Similarly, behavioral items 2 through 7 and 11 are all important in preventing dental caries. Drinking fluoridated water each day is a most desirable practice. If you are unable to do so, you are penalized 20 points. The penalty is a harsh one if your community does not fluoridate its water supply. But most of us have a chance to vote for fluoridation and should make every effort to support such legalization.

Eating between meals provides food for bacteria in your mouth (unless you brush your teeth after eating and snacking). When bacteria increase because of the availability of food, then there is a possible increase in dental plaque. This obviously increases your risk of dental caries. Everyone can cut down munching between meals. See Chapter 6 for suggestions on modifying eating between meals.

Bad breath or halitosis may occur for numerous reasons. Persistent bad breath may indicate poor dental habits.

Your score indicates the quality of your dental health. You can do something about improving it.

It is important to react to this inventory before proceeding to the subsequent steps of the oral hygiene behavior-modification module. You want to find out the status of your dental habits now. Doing so gives you a baseline; that is, it gives you a reference point at the beginning. You can compare your dental health 1 week, 1 month, and 1 year later with your initial score on this inventory. You can also relate such scores to how successful you were in cutting down dental plaque.

ORAL HYGIENE

Clean, sparkling teeth are the most important part of your face and mouth appearance. Healthy teeth will contribute to keeping you looking youthful. They also maintain your self-esteem, make you feel good about yourself, and help you to mix socially with others. A beautiful smile is buttressed by clean, sparkling teeth. Together they help sell your ideas or products, and make you more socially acceptable. A person's success in life may often be influenced by the attractiveness of one's teeth. On the other hand, dental diseases lead to facial deformities, mouth odors, skin wrinkles, and premature signs of aging. People often view the loss of teeth as the loss of youth. However, with proper oral hygiene and maintenance, teeth should never be lost.

The formation of healty teeth begins before pregnancy. The prospective mother should be on a nutrient-balanced diet 3 to 6 months before pregnancy so as to bolster the woman's nutrient reserves and general level of well-being. Thereafter, the pregnant woman's state of well-being and diet merely add to the preconception foundation for hard, resilient, and healthy teeth. The body cells responsible for tooth production during preg-

nancy need complete nutrition. Permanent teeth, for example, begin their existence 5 months before a child is born and not at age 5 to 8 years (27:117–125;28:83). Dentists have observed that the children of women who followed inferior diets during pregnancy grow up with teeth that are highly susceptible to decay. Once a child is born, a diet consisting of refined sugar-flour foods increases the susceptibility to dental caries. Thus the best way to prevent dental caries is for a prospective mother to be nutrient-healthy before and during pregnancy.

Just as the foundation for good teeth begins with the mother's diet before pregnancy, so good oral care is the foundation for healthy teeth and mouth once a child is born. Almost everyone in North America has trouble with teeth (see Figure 12.1). Ninety-five percent have some decayed teeth, and one in five has no teeth at all (24:160). Millions of persons gargle with mouth washes in the hopes of ensuring an esthetic and pleasant breath, and thereby enhancing their social and love life. It is unfortunate that most persons are motivated to brush their teeth to control their bad breath and not to prevent dental caries.

Dental problems prevail for two basic reasons—ig-

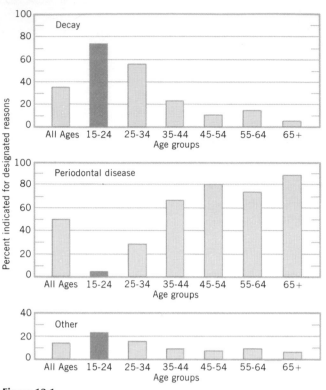

Figure 12.1

Comparison of the incidence of decay, periodontal disease, and other dental problems for various age groups. College-age persons (15 to 24) are highly susceptible to decay or dental caries. The incidence of periodontal disease increases after age 35. (With permission from W. Pelton, E. Pennell, and A. Druzina, *Journal of the American Dental Association*, 49:441, 1954. Copyright by the American Dental Association. From W. Nolte, *Oral Microbiology*, St. Louis: The C. V. Mosby Co., 1977, p. 492.)

norance and laziness — about cleaning teeth. Many have learned ineffective or outmoded techniques for oral hygiene.

There are three basic ways to reduce the risk and incidence of caries in children, teenagers, and adults: (1) reduce bacteria, (2) reduce bacterial food by reducing dietary refined sugars (sucrose), and (3) strengthen the tooth against the effects of bacterial plaque.

Mouth washes are ineffective in reducing bacteria in the mouth and are a waste of money. Toothpastes also contribute very little to bacterial control. But brushing and rinsing the mouth with water after every meal is a good way to keep the bacterial population at a low level and in check. The key to controlling dental caries is the continual breaking up of fertile bacterial areas between and around the teeth and gums. Brushing by vibrating the toothbrush along the tooth-gum line for 3 to 5 minutes at least once a day, along with regular dental flossing disorganizes bacterial colonies. This disrupts bacteria from producing waste acids (toxins), which combine with

saliva to produce strong acids that can eventually dissolve tooth enamel and cause cavities or dental caries. The strong bacterial acids can also irritate the gums, causing periodontal disease. Brushing also breaks up bacteria and stops the bacteria from forming large colonies or plaques (see Figure 12.1). When plaque accumulates over a long period of time, it may harden to become calculus or tartar. Calculus dams up the toxins produced by bacterial plaque, thereby aggravating the gums, irritating the gums, and causing the gums to swell, eventuating in periodontal disease.

Bacteria can also be reduced by cutting off their food supply. Eliminating refined sugar (sucrose) and refined flour products, such as soft drinks, pastries, candy, chocolate bars, ketchup, and desserts will greatly reduce the food supply of bacteria (see Figure 12.2). Bacteria begin digesting sucrose immediately, and toxic acids are formed 5 minutes after sweet foods are eaten. Harmful acid levels build up within 15 minutes of ingesting sucrose foods. Consequently, it is most important to brush the teeth, gums, tongue, and all the mouth and rinse thoroughly with water immdiately after eating sugar foods.

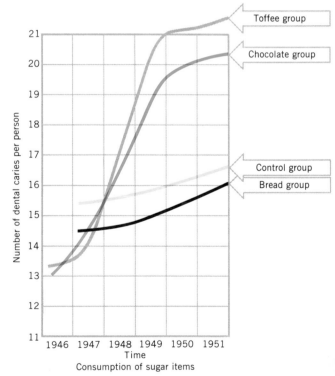

Figure 12.2.

Eating sugar foods increases dental caries. Data from the Cipeholm study. (From E. A. Sweeney (ed.), *"The Food That Stays: An Update on Nutrition, Diet, Sugar, and Caries,* Medcom Inc., 1977. Adapted from Briggs, George M., and Calloway, Doris Howes, *Bogerts' Nutrition and Physical Fitness*, Philadelphia: W. B. Saunders, 1979, p. 547.)

Many dentists feel that one can strengthen the tooth against bacterial plaque. Dr. Aslander perceives dental caries as a deficiency disease and not a bacterial infection (1:44–47). He perceives the nourished tooth as being immune against dental caries. Only nutrient-starved teeth are attacked by disease. Just as mineral deficiency contributes to tooth decay, so a deficiency of fluorine and molybedenum in the regular diet makes teeth especially sensitive to dental caries (1:49). Adequate dental nutrition can be aided by a dental checkup every 6 months and drinking fluoridated water. Adding one part fluoride to 1 million parts of drinking water cuts dental decay in children and teenagers by one-half.

WHAT TO DO ABOUT BAD BREATH (HALITOSIS)

Almost everyone has bad breath (halitosis) at one time or another. However, a clean, healthy mouth gives a fresh, clean, non-odor breath. For years advertisers have taken advantage of this with a barrage of advertising for mouthwashes, breath sweeteners, and toothpastes.

Bad breath may be caused by (26):

Food you eat (garlic or onions).
Tobacco smoking or chewing.
Drinking alcoholic beverages.
A dry mouth and throat, as when you wake up in the morning.
Poor flow of saliva.
Stomach indigestion.
Poor nutrition.
Poor mouth hygiene (sugar fermentation).
Tooth-gum infections.
Infected tonsils.
Lung infection.
Diabetes.
Liver disease.

Brushing with a toothpaste or using a mouth wash may be temporary and ineffective ways of dealing with halitosis. Drinking plenty of water will help control bad breath. If bad breath persists, see your doctor or dentist or both so that you can identify the cause.

WAYS TO MAINTAIN ORAL HYGIENE

1. Brush your teeth properly a minimum of 3 or more minutes after each meal (or at least once a day).
2. Use a soft bristle toothbrush.
3. Floss each day the adjacent surfaces of teeth that brushing cannot clean.
4. Drink plenty of water and rinse your mouth out each time. Doing so reduces bacterial content in the mouth.
5. Do not crack nuts or hard objects with your teeth.
6. Massage the gums each day with a toothbrush while brushing and also with your fingers.
7. Have a dental checkup every 6 months.
8. Avoid drinking extremely hot or cold liquids.
9. Eat a balanced nutrient diet each day.
10. Avoid tobacco smoking and/or chewing.
11. Drink fluoridated water.
12. Do not eat refined sugar (sucrose) products.
13. Assess your oral hygiene habits (for plaque) regularly—once a month.
14. Avoid playing body contact sports that may injure your teeth.
15. See a dentist immediately whenever you have injured your teeth and/or mouth.

BEHAVIOR MODIFICATION TECHNIQUES

You should periodically evaluate your tooth-brushing techniques. It is possible that the oral habits you learned and/or developed while young are not very effective today in keeping your teeth clean and free from dental plaque. The following sequence of steps is suggested to help you assess your oral hygiene:

Step 1. React to the "Dental Habits Inventory." This inventory helps you to assess your present dental habits.

Step 2. Identify and locate the different teeth in your mouth (Figure 12.3). This helps you to score the amount of plaque on a tooth.

Step 3. Study the technique for scoring the amount of plaque on a tooth (Figure 12.4). The red-dye disclosing tablet provides an immediate visual picture of those tooth and gum areas that require special attention. Brushing and flossing the dyed areas until the pink-red color disappears helps to temporarily cleanse the teeth of plaque (see Figure 12.5). This is a temporary removal. You may need to brush more than once a day to disrupt bacteria from forming dental plaque. The more bacteria you have in your mouth, the more often you may have to brush your teeth and mouth.

Step 4. Chew the disclosing tablet (an erythrosin dye-

DENTAL PLAQUE RECORDER

Name _____ Date _____ Age _____

Name of Tooth	Side	Tooth Area With Plaque (Stained Pink-Red)				Total
		0	1	3	5	
Molar	Right					
	Left					
Cuspid	Right					
	Left					
Bicuspid	Right					
	Left					
Incisor	Right					
	Left					
Other	Right					
	Left					
	Total					

A. Check (✔) one of the statements below that best explains the circumstances under which this evaluation was performed:

_____ 1. Initial examination (no brushing or flossing) + disclosing tablet
_____ 2. Brushing alone + disclosing tablet
_____ 3. Brushing + toothpaste + disclosing tablet
_____ 4. Dental floss alone + disclosing tablet
_____ 5. Brushing + dental floss + disclosing tablet
_____ 6. Brushing + toothpaste + dental floss + disclosing tablet

B. Length of time to brush all teeth [check (✔) one]:

_____ 1. One minute or less
_____ 2. Two minutes
_____ 3. Three minutes
_____ 4. Four minutes
_____ 5. Five minutes

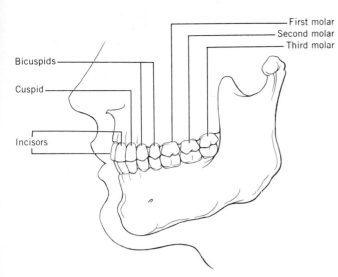

Figure 12.3.
A side view of the locations and names of teeth in the upper and lower jaws.

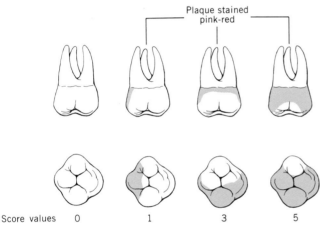

Figure 12.4
Technique for location and scoring the amount of plaque on a tooth. The amount of plaque is scored by the numerical values of 0, 1, 3, and 5. The score values are 0 = no plaque (tooth is white); 1 = plaque found medically between teeth only; 3 = plaque found either on crown (top) of tooth or around the neck (near the gum) of the tooth; and 5 = plaque found on most of the tooth.

disclosing tablet) or use any suitable disclosing solution. The dye stains pink-red those parts of your teeth and tongue that have high dental plaque deposits. Disclosing tablet and/or solutions can be obtained without prescription from your local pharmacy.

The disclosing tablet contains a harmless dye. It will wear off in about an hour, but that is long enough to enable you to assess how well you brush and/or floss.

After chewing the tablet and swishing it around in your mouth for about 30 seconds, you may spit it out or swallow it.

Step 5. Score the amount of plaque on your teeth. (see Figure 12.4).

Step 6. Record your plaque scores (the amount of dental plaque on your teeth) on the "Dental Plaque Recorder." You will need to duplicate a copy of this recorder each time you evaluate your dental plaque. It is suggested that you begin by taking a sample of four teeth on one side of your jaw first; later, you can check the teeth on both sides of your mouth, as well as the teeth in the upper and lower jaws. Identify an incisor, a cuspid, a bicuspid, and a molar tooth. The left vertical column in the recorder lists these teeth.

Step 7. Brush away the red-stained plaque areas on your teeth and gums. Look in a mirror to identify stain plaque areas.

Step 8. Record your dental plaque scores—the *vertical column* at the top of the recorder has the numbers 0, 1, 3, and 5. These numbers are the scores assigned to the amount and location of dental plaque on each tooth. (Refer to the illustration and scoring in Figure 12.4). If your tooth is dyed pink-red and has a score of 3, as in Figure 12.4, then record a check in the vertical column 3 opposite that tooth. Similarly, record your scores for the amount of dye on the other teeth. Add the score for each vertical column. The total gives the amount of dental plaque found on each selected (sample) tooth.

By adding the checks in the horizontal column for each tooth, you get a total plaque score for each tooth. This suggests how effective your brushing-flossing technique is. A score of 4-5 for a tooth means that most of the tooth is covered with plaque. A score of 3-4 for a tooth means that there is plaque on either the crown or neck of the tooth or both. A score of 1 means that there is plaque only on the side of the tooth facing another tooth. A score of 0 implies excellent brushing-flossing technique.

By adding your total scores for all four teeth, you get a grand dental plaque score for each day. This grand score may be plotted on a graph to give you an analysis of your progress in maintaining your oral hygiene.

If an analysis of the recorder indicates high scores for a tooth or teeth, you should concentrate on doing a more thorough job of brushing that part of the tooth or teeth. If the dental plaque does not disappear, then you should sequentially:

1. Brush and floss longer (brush more than 2 minutes each time).
2. Brush and floss more often (three or more times a day).
3. Seek advice from your dental hygienist or dentist.

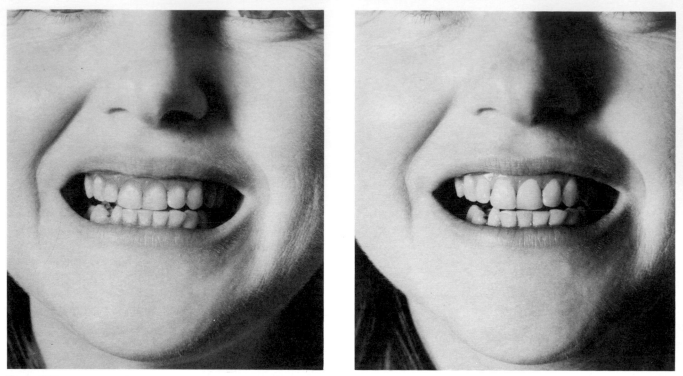

Figure 12.5
The use of a disclosing stain to show dental plaque. Left, plaque is made visible by the stain. Right, after adequate brushing and flossing the plaque is removed.

You should evaluate how effective your new brushing technique is by repeating Steps 4 through 9 each time you modify your brushing technique.

Step 9. Evaluate your brushing technique as suggested in Step 5. Repeat the procedure once a week, modifying or changing your brushing technique as needed to cut down the amount of dental plaque.

A simple and quick check for plaque is to feel if the tooth surfaces feel rough; if it does, then you have *not* removed the dental plaque. If the tooth surfaces feel smooth, then you have removed the dental plaque. You need to brush long enough to remove the dental plaque.

Step 10. Evaluate your flossing technique and frequency. Step 5 will help you to assess whether you are flossing properly and/or often enough. Beside using the

disclosing pill, you can also tell whether you are flossing long enough by the sound the floss makes against the side of the tooth. If it causes a screechy sound, then the plaque has been removed or disorganized. If there is no screechy sound, then the plaque is still on the tooth surface, and you should floss until you can hear the screechy sound.

Step 11. Rinse your mouth after brushing and flossing your teeth, and especially when munching between meals.

Step 12. Plot a profile graph to summarize your progress. Compare each week or month.

Step 13. Modify oral hygiene as suggested by this analysis.

SKIN

Your skin can make you look younger or older than your actual years, and what it does for you often depends on how well you treat it. How your skin looks may also affect your social standing and your popularity with the opposite sex. Healthy skin radiates and glows and makes you attractive and young looking. Healthy skin is very

important to your self-esteem and self-confidence. Let us look at how the skin functions so we can know how to best care for it.

The skin is the largest organ in the body. It acts as a radiator and helps control body temperature and fluid loss. Sweat glands secrete sweat and oil, which keep the skin moist. Skin also acts as a barrier against external injury and blocks the entry of germs into the body.

The skin has special sensory cells that are sensitive to pain, heat, cold, and touch. Often, the sensory cells will become inflamed when overstimulated by chemicals, such as detergents, gasoline, soap, and strong acid or base materials. Constant overexposure to the sun dries out and irritates the skin, eventually wrinkles the skin, and can cause cancer.

Your skin mirrors the state of health of your inner body. A metabolic or physiological disorder of the organs will often cause a rash, infection, hypersensitivity or inflammation in the skin. On the other hand, a healthy skin radiates optimal well-being. As should be anticipated, diet greatly affects the condition of the skin. Fresh vegetables and fruits supply the vitamins and minerals needed to keep the skin healthy. Vitamins A, riboflavin (B$_2$), pyridoxine (B$_6$), PABA, C, D, and E, zinc, and sulfur are essential for healthy skin.

The skin is covered with many organisms, both harmful and harmless, and it has its own way of dealing with germs. On a clean and healthy skin, the harmless organisms synthesize antibiotics against disease-causing bacteria. Sebaceous glands, just under the skin and alongside hairs, secrete an oily substance (sebum) through the pores and onto the skin surface to keep the skin soft and pliant.

The skin has pores to help it breathe. Dirt or covering the skin continuously with oils or cosmetic makeup interferes with the skin pores being able to breathe. Similarly, when the skin is dirty, and the normal proportion of harmless bacteria is upset, or when the skin is damaged, disorders and infections may occur. Without regular washing, the skin can become covered with dirt, bacteria, fungi, and flakes of dead skin that also become trapped in an oily sebum. When this happens, the skin pores become blocked and harmful bacteria can multiply. Infections, such as boils, pimples, and blackheads, can develop. Fungi settling on dirty skin can cause rashes like athlete's foot and ringworm.

Skins can suffer from infection and diseases just like any other body organ. Nearly everyone's skin at some time will have pimples, blackheads, whiteheads, or acne. Acne is an inflammation of the sebaceous glands and occurs most often between puberty and young adulthood, but can occur at any age. Although the cause of acne is not completely understood, it is initially caused by the secretion of large amounts of the male sex hormone, androgen. Acne can also occur in a young female when her body does not make enough estrogen to counterbalance its production of male hormone. Other causative factors related to acne are heredity, presence of cornycbacterum acne, emotional stress, certain cosmetics, and drugs. Foods (chocolate, nuts, greasy hamburgers) are not a cause of acne in most persons; nor are masturbation, sexual intercourse, or lack of it. Although there is no known cure for acne, control is always possible. One can prevent acne by eating a balanced diet regularly, cleansing the skin with soap and water, and wearing clean clothes. Seek help for infected skin from a doctor just as you would for any other disease or health problem. If untreated, acne can leave both psychological and physical scars.

Some parts of the body need more attention than others — especially the armpits, the genital areas, and the anal area. These are regions that contain the largest amount of hair, have high populations of bacteria, and have special sweat glands, called apocrine glands that produce a milky secretion concerned with sexual attraction. These body areas are poorly ventilated, become moist with sweat, and provide fertile breeding grounds for bacteria. The bacteria feed on the oil in the secretions, and their metabolic waste products become oxidized, causing body odors. It becomes necessary, especially in warm weather, to wash these areas so that trapped skin moisture does not allow rashes to occur.

How often you bathe or shower depends on your rate of sweating, your level of activity, the weather, the "dustiness" of your environment, and how you dress. It usually takes about 8 to 10 hours before enough sweat is excreted (in the armpits) for bacteria to produce enough waste so that body odors are detectable. When body odors are detectable, you can use a deodorant that contains an antibiotic that kills the odor-producing bacteria, as well as a perfume to mask the odors. Antiperspirants are even more effective against body odor because they contain aluminum or zinc salts that block sweat ducts and slow down the rate at which bacteria multiply. Some persons may be allergic to the chemicals in soaps, deodorants, and antiperspirants. A person should not rely on perfumes, deodorants, or antiperspirants to control body odors for too long. There is no substitute for bathing or showering with soap at least once a day. Hands should be washed before handling and preparing food, and after going to a lavatory.

Genital skin in males and females produce a white, cheesy substance called smegma (see Figure 12.6). A waste product of skin, it accumulates under the foreskin and behind the glans on the male penis. Men should retract the foreskin (prepuce) and wash the accumulated smegma away each day. Smegma does not accumulate in circumcised males.

Smegma may also accumulate under the clitoral margins or between the labia minora and majora in women. The vagina normally discharges a small amount of clear, white substance each day. This is a natural cleansing action.

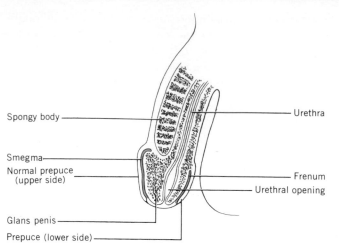

Spongy body

Smegma

Normal prepuce
(upper side)

Glans penis

Prepuce (lower side)

Urethra

Frenum

Urethral opening

Figure 12.6
Smegma excreted under the prepuce of the penis. (Ref. Health by J. Mayer, p. 113.)

Daily washing with soap and water is the best way to keep the vulva and genital area clean. Vaginal douches should not be necessary if the woman washes the genital area with soap and water each day. Vaginal deodorants often irritate the vaginal area, causing vaginitis.

Healthy skin on all parts of the body perspires. Undergarments and socks absorb perspiration. Clothing next to the skin should be changed daily to minimize unpleasant body odors, and to avoid fungal or bacterial infections. Bed sheets and night clothes should also be changed often. Cotton socks are good sweat absorbers but need to be changed daily if one is to avoid athlete's foot.

Fingernails and toenails are made of keratin, a protein substance. The average nail grows about 0.3 centimeters (0.1 inch) a month. Nails are extensions of the skin and protect the ends of our extremities. The condition of your nails reflects your general state of health, as well as your diet. Brittle nails may mean that you are not getting enough calcium and sulfur in your diet. Excessive use of nail polish remover and strong soaps and detergents may tend to dry out nails and cause layers to separate.

Many women use cosmetics. Such beauty aids as lipstick, face powder, eye shadow, mascara, and so on, are not good for the skin. Many cosmetics have an oil base and plug up skin pores, causing rashes and acne cosmetica. If you must use beauty aids, use water-based cosmetics.

Each woman should remember that she has natural beauty. It should be mentally satisfying to know that a woman's natural beauty is long-lasting and genuine, as compared to superficial makeup beauty. Sound nutrition and daily skin and body care are the best ways to have attractive and healthy skin.

SUNBURN, AGING, AND SKIN CANCER

Many young persons are sun worshippers. They like to go snow skiing on the sunny mountain slopes in the winter, or play and bask in the sun during the summer. Although discrete tanning brings on a feeling of well-being and enhances one's appearance, continued overexposure to sunlight can cause skin burn, wrinkling, premature aging of the skin, and skin cancer. Suntanning causes the skin to synthesize the protective dark pigment melanin. Melanin gives one a dark skin and screens the dangerous ultraviolet rays that burn the skin. Those most susceptible to sunburns and skin cancer have light skin, blue eyes, light hair, freckles, and skin that is hypersensitive to ultraviolet light (sun). (see Figure 12.7.)

To avoid sunburn and reduce the risk of sunburn and skin cancer, you should (29):

1. Stay out of the noonday sun—go out before 10 A.M. or after 2 P.M.
2. Build up a tan gradually without burning.
3. Have short exposures to the sun until a tan is developed.
4. Begin with a 15-minute exposure the first day and increase the time thereafter—not over 5 minutes each day.
5. Expose all parts of your body gradually so that the face and back does not get the full blast.
6. Be aware that ultraviolet rays are reflected from the sand and water and can cause a sunburn even though you may be under a sunshade.
7. Use a practical ultraviolet screen or suntan lotion. The best screening lotions contain PABA.
8. Eat a balanced, nutritious diet that contains high amounts of vitamins B_6, PABA, A, C, E, and zinc. Upon exposure to the sun, the skin can synthesize vitamin D.
9. Cover up after a moderate exposure to the sun.
10. Do *not* apply baby or olive oil, as these oils increase the damage to the skin.
11. Reapply suntan lotion often, especially if you perspire a lot or go for a swim (the protective lotion will rinse off).

HAIR

Hair covers all parts of the body, except for the lips, palms of the hands, soles of the feet, and the external genitalia. Most of the hair is so fine that it is virtually invisible. Body hair is thought to act as a protective cover and helps keep the body warm and somewhat moist.

Women in North America are very conscious of being attractive and beautiful. They shave the hair on their

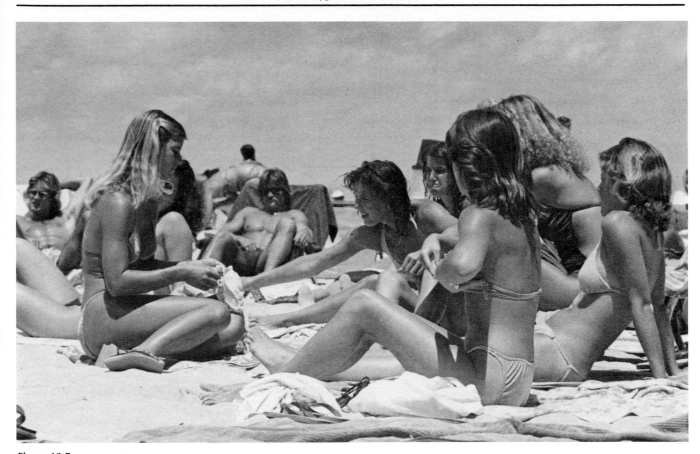

Figure 12.7
Suntanning. What kind of suntan lotion should the people in this photo use? How much sun exposure per day should one receive?

legs, often causing skin rashes and infections. Excess hair, or hirsutism, is hereditary, and only electrolysis (burning of hair papilla with an electric needle inserted into each hair follicle) is permanent. Electrolysis is a tedious, expensive, and uncomfortable process and can cause permanent scars. It is not recommended.

Most of the body hair is on the scalp. Scalp hair reflects the general state of your health and diet. Growing at a rate of about half-an-inch (1.25 centimeters) a month, it drops out after 3 years. About 100 hairs a day are shed from the scalp, and all are normally replaced by new ones.

The best way to maintain a head of healthy hair is to keep it clean. Daily brushing and scalp massage with the fingertips removes dust and dirt, spreads oil along the hair shaft, and stimulates blood circulation. However, over-vigorous brushing will damage the hair cuticle and break it. Another way to damage hair is by washing it with alkaline soaps or shampoos. Too much sea, sun, chlorinated pool water, bleaching and coloring, as well as permanent waving will break down the keratin pro-

tein into smaller peptide and amino acids that wash away, causing the loss of hair strength and elasticity. The ends of hair shafts also split so that hair ends look frizzy.

Hair should be washed every 4 to 10 days; oily or greasy and dirty hair needs to be washed more frequently. Use a shampoo, rather than a soap which tends to produce a scum and kill the glossy appearance of hair.

Always clean your brush and comb when you wash your hair.

Many people suffer from dandruff, flakes of dead greasy skin. Dandruff is caused by overactive or underactive oil-producing (sebaceous) glands in the scalp. It can usually be treated successfully by washing the hair several times a week with medicated shampoo until the condition clears up.

Many people put hair lotions and oil dressings on their hair, which tend to clog up the openings of the glands and encourage dandruff.

Baldness is usually inherited and affected by the male sex hormone testosterone. Many men and some women

291

suffer from baldness. Baldness in women is commonly the result of some disease that destroys the hair follicles. It can also be brought about by injury to the hair follicles —by excessive bleaching, pulling the hair into tight ponytails, or using curlers.

WAYS TO MAINTAIN YOUR SKIN AND HAIR

The best beauty and cosmetic care for healthy skin and hair is dependent on good hygienic habits:

1. Eating a well-balanced nutritious diet.
2. Getting lots of exercise.
3. Getting plenty of fresh air.
4. Massaging to promote blood circulation.
5. Getting intermittent rest.
6. Getting plenty of sleep.
7. Having frequent and regular washings.
8. Avoiding overexposure to the sun.
9. Avoiding exposure to toxic chemicals and X-rays.

WHERE TO GO FOR INFORMATION

1. Local public health department.
2. Campus health services.
3. A local dermatologist.
4. Your dentist.

CONTROVERSY □ CELLULITE

Eight out of ten women of all weights and ages are marred by unattractive, dimpled, rippling masses of flabby skin just below the skin surface (22:17). These unsightly and embarassing lumps and skin ripples ruin a woman's figure, mar her appearance, destroy her self-confidence, and can even cause depression (see Figure 12.8). Such women cannot wear clothes they like, and are embarrassed to go to a beach, play sports, or appear in front of a husband or lover without feeling ugly and unattractive. Nicol Ronsard describes this skin disorder as cellulite (22). This skin disorder is nature's way of telling a woman that her life style is threatening her well-being.

Although the condition of cellulite is very controversial in this country, research in Sweden and Europe has added credulence to cellulite (30). Dr. George Bray[1] (30), professor of medicine at the University of California, Los Angeles, and an authority on obesity, explains the disorder as probably arising when fat deposits in the various skin areas are removed at slower rates than from other body areas. Nicol Ronsard, in her book *Cellulite* (1978), perceives cellulite as being formed when the waste removal process of the body is slowed down in cellulite-prone areas, such as the thighs, hips, abdomen, knees, and ankles. As a result, connective tissue get saturated with water and wastes. Wastes seem to be locked into the connective tissue. The whole water-waste connective tissue thickens, hardens, and forms pockets that bulge and give the skin a ripple or orange peel texture. These pockets of "fat-gone-wrong" act like sponges to absorb more water, causing the affected skin area to blow up and bulge.

Although medical doctors may have difficulty recognizing and treating cellulite, women in everyday life can easily distinguish cellulite from fat. Squeeze the skin tissue between the thumb and index finger or between the palms of both hands. Regular fat, when squeezed, is smooth in texture. Cellulite skin ripples and looks like an orange peel and is sensitive. In the advanced stage, cellulite skin is flabby (see Figure 11.1).

Many conditions are suspected of contributing to the cellulite disorder. The female hormone, estrogen, causes body tissues to retain water, indirectly contributing to the disorder. Women, using birth control pills (estrogen) aggravate cellulite. Emotional tension and stress can also initiate this disorder. In general, neglect of the body, as exemplified by such poor health habits as the lack of continuous physical activity; excessive ingestion of alcohol, tea, coffee, cola drinks, chocolate, fats and fried

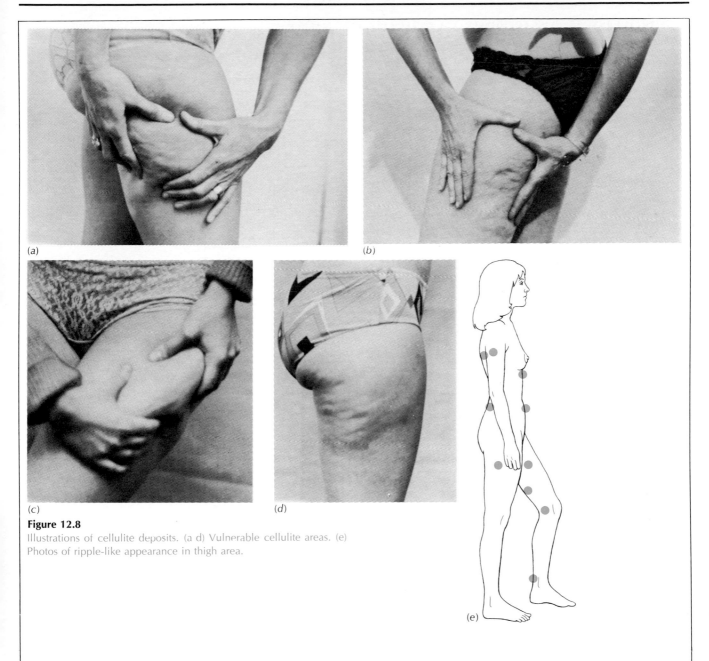

Figure 12.8
Illustrations of cellulite deposits. (a d) Vulnerable cellulite areas. (e)
Photos of ripple-like appearance in thigh area.

foods; too many pills and medications; and cigarette smoking all contribute waste products that can be deposited in connective tissue when the circulatory and excretory systems are sluggish. Cellulite appears after the body has been abused for some time by a faulty life style. All women are especially prone to this condition.

How susceptible are you to cellulite? You can look at your naked body in a mirror and examine your skin for ripples and flabbiness. You may want to confirm your observations by responding to the inventory that follows. It will help you to assess your predisposition to cellulite.

[1] Private communication with Dr. George A. Bray, Professor of Medicine at UCLA School of Medicine: "The basic observation is that the rate at which fat depots are removed from some regions of the body is faster than others. Moreover, the influence of various hormones in fat mobilization differs with fat from different parts of the body. Thus, today, I have to conclude that there are important regional metabolic differences in fat, which might be called cellulite." (January 19, 1979).

CONTROVERSY □ SUSCEPTIBILITY TO CELLULITE INVENTORY

DIRECTIONS   Check the column that best describes your behavior.

	10 Always	7 Often	3 Sometimes	0 Never
1. How often do you eat the following foods?				
Refined white sugar (sucrose)				
Puddings and pies				
Pastry and cookies				
White bread				
Canned foods (peas, corn, etc.)				
Ketchup				
Salt food on your plate				
Fats (cream, butter, margarine, and dips)				
Pork (sausage and bacon)				
Cold meats (hot dogs and sausage)				
Sundaes, ice cream, and milkshakes				
Salted nuts				
Popcorn				
T.V. dinners				
French fries, potato chips, and pretzels				
Pizza				
2. Do you sit down for long periods of time each day?				
3. Do you feel muscle tension in the neck and shoulder-joint areas?				

	10 Always	7 Often	3 Sometimes	0 Never
4. Do you cross your legs at the knees?				
5. Do you wear tight underwear or a girdle?				
6. Do you smoke cigarettes?				
7. Do you smoke marijuana?				
8. Do you drink alcoholic beverages (beer, wine, or cocktails)?				
9. Do you use birth control pills?				
10. Do you take prescribed medications?				
11. Do you live or work in a polluted environment?				
12. Did your mother and sisters have flabby skin?				
13. Do you crash diet to lose body weight?				

	10 Never	7 Sometimes	3 Often	0 Always
14. Do you eat a lot of fresh fruit and fresh, green, leafy vegetables each day?				
15. Do you eat bran, wheat germ, fresh vegetables, and other fiber foods each day?				
16. Do you cause skin perspiration two or more times a week by exercising or taking a sauna?				
17. Do you exercise vigorously 1 hour or more four or more times a week?				
18. Do you drink 8 glasses of fluids (water) each day?				

	10 Always	7 Often	3 Sometimes	0 Never
19. Do you take a hot bath one or more times a week?				
20. Do you snooze for half-an-hour in the late afternoon each day?				
21. Do you get the proper amount of sleep each day?				
22. Do you rest, relax, and do nothing for half-an-hour each day?				
23. Do you have an easy bowel movement one or more times each day?				
24. Vary from very much physical activity to very little or no physical activity?				
25. Do you use diuretic pills (promote water loss)?				
26. Has your body weight been changing?				
27. Do you have wide hips and bulging thighs?				
28. Are you overweight or obese?				
29. Do you drink coffee?				
Subtotal				

INTERPRETATION

Score Range	Risk of Cellulite
200+	Very high
131–199	Above average
81–130	Average
50–80	Below average
0–49	Very low

BEHAVIOR MODIFICATION

Cellulite can be both prevented and treated successfully. A health-oriented life style is the best way to prevent it (22:27). Ronsard suggests the following treatment (22:27–39).

1. *A purifying diet.* One should eliminate toxic-residue foods such as refined, white sugar (sucrose); refined white flour products (pastry and bread); canned foods; fats; and other empty calorie foods. The anticellulite diet is designed to help rid the body of toxic wastes. Purification and elimination are its primary goals, not weight loss. (When a woman is both overweight and has cellulite, she should lose weight first.) Eating a balanced diet of vitamins, minerals, and amino acids is essential.

2. *Proper elimination.* Avoiding constipation, activating perspiration, and increasing the volume of urine help to prevent cellulite. A high-fiber diet, lots of exercise, and drinking lots of water will promote a regular bowel movement and flush out the wastes in the kidneys. Unfortunately, most women with cellulite seldom drink water (22:74).

3. *Exercise.* Regular exericse stimulates the circulation, breathing, digestion, and elimination; stimulates the metabolism; and helps the skin to perspire. It helps replace cellulite with good muscle and fiber tissue. Most important of all, exercise relieves tension and anxiety. Exercising vigorously for an hour or more each day will help prevent cellulite.

4. *Massage.* This treatment stimulates blood and lymphatic circulation and unclogs the lymphatic vessels so that waste materials can be flushed out. Rub, stroke, knead, and wring the lumps and bulges for about 20 minutes. Stroke deeply in the direction of the heart.

5. *Relaxation.* One must learn the art of relaxation, which relieves stress and tension. The best way is to relax your mind through your body. For example, loosen stiff neck muscles, exercise vigorously, take a hot bath, snooze for half-an-hour in the late afternoon, and/or do nothing for half-an-hour each day.

6. *Breathing and oxygenation.* Breathing large amounts of oxygen into the body helps to ''get rid of cellulite-causing wastes.'' Vigorous exercise is a great help in promoting blood circulation and increasing the oxygen supply to cellulitic areas.

All of these ways must be used together if one is to treat and prevent cellulite. Do not allow cellulite to spoil your physical appearance and personal beauty.

PART D

DISEASES AND DISORDERS—CONSEQUENCES

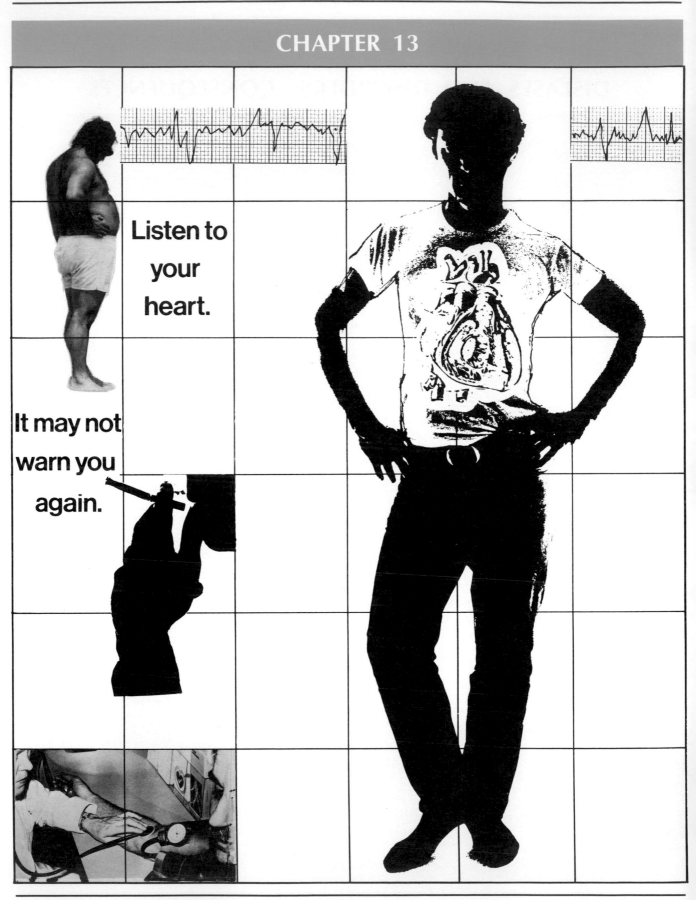

CHAPTER 13

Listen to your heart.

It may not warn you again.

CARDIOVASCULAR DISEASES

Do younger people get heart disease and/or high blood pressure? What causes both of these disorders? Are cardiovascular diseases related to one's life style? Can you prevent a heart attack? These and other questions will be answered in this chapter.

What is your risk of a heart attack, stroke, or high blood pressure? To find out, react to the "Susceptibility CVD Inventory." It will make you aware of the factors in your life style that contribute to cardiovascular diseases and disorders (CVD) and help you find out how susceptible you are to CVD.

☞ SUSCEPTIBILITY TO CVD INVENTORY[1]

DIRECTIONS: 1. Circle the number in the columns that most closely applies to you.
2. Be honest.
3. React to all statements.

SUSCEPTIBILITY TO CVD INVENTORY[1]

Factors	A	B	C	D
	Age in Years			
I. Age	40+	30–39	21–29	10–20
1. Years	15	10	3	0
II. Heredity—Family History	Fathers or Mothers	Grandparents	Other Blood Relatives	None
2. Suffering or dying from stroke	10	7	4	0
3. Suffering or dying from high blood pressure	10	7	4	0

[1] I am grateful to Dr. Jerre Nelson, Internist and Geriatrician, Chairman Hypertension Task Force Committee, San Diego County Heart Association, for reacting to and making suggestions for improving the initial draft of this instrument.

	Fathers or Mothers	Grandparents	Other Blood Relatives	None
4. Suffering from diabetes	5	3	1	0
5. Suffering from elevated cholesterol	5	3	1	0
6. Suffering from low thyroid function	5	3	1	0
7. Suffering from heart attack or heart condition	10	7	4	0
8. Suffering from hardening of arteries (arteriosclerosis)	10	7	4	0
9. High strung or very tense	5	3	1	0
Subtotal	+	+	+	

	Frequency			
III. Medical Checkups	Never	Once in 5 Years	Every 1–3 Years	Each Year
10. Frequency	15	12	5	0

IV. Diabetes	Have None	Parents Have	Never Had Glucose Tolerance Test	Test Negative and No Family History
11. Diabetic history	5	3	1	0

V. Smoking Cigarettes per Day	10+	5–9	1–4	1–6 Months or Do not Smoke
12. Number of years smoking	30	20	10	0

	Frequency			
V. Smoking Cigarettes per Day (cont'd)	30–40	11–29	5–11	Ex- or Nonsmoker

13. Number of cigarettes you now smoke per day	30	20	10	0
	10–14	15–19	20 or over	Ex-or Nonsmoker
14. Age you started smoking	20	15	8	0
VI. Occupation	Inactive	Some Activity	Moderate Activity	Very Active
15. Kind of physical work you do for 8 hours each day	10	9	3	0
	Very High Hate Job	Moderate Tolerable Job	Low It Is OK	None Like Job Very Much
16. Potential for emotional stress in work	10	7	3	0
VII. Exercise	0	1–2	3–4	Daily
17. Frequency of exercise or workout per week	40	25	5	0
	0–10 Min.	11–20 Min.	21–40 Min.	41+ Min.
18. Length of exercise or workout periods (including warmups)	20	10	3	0
	Your Performance Effort			
	0–¼	⅓	½	¾ or All Out
19. Intensity with which you perform the entire workout	10	7	4	0
	Pounds over Standard Weight			
VIII. Weight	26+	11–25	4–10	0±3
20. Body weight	20	15	8	0
IX. Alcohol	6+	3–5	1–2	0
21. Number of drinks (1 oz) you now drink per month	10	7	3	0

	Often You Eat			
X. Fiber in Diet	Never	Once a Week	1–3 Times per Week	Daily
22. Use bran in cereals	20	10	5	0
23. Eat fresh vegetables and fruit	20	10	5	0
XI. Excess Calories	Each day	2–4 Times per Week	1–2 Times per Week	0 Times per Week
24. Often you overeat (feel stuffed) after a meal	20	10	5	0
XII. Sugar	2–3 Times a Day	Once a Day	1–3 Times per Week	Never
25. Use granular white sugar or syrup with tea, coffee, and cereal	20	10	5	0
26. Drink soft drinks	20	10	5	0
27. Eat pies, cookies, puddings, and pastries	20	10	5	0
	Percent Fat in Diet			
XIII. Fat Intake	31+	21–30	11–20	0–10
28. Animal fat intake per week (see "Behavior Modification Module 1" for estimating this value)	50	40	15	0
	Frequency per Week			
XIV. Eating Habits	6+	4–5	2–3	0–1
29. Restaurants and fast-food restaurants	10	7	4	0
	Percent Milligrams			
XV. Cholesterol	280+	231–279	201–230	−200

30. Cholesterol (blood serum)	50	40	15	0

	Upper Reading			
XVI. Blood pressure Readings	161+	141–160	121–140	120 or less
31. Blood pressure	50	40	15	0

	How Often You Eat Food Item			
XVII. Foods Eaten	Each Day	3–4 Times per Week	1–2 Times per Week	0 Times per Week
32. Butter or cream	5	3	1	0
33. French fries or potato chips	10	7	4	0
34. Hamburger or steak	10	7	3	0
35. Bacon or pork	10	7	4	0
36. Eggs	10	8	5	0
37. Luncheon meats (bologna)	5	3	1	0
38. Pies, cookies, cake or chocolate bars, or candy	5	3	1	0
39. Ice cream or whole milk	5	3	1	0
40. Cheese	5	3	1	0
41. Pizza or spaghetti	5	3	1	0
42. Salt on food	50	40	15	0
	+	+	+	

	A	B	C	D
	Frequency			
XVIII. Stress	Usually or Always	Often	Sometimes or Seldom	Never
43. Participation on athletic teams in high school or college	5	3	1	0

	A	B	C	D
		Frequency		
	Usually or Always	Often	Sometimes or Seldom	Never
44. Assume the role of captain or leader of team(s)	5	3	1	0
45. Go to night school while working	5	3	1	0
46. Dissatisfaction with present job	5	3	1	0
47. Feel ambition to be great and successful	5	3	1	0
48. Strive for advancement	5	3	1	0
49. Active in community service clubs	5	3	1	0
50. Are you hard-drivng and aggressive?	5	3	1	0
51. Strive for admiration and respect of your friends and co-workers	5	3	1	0
52. Play sports with an all-out effort	5	3	1	0
53. Enjoy competition in your work	5	3	1	0
54. Competition brings out the best in you	5	3	1	0
55. Irritation when delayed by a car in front of you	5	3	1	0
56. Get upset or angry easily	5	3	1	0
57. Bottle up anger inside of you	5	3	1	0
58. Tendency to drive your car fast	5	3	1	0
59. Work best under pressure (of deadlines)	5	3	1	0
60. Are punctual for appointments	5	3	1	0
61. Waiting for others bothers you	5	3	1	0
62. Do something else while eating or watching TV	5	3	1	0
63. Become irritated if you have to wait in line at the bank, movies, and so on	5	3	1	0
64. Strive for perfection	5	3	1	0

65.	Eat fast	5	3	1	0
66.	Get less than 6 hours sleep a night	5	3	1	0
67.	Talk and move rapidly	5	3	1	0
68.	Lack patience for others who move or think slowly	5	3	1	0
	Subtotal	+	+	+	

		Frequency			
XIX. Symptoms		Several Times in Past: Year	2–3 Years	3–5 Years	Never
69.	Bothered by recurring pain or discomfort in your chest	5	3	1	0
70.	Feel faint or get dizzy spells	5	3	1	0
71.	Usually get short-winded on exertion such as climbing stairs or walking around the block	5	3	1	0
72.	Aware of your heart beating rapidly or irregularly or very slowly	5	3	1	0
73.	Get frequent pain in your legs when you walk	5	3	1	0
74.	Have enlarged or protruding (varicose) veins in your legs	5	3	1	0
75.	Fingers or toes change color or become painful in cold weather	5	3	1	0
76.	Get pain in left arm	5	3	1	0
77.	Have high blood pressure	10	8	5	0
78.	Take medicine(s) for heart or blood pressure	10	10	7	0
79.	Swollen ankles	5	3	1	0
	Subtotal	+	+	+	
	Total score				

SCORING

Add the scores for each section. The total is your susceptibility to cardiovascular diseases/disorders.

INTERPRETATION

Classify your total score into the score range below:

Score Range	Degree of Susceptibility
300+	*Extreme susceptibility*
201–299	*High susceptibility*
130–200	*Above-average susceptibility*
101–129	*Average susceptibility*
0–100	*Low susceptibility*

This inventory should make you aware of the factors contributing to your chances of suffering a heart attack. This instrument should provide you with an opportunity to screen yourself as a present heart attack possibility.

Your total score is an estimate of your risk of a heart attack in the near future if you continue to live as you do. At best, this type of assessment prediction is crude and approximate but it does identify your chances of being a high-risk candidate for a heart attack. If you should identify yourself as a high-risk candidate, recheck your reactions and scoring for possible mathematical error. Then discuss the results of this assessment with your instructor, nurse, or doctor. A thorough medical examination and assessment may be in order.

Another suggestion, as a follow-up, would be to refer to other interrelated chapters of this text, such as the assessment of your eating and exercise habits, weight control, heredity, and so on, and study how you score in the appraisal of these health areas. Perhaps you should seriously modify or alter these habits and behaviors, thereby making you less susceptible to CVD.

Read the remainder of this chapter for more information on cardiovascular diseases.

The number one killer of Americans today is heart disease. About 53 percent of all deaths each year come from heart diseases, primarily heart attack, stroke, and hypertension (high blood pressure) and the death rate from these diseases appears to be increasing. Many people consider heart disease to be a problem found only in the old—an unfortunate aspect of our increased longevity. They assume that nothing can be done about such diseases of old age. But is heart disease inevitable? Is there something you can do now, while young, to keep from dying of heart disease when you get older? All evidence seems to point to the idea that you *can* prevent heart disease if you are able to control certain risk factors.

ARE YOU SUSCEPTIBLE TO HEART ATTACK?

Are college-aged persons susceptible to cardiovascular disorders (CVD), especially high blood pressure, heart disease, and stroke? Only about 5 percent of college-aged young persons suffer from CVD. Although most young men and women do not die from a heart attack while young, the real danger for them is incubating a heart attack or stroke now. Many incubate a heart attack over a period of 5 to 20 years by leading a high-risk-to-CVD life style. Putting it in another way, although you do not suffer from a heart attack or stroke now, your body is slowly developing physiological changes that could eventuate in a heart attack or stroke in 20 years' time. There is ample evidence (47:516) that many 15 to 25-year-olds have cardiovascular systems that have already initiated cardiovascular diseases. (See Figure 13.1.) Evidence of this has come from autopsies of Korean and American servicemen killed in the Korean War. These autopsies showed that 15.3 percent of American soldiers (average age 22.1) had atherosclerosis, while most Korean soldiers did not (47:516). Follow-up autopsies of American soldiers in the Vietnam War corroborated these findings and also the conclusion that cardiovascular disorders are initiated in childhood and are incubated for many years thereafter. We can speculate that heart disease will strike you at a much earlier time in life than it would your parents. Without any doubt, cardiovascular diseases are a most relevant health and life problem. How you live now sets the stage and predisposes you to CVD, probably before the age of 50.

What causes heart disease? Why has it become such a major killer in our society? What are the risk factors? How can you start now to prevent heart disease in later life? We will answer these questions after we briefly examine the nature of the normally functioning cardiovascular system.

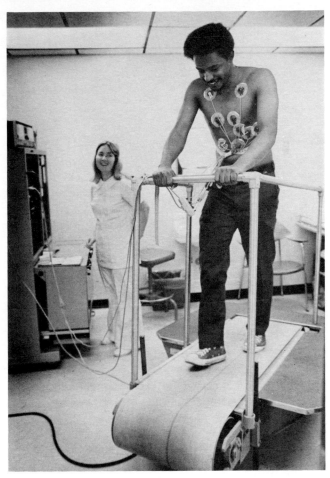

Figure 13.1

A treadmill test should be taken by those whose heart condition is in doubt. The treadmill provides physical stress on the heart, causing the heart to cope with the stress. The EKG machine monitors the heart's reaction to work or physical stress.

OPTIMAL CARDIOVASCULAR FUNCTIONING

The cardiovascular system (heart and blood vessels) of the human body is a pipeline through which blood is pumped to every cell. The system delivers nutrients, oxygen, and hormones to the cells and carries away waste products such as carbon dioxide. If a cell does not receive a continuous supply of blood, it dies—from the lack of nutrients, the lack of oxygen, or an excess of toxic wastes.

The cardiovascular system is obviously vital to human life. If a main artery is severed, an individual can bleed to death within 2 minutes. If a clot blocks the supply of blood to the heart muscle (myocardium), a part of the heart muscle dies (heart attack) and the functioning of the heart itself is threatened.

For the cardiovascular system to be in top operating condition, it needs constant maintenance: a balance of

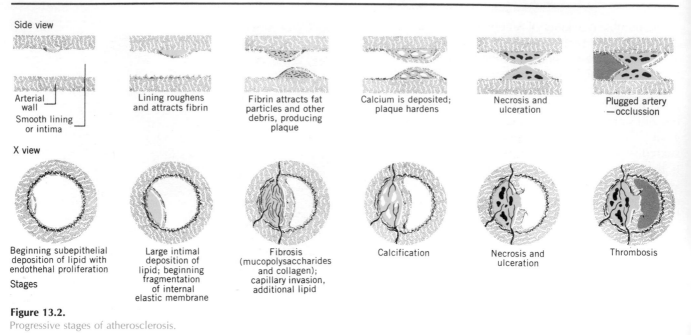

Side view

Arterial wall
Smooth lining or intima

Lining roughens and attracts fibrin

Fibrin attracts fat particles and other debris, producing plaque

Calcium is deposited; plaque hardens

Necrosis and ulceration

Plugged artery —occlussion

X view

Beginning subepithelial deposition of lipid with endothelial proliferation
Stages

Large intimal deposition of lipid; beginning fragmentation of internal elastic membrane

Fibrosis (mucopolysaccharides and collagen); capillary invasion, additional lipid

Calcification

Necrosis and ulceration

Thrombosis

Figure 13.2.
Progressive stages of atherosclerosis.

nutrients, physical activity to exercise the heart muscle, and sufficient rest and sleep. A cardiovascular system that is in top condition shows a number of important characteristics. For one thing, a low resting pulse rate is a good sign of cardiovascular fitness. In sedentary people, the resting heart rate can exceed 100 beats per minute, whereas in highly conditioned athletes the rate is likely to be 40 to 50 beats per minute. In the conditioned person, a resting heart rate of 60 to 80 beats per minute can be accelerated to 150 to 180 beats per minute in an active state and then quickly decelerated to the resting rate. The unconditioned heart takes much longer to recover.

Another sign of a well-functioning cardiovascular system is a low resting blood pressure. Normal blood pressure is 120/80 (blood pressure readings will be explained a little later in the chapter). A blood pressure in the range of 115/75 to 130/85 indicates that the main arteries are flexible and elastic with little or no blockage. The optimally functioning cardiovascular system also carries a higher blood volume that a less-fit system, and distribution of blood to all parts of the body is at maximum efficiency.

The cardiovascular system services all other systems in the body; if it functions poorly, the other systems cannot function optimally either. Fortunately, the functioning of the heart and blood vessels can be improved, primarily through exercise and dietary changes, as we shall discuss shortly. The cardiovascular system is probably the most important body system.

TYPES OF HEART DISEASE

Now that we have become aware of the optimal functioning of the cardiovascular system, let us look at some things that can go wrong with it. There are quite a few disorders that can disrupt cardiovascular functioning, but here we will concentrate on the major problems that are responsible for the high heart disease death rate: atherosclerosis, heart attack, high blood pressure, and stroke. All are interrelated.

Atherosclerosis

The term *atherosclerosis* refers to a condition that occurs when fatty deposits narrow the arteries and reduce or block the flow of blood through them (see Figure 13.2). These fatty deposits, called *plaque,* may become so thick that the artery becomes entirely blocked, or pieces of plaque may break off, travel through the bloodstream, and eventually plug up a smaller blood vessel. If the blockage or plugging occurs in a coronary artery (one that feeds the heart muscle), a heart attack occurs. If the obstruction is in a brain blood vessel, stroke occurs. If the blockage is in the lower extremities, gangrene can develop.

When plaque deposits harden, the arteries lose their elasticity (arteriosclerosis) and the heart must work harder to pump blood through the system. Thus the heart carries an extra burden, and blood pressure is elevated. Unfortunately, there are no outward symptoms of atherosclerosis; people usually find out that they have clogged arteries only after they have suffered a heart attack, stroke, or similar major consequence.

Although medical science is still not sure what causes atherosclerosis, a number of factors seem to be involved. Statistical studies have shown that people who eat a high-fat diet, live a sedentary life, drink alcohol, smoke cigarettes, or experience a great deal of social or emotional stress are those most likely to develop atherosclerosis. These and other factors associated with atherosclerosis will be discussed in the section on risk factors.

Heart Attack

A heart attack does not happen without precursory behavior. The conditions for an attack have been brewing for many years. Figure 13.3 illustrates how a heart attack develops in a typical American male from age 21 to 58.

A heart attack occurs when part of the heart muscle (myocardium) dies. Such destruction of myocardial tissue is called a *myocardial infarction,* and the affected tissue is called an *infarct.* As already mentioned, atherosclerotic deposits can build up and block coronary arteries, preventing the heart muscle from getting oxygen, thereby causing a heart attack (1). But heart attacks can have other causes as well (3). Sometimes a blood clot, or *thrombus,* a floating clot formed elsewhere in the body, will travel to the heart's artery and clog the artery, causing embolism. The result may be pain in the chest (a symptom referred to as *angina pectoris*), or a full-fledged heart attack (in this case called a *coronary thrombosis*). If heart attack damage is mild (the infarct is small), the heart continues to function, and scar tissue forms over the dead area. New blood vessels develop to compensate for damaged or blocked vessels. Such *collateral circulation* is the heart's adaptive approach to the crisis. If damage to the heart tissue is massive and the coronary blood supply is not immediately restored, the heart dies, and so does the patient.

Sometimes people who suffer a heart attack survive the episode only to succumb to new problems created by the heart attack. For example, a heart attack may throw off the rhythm of the heartbeat, and the heart may beat erratically and uncontrollably. Such irregular heartbeat is called *fibrillation* and is fatal unless stopped. A heart attack victim with this problem must immediately be hooked up to a defibrillator, a machine that applies electric shock to the heart in order to try to restore the regular heartbeat. Heart attack victims are also subject to *heart block,* a slowing of the heartbeat caused by damage to the heart's pacemaker. If the damage turns out to be permanent, the person can be fitted with an artificial pacemaker.

Some people experience heart attacks without realizing it. Minor heart attacks are characterized by shortness of breath, sweating, blueness of the lips and fingertips,

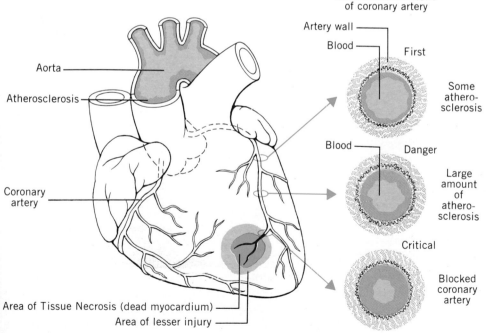

Figure 13.3.

Illustration of a etiology of a heart attack. Myocardial infarction occurs when the central area (+++) around the blocked artery actually dies (necrosis). Atherosclerotic deposits have blocked the coronary arteries' right side views, preventing the heart muscle from getting enough oxygen, which causes a heart attack.

pale complexion, fatigue, possible faintness or dizziness, and irregular heartbeat. These symptoms may subside and return. More often than not a minor attack is a sign of a major heart attack to come. The symptoms of a major heart attack are more obvious. They include the symptoms of a minor attack (but more pronounced) plus a sensation of tightening in the chest, heavy pressure behind the breast bone, pain sometimes radiating to the shoulder, back, neck, arm, or hand, and physical collapse.

High Blood Pressure. High blood pressure is a "silent" health problem, in that there are no obvious symptoms. Yet 23 million Americans have this problem and many die of it.

Blood pressure is the force exerted against the walls of the blood vessels by the blood flowing through them. The pressure is maintained by a complex system of nerve signals and hormonal messages that control the width of the blood vessels, primarily the arterioles (smaller branches of the arteries). Blood pressure in the arteries is normally expressed in millimeters of mercury. The measurement consists of two numbers. The higher of the two is recorded during the heart's pumping stroke, or systole, and is called the *systolic blood pressure*. The lower number represents the pressure prevailing while the heart relaxes between beats and is called the *diastolic blood pressure*. When measured in relaxed, resting, young person, normal systolic pressure is around 120 millimeters of mercury, and normal diastolic pressure is around 80. This is expressed as 120/80. (See Figure 13.4.)

When a person has a blood pressure of 140/90 or higher, he or she is said to have high blood pressure, or *hypertension* (see Figure 13.5). Although we do not know the exact cause of hypertension, atherosclerosis is definitely a factor that aggravates this condition. Atherosclerosis becomes arteriosclerosis when the arteries lose their elasticity and the blood passageway becomes narrow, causing a rise in blood pressure. High blood pressure is a serious disorder because it can lead not only to heart attack but to damage of the kidneys and other organs as well. Fortunately, most cases of hypertension can be controlled through exercise, diet, cessation of smoking and medications. The main problem is discovering those persons with the condition in the first place. (See Chapter 2 for more information on the interpretation of blood pressure.)

Stroke

A stroke is damage to the brain tissue caused by clogging of, or hemorrhage in, blood vessels feeding the brain (see Figure 13.6). One type of stroke, *cerebral thrombosis,* is caused by a blood clot in the brain, while a *cerebral embolism* is caused by the clogging of a brain artery

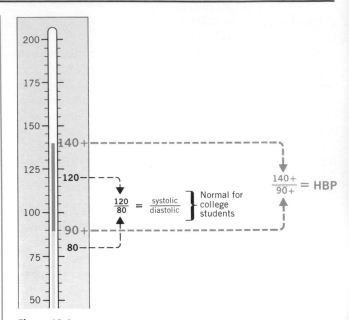
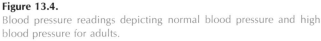

Figure 13.4.
Blood pressure readings depicting normal blood pressure and high blood pressure for adults.

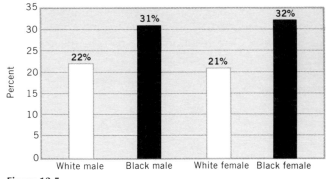

Figure 13.5
Hypertension prevalence by sex and race, U.S. adults age 18 and over: 1977 estimate. Black males and females have a higher incidence of hypertension than white males and females. Reprinted with permission from *Heart Facts: 1980,* American Heart Association, p. 20.

with an embolus, or piece of material (such as atherosclerotic plaque), that floats to the brain artery. *Cerebral hemorrhage* is the term used for a stroke caused by the bursting of a blood vessel in the brain.

Small strokes, in which only a small area of brain tissue has been affected, cause temporary paralysis or malfunctioning of particular body systems controlled by that area of brain tissue. That is, the person may experience a temporary numbness in some part of the body, a temporary loss of speech or of the ability to understand speech, momentary dizziness or double vision, or loss of balance. Massive strokes, on the other hand, can cause permanent paralysis to parts of the body, loss of speech or vision, other major malfunctions, and even death.

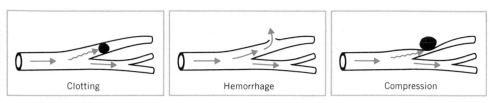

| Clotting | Hemorrhage | Compression |

Figure 13.6

How strokes occur. (With permission from *Facts About Strokes*, 1968, by the American Heart Association.)

RISK FACTORS

Atherosclerosis, heart attack, hypertension, and stroke all seem to be associated with the life style prevalent in Western nations (7;8;11;12;13;14;16;19;20;24). People in the Western world, with their high-fat diets, sedentary habits, and social-emotional pressures show a much higher rate of heart disease than people in the undeveloped countries of the world. What is it about the Western life style that seems to make us more prone to cardiovascular diseases? For one thing, we live longer than people in the undeveloped nations. Cardiovascular disease is initiated in early childhood and is incubated for 20 to 30 years, and we happen to live long enough for the bad effects to eventually be expressed. But heart disease is by no means inevitable for everyone in the industrialized world; some people are more prone to clogged arteries than others. Those who do suffer heart disease have been studied extensively and compared with people without heart disease in order to determine what causes such disorders. The findings of these studies have been summarized in Figure 13.7. People with high blood pressure are four times more likely to suffer heart disease than those with normal blood pressure. Smokers have twice the risk of heart disease as nonsmokers. Women who smoke and use birth control pills increase the risk of heart disease six-fold when they reach the age of 40.

In addition to these aspects of life style that increase heart disease risk, there are several uncontrollable factors that can predispose one to cardiovascular disease; these factors include heredity and metabolic disorders such as diabetes and hypothyroidism (see Figure 13.6). Furthermore, risk factors tend to multiply one's chances of developing heart disease—the more risk factors in one's life, the greater the chances one will develop atherosclerosis and run the risk of heart attack and stroke.

How do the controllable factors, the elements of the American life style that correlate with heart disease, contribute to atherosclerosis? Let us examine some of the major risk factors—diet, inactivity, smoking, and stress—to discover their roles in the development of today's major killer disease.

Diet

Diet itself is a major predisposing factor to premature cardiovascular disorders (CVD). A high-fat, refined-sugar and/or cholesterol diet, as well as an excess of calories, collectively contribute to CVD. A major controversy exists over vitamins C and E and their use in the prevention and treatment of heart disease. Doctors Evan and Wilfred Shute have treated over 30,000 cardiac patients with vitamin E therapy (17:17). Also, since 1950, Dr. Oschsner has prescribed vitamin E to his patients against postsurgical blood clots (36:96–98). Adequate amounts of vitamin C lead to increased rate of destruction of cholesterol from the bloodstream; vitamin C maintains vascular integrity. In other words, vitamin C keeps the arteries clean and blood free-flowing. In addition to vitamins C and E, minerals are related to heart disease (44). Selenium in trace amounts in the diet appears to prevent the breakdown of heart muscle. Chromium and manganese deficiencies contribute to atherosclerosis, while a zinc deficiency and an imbalance of sodium/potassium ratio contribute to hypertension. A high-salt (sodium) diet is highly related to hypertension. Alcohol, when used in excess, may damage the myocardium and make it more irritable. Finally, research on fiber and heart disease in England in 1977 found that men with high dietary fiber intake had the lowest incidence of heart disease (16).

Coffee is no longer implicated as a contributing risk factor (27).

Many metabolic disorders are associated with cardiovascular disorders. The most publicized is, of course, cholesterol metabolism.

Cholesterol is a fatty substance found in most body cells and is essential to human life. It is manufactured by the liver, as well as ingested in the diet (refer to Chapter 6 for more information). Cholesterol has been implicated in atherosclerosis because it is found in atherosclerotic plaque (Chapter 6) and because statistical studies have shown a relationship between high blood pressure, cholesterol level, and heart disease. Recent research has identified two kinds of cholesterol: bad and good. Their relationship to atherosclerosis was discussed

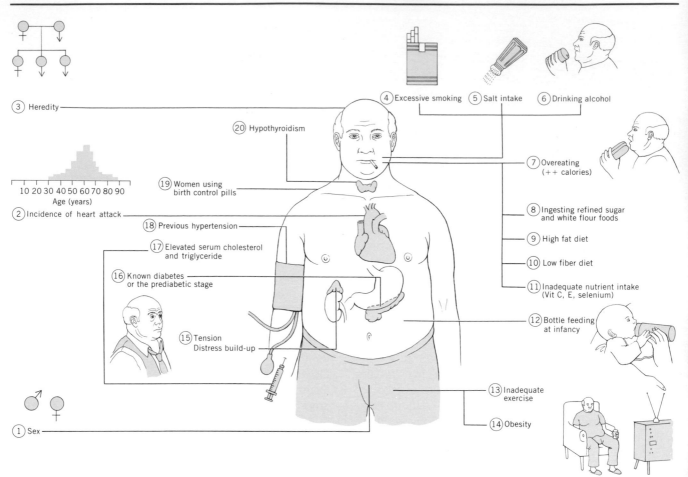

Figure 13.7

Life-style factors contributing to the risk of cardiovascular disorders. Cardiovascular disorders (CVD) are a consequence of life style. This illustration summarizes the multi-factorial causes of CVD. Many health habits, initiated in early childhood by parents, are precursors to CVD. CVD may remain asymptomatic and build up in youth, and then erupt in middle age (symptomatic).

in Chapter 6. Although the cholesterol theories are still highly speculative, many physicians are now advising patients with cardiovascular problems to go on low-fat as well as cholesterol diets. This means cutting out or reducing the intakes of such high-cholesterol foods as eggs, animal fat, butter, cheese, steak, and certain seafoods.

Related to cholesterol is the presence of fats in the diet. Specifically, *saturated fats*—those solid at room temperature such as butter and lard—have been accused of elevating blood cholesterol level and contributing to the buildup of plaque on artery walls. On the other hand, *unsaturated fats*—those liquid at room temperature such as vegetable oil—may be involved in reducing the blood cholesterol level. Thus doctors also advise their heart patients to go on diets low in fats, emphasizing the consumption of unsaturated fats over saturated ones.

Another risk factor related to diet is *obesity*. Obese people tend to have high blood fat levels, high blood

sugar levels, elevated blood pressure, and often diabetes. All these conditions increase the individual's heart disease risk. When the obese person sheds pounds and reaches a normal weight, the risk is greatly reduced. Furthermore, weight loss usually involves a low-fat diet, which also helps reduce the risk.

Inactivity

Americans are, in general, a sedentary group of people. We drive two blocks to the store rather than walk. We sit all day at work or at school and then go home and sit in front of the television set. We have lots of heart attacks. It is not that lack of activity actually *causes* heart attacks; rather, regular physical activity helps to *prevent* heart attack. By "regular physical activity" we mean sustained endurance exercise such as running and swimming (see Chapters 5 and 6). This type of exercise is beneficial to the cardiovascular system because it strengthens the heart muscle, increases the circulating blood volume, prevents atherosclerosis formation in the arteries, increases the blood supply to the heart muscle, lowers blood pressure, lowers heart rate, lowers blood cholesterol and triglyceride, increases low-density lipoprotein levels, increases the endorphin level to give a natural high, and aids in weight reduction.

Regular exercise is not guaranteed to prevent athero-sclerosis and heart attack, but it does provide obvious benefits to the cardioovascular system and to other body systems as well. (See figures 13.8 and 13.9.) If you wish to undertake such an exercise program, consult Chapter 5. But note that no one should begin a vigorous exercise program without first seeing a doctor for a complete physical checkup.

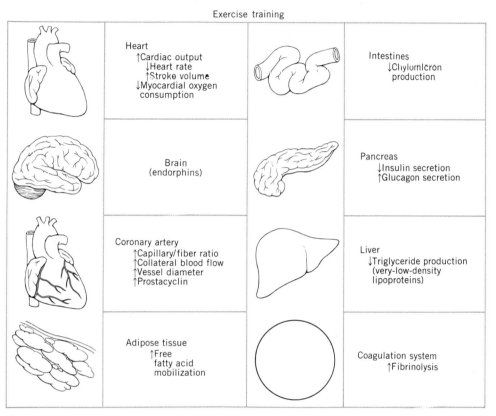

Exercise training

Figure 13.8.

Cardiovascular and metabolic adaptations that theoretically occur with exercise training. Arrows indicate increase or decrease effects. (Adapted from Christine Simonelli and R. Phillip Eaton, "Cardiovascular and Metabolic Effects of Exercise," *Postgraduate Medicine*, February 1978, p. 72.)

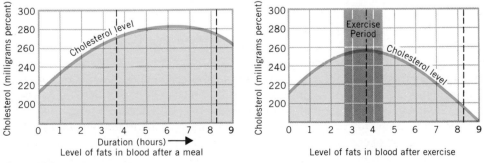

Figure 13.9.

Effects of exercise on fats in blood. Exercising 2 to 3 hours after a meal decreases fat concentration in blood.

Smoking

Cigarette smokers have twice the risk of heart attack as nonsmokers. Furthermore, they are more likely to die of heart disease at younger-than-average age, in their forties and fifties. What is it about cigarettes that can have such an adverse effect on the heart? Nicotine is, of course, a poisonous substance. In the human body, it is known to contract peripheral arteries (the smoker's hands and feet are often cold), to increase the heart rate, to elevate blood pressure, and to deplete vitamin C, which is important in keeping the artery walls strong and flexible. Furthermore, the carbon monoxide in cigarette smoke reduces the oxygen-carrying capacity of the blood so that less oxygen is delivered to the important heart muscle itself. Fortunately, the risk can be totally reduced by simply stopping smoking. Those who have quit smoking have a heart attack frequency comparable to that of people who have never smoked.

Stress

In times of emotional stress, the heart beats faster, blood pressure rises markedly, and blood cholesterol levels fluctuate wildly. According to one theory, if such stress is not immediately dissipated, long-term negative effects on the heart and other systems will occur. Related to this theory is the heart disease personality theory (4;5). This theory suggests that there is a specific heart-attack-prone personality (Type A behavior) characterized by competitiveness, a high degree of anxiety, striving for achievement, aggressiveness, haste, and a sense of urgency (see Figure 13.10). Although stress itself may indeed contribute in some way to heart disease, studies have failed to support the idea that a specific achievement-oriented personality is more likely to be heart-attack-prone.

MULTIPLE FACTORS

Medical science is still a long way from fully understanding what causes cardiovascular disease. Certainly, there are many elderly people alive today who boast of high-fat diets, smoking, drinking, and so on, and somehow elude the dread heart attack. Nevertheless, statistics not only show that diet, exercise, smoking, and high blood pressure are related to heart attack, but that these factors can amplify each other. For example, a person with high blood pressure has up to seven times the risk of heart attack of someone with lower blood pressure, but that risk is then doubled if the person also smokes. Also, there may be other related risks that have yet to be discovered.

REDUCING THE RISK

What is the likelihood of your developing atherosclerosis, having a heart attack, or suffering a stroke? You can get a rough idea by responding to the inventory at the beginning of this chapter. Another approach is to get a thorough medical checkup that includes tests of your blood pressure, blood fats, and blood sugar. You can also have your health risk profile done, which gives you a computer printout identifying high- and low-risk factors in your life style that predispose you to cardiovascular disease.

Whatever method you use, you will probably find that in certain aspects of your life your behaviors put you in a high-risk category (see Figure 13.11). If you place a high priority on your optimal well-being, you will want to make some changes in your life style to reduce that heart attack risk. Note too that your risk of cardiovascular disease increases with the number of predisposing factors in your life style. The more uncontrollable factors in your life (genetic predispositions, diabetes, or hypothyroidism) that increase your risk, the more important it is for you to do something about the controllable factors (see Figures 13.12 and 13.13).

WAYS TO MAINTAIN A HEALTHY CVS

1. Stop smoking cigarettes or decrease the number of cigarettes you now smoke and try not to inhale the smoke (see Chapter 9) for suggestions on how to break the smoking habit).

2. Start a program of regular endurance exercise (especially if you are a smoker (see Chapter 5). Become more physically active—take the stairs instead of the elevator, walk or bicycle to the store instead of driving, and so on. (See Figure 13.14.) "You are as old as your arteries."

3. If you are overweight, undertake a weight reduction program that will help you adjust your caloric intake to appropriate levels (see Chapter 7).

4. Lower your fat intake, particularly the saturated fats, such as fried foods, fatty meats, cold cuts, and dairy products rich in fats.

5. Eat a diet high in fresh fruits and vegetables and low in refined sugar products (cakes, cookies, candy, and so on).

6. Cut down on your salt intake. Americans eat much more salt than their bodies need, and salt is involved in high blood pressure (see Chapter 6).

7. Reduce your intake of alcoholic beverages. Many studies have indicated that alcohol consumption aggravates the cardiovascular system and multiplies other risk factors.

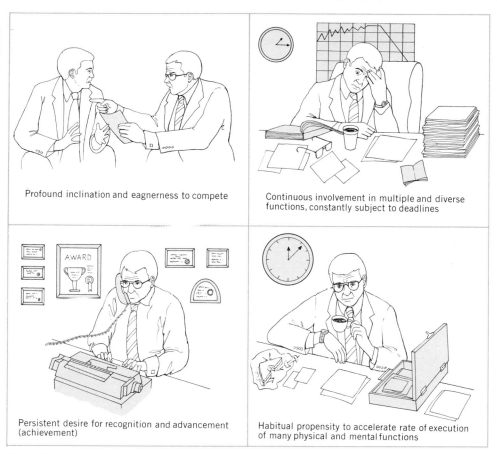

Figure 13.10.

Characteristics of a heart attack personality.

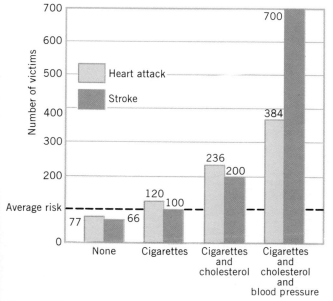

Figure 13.11.

Increase in the danger of heart attack and stroke with the number of risk factors present. The figures in the chart refer to the number of victims in the study sample. (With permission from Dr. William B. Kannel, Director of Framingham Heart Study, Department of Medicine, Boston University, Boston, Mass.)

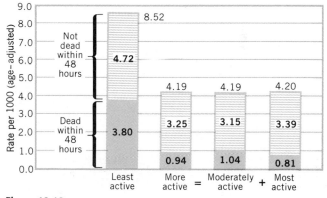

Figure 13.12.

Physical activity increases the survival rate of men suffering their first heart attack (myocardial infarction). Those least active died within 48 hours. (With permission from Sam Shapiro et al., "Incidence of Coronary Heart Disease in a Population Insured for Medical Care (HIP)," *American Journal of Public Health,* Supplement, Part II, June 1969.)

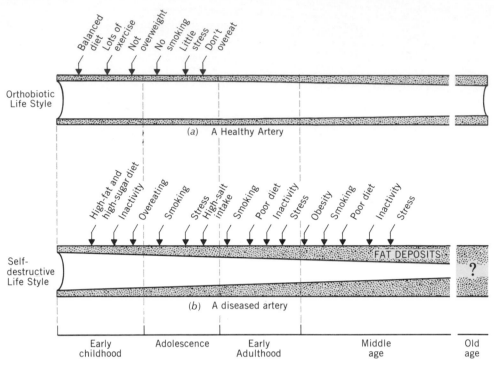

Balanced diet · Lots of exercise · Not overweight · No smoking · Little stress · Don't overeat

Orthobiotic Life Style

(a) A Healthy Artery

High-fat and high-sugar diet · Inactivity · Overeating · Smoking · Stress · High-salt intake · Smoking · Poor diet · Inactivity · Stress · Obesity · Smoking · Poor diet · Inactivity · Stress

Self-destructive Life Style

FAT DEPOSITS

?

(b) A diseased artery

| Early childhood | Adolescence | Early Adulthood | Middle age | Old age |

Figure 13.13

Effects of two contrasting life styles on the cardiovascular system. A health promotion or orthobiotic life style (top), comprised of stress management, (a) low-salt, low-fat, no-sugar, high-fiber, and balanced-nutrient diet, a low caloric intake, no smoking, nondrug misuse, and regular physical activity, keeps the arteries in a youthful working condition throughout life. A self-destructive life style (bottom), initiated in early childhood and continued into later age, accelerates the aging of the arteries (illustrated by narrowing of the blood passageway). A person may be chronologically young but physiologically old.

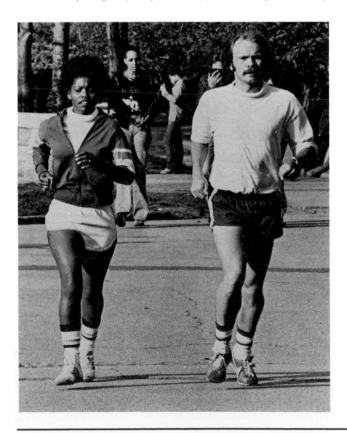

Figure 13.14

Jogging is an excellent exercise to maintain a healthy cardiovascular system and prevent cardiovascular disorders, including high blood pressure and heart disease.

8. Have regular medical checkups to detect hypertension and early signs of atherosclerosis.

9. Examine the stresses in your life and determine whether you can reduce the stress level by making changes in your work, your school, your interpersonal relationships, your living conditions, or other stressful aspects of your life (see Chapter 3).

10. Learn to relax. When you study or work, allow for short breaks every hour to stretch, or rest, or meditate. If you are involved in tense work, allow a few minutes to "let off steam" through vigorous physical activity.

11. Program time for yourself. Schedule time each day to look after your physical and emotional needs. This time could be devoted to exercise, relaxation, grooming, taking a nap—whatever you need.

12. Enroll in a course on emergency cardiopulmonary resuscitation. You can learn how to administer life-saving help to heart attack victims, and you will know what to do should you ever a suffer a heart attack yourself.

BEHAVIOR MODIFICATION TECHNIQUES

Refer to earlier chapters on emotional well-being, physical fitness, nutrition, and weight control for ways to modify or change those habits and behaviors that predispose you to cardiovascular disorders.

Where to go for More Information

1. Your local chapter of the American Heart Association, or write American Heart Association, 44 E. 23rd Street, New York, N.Y. 10010.

2. Write to: Heart Information Center, National Heart Institute, Bethesda, Md. 20014.

3. Your campus health center.

4. Your family doctor.

5. Your public health department.

6. Your health education instructor.

7. Your campus or community library.

Further Readings

Leonard, Jon N., J. L. Hofer, and N. Pritikin, *Live Longer Now,* New York: Grosset, 1977.

U.S. Senate Select Committee on Nutrition and Human Needs of the United States, "Diet Related to Killer Diseases III," Washington, D.C., U.S. Government Printing Office, March 24, 1977.

Williams, Roger, *Nutrition Against Disease,* New York: Bantam Books, 1973.

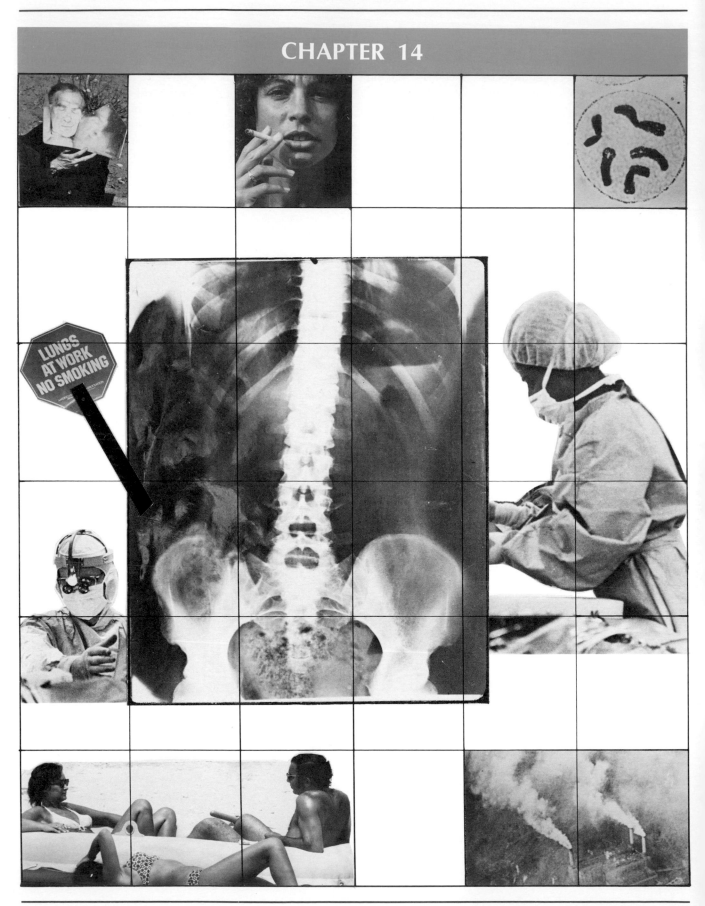

CHAPTER 14

CANCER

Cancer is the second leading cause of death in the United States (after cardiovascular disease). About one in every four Americans suffers from this disease at some time in his or her life. In 1978 alone, 700,000 new cases were reported. Of these who contract cancer, more than half die from it (36). No wonder the word "cancer" has become frightening.

Cancer strikes primarily in the older age groups, but there are several types of cancer that can affect people at any age. The cancers that most frequently affect college-age individuals include leukemia; Hodgkin's disease; and cancers of the breast, uterus, and brain. But even the cancers that strike older people can begin in the first 30 years of life, for cancer can take many years to develop and begin to exert its harmful effects. For these reasons, it is important for young people to be knowledgeable about both the warning signs of cancer and behaviors that are conducive to cancer development. A knowledge of factors associated with cancer can allow the individual to adopt a life style that will help him or her reduce the risk of ever having cancer.

In this chapter we will focus on the nature of cancer, what is thought to cause it, what sorts of behaviors are related to cancer development, and the behavioral changes people can make to reduce cancer risk.

React to the appropriate inventories on cancer to assess your susceptibility to cancer and to make you more aware of the factors causing cancer.

☞ SUSCEPTIBILITY TO CANCER INVENTORY[1]

DIRECTIONS: This is not a test. Five separate instruments, similar in format, have been designed to assess susceptibility to cancer at a specific cancer site.

Statements on the left side of the page in each instrument describe variables related to a specific site.

Circle the number on the right side of the statement that you feel best describes your behavior on how it relates to you.

Be honest in your responses.

Important: react to each statement.

[1] The five following instruments were designed with the help of Dr. Sidney Saltzstein and members of the American Cancer Society, San Diego chapter.

SUSCEPTIBILITY TO LUNG CANCER (FOR MALES AND FEMALES)

	A	B	C	D
	50–60	61+ or 40–49	25–40	Under 25
1. Age (at present)	10	5	0	0
2. Number of years smoking cigarettes (or as exsmokers)	10+ Years	5–9 Years	1–4 Years	Few Months or Do Not Smoke
	40	30	15	0
3. Number of cigarettes you now smoke per day	30–40	11–29	5–10	Do Not Smoke or Exsmoker
	20	15	5	0
4. Age you started smoking	10–14	15–19	20–24	25+ or Do Not Smoke or Exsmoker
	10	7	3	0
5. Number of years working in coal mine or rock quarry	20 Years	10–19 Years	1–9 Years	Few Months or Never
	10	7	4	0
6. Number of years working in asbestos factory	20 Years	10–19 Years	1–9 Years	Few Months or Never
	20	15	5	0
7. Number of years working in other jobs such as sandblasting, tunneling, fiberglass, or grain elevator	20 Years	10-19 Years	1–9 Years	Few Months or Never
	5	3	1	0
8. Number of years working in chromium plating factory	20 Years	10–19 Years	1–9 Years	Few Months or Never
	5	3	1	0

	A	B	C	D
	Yes	—	—	No
9. Unexplained chronic coughing	5	—	—	0
	5+	3–4	1–2	None
10. Repeated episodes of respiratory infections (flu, pneumonia, or bronchitis) in past year	5	3	1	0
	Always	Often	Sometimes	Never
11. Feeling shortness of breath	5	3	1	0
12. Feeling tired or exhausted	5	3	1	0
13. Wheezing (chest) while breathing	5	3	1	0
Total				

SUSCEPTIBILITY TO BREAST CANCER (for females only)

	A	B	C	D
	45–64	25–45 or 65–75	21–24	Other
1. Age	10	7	4	0
	Never	Once per Year	2–3 Times per Year	Each Month
2. Frequency of self-examining your breasts	25	20	10	0
	Grandmother	Mother	Sister or Aunt	None
3. Heredity—relatives who had or were treated for breast cancer	10	10	5	0
	Never	Less than Every 3 Years	Every 2–3 Years	Yearly
4. Frequency of doctor's examining your breasts	10	7	4	0

	A	B	C	D
5. Income—check *one* only (a) *Family* income per year (b) *Single* income per month	$9000 $400 or less	$10,000– $14,000 $500– $700	$15,000– $19,000 $800– $900	$20,000 $1000+
	5	3	1	0
	—	Jewish	—	Other
6. Your religion	—	3	—	0
	Yes	—	—	No
7. Discharge or fluid and/or blood from nipple	5	—	—	0
	Yes	—	—	No
8. Lump in breast not examined by doctor	5	—	—	0
Total				

SUSCEPTIBILITY TO CERVICAL (UTERAL) CANCER (for females only)

	A	B	C	D
	35–54	25–34 55–65	18–24	Other
1. Age	20	15	5	0
	Never	Over 2 Years Ago	Once in Past 2 Years	Once or No Times a Year
2. Frequency of having Pap smear test	20	15	5	0
	Always	Often	Sometimes	Never
3. Vaginal bleeding between periods or during or after sexual intercourse	15	12	5	0
4. Foul vaginal discharge	5	3	1	0
	16 Years or Under	16–18	19–20	20 Years or Over
5. Age you began intercourse	10	7	3	0
	10+	6–10	2–5	0–1
6. Number of different sexual partners	5	3	1	0

	A	B	C	D
7. Number of times you have had syphilis or gonorrhea	6+	2–5	1	0
	5	3	1	0
	Catholic	Protestant	Other	Jewish
8. Your religion	3	3	3	0
9. Income—check *one* only (a) Family income per year or	$9000	$10,000– $14,000	$15,000– $19,000	$20,000
	$400 or less	$500– $700	$800– $900	$1000+
(b) Singles income per month	5	3	1	0
Total				

SUSCEPTIBILITY TO ENDOMETRIAL (UTERAL) CANCER (for females only)

	A	B	C	
1. Age	50+	45–49	—	−44
	10	7	0	0
2. Heredity—relatives who had or were treated for endometrial cancer	Sister	Mother, Grandmother	Cousin	None
	10	7	3	0
3. Menstrual history	Finished Menopause	In Menopause	—	Other
	10	5	—	0
4. Menstrual history—regularity	Always Irregular	Occasionally Irregular	—	Regular
	10	5	—	0
5. Number of pregnancies	0	1	2	3+
	5	3	1	0
6. Obesity—number of pounds overweight	25+ lbs. Overweight	11–24 lbs. Overweight	5–10 lbs. Overweight	Skinny
	5	3	1	0

	A		B		C	
	Yes	—		—		No
7. Are you a diabetic?	5	—		—		0
	Yes	—		—		No
8. Do you have hypertension?	5	—		—		0
	Yes	—		—		No
9. Vaginal bleeding after menopause	15	—		—		0
Total						

SUSCEPTIBILITY TO RECTAL (COLON) CANCER (for males and females)

	A	B	C	D
	65–76	45–64	35–44	Under 34
1. Age	10	7	3	0
	More Than Once a Month	Once in 2 Months	Once in 3 Months	Never
2. Frequency of bleeding from rectum	20	15	10	0
	Frequently	Occasionally	Rarely	Never
3. Bowel movement—black in color	20	10	3	0
4. Change in bowel habits	5	3	1	0
	1–2 Times per Month	1–2 Times in Past 6 Months	Once in Past 6 Months	Never
5. Pus or mucus in bowel movements	5	3	1	0
	Never	Once Every 5 Years	Once Every 2–3 Years	Once a Year
6. Frequency of medical examination of rectum	10	7	3	0
Total				

SCORING

1. Score each cancer instrument separately.
2. For each cancer site, add all your circled responses in each of the four columns (A, B, C, and D).
3. Total the scores of all four columns. This is your susceptibility score.

INTERPRETATION

The purpose of the five cancer-site inventories is to help you to (1) become aware of those habits, behaviors, and situations that make you prone to cancer, and (2) identify your susceptibility to cancer in various parts of the body.

You should be aware that many variables work collectively to cause cancer. Cancer can strike one person and not another, even though both may have the same genetic and environmental backgrounds. Then too, there are many facts that we just do not know about cancer yet.

The variables associated with a cancer site vary and may not be interrelated to another cancer site. It is for these reasons that five separate instruments were designed. The five cancer sites were selected over other cancer sites on the basis of mortality statistics.

The weighing of statement items vary for each cancer site. Some variables contribute more to one site than to others and this is implied in the numerical values for each statement. For example, cigarette smoking is the most important causative agent in lung cancer and receives almost half of the total points in the lung cancer instrument.

Should your chances of cancer be above average, you should discuss the results of this assessment with your health science teacher, nurse, or doctor.

There are separate score ranges for estimating just how susceptible you might be to each of the five cancer sites.

Refer to the following score ranges to classify your scores.

1. Lung Cancer

   (a) *For nonsmokers:*

Score Range	Degree of Susceptibility
0–5	Low
6–17	Moderate
18–50	High
51+	Extremely high

   (b) *For smokers and (ex-smokers):*

Score Range	Degree of Susceptibility
23–25	Moderate
26–35	Above moderate
36–54	High
55–90	Very high
90+	Extremely high

2. Breast cancer:

Score Range	Degree of Susceptibility
0	Low
1–5	Below average
6–16	Moderate
17–60	High
61+	Very high

3. Rectal (colon) cancer:

Score Range	Degree of Susceptibility
0–10	Low
11–20	Moderate
21–40	High
41+	Very high

4. Cervical cancer:

Score Range	Degree of Susceptibility
0–10	Low
11–20	Moderate
21–40	High
40+	Very high

5. Endometrial cancer:

Score Range	Degree of Susceptibility
0–5	Low
6–25	Moderate
26–35	High
36+	Very high

WHAT IS CANCER?

Cancer is a general term for a condition that results when a group of cells begins to grow abnormally and the cells no longer fulfill their normal body functions. The body is constantly producing new cells for the purpose of growth and repair—about 500,000 million new cells each day. It does so by cell division. When this process proceeds correctly, the new cells show the same characteristics as the tissue in which they originated. They stay in the tissue and stop growing after reaching a certain size. When a cell goes berserk in its growth and no longer resembles the original tissue, it has become cancerous.

A cancer cell may be distinguished from a normal cell by its nucleus, which is usually larger than normal (see Figure 14.1). The earliest detectable sign of cancer is an increase in the number of chromosomes in the nucleus, and these chromosomes are abnormally shaped and otherwise irregular. At first, a group of cancerous cells stays in the tissue and competes for the nutrients needed by the healthy cells. The mass of cells may develop into a *tumor,* which is a piece of tissue that grows persistently without serving any useful purpose. *Benign* tumors are noncancerous growths that are encapsulated by a fibrous membrane that prevents them from invading surrounding tissues (see Figure 14.2). Although many benign tumors are harmless, some can grow in bone tissue,

the brain, or other vital areas and interfere with normal functioning. *Malignant* tumors are cancerous growths. They can invade surrounding tissues and spread to other parts of the body. Cancer cells can be shed from the initial growth area and carried by the blood or lymph to other sites in the body; such spreading of cancer from one part of the body to another is called *metastasis.* Figures 14.3 & I, II, III, and IV show the normal lung and then the progressive development of cancer in the lung.

Cancers are classified according to the primary tissues in which they develop. Cancers that grow on inner membranes (epithelial tissues) are called *carcinomas.* Carcinomas include cancers of the bronchial tubes and lungs, uterus, colon, rectum, mouth, pharynx, and gastrointestinal tract. Cancers that arise in connective tissue, such as bone and muscle, are referred to as *sarcomas.* Cancer of blood-forming tissues is called *leukemia.* Cancers on the skin are termed *melanomas.*

The kinds of cancers people get vary with sex as well as with age. Figure 14.4 shows which cancers are most likely to strike men and women and which ones are the greatest causes of death. As shown in the figure, men are most likely to contract cancers of the lung, prostate, and colon and rectum, whereas women are more subject to cancers of the breast and uterus, as well as colon and rectum. Lung cancer is by far the greatest killer in men, while breast cancer has the highest death rate in women.

Cancer progresses slowly and exerts its effects in a

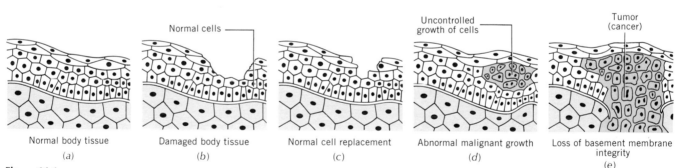

Normal cells

Uncontrolled growth of cells

Tumor (cancer)

| Normal body tissue (a) | Damaged body tissue (b) | Normal cell replacement (c) | Abnormal malignant growth (d) | Loss of basement membrane integrity (e) |

Figure 14.1
Process of cancer. Cancer is the uncontrolled growth of cells.

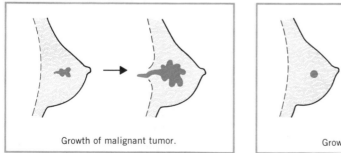
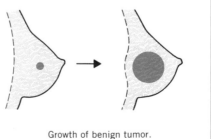

Growth of malignant tumor.

Growth of benign tumor.

Figure 14.2
Illustrating malignancy and benign tumors.

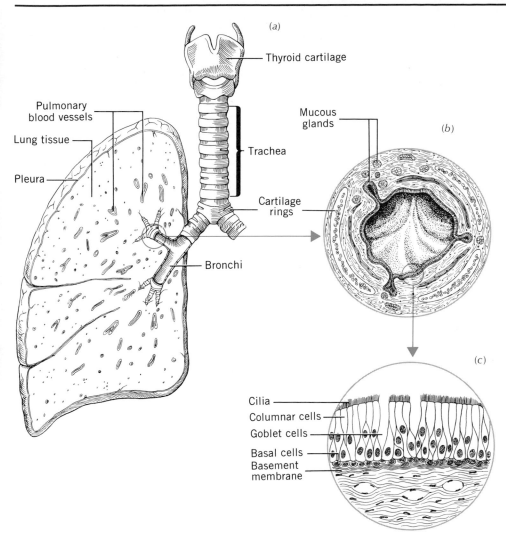

(a) Thyroid cartilage

Pulmonary blood vessels

Lung tissue

Pleura

Trachea

Mucous glands

(b)

Cartilage rings

Bronchi

(c)

Cilia
Columnar cells
Goblet cells
Basal cells
Basement membrane

Figure 14.3

I. The Normal Lung

Cancer is a disease of "runaway cells" that multiply unchecked and uncontained. Lung cancer most often starts in the lining of the *bronchi* (large air tubes). This figure shows a normal right lung with *bronchi* (D) that supply it with air. The tissue and cells that line the bronchi are shown greatly enlarged. Figures 14.2, II, III, and IV, show how these tissues and cells progressively change to produce the growth called cancer.

The wall of a normal bronchus is shown in goblet cells (J) and deeper grands, Near circle above. The "hairs" at top are cilia at basement membrane (K) are basal (H) which are attached to columnlike cells (L). A precancerous condition may cells (I) Cilia propel inhaled particles to exist when basal cells multiply, atypical ward the throat in the mucus secreted by cells appear, and cilia disappear.

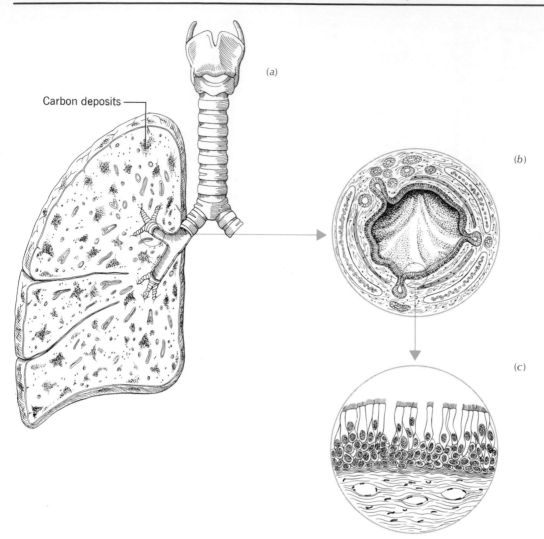

(a)

(b)

(c)

Carbon deposits

Figure 14.3

II. The Attack.

Smoke and other air pollutants are inhaled into the trachea, travel down the bronchi, and eventually reach lung tissue, darkening it with black carbon and other deposits. On the way, almost all pollutants irritate the bronchi to some extent. Some actually may be *carcinogenic* (cancer causing) and act as triggers for the wanton process of cell division that eventually results in a full-blown case of cancer.

Pathologists regard the cell picture, *above,* as the first stage in the development of lung cancer. Additional rows of basal cells have crowded and displaced columnar cells. The cell nuclei take a darker stain and are irregular in size. The cilia function less efficiently in moving heavy secretions from the bronchi toward the throat. Breathlessness and a persistent cough are signs that trouble lies ahead.

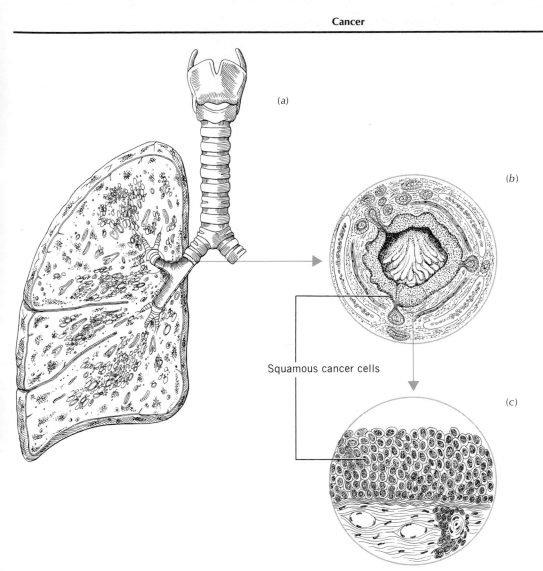

(a)

(b)

(c)

Squamous cancer cells

Figure 14.3

III. The Invasion.

Because of a loss of cilia, secretions move sluggishly. The walls of thousands of tiny *alveoli* (air sacs) rupture, and air becomes trapped. The affected lung tissue enlarges, and the rest of the lung becomes involved. The patient becomes a ''lung cripple'' as the area of breathing surface inside the lung diminishes greatly. This condition, *emphysema,* is present in most lung cancer cases. The lung still is in a precancerous state.

The ongoing process of cell division and multiplication continues in willy-nilly fashion. The columnar cells and their cilia have been displaced by abnormal *squamous cancer cells* (O). Many bizarre cell forms, including those that are about to divide, are seen. The ''runaway'' basal cells already are beginning to penetrate the basement membrane. An invasion of the deeper tissue is about to begin.

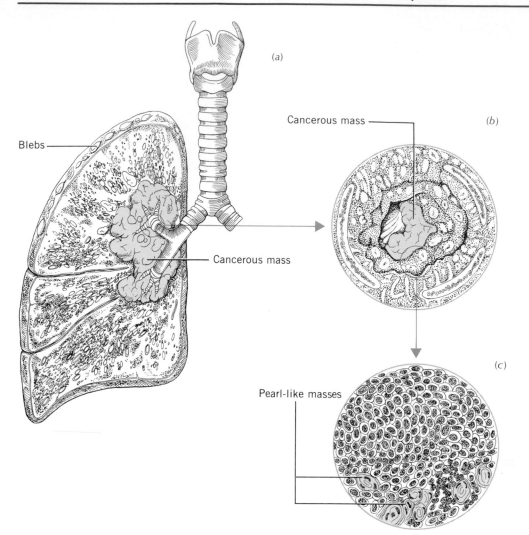

Figure 14.3

IV. The Conquest.

Because of emphysema, many pockets of trapped air, called *blebs* (P), appear on the surface of the darkened lung. A grayish mass of cancerous tissue (Q), composed of squamous cancer cells, has partly blocked the bronchus and spread to surrounding tissue. The patient's only hope—a small one—is the removal of the lung before cancer cells enter the lymphatic vessels and spread to organs elsewhere in the body.

Squamous cancer cells (O) completely line the bronchial wall. Numerous hard, *pearl-like masses* (R), made of keratin, have been deposited in the cancerous tissue. With the cancer unchecked and uncontained, the conquest is all but complete. Cancer, blocking the bronchus, also deprives the alveoli of oxygen and makes them ripe for infection by bacteria, which flourish in defenseless tissue.

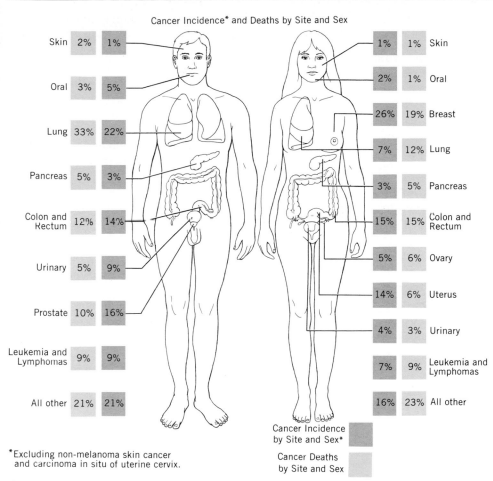

Cancer Incidence* and Deaths by Site and Sex

	Male			Female	
Skin	2%	1%	1%	1%	Skin
Oral	3%	5%	2%	1%	Oral
			26%	19%	Breast
Lung	33%	22%	7%	12%	Lung
Pancreas	5%	3%	3%	5%	Pancreas
Colon and Rectum	12%	14%	15%	15%	Colon and Rectum
			5%	6%	Ovary
			14%	6%	Uterus
Urinary	5%	9%	4%	3%	Urinary
Prostate	10%	16%			
Leukemia and Lymphomas	9%	9%	7%	9%	Leukemia and Lymphomas
All other	21%	21%	16%	23%	All other

Cancer Incidence by Site and Sex*

Cancer Deaths by Site and Sex

*Excluding non-melanoma skin cancer and carcinoma in situ of uterine cervix.

Figure 14.4
Estimates of cancer incidence and death by site and sex for 1978. Source: American Cancer Society. Reprinted with permission from the American-Cancer Society.

number of ways. Because cancer cells rob nutrients from normal cells, the body actually becomes malnourished and begins to waste away. The victim loses appetite and weight and is physically weak. Cancer of specific organs impairs the functioning of those organs, and this is especially harmful in the case of the blood-producing tissues such as bone marrow. Cancer of the blood-producing tissues reduces not only the number of available red blood cells but the important white cells that fight infection, leaving the individual vulnerable to viral and bacterial diseases. In fact, many leukemia victims actually die from other diseases because their body has no resistance. Many cancer patients also suffer from anemia because red blood cells are unable to supply sufficient oxygen to the body. Thus cancer causes death by damaging vital organs, much as a bullet causes damage to the heart and circulatory system.

The general symptoms of cancer include fatigue, weight loss, loss of appetite, and skin pallor. Specific symptoms include the well-known seven warning signals of cancer.:

1. A change in bowel or bladder habits.
2. A sore that does not heal.
3. Unusual bleeding or discharge.
4. Thickening or lump in breast or elsewhere,
5. Indigestion or difficulty in swallowing.
6. Obvious change in a wart or mole.
7. Nagging cough or hoarseness.

Note that these symptoms do *not* mean that one has cancer; they are simply indications that one should see a doctor for a complete examination.

WHAT CAUSES CANCER?

The exact cause of cancer is still unknown. Various theories have been advanced to explain how normal cells go wild. Here we will concentrate on environmental factors that have been statistically linked to cancer and on a few of the many theories as to how cancer develops.

Environmental Carcinogens

Prolonged irritation of human tissue, such as the exposure of lung tissue to cigarette smoke, or the rubbing of sensitive skin by rough clothing, may trigger normal body cells to begin uncontrolled growth. Substances that are known to initiate uncontrolled growth are called *carcinogens*. Known carcinogens range from sunlight and radiation to cigarette smoke, soot, and arsenic (see Table 14.1). The World Health Organization estimates that about 80 percent of all human cancers are caused by such environmental factors. A high incidence of bladder cancer, for example, has been found in dye and rubber workers; lung cancer has a high rate in asbestos, cotton, and uranium workers (see Figure 14.5); and liver cancer has been observed in workers who handle the plastic polyvinal chloride.

Many of the occupational carcinogens do their work in combination with other noxious agents. Asbestos workers, for example, are much more likely to develop lung cancer if they also smoke. In fact, smoking seems to amplify the effects of many other inhaled carcinogens. Just living in polluted cities greatly increases the chances of smokers contracting lung cancer.

How carcinogens work their effects is not known although the details are not totally mysterious. Take lung cancer, for example. Components in cigarette smoke paralyze the hairlike cilia that normally sweep harmful materials out of the lungs. The underlying bronchial tissue is then left open to the irritating substances in the tobacco smoke. The irritation produces an increase in the number of underlying basal cells, and these cells begin to pile up and take on abnormal shapes. Continued irritation intensifies the condition, which can eventually become cancerous.

Table 14.1

Cancer-Causing Substances, Where They Are Found in the Environment and the Cancers They May Cause

Carcinogenic Substances	Where Found	Cancers They May Cause
1. Alcohol	Alcoholic beverages	Mouth, lip
2. Biological		
(a) Aflatoxin (common mold)	Moldy vegetables, fruits, nuts, and seeds	Liver, bladder
(b) Irritation	Tight clothing, exposure to chemicals and sunlight	Skin
(c) Malonaldehyde	Fat in meats	Stomach, colon, rectum
(d) Benz(a)pyrene	Charcoal-broiled sausage, beefsteak, and hamburger	Colon, rectum
3. Coal tars	Tobacco and marijuana smoke	Lungs, mouth, bladder, esophagus, larynx
4. Diet food		
(a) Fat	Beef meat, cold meats, bacon, diary products	Breast, colon, rectum
(b) Refined white sugar (sucrose)	Candy, pastry, desserts, canned foods, ketchup as sweetener	Colon, breast, uterus, ovaries, pancreas
(c) Refined white flour	White bread, pastry	Colon, rectum, prostate, breast, bladder, liver
(d) Saccharin	Soft drinks, canned food, sweeteners	Bladder, liver

Carcinogenic Substances	Where Found	Cancers They May Cause
(e) Some food additives and preservatives, diethylstibestrol (DES) (synthetic estrogen), nitrites, and dyes	Meats, canned and dried foods	Bladder, liver, kidney, pancreas
5. Drugs	Birth control pills and synthetic estrogens (DES)	Vagina, cervix, uterus, testicles
6. Industrial		
(a) Asbestos	Asbestos plants, insulators, mechanics	Lungs
(b) Benzene (solvent)	Mechanics, garages, dry cleaners	Skin, bone marrow, leukemia
(c) Benzidine (rubber)	Rubber factories, tire-retread shops	Bladder
(d) Coal products		
(1) Asphalt	Roofing and paving industries	Lung, bladder
(2) Coal dust	Mines	Lungs
(3) Cotton dust	Cotton industries	Lungs
(4) Azo and analine dyes	Textile mills	Liver
(5) Arsenic	Mining and smelting industries	Skin, lungs, liver
(6) Nickel, cadmium, copper	Metal, alloys, and plating industries	Lungs, nasal sinuses
(7) Mercury and sulfur	Paper-pulp mills	Lungs, liver
(8) Vinyl chloride	Plastics industries	Liver, brain
7. Some pesticides	Pesticide industries, crop dusters, and farms	Lungs, liver, bone
8. Radiation		
(a) X rays	Medical and dental offices	Skin, leukemia
(b) Uranium or radium	All mines—nuclear power plants	Thyroid
(c) Ultra-violet irradiation	Sunlight	Skin

Dietary Factors

The food we eat and the beverages we drink contain so many chemicals that it is no wonder that we have begun to worry about potential carcinogens in our diets. Many scientists estimate that 75 percent of new cases of cancer are related to eating, smoking, and drinking habits. It has been found, for example, that normally harmless nitrites in some foods and water supplies can combine with the amines in the stomach to form carcinogenic nitrosamines. Another carcinogen, malonaldehyde, is formed from a breakdown of unsaturated fat in beef and other meats when natural antioxidants are low or missing. Malonaldehyde is suspected of causing stomach, colon, and rectal cancers (31). Potentially carcinogenic chemicals (diethylstibestrol) fed to cattle to "beef" them up sometimes remain in the meat and find their way to the dinner table.

The general high-fat diet of most Americans has been implicated in some cancers. For example, a fatty diet in women is suspected to overstimulate hormone production or disrupt normal hormone balance, indirectly causing breast cancer. According to testimony at the 1976

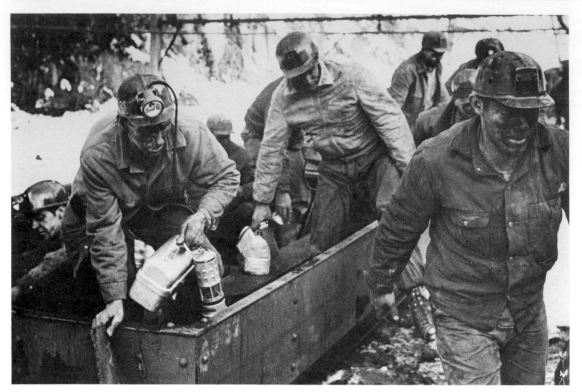

Figure 14.5.
Coal miners inhale coal dust and are highly susceptible to an occupational lung disease called black lung disease. Many miners also die from lung cancer.

hearings of the Senate Select Committee on Nutrition and Human Needs, dietary factors are correlated to more than half of all cancers in women and at least one-third of all cancers in men (26).

Dietary factors can also be helpful in cancer prevention. Areas of United States deficient in molybdenum have high rates of esophageal cancer (1:176–178). For example, breast cancer death rates are lower in areas with adequate or high dietary selenium supply than in areas low or deficient in this trace element (32) (see Figure 14.6). Among other nutrients suggested as possible "protectors" against cancer are vitamins A, C, and E; and the minerals molybdenum, zinc, copper, and manganese (32:224). Furthermore, a high-fiber diet is associated with the reduced incidence of colon cancer. Theoretically, because fiber aids in moving food through the digestive tract and in preventing constipation, wastes are prevented from forming carcinogens that irritate the sensitive tissues lining the colon (13;32:213). Such nutrients are often lacking in our diets because they are removed through the milling of whole grains and bleaching of flour with chlorine (1:179). Boiling or simmering beef and other meats with water will steam away malonalde-

hyde, thereby removing this carcinogen from the meat (31). Recent research strongly suggests that we avoid charcoal broiling or frying steaks and hamburger to avoid forming the carcinogen benso(a)pyrene.

Drugs

Some medications that we take may be potential carcinogens. Several studies have suggested that the use of estrogens by middle-aged women to alleviate the symptoms of menopause increase their risk of uterine cancer. Researchers at the University of Washington reported that the risk of cancer was nearly five times higher among those who took the hormone than among those who did not (40). A major unresolved question is whether birth-control pills also pose a cancer risk. Estrogen, a constituent of the pill, has been shown to cause breast cancer in experimental animals.

A disturbing finding in this area is the fact that an artificial estrogen, diethylstilbestrol (DES), can cause cancer in the children of the user. That is, women who took the drug in early pregnancy produced daughters who were susceptible to an often fatal vaginal cancer.

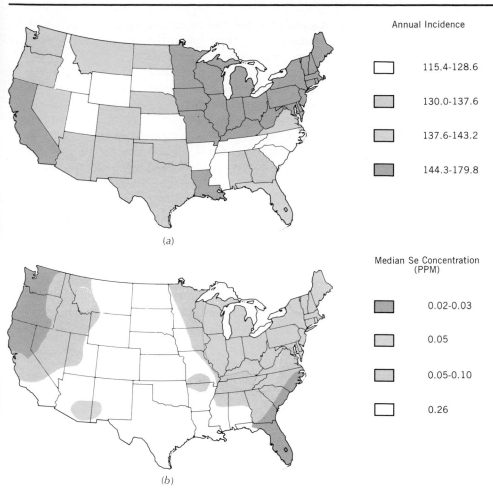

Annual Incidence

☐	115.4-128.6
▨	130.0-137.6
▨	137.6-143.2
▨	144.3-179.8

(a)

Median Se Concentration
(PPM)

▨	0.02-0.03
▨	0.05
▨	0.05-0.10
☐	0.26

(b)

Figure 14.6

Relationship of selenium in sales and incidence of cancer rates by state for 1959. (a) The cancer incidence rates for the continental United States, 1959. (b) Median selenium concentrations (ppm) in grains and forage crops in the continental United States. From G. N. Schrauzer, *Inorganic and Nutritional Aspects of Cancer*, New York: Plenum Press, 1970, p. 326.

The sons of DES users are more prone to undescended testicles, testicular cancer, epididymal cysts, problems in urination, and lower sperm counts than non-DES-exposed men. Diethylstibestrol was given to about 2 million women after World War II on the theory that it would prevent miscarriage (40).

Radiation

Another known producer of cancer is radiation, including sunlight and ultraviolet radiation as well as X rays, radium, and atomic radiation. The high doses of radiation used to treat childhood tonsilitis and thymus glands in the 1940s and 1950s has resulted in an increased incidence of thyroid cancers. Survivors of the atomic bombings of Hiroshima and Nagasaki have shown a sig-

nificantly higher than average incidence of leukemia and cancers of the breast, skin, bone, bowel, and brain. It appears that the irradiation of men and women during their reproductive years also increases the likelihood that their offspring will develop leukemia. See Chapter 21 for more information about the hazards of radiation.

Heredity

Up to this point we have discussed environmental factors contributing to cancer, but hereditary contributions should not be overlooked. Genetic factors are thought to be involved in several cancers. For example, people with very light skin may have inherited a condition that makes them particularly susceptible to skin cancer. A few very rare cancers have specific genetic causes although, for the most part, heredity plays a minor role in the more common forms of cancer. Nevertheless, if more than one person in your family has had a specific type of cancer, you should be especially alert to any symptoms of this disease in yourself or in members of your immediate family. The appearance of cancer before menopause probably indicates that a woman carries more of the susceptibility genes than if it appeared after menopause. If a woman has breast cancer before menopause, her daughter's chances increase to one in 15, or three times the average (44).

THE VIRUS THEORY

What makes a good cell go bad? According to one theory, viruses may be the cause. The viral theory suggests that all human beings carry in their bodies viruses with cancer-producing potential. These viruses remain harmless until some inside factor (low vitamin C, E, and selenium levels) (28:43) and/or outside factor (carcinogens or radiation) activates them, and they begin invading individual cells and altering the cells' functioning. Although this theory has yet to be proved, it is known that viruses are definitely involved in several cancers in other animals. Research is currently aimed at finding viral bases for human leukemia, Hodgkin's disease, breast cancer, and cancers of the uterus and cervix. Some women have developed cancer of the cervix or the uterus after they had a virus-caused venereal infection known as herpes II (see Chapter 16 for more information).

IMMUNE THEORY

Another approach to understanding the causation of cancer is the immune theory, or the idea that cancer is a result of defects in the body's immune system. This theory suggests that cancer cells appear from time to time in almost everyone, but the immune system destroys them before they can spread. We never know that they appeared. Cancer cells change chemically, and the body recognizes them as being different from normal cells. Cancer cells stimulate the body to produce antibodies and leucocytes that attack them; then huge, wandering cells (megacytes) gobble them up. When this immune mechanism breaks down, possibly due to low amounts of vitamin C in leucocytes, cancer grows unchecked. Carcinogens are suspected of disrupting the immune mechanism. This theory also explains why cancer is more frequent in older people. Physiologically, the immune system becomes less efficient with the passage of years. A person of 60 can produce only about one-half the number of antibodies that a person of 15 produces (44). Thus, when the immune system breaks down, cancer grows unchecked.

Based on this immune theory, Dr. Thelma Arthur of the Arthur Test and Research Center of Chula Vista, California, has perfected a test (Arthur Morphologic Immunostatus Differential), which is reputed to be 98.6 percent accurate in detecting early untreated cancer (4;10). It also detects a person's susceptibility to cancer by analyzing the morphology of white blood cells. Since the level of white blood cells is highly correlated to one's immunity level, this test is supposed to tell the physician what the status of the patient's immunity is before cancer strikes. Although high cancer risk persons should be able to use the test to detect and monitor annually their susceptibility to cancer, this test has not been recognized by the medical profession and the American Cancer Society. Although presently controversial, this test is mentioned as an example of how a theory can lay the groundwork for disease monitoring, testing, and treatment.

A cancer intervention treatment, one of building self-immunity through hope, praying, and self-hypnosis, is also based on the immune theory of cancer (see Figure 14.7).

THE CANCER PERSONALITY

A number of researchers have suggested that certain personality types are more susceptible to certain kinds of cancer, especially cancers of the face, breast, and cervix (35). Such "cancer personalities" are characterized by feelings of helplessness, incompetence, despair, and depression. They have a history of loss, usually beginning with cold, neglecting parents who rejected them. Highly susceptible to stress, they rarely show their emotions. It has been suggested that such people have been denied fulfillment of an inborn need for tenderness and closeness with others; if they continue to experience such denial, they are likely to develop cancer. Although this theory is highly speculative, it does suggest that high-risk-of-cancer persons need to learn how to deal with "distress" in their lives.

CAN CANCER BE CURED?

No matter what turns out to be the cause of cancer, our greatest concern at the moment is treating those who are already afflicted with the disease and having healthy persons develop preventive habits. Unfortunately, there is no known "cure" for cancer although cancers are considered cured after 5 years if they are destroyed or removed from the body. Current methods of cancer treat-

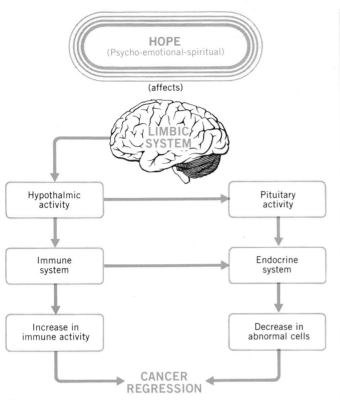

Figure 14.7

Theoretical explanation of how hoping or praying and self-hypnosis pschophysiologically intervene to fight cancer. Hoping or praying for about 2 to 3 weeks appears to gradually stimulate the hypothalamus to send chemical messengers to the pituitary gland and to slowly activate the immune system. These, in turn, eventually activate autoimmunity and the self-defense system to fight cancer cells, causing regression of cancer. (Adapted from Carl O. Simonton, *Getting Well Again*, Los Angeles: J. P. Tarcher, 1978.)

Table 14.2

Comparison of Projected Cure Rate with When Treatment Is Begun. The Earlier Cancer Is Discovered and Treatment Begun, the Greater the Chances of Successful Cure

Percent Cure Rate	Time Lapse Before Treatment
75–100	Within 1 year
50–75	1–2 years
25–50	2–3 years
0–25	4–5 years

The success of any cancer treatment is gauged by the patient's survival for at least 5 years without the cancer's recurring. The earlier a cancer is discovered and treatment is begun, the greater the cure rate (see Table 14.2). At least half of all cancers develop in parts of the body that can easily be examined by a physician; because of this, 70 percent of all cancers can be "cured" if diagnosed and treated early. Thus it cannot be stressed enough for individuals of any age to have regular checkups and to see a doctor at the appearance of any of the seven cancer warning signals. Furthermore, women should have an annual Pap smear, in which cells are scraped from the cervix and checked for any irregularities. Women should also conduct monthly breast self-examinations (see Figure 14.8), especially since breast cancer is the number one cause of cancer deaths in women. Doctors estimate that almost twice as many people could be saved from cancer death as are currently saved if one thing would happen: people would go to their doctor at the first sign of a problem rather than ignore it and hope it will go away (see Figure 14.9).

WAYS TO MAINTAIN AN ANTI–CANCER LIFE STYLE

Early diagnosis and treatment are the best weapons we have against cancer. But it is, of course, preferable not to get cancer in the first place. Fortunately, even though we are not sure what causes cancer, we do know that behaving in certain ways can help reduce one's chances of ever contracting this deadly disease (see Table 14.3). Here are a few suggestions of things you can do to reduce your cancer risk:

1. If you smoke, quit. Around 80 percent of all lung cancers and 17 percent of all cancer deaths would be prevented if no one smoked cigarettes (10:36).

2. Choose to live in a community with very little or no air pollution.

ment include the surgical removal of malignant tissue (such as a cancerous tumor), radiation therapy (X rays and cobalt treatment) to destroy cancerous cells without removing tissues, chemotherapy (use of drugs) to retard or even reverse cancer growth, and combinations of these methods. Radical mastectomy involves removal of not only the cancerous breast, but also nearby lymph nodes under the arm and the muscle tissue on the chest. Because radical mastectomies result in physical disfiguring, the loss of self-image, and no assurance that cancer will not reappear again, such operations are highly controversial.

The three standard treatments for cancer—surgery, radiation, and chemotherapy—have improved cancer survival rates by only 1 percent in the past 30 years (36). Thus conventional medical approaches to cancer have been a failure.

(a) LOOKING

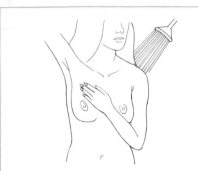

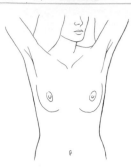

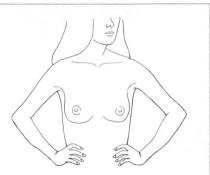

In the shower:
Examine your breasts during bath or shower; hands glide easier over wet skin. Fingers flat, move gently over every part of each breast. Use right hand to examine left breast, left hand for right breast. Check for any lump, hard knot or thickening.

Before a mirror:
Inspect your breasts with arms at your sides. Next, raise your arms high overhead. Look for any changes in contour of each breast, a swelling, dimpling of skin or changes in the nipple. Then, rest palms on hips and press down firmly to

flex your chest muscles. Left and right breast will not exactly match — few women's breasts do. Regular inspection shows what is normal for you and will give you confidence in your examination.

(b) FEELING (palpation)

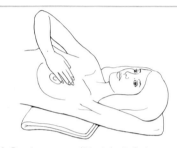

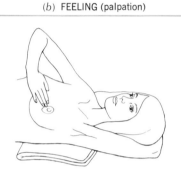

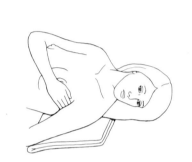

3. From here on you will be trying to find a lump or thickening. Lie down on your bed, put a pillow or a bath towel under your left shoulder, and your left hand under your head. With the fingers of your right hand held together flat, press gently against the breast with small circular motions to feel the inner, upper portion of your left breast, starting at your breastbone and going outward toward the nipple line. Also feel the area around the nipple.

4. With the same gentle pressure, feel the low inner part of your breast. Incidentally, in this area you will feel a ridge of firm tissue. Don't be alarmed. This is normal.

5. Now bring your left arm down to your side and, still using the flat part of the fingers of your right hand, feel under your left armpit.

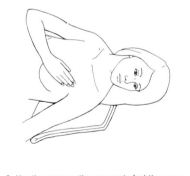

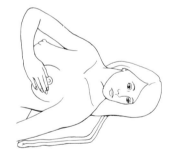

6. Use the same gentle pressure to feel the upper, outer portion of your left breast from the nipple line to where your arm is resting.

7. And finally, feel the lower outer portion of your breast, going from the outer part to the nipple.

8. Repeat the entire procedure, as described, on the right breast using the left hand for the examination.

Your own doctor may want you to use a slightly different method of examination. Ask him to teach you that method.

Examine your breasts every month, about one week after each menstrual period. Be sure to continue these checkups after your time of menopause.

If you find a lump or thickening, leave it alone until you see your doctor. Don't be frightened. Most breast lumps or changes are not cancer, but only your doctor can tell.

Figure 14.8

Procedures for breast self-examination (a) looking (b) feeling or palpation. Source: American Cancer Society.

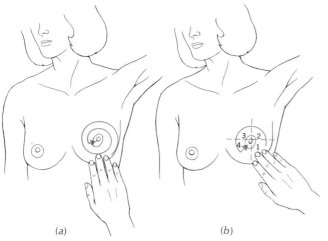

Figure 14.9
Technique of medical breast examination. A, Starting at the periphery and working toward the nipple in ever-decreasing concentric circles. B, Examining each quadrant separately in sequence. Reprinted with permission from O'Donnell et al, *Early detection and Diagnosis of Cancer.* St. Louis, The C. V. Mosby Co., 1962, p. 63.

3. Avoid exposure to carcinogenic chemicals and fumes at work and in your home.

4. Use suntan products with a strong sunscreen (PABA) that will help block out the sun's harmful rays. Do not overexpose yourself to the sun.

5. Make sure you are getting adequate fiber in your diet.

6. Cut down on fats, sugar, and refined white flour products in your diet and avoid overeating.

7. Make sure you are getting a balanced diet that contains all essential vitamins and minerals in adequate quantities.

8. If you identify with the "cancer personality," see a counselor or therapist about dealing with the stresses in your life or the depression you feel. Assume a positive optimistic attitude toward life.

9. Keep your body clean, paying special attention to areas with sensitive tissues, such as the mouth and genitals.

10. Avoid unnecessary exposure to X rays or other types of carcinogenic radiation. Avoid submitting to X-ray machines that emit 2.5 or more roentgens.

11. Assume a self-care attitude; only you can prevent cancer.

12. Continuously bolster your immunity level. When having a medical checkup, ask the doctor to give you a CBC test with the Arthur Morphologic Immunostatus Differential (AMID) test (4;10). You can bolster your immunity in the same way you can prevent the common cold or influenza: get adequate rest and sleep, avoid or

resolve stress, and maintain a positive and optimistic attitude and outlook on life. Having hope, confidence, and high spiritual faith can elevate autoimmune chemicals in the body. You may want to supplement your diet with vitamins and minerals.

13. Check your hereditary tree. How many relatives have cancer or died from it?

14. Have at least one bowel movement each day.

15. Exercise regularly to promote oxygenation of all body cells.

16. Learn to cook meats in noncancerous ways. The cooking temperature, type of fuel used, and fat content of meat all affect the amount of benzo(a)pyrene formed. Avoid charcoal broiling; barbecuing; and pan-frying steaks, sausages, and hamburger. Use an electric or gas broiler with the heat source above the meat.

17. Give your body regular self-examinations.

Ask the physician to give you a comprehensive cancer checkup. Both of you should screen for precancerous conditions (see Figure 14.9). A regular checkup is important to insure overall good health, and vital to finding cancer early so that it is treated promptly. Following are some of the ways you, a nurse, or a physician can check for signs of the disease.

Skin

Check the skin visually and by palpation, searching for abnormal discolorations, keratosis or small skin thickenings, swelling, sores, lumps, or other conditions that might signal cancer.

Head and Neck

Examine the face inside and out for abnormalities in color and contour. The lips are palpated for firm spots.

Palpate the series of lymph nodes on both sides of the neck at the same time, comparing them for signs of enlargement. The larynx also is palpated for immobility or enlargement. The entire thyroid is palpated for size, consistency, and tenderness. Part of this examination involves swallowing.

Inside the mouth, the inspection includes the hard and soft palates, cheeks, and floor of the mouth, as well as the tongue. With a laryngeal mirror, inspect the larynx, pharynx, and tonsillar area. Pull your lower lip down and look at your gums. See anything funny? Put your finger on it—is it hard or mushy? Are there any white patches or bleeding cracks? If you catch mouth cancer before it gets bigger than a penny, you have a good chance of curing it. Mouth cancer is painless, silent, and comes from years of irritation due to smoking and drinking.

Table 14.3

Cancer Prevention (What you can do for yourself.)

Skin

1. Self-examination for keratosis change in color or size
2. *Limit* ultraviolet exposure—*avoid* 10:00 A.M. to 2:00 P.M. sun
3. Use PABA (ultraviolet-screen tanning lotion)
4. Eat a balanced diet—Vitamins B_6 PABA, A, C, D, E, and zinc and molybdenum
5. Avoid tight, irritating clothes and skin irritation

Kidney—Bladder

1. Avoid Xrays and radiation
2. Avoid ingesting chemicals, e.g., aniline dyes, red dyes (No. 3), and yellow butter dye
3. Eat a balanced diet
4. Drink plenty of liquids

Rectal—Colon

1. Low fat diet
2. High-fiber diet
3. Avoid cold-cut meats (contain nitrates)—e.g., bologna and hot dogs
4. Bowel movement at least once a day
5. Eat balanced nutrient diet
6. Exercise—no constipation
7. Regular medical checkup or proctosigmoidoscopy
8. Guaiac test for blood in stools
9. Boil meats

Breast Cancer

1. Monthly self-examination
2. Low fat diet (10%)
3. Moderate selenium intake
4. Eat balanced diet as for skin
5. Do not use birth control pills—high in estrogen
6. Positive attitude
7. Do not eat refined sugar
8. High-fiber diet
9. Adequate iodine intake

Prostate

1. Adequate zinc intake
2. Regular sexual activity
3. Eat balanced diet
4. Annual medical exam and self-palpation
5. Avoid sugar and pastry

Liver

1. Avoid X rays
2. Avoid chemicals in food and drink, e.g., dyes
3. Avoid smelter fumes—industry
4. Avoid plastics fumes, e.g., airplane glue and vinyl chloride
5. Avoid aerosol sprays

Leukemia (Blood)

1. Avoid radiation and X rays
2. Eat a balanced diet

Cervical—Uterine

1. Avoid high-estrogen birth control pills
2. Eat a balanced diet
3. Wash regularly
4. Annual pap smear test
5. Avoid synthetic estrogens, e.g., DES
6. Avoid sugar, pastry, and sweets
7. Avoid X-ray overexposure
8. Avoid venereal diseases
9. Establish regular menstruation
10. Prevent vaginal bleeding

Lung

1. *No* cigarette smoking
2. Do not inhale polluted air or tar fumes.
3. Wear protective mask when spraying, painting, or dusting or using pesticides
4. Do not work in coal mine, or cotton, asbestos, chemical, or plastics industries
5. Eat a balanced diet, especially anti-oxidants, vitamins C, E, B_6, selenium, vitamin A - epithelium protection
6. Exercise regularly
7. Avoid respiratory infections and aerosol sprays
8. Avoid occupational high-risk jobs (No. 4)
9. Positive mental attitude
10. Vial Sputum test after age 40

Source: Compiled by the author from a review of cancer literature.

Breast

The cervical lymph nodes are gently palpated for signs of enlargement. Then inspect the breasts with your arms raised and lowered. Look for irregular contours, skin dimpling, and other changes.

The breasts are then palpated, using a rotary pattern, while the woman first is seated, then is lying, in both positions with her arm behind her head. The nipples are checked for discharge.

Finally, the woman's axillary lymph nodes, in the armpits, are examined and palpated. Do this once a month. Ninety-five percent of women discover their own breast cancer.

Ask your doctor to give you a graphic stress telethermometry (GST) test. It measures minute temperature differences in the body and on the skin surface. Since tumors are hotter than normal body tissues, the differences in temperature are detected by the GST test (25:6).

Chest

The physician listens to the lungs functioning through a stethoscope, and may advise a chest X ray and/or sputum test, especially for smokers.

Pelvic

The physician examines and palpates the external pelvic tissue, and then uses a speculum while visually inspecting the interior of the vagina and uterine cervix. During this last step, a Pap test is performed, in which a cervical smear is taken for miscroscopic study.

The physician then palpates the pelvic organs from within and without.

Women at high risk of endometrial cancer should have a sampling of endometrial tissue taken for examination.

Colon and Rectum

A routine physical usually includes a digital examination of the rectal area and a guaiac (hemocult) test for invisible blood in the stool. In men, a physican can check the prostate gland through the rectal wall (see Figure 14.10). Another common test is the "procto," a visual inspection of the rectum and lower colon with the lighted sigmoidoscope. Your physician can help you take the Hemoccult slide test to detect colon and rectal cancer. If microscopic amounts of blood are found in the stool—a warning of possible tumor—then your doctor can carry out follow-up tests to confirm this test. Information about this inexpensive test can be obtained from your local cancer society.

Testicles

Males should palpate their testicles for lumps or swellings every 6 months (see Figure 14.11)

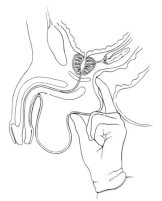

Rectal Examination of the Prostate

Figure 14.10
Finger palpation for prostate cancer by inserting finger into the rectum.

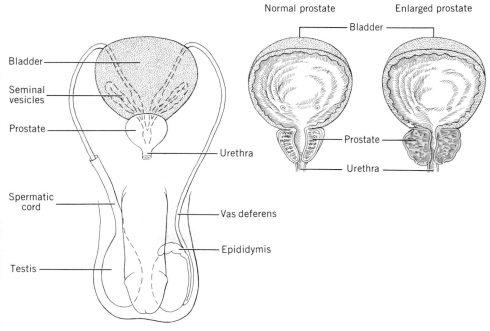

Figure 14.11
Internal genitalia and bladder of the male; prostatic hypertrophy. (From Dowling and Jones, *That the Patient May Know,* Philadelphia: Saunders.)

Other Tests

Test also may be routinely performed on urine and blood samples. If any of the previous examinations indicate an abnormal condition, the physician may recommend more extensive tests.

Because cancer is such a major killer in America, it is important for everyone to be aware of the warning signs in themselves and those close to them. It is also important to develop a personal life style that will reduce the risk of cancer. In this sense cancer is often self-inflicted. Many indulge in harmful pleasures and self-destructive behaviors that increase the likelihood of cancer (e.g., cigarette smoking, and eating nitrate-preserved bacon, ham, and hot dogs). One also needs to learn to manage distress effectively, ingest a balance of nutrients, and have an optimistic outlook on life. In addition, everyone concerned about cancer should keep up with current findings in this heavily researched area. Researchers are continuing to discover carcinogenic substances in our environment—substances we should be aware of and avoid. They are also making progress in finding screening tests and more effective treatments for cancer such as successful chemotherapies for leukemia.

Despite all these research efforts, cancer is still a poorly understood disorder—one that is wide open to quackery. Each year desperate cancer victims spend untold sums of money on quack treatments, meanwhile putting off medical treatment from qualified physicians. Thus quackery is by no means harmless, for the growing cancer becomes more resistant to legitimate methods of treatment. Unfortunately, this situation will continue until medical science can give us a better idea of what cancer is and what can be done to cure and prevent it.

WHERE TO GO FOR MORE INFORMATION

1. Your local chapter of the American Cancer Society.
2. Your campus health center.
3. Your family doctor.
4. Your public health department.
5. Your campus or community library.
6. Write to:
   American Cancer Society
   777 Third Avenue
   New York, N.Y. 10017
7. Write to:
   National Cancer Institute
   900 Rockville Pike
   Bethesda, Md. 20014

8. Write to:
   (a) Carcinogen Information Program (CIP Bulletin)
       Centre for Biology of Natural Systems
       Washington University
       St. Louis, Mo. 63130
   (b) Cancer Couseling & Research Center
       Suite 710
       1300 Summit Avenue
       Fort Worth, TX 76104

For cancer counseling, supportive educational help, temporary care and sympathy, and information on how to live with cancer:

1. American Cancer Society.
2. Reach to Recovery (for mastectomy patients).
3. Cancer Inco Service
   1825 Connecticut Avenue, N.W.
   Suite 218
   Washington, D.C. 20009
4. Breast and Cancer Advisory Center
   P.O. Box 422
   Kensington, Md. 20795
5. Cancer Care Inc.
   One Park Avenue
   New York, N.Y. 10016 (Try local chapter)
6. Lynn Ringer
   Can Surmount Program
   1850 Williams Street
   Denver, Colo. 80218
7. Cancer Counseling and Research Center
   1300 Summit Avenue, Suite 710
   Fort Worth, Tex. 76102
8. Hospice, Inc.
   765 Prospect Street
   New Haven, Conn. 06511
9. Make Today Count
   218 S. Sixth Street
   Burlington, Iowa 52601
10. Shanti Project
    1137 Colina Avenue
    Berkeley, Calif. 94707
11. DES Action
    Long Island-Hillside Medical Centre
    Lakeville Road
    New Hyde Park, N.Y. 11040

Further Readings

Cancer Facts and Figures, lastest ed., New York: American Cancer Society, 1980.

Pelletier, K. R., *Mind as Healer, Mind as Slayer* (A holistic approach to preventing stress disorders), New York: Delacorte, 1977.

Rosenbaum, E. H., *Living with Cancer* (A guide for the Patient, Family, and Friends), New York: Praeger, 1975.

Schrauzer, G. N., *Inorganic Nutritional Aspects of Cancer,* New York: Plenum Press, 1978.

Simonton, Carol O., *Getting Well Again,* Los Angeles: J. P. Tarcher, 1978.

U.S. Select Senate Committee on Nutrition and Human Needs, *Nutrition and Cancer,* Washington, D.C., U.S. Government Printing Office, July 27, 28, 1976.

Williams, Roger J., *Nutrition Against Disease,* New York: Bantam Books, 1973.

CONTROVERSIAL □ THEORIES

A couple of theories of cancer causation have become controversial, partly because of the "illegal" treatments they entail. One theory suggests that cancer is caused by the cellular starvation of oxygen. Dr. Felix Warburg, who received a Nobel prize for showing that malignant growth can be retarded by oxygenating tumor masses, has suggested that the primary cause of cancer is the replacement of oxygen respiration by sugar fermentation in normal body cells (21). All body cells meet their energy needs through aerobic processes (respiration), whereas cancer cells meet their energy needs in great part by anaerobic processes (fermentation). Without oxygen, a cell will die. Some cells switch their metabolism in order to survive, and they become malignant. However, if a cell is able to withstand oxygen deprivation, it is less likely to become malignant. Pangamic acid (often referred to as "vitamin B_{15}"), according to Russian studies, retards the destruction of the cell when there is a lack of oxygen (39). This chemical is thought to improve the oxygen distribution system in the body. It should be noted, however, that B_{15} is not legally available in most states.

Another controversial theory was formulated at the turn of the century by Beard, an English physician (22). The so-called trophoblastic theory suggests that cancer is the result of "misplaced" cells produced during early cell division in prenatal development. Such cells, called trophoblasts, normally establish a foothold for the fertilized egg in the uterine wall and form the chorion. Around the fifty-sixth day of pregnancy, the umbilical cord matures and the trophoblasts are no longer needed. Some of these cells are discarded and the rest are scattered in various parts of the body of the fetus. Eventually the cells are destroyed by pancreatic enzymes. According to this theory, malfunctioning of the pancreas may allow many of the cells to survive, and any surviving trophoblasts invariably become cancerous.

The trophoblast theory was used by Ernest T. Krebs, Jr., as a basis for his assertion that laetrile (also called "vitamin B_{17}") is a cancer preventative (8). He suggests that laetrile works by surrounding cancerous cells and releasing a minute amount of cyanide that diffuses into the cell and paralyzes it. Laetrile does not affect normal cells because they contain an enzyme that destroys cyanic acid, an enzyme not found in cancer cells. Krebs says laetrile works best when the tumor is small and new (22). Both the trophoblast theory and laetrile therapy are based on the idea that cancer is basically the result of a pancreatic deficiency. Laetrile therapy is illegal in most of the United States (47), and the trophoblast theory has gained very little acceptance among the medical profession in this country.

Should you or your doctor wish to get more information about the Arthur Morphologic Immunostatus Differential Test (AMID), you can contact: Arthur Test and Research Inc., 401 H Street, Chula Vista, Calif. 92010; or Aid Laboratory, 605 South Sherman, Suite E, P.O. Box 2407, Richardson, TX 75080.

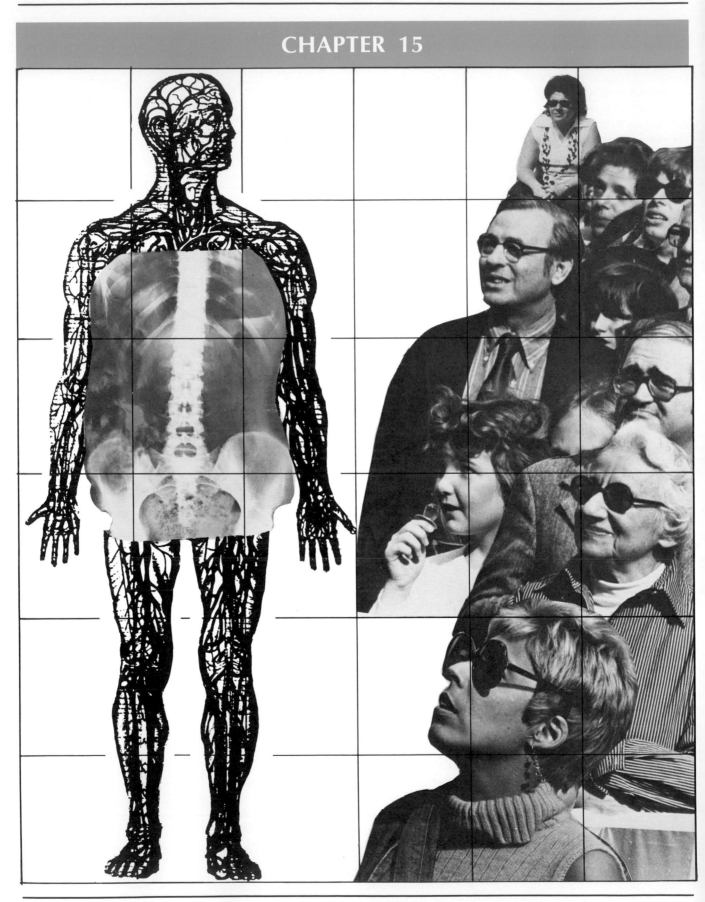

Debbie is an attractive college sophomore. Since moving into her dormitory in the fall, she has been constantly sneezing and experiencing colds. Since these symptoms got worse last week, she went to the campus health center for medical help. She was a given a thorough medical checkup, including blood chemistry tests.

To her amazement, the doctor told her that she had syphilis and probably an allergy of some sort. Her red and white blood cell counts were also very low. Debbie had never paid much attention to syphilis, much less allergies. She wondered whether the boy with whom she had intercourse several months ago gave her the syphilis infection. Did this infection have anything to do with her allergy? Should she reveal his name to the doctor? Or should she inform her former lover that he had syphilis and that he should seek medical help immediately?

Debbie's concerns about syphilis and allergy are the nature of this chapter. In addition to these disorders, this chapter also discusses disorders and infections that people of all ages may get or have—arthritis, diabetes, respiratory infections, and other venereal diseases.

Respond to the inventories and checklist that follow before proceeding to read this chapter.

☞ SUSCEPTIBILITY TO ARTHRITIS INVENTORY

INSTRUCTIONS Circle the number on the right side that you feel best describes your situation.

	Relatives			
	Mother Father	Sisters Brothers	Aunts Uncles Grandparents	None
1. Heredity—relatives who had, or were treated for, arthritis, rheumatism, or gout	50	40	20	0
	Age			
	40+	40–30	30–20	20–0
2. Age—female	60	40	20	5
male	20	10	5	1

	Never	1–2 Times per Week	3–4 Times per Week	Daily
3. Amount of physical activity — frequency of exercise	25	20	5	0
	0–30 minutes	30–45 minutes	45–60 minutes	1–2+ hours
Length of exercise or activity per frequency	15	10	3	0
	5+	3–4	1–2	Never
4. Number of times bones have been broken in your lifetime	10	7	3	0
	Number of Years			
	10+	5–9	2–4	1–0
Playing (body-contact) sports	10	7	1	0
	Pounds			
	50+	25–49	10–24	0
5. Overweight	30	20	10	0
	None	½–1 Hour	1–2 Hours	2+ Hours
6. Amount of rest per day from all activity	10	7	2	0
	Hours			
	4–5	5–6	6–7	8+
7. Amount (hours) of sleep per day	10	7	3	0
	Number of drinks per week			
	10+	6–9	5–1	0
8. Drinking alcoholic beverages	25	20	10	0
	Never	Once a Week	3 Times per Week	1–2+ Times per Day
9. Diet—eat fresh fruits and vegetables (minerals, vitamins C and A)	30	10	3	0

	Never	1–2 Times per Week	3 Times per Week	1–2 Times per Day
Drink whole or skim milk; eat cheese (minerals and vitamins)	10	7	3	0
B vitamins	20	15	5	0
	Always	Often	Sometimes	Never
10. Emotional stress				
Work stress or crises	25	20	5	0
Home or family stress	10	7	3	0
Crises of living	15	10	5	0
11. Rash—skin or face	30	20	5	0
12. Pain or stiffness in joints	75	50	25	0
13. Climate (live in cold)	10	7	3	0
14. Dampness (live in damp weather)	10	7	3	0

INTERPRETATION

	Degree of Risk
250+	*High*
250–100	*Average*
99–0	*Low*

Read the section on arthritis for more information.

☞ ARE YOU A DIABETIC? CHECKLIST

	Yes	No
Are you over 40?		
Any diabetics in your family?		
Are you overweight?		
Any sudden weight loss?		

	Yes	No
Are you constantly thirsty?		
Do you eat excessively?		
Do you urinate frequently?		
Do you tire easily?		
Do wounds heal slowly?		
Any pain in fingers or toes?		
Any changes in vision?		
Does skin itch frequently?		
Are you often drowsy?		
Have you had any babies weighing over 9 pounds at birth?		
Do you have a craving for sweets?		
Total		

INTERPRETATION:

Every "yes" you checked on the quiz raises the possibility that you could be a "hidden diabetic."
  Read the section on diabetes for more information.

☞ SUSCEPTIBILITY TO RESPIRATORY DISEASES

DIRECTIONS   Circle the number in the vertical column that best describes your behavior or habit.

	Frequency of Occurrence			
	Usually	Often	Seldom	Never
A. Symptoms				
1. Shortness of breath, as after climbing stairs	10	7	3	0
2. Coughing up sputum	15	12	4	0
3. Sore throat (irritation)	10	8	3	0

	Frequency of Occurrence			
	Usually	Often	Seldom	Never
4. Glands swell in neck	5	3	1	0
5. Running nose (sniffles)	5	3	1	0
6. Fever	10	7	3	0
7. Feeling tired at end of day	5	3	1	0
8. Poor physical endurance	5	3	1	0
B. Behavior				
9. Smoking 10 or more cigarettes a day	20	15	5	0
10. Live in an air-polluted community	5	3	1	0
11. Work with chemicals, grain, dusts, or metallic vapors	5	3	1	0
12. Use aerosol hair sprays or deodorants	10	8	3	0
13. Use or work with pesticide sprays	5	3	1	0
14. Have dog or cat as pet	5	3	1	0
15. Have carpet on the floor	5	3	1	0
16. Have children under 5 years of age or come in contact with them	10	7	4	0
17. Work with children ages 6–12	10	7	3	0
18. Come in contact with people all the time	10	7	3	0
19. Eat an unbalanced diet	10	7	3	0
20. Do not get enough rest	5	3	1	0
21. Get less than 8 hours sleep per day	5	3	1	0
22. Become overfatigued	5	3	1	0
23. Drink alcoholic beverages	5	3	1	0
24. Get feelings of depression	10	8	3	0
25. Feel life is not worth living	5	4	1	0
26. Live a sedentary life style	10	8	4	0

	Frequency of Occurrence			
	Usually	Often	Seldom	Never
27. Use hand when sneezing	5	3	1	0
28. Inhale air full of cigarette smoke	15	12	5	0
29. Become irritated at others	5	3	1	0
30. Have deadlines to meet	5	3	1	0
31. Have many crises or problems to solve	10	8	3	0
32. In company of friends or relatives suffering many colds or infections	5	3	1	0
33. Work or live in an air-conditioned office or house	5	3	1	0
34. Visit sick relatives	5	3	1	0
Total				

SCORING

1. Add the numbers you circled. This is your susceptibility score.

INTERPRETATION

Classify your score in the appropriate score range.

Score Range	Susceptibility to Respiratory Diseases
0–35	*Exceptionally low*
35–65	*Some*
66–90	*Average*
91–130	*High*
131+	Extremely high

Your susceptibility to respiratory diseases depends on many things, some of which are included in the behavioral variables. A few factors, like smoking cigarettes, being exposed to people, eating poorly, and feeling depressed collectively make one highly susceptible to respiratory infections. Some, like living in an air-polluted environment, having a pet, and not getting enough rest, are probably of lesser importance. There is an obvious vocational risk, for example, when working in a chemical or dust environment. Miners inhale fine dusts that irritate the lungs, causing miner's lung disease.

People differ in their ability to resist respiratory infections: Your behavior and life style can help to protect your body against infection.

If you are susceptible to respiratory infections, you should identify those behavioral items you circled that have weighted values of 10 or more points. By eliminating these behaviors, you can lower your susceptibility to respiratory infections.

ARTHRITIS

Arthritis is an umbrella used for up to 100 different kinds of rheumatic disorders. Although it is most commonly a chronic, disabling, systemic inflammation of the joints, arthritis also can affect connective tissue throughout the body. When this happens, the victim may have fever, get tired easily, have a poor appetite, lose weight, and have anemia, as well as the usual general symptoms of arthritis:

1. Pain and stiffness in joints on arising.
2. Pain and tenderness in one or more joints.
3. Pain and stiffness in the neck.
4. Lower back, knees and other joints.
5. Lengthy sensations in the fingertips, hands, and feet.
6. Recurrence of these symptoms periodically.

More than 50 million Americans suffer from some form of arthritis, with about 32 million arthritics requiring medical aid to relieve their pain and discomfort (1). (See Figure 15.1.) It can and does occur at all ages, affecting infants, children, teenagers, young persons, and middle-, and older-aged persons.

Arthritis takes many forms (see Figure 15.2):

1. Rheumatoid arthritis. This is an inflammation of the joints primarily, but it can also cause disease in other organs such as lungs, heart, spleen, and skin. It tends to subside and flare up unpredictably. It can occur at any age but often begins between the ages of 20 to 35 years. Women are affected three times more often that men.
2. Osteoarthritis. This is a wear-and-tear disease of the joints that comes with getting older.
3. Ankylosing spondylitis. This is a chronic inflammatory arthritis of the spine. It usually begins in the teens or early twenties.
4. Systemic lupus erythematosus (SLE arthritis). It damages joints and organs through the body. A skin rash on the face is a common mild form of this disease. Women are affected more often than men.
5. Gout (gouty arthritis). An inherited disorder with a nutrient-deficiency component, it usually inflames the big toe in men. Deposits of urate crystals in and around joints make gout very painful.

The exact cause of arthritis is unknown. However, it does seem to run in families. Persons may inherit a predisposition to one of the disorders. The biochemical makeup and metabolism of their bodies may make them more susceptible than others. Age, trauma, abnormal abuse of the body, diet, impaired blood supply to the joints, and emotional upsets, tensions, and crisis of living may also contribute partially to an arthritic condition. Although the various forms of arthritis cannot be cured, the inflammation of the surrounding tissues and the discomfort can be reduced by aspirin, sulindac, and other drugs; local heat; rest; exercise; managing stress; nutritious diet; and the loss of excess weight. Of these the two most important are exercise and diet.

The nature of arthritis is such that people with this condition will look anywhere for relief and help. As a result, this disorder makes it victims most vulnerable to misconceptions and quackery.

Interact with the Arthritis Inventory to determine your susceptibility to arthritis.

WAYS TO REDUCE THE RISK OF ARTHRITIS

1. Exercise all joints and parts of the body regularly.
2. Eat a well-balanced nutrient diet.
3. Avoid ingesting foods that have chemical preservatives.
4. Avoid exposing your body to long-term physical trauma.
5. Avoid getting emotionally upset.
6. Learn to cope with the crises of living.
7. Maintain a normal body weight—avoid becoming overweight or obese.

DIABETES

Diabetes is a major American health problem—a metabolic disorder that kills 300,000 people annually (25:1). More than 10 million have it, although only 5 million know they have it, while millions more are genetic carriers of this disorder.

Diabetes is a malfunction of the complicated system of physiological controls designed to supply the body with the right amounts of available fuel at the right times. In the normal body, starchy and sweet foods are broken down in the intestine to a simple sugar called glucose. Glucose circulates in the blood and enters cells all over the body to be used as energy or stored as glycogen in the liver and muscles, or stored as fat to be burned later to produce energy. In the diabetic, glucose cannot enter the cells as in a nondiabetic person and accumulates in the blood (25:5). The level of glucose in the blood depends on adequate amounts of insulin, a hormone or chemical messenger made in the pancreas. Insulin allows the cells to absorb glucose for energy. Insulin also promotes the storage of glucose as well as breaking-down stored fat and converting it into glucose when the level of glucose from food drops. Insulin actually main-

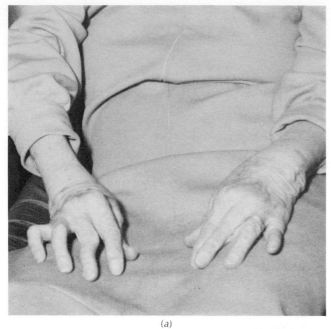

(a)

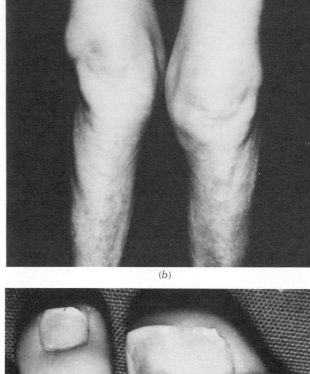

(b)

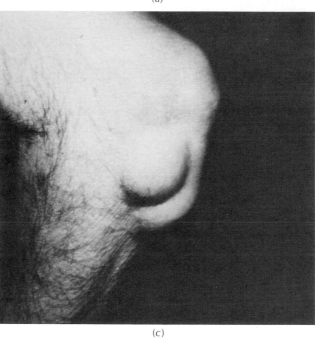

(c)

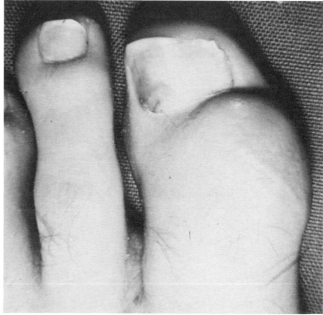

(d)

Figure 15.1
Symptomatic illustrations of different forms of arthritis. (a) Rheumatoid arthritis, (b) Muscle atrophy, (c) Rheumatoid nodules, and (d) Gout

tains a minimum blood sugar level, thereby ensuring adequate nourishment at all times for the brain and red blood cells. As would be expected, the high level of glucose buildup in the bloodstream results in the kidney filtering it out into the urine.

There are two kinds of diabetics (25:5). In growth-onset or juvenile diabetes (before age 20), the pancreas cannot secrete enough insulin, resulting in a pile-up of excess glucose in the blood. In the adult type of diabetes or maturity-onset diabetes (usually over age 40), the pancreas malfunctions to secrete too much insulin, resulting in hyperglycemia. Disrupting the work of insulin is overeating or excess body weight. Overweight reduces the number of insulin receptors or cell sites where insulin must bind to allow glucose to enter the body cell. These insulin receptors return to normal func-

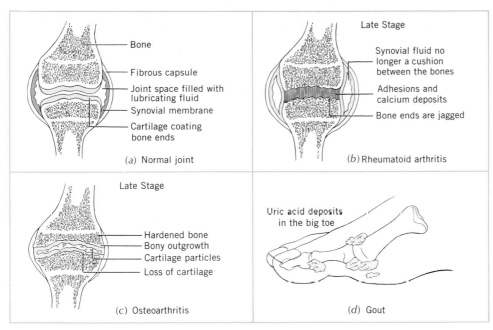

Figure 15.2
Anatomical illustrations of different kinds of arthritis.

tioning when the body weight returns to normal. Obesity also forces the fat person's pancreas to secrete excess insulin, thereby further disrupting physiological control of cellular fuel.

Diabetics have a predisposition to other diseases, disorders, and health complications (see Figure 7.6 in Chapter 7). Heart attacks occur two to four times more frequently in diabetics than in nondiabetics of the same age and sex (25:3). Diabetics are 17 times more prone to kidney diseases and 25 times more prone to blindness than nondiabetics (25:3). Diabetics also have a predisposition to vascular diseases such as gangrene in the legs and feet. Diabetes lessens the chance of successful pregnancy. It shortens life expectancy.

Diabetics can live normal lives, but they need to control their disorder with a proper diet and regular exercise (19:25). Although many doctors still prescribe drugs and a low carbohydrate diet, research strongly advocates a complementary diet and exercise programs. The emphasis in the diet for maturity-onset diabetics consists of restricting the total caloric intake to a level matching his or her ideal body weight and also allowing liberal allowances of starches but restricting sweets, sugar-rich pastries, and fats (see Chapter 6).

Diabetes runs in families (see Figure 15.3). A person inheriting this tendency may not show the disease until 40 years of age. Often diabetes may develop suddenly during an illness, during pregnancy, or when the predisposed person becomes overweight or obese. Over-

weight women entering menopause are especially vulnerable to diabetes. Most adults carrying a hereditary tendency for the maturity-onset form can avoid the disease entirely by merely controlling their food consumption, body weight, and exercising.

WAYS TO MAINTAIN A DIABETES-FREE LIFE STYLE

1. Eat a balanced nutrient diet.
2. Exercise regularly.
3. Avoid eating refined sugar and refined white flour foods such as pastries, sweets, soft drinks, and candy. Substitute more complex starch foods such as whole grain cereals and breads, fresh, green leafy vegetables, and fresh fruits.
4. Avoid alcoholic beverages.
5. Avoid smoking cigarettes.
6. Avoid becoming overweight or obese. This is especially important for women having a genetic predisposition to diabetes.
7. Know if you are a likely carrier.

BEHAVIOR MODIFICATION TECHNIQUES

A diabetic must be under the supervision of a medical doctor when modifying habits and/or behaviors.

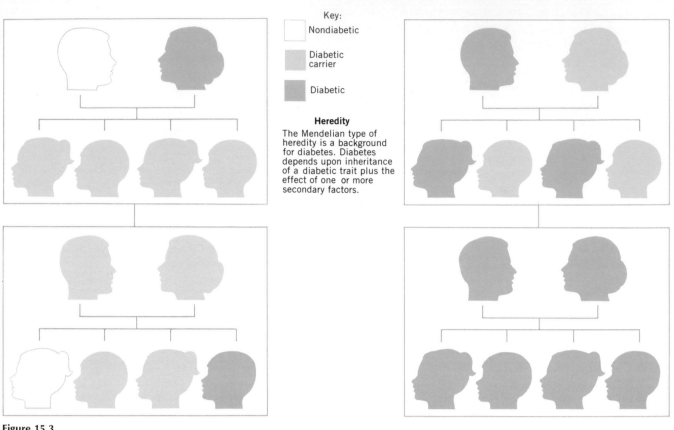

Key:

☐ Nondiabetic

▨ Diabetic carrier

▨ Diabetic

Heredity

The Mendelian type of heredity is a background for diabetes. Diabetes depends upon inheritance of a diabetic trait plus the effect of one or more secondary factors.

Figure 15.3

Diabetes is an hereditary disorder that prospective marriage partners should know about. (Courtesy of Eli Lilly and Co.)

COLDS AND INFLUENZAS

The most common infection of the respiratory system is the cold. Influenzas are also common. Numerous habits, such as inhaling cigarette smoke and air pollutants, lack of rest, overwork, lack of exercise, stress overload, poor nutrition, and poor mental attitude lower one's resistance to respiratory infections.

There is no known vaccine to ward off a cold or influenza. Taking superdoses of vitamin C, as professed by Linus Pauling and advocates of orthomolecular medicine, is not the complete answer. The human body fights infection best when a balance of all vitamins, minerals, and amino acids are all present in the body in adequate amounts. Medical science has not progressed far enough to give us the best way to prevent and treat colds and influenzas. After setting aside the nutritional controversy and lack of medical insight, the best way to prevent a cold or flu is to get plenty of rest and sleep, drink plenty of fluids, get proper nutrition, and maintain a positive emotional and psychological predisposition. Following this procedure lets your body fight the infecting cold viruses in a natural way. Taking antibiotics does not help to fight the infection, and other medications only alleviate symptoms.

LEGIONNAIRE'S DISEASE

A new respiratory disease aroused national alarm and fear in 1976 when 29 people died in July after attending an American Legion Convention in Philadelphia; hence its name "Legionnaire's Disease" (6;9;10). It became a mystery illness because epidemiologists and public health doctors were unable to identify the real cause of this disease. Today, the disease is still baffling physicians and the public at large, but we are making headway in trying to unravel the mystery.

Legionnaire's Disease (Legionella pneumophila) is caused by a long-lived bacteria in certain surroundings. It is capable of surviving in tap water for over a year. It is suspected that the organism usually lives in the soil. Air conditioning cooling-tower water was suspected as one of the places the Legionnaire's Disease bacteria live. However, these organisms do not survive in cooling-tower water for longer than 48 hours.

There is no evidence of direct person-to-person spread. Many of the cases of Legionnaire's Disease have occurred in persons already weakened by underlying disease or made more susceptible by drugs that suppress their immune systems.

The symptoms are identical to that of influenza and pneumonia, and include respiratory problems, diarrhea, high fever, headache, and severe pneumonia that does not culture the usual bacteria and does not respond to penicillin.

From 1976–1978, about 453 cases of infection with Legionnaire's Disease bacterium (LDB) have been confirmed in the United States. The majority of these cases have been in eastern and midwestern states. Death has occurred in about 20 percent of those infected.

This disease went unrecognized until 1976. Many deaths from pneumonia prior to 1976 were probably diagnosed incorrectly. We now suspect that many people who died from pneumonia probably died from Legionnaire's Disease. Hopefully, medical science will soon provide us with an LDB vaccine, together with an understanding of this mysterious disease.

EMPHYSEMA

Emphysema attacks those persons whose lungs had been exposed for long periods of time to irritation from chronic bronchitis, cigarette smoking, air pollution, and other chemical irritants such as coal dust. It also attacks glass blowers. Although it is most common among the elderly, it is probably initiated during youth.

In emphysema the thin walls of the tiny air sacs (the alveoli) lose their elasticity and rupture, resulting in large, nonfunctioning air spaces (see Figure 15.4). Breathing becomes progressively more difficult as the victim attempts to squeeze trapped air out of the lungs. Exchange of oxygen for carbon dioxide is impaired, necessitating more rapid breathing. Eventually, the air spaces fill with used air and produce the barrel-chest so typical of this disease. As the alveoli deteriorate, the passage of blood through the lungs is impaired and the heart must work harder in order to pump the blood. Heart failure often results from emphysema.

The best way to prevent emphysema is not to smoke, avoid polluted air, and exercise regularly throughout life.

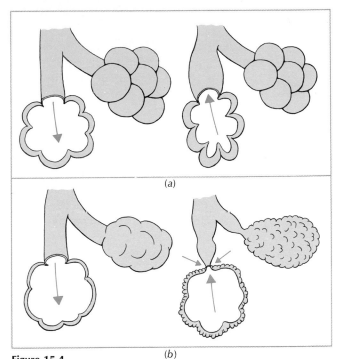

(a)

(b)

Figure 15.4
Illustrations contrasting healthy alveoli (a) dilating during inhalation and constricting during exhalation, with an emphysematic alveoli; (b) where air may enter the open space of the ruptured alveoli but may be poorly expelled.

ASTHMA

Asthma is a disorder that results in difficult breathing. The symptoms of an attack include sneezing, shortness of breath, and choked breathing. The choked breathing is caused by a swelling of the membrane that lines the bronchioles, a spasm or constriction of the bronchiole tubes, and mucous blockage of the tubes.

There are two types of asthma: extrinsic and intrinsic. The extensic type is caused by a reaction to substances called allergens (pollen, dust, animal hair, and certain foods). About 75 percent of people having asthma are allergic to one or more substances. Asthma may come on suddenly and disappear just as suddenly. When no allergens are identified in the asthmatic, the intrinsic type is suspected. Many such cases of asthma are associated with bacterial infections.

The cause of asthma is thought to be related to a chemical deficiency that causes clogged air passages and swollen mucous membranes. Heredity is also thought to be important. In some cases, attacks are often brought on by, or made worse by, emotional stress. Drugs such as aminophylline and adrenalin, are often prescribed to relax muscles and help keep air passages open.

ALLERGIES

Many persons suffer from headaches, tension, depression, upset stomachs, fatigue, and irritability. On the surface, these symptoms appear to be related to emotional disorders, but many doctors are now aware that they may be symptoms of an allergy.

Allergy is hypersensitivity to a specific substance, which, in a similar quantity, does not bother other people (5:3). There are millions of people with allergies, most of whom are not aware that they have allergies. Many conditions, such as asthma, skin rash, and hay fever, are publically recognized allergies. But few persons are aware that allergies often masquerade as bronchitis, colds, headaches, depressions, and emotional disorders, or that the food they crave the most, or eat regularly, may often be allergic to their bodies. Most allergic persons have multiple allergies that affect various parts of their bodies at different times in their lives.

Allergies tend to run in families. Often lack of a metabolic enzyme causes an allergy to flare up. The tendency to develop an allergy is often related to the body's inability to protect itself against harmful germs and other foreign substances. Human bodies develop antibodies in an effort to destroy the body invaders or allergens. Developing an allergy resembles, to a certain degree, developing antibodies against germs. Thus, when you develop an allergy, you develop antibodies against a specific allergen. For example, if you are allergic to cat dander and are exposed to a houseful of cats, the cat antibodies in your system immediately "pounce on" the cat-dander allergen. Your body reacts by releasing chemical substances such as histamine, SRS-A, bradykinin, and prostaglandins, which, in turn, irritate or injure different tissues found in almost all parts of your body. The symptoms vary, depending on many factors, including your age, the severity of your allergic sensitivity, the physical state of your body, and the amount of allergen to which you are exposed.

Allergies are caused by sensitivity to something you eat, breathe, or touch (5). In addition, infections, emotional stress, and weather change can trigger or aggravate an allergy that is latent, hidden, or asymptomatic. You can be allergic or become allergic to any of the following substances (5):

1. Ingestants (what you eat or take into your body).
   (a) Foods. Allergic reactions to something you eat can make you sneeze, wheeze, swell, or itch. Unsuspected food allergy can give you a variety of delayed symptoms, including headache, abdominal pain, and nervous system symptoms. Among the most common causes of food allergy are milk, wheat, chocolate, sugar, corn, cola, egg, citrus, the pea-
   bean family, fish, beef and shellfish. Food coloring and food additives can also cause allergic reactions. The more often you eat a food, and the larger the quantity of food you eat, the greater the chances of developing symptoms of a hidden allergy to that food. Food allergies are usually "hidden allergies." The usual symptoms are nasal congestion, stomach ache, headache, irritability, fatigue, as well as other general body symptoms.
   (b) Drugs. Almost any drug or chemical can cause any variety of allergic reactions. Such drugs include aspirin, penicillin, or other antibiotics; pain relievers; tranquilizers; and sedatives.

2. Inhalants.
   (a) Plants. Pollen grains from trees, grasses, and shrubbery can make your eyes water and run—an allergic reaction called hay fever. If your condition gets worse from late August until fall, you are probably allergic to ragweed pollen. If you have trouble in the spring or summer, you are probably allergic to mold or grass pollen. If your trouble comes early in the spring, you are probably allergic to tree pollen.
   (b) Molds. If you sneeze, get a headache, or get watery eyes when cleaning the basement or a musty closet, you may be allergic to molds. Molds (mildew or fungus) are tiny forms of plant life that are found everywhere. Indoor molds in windy and/or damp, rainy areas cause year-round symptoms. A change in air circulation and/or temperature can also cause a short-term allergic reaction.
   (c) Animal danders. Cats, dogs, horses, cattle, ducks, chickens, and other pets deposit their dander (waste skin cells) around the house causing an allergy to flare up in susceptible persons.
   (d) House dust. House dust particles cause symptoms in many allergic persons. Such dust can bring on early asthma or cause you to "keep a cold." House-dust-sensitive persons experience more trouble when they stay indoors a lot and when forced-air furnaces are operating.
   (e) Chemical inhalants. Strong fumes and odors bother some people. Chemical substances in paint, perfume, tobacco smoke, smog, plastic, printing ink in newspapers, fabric slip-cover odors, hair sprays, deodorants, room-freshener sprays, and insect bomb sprays can cause allergic symptoms.

(f) Miscellaneous other inhalants. Other substances, such as wool, silk, cottonseed, rice and corn powders, talcum powder, cereal grain dust, and insect dust (disintegrating insect bodies), can cause allergic reactions.

3. Substances that enter your body through your skin. Most persons are aware that poison ivy and poison oak can cause a skin rash, fever, and other allergy symptoms. A rash may also develop from wearing clothing washed in a particular type of soap. Bee, hornet, wasp, and spider stings, as well as snake bites, cause allergic reactions. Stingrays and jelly-fish bites, while bathing in ocean waters, can also cause discomforting reactions.

4. Other nonspecific factors. These factors may trigger or aggravate your allergic symptoms:

(a) Your physical environment. Heat, cold, weather change, humidity, and atmospheric pressure may influence your allergy. Barometric pressure change may precipitate an attack of asthma, headache, or muscle-joint pains. Light-skinned persons are hypersensitive to sunlight.

(b) Infections. Infections may make an allergy worse. Persons who continuously "have a cold" all winter probably suffer from combined allergy and infection. Respiratory infection may occur more frequently in an allergic person.

(c) Psychological and emotional factors. Emotional upsets can trigger or aggravate illnesses, as well as allergies, in individuals who have already been specifically sensitized to dust, pollen, mold, food, and allergens. However, doctors disagree on the importance of emotions in causing allergic diseases.

Common complaints, signs, and symptoms of allergy (5) are as follows:

1. Overall symptoms—the person looks pale and feels tired; has muscle aches, stiff joints, enlargement of lymph glands, as in the neck; has a low-grade fever (37–37.6° Celsius or 99–99.8°F). The hands may feel "puffy" and swollen.

2. Skin—rash; welts; hives; scaly, dry, itchy, and burning skin; excessive sweating; eczema; urticaria (hives); and contact dermatitis.

3. Mouth—rash on tongue, canker sores, excess drooling, itching of the roof of the mouth, and puffiness or stinging of the lips.

4. Nose-throat—itchy nose, running (clear discharge) or stuffed-up nose, clearing throat a lot, having excess mucus.

5. Ear—repeated rubbing or scratching of the ears; repeated ear infections; ears that ring, buzz, or hurt; vertigo or dizziness.

6. Eye—itchiness and burning sensation; red, bloodshot eyes; puffy eyelids, bags or dark circles under eyes, blurred vision.

7. Chest—chest feels tight, coughing, wheezing, coughing up phlegm, shortness of breath.

8. Digestion—stomach ache, diarrhea, constipation, bloated feeling, excessive gas (flatulence).

9. Circulatory—cold hands, fast pulse, pale skin, elevated blood pressure.

10. Nervous—hyperactivity, irritability, restlessness, clumsy and uncoordinated, disrupted sleep, dopey or drowsy feeling, depression, inability to concentrate.

11. Urogenital—frequent urination, burning sensation during urination, frequent urinary infections, itching and/or extra secretion of mucus from vagina.

BEHAVIOR MODIFICATION TECHNIQUES

What to do if you have or suspect that you have an allergy (5:18–24):

1. Keep a diary, a record of the time of day, month, year when you suffer from an allergy and the symptoms.

2. Make a family history of allergy in your relatives.

3. Get a physical-laboratory examination from a good allergist.

4. Get allergy, scratch intradermal skin, food, gastric, and radioallergosorbent (RAST) tests. The RAST test determines the levels of antibodies for specific allergic substances present in the bloodstream from a blood sample.

5. Get desenitization shots for those things you are allergic to.

6. Try elimination diets with the pulse test for allergy. This is the best way to find out if you are allergic to food. Simply remove a single food from your diet for one to three weeks. If your symptoms disappear, or improve, then you may be allergic. When the symptoms reappear upon eating the food again, your suspicions of allergy about the food are comfirmed. Keep eliminating foods, one at a time, until you have checked all foods. Start

with foods and drinks you eat/drink the most or crave for.

7. Eat a variety of foods and don't eat the same food all the time. Although you may not have allergic symptoms now, the symptoms to the food you eat often could surface later on in life.

8. Observe and manipulate your surroundings. Just as you eliminate one food, try eliminating dust, feathers, dogs, cats, smoke, perfumes, sprays, etc. Try to identify what it is that seems to trigger or aggravate your symptoms.

9. Get medicine (such as antihistamine decongestant and asthma sprays) that can make you more comfort-able, and lessen the severity and duration of your symptoms.

10. Take extra amounts of vitamin C (refer to Chapter 6).

11. Keep your house/room dust free.

12. Avoid fumes and strong odors.

13. Get a pet that will not cause an allergy.

14. Stay away from barns or grain elevators.

15. Avoid insect powders and sprays.

16. Avoid chilling.

17. Stay away from heavy pollen exposure.

18. Air condition your home.

19. Learn as much as you can about allergies.

SEXUALLY TRANSMITTED DISEASES

Venereal diseases (VD) are transmitted by direct skin-to-skin contact during sexual intercourse or other intimate contact. The term *venereal* is derived from Venus, the ancient Roman goddess of love. Most of these diseases have been around for thousands of years. Although basically easy to detect and diagnose, and in most cases treat, venereal diseases are difficult to prevent and stamp out. Social and cultural factors, along with sex being private and personal, create embarrassment and guilt, thereby interfering with bringing these diseases under control.

The most prevalent venereal diseases include gonorrhea, syphilis, vaginitis, trichomonos vaginalis vaginitis, candida albicans vaginitis, lymphogranuloma venereum, herpes genitalis, and pubic lice (crabs).

Each of these diseases is caused by a separate distinct type of infecting microorganism. Therefore, an individual may be infected with two or more of these microorganisms at the same time and display signs and symptoms of both diseases simultaneously. The symptoms may often be hidden and nonobservable, as in women. Reinfection is also possible everytime one has a new sexual experience, as immunity to venereal disease usually does not occur.

In the United States VD is transmitted every 11 seconds, and 75 percent of all cases are in young people between the ages of 15 to 30 (23). The U.S. government has done many things to encourage people to be treated. It is not legal for anyone over 12 to be treated without parental consent. Clinics have been set up to treat infected persons at no cost. Recent VD screening programs have been a big factor in reducing gonorrhea.

Although there are numerous concerns and suggestions voiced about controlling these diseases, one thing is certain: many persons are not going to stop having sexual relations for fear of getting venereal disease. In order to protect your body from such diseases and detect early signs of these diseases, you should know something about the anatomy and physiology of your body, as well as the nature of these infections. You should become knowledgeable about the male and female reproductive systems.

GONORRHEA

Gonorrhea, the most common of all venereal diseases, is caused by the diploid bean-shaped bacteria, gonococcus. Outside the human body the gonococcus dies within a few minutes. Thus it is impossible to catch gonorrhea from toilet seats, towels, cups, and so on, that have been used by an infected person. Gonococcus grows well only in mucous or moist membranes, such as the mouth and throat, eyes, the vagina, cervix, anal canal, and the urethra (the tube from the bladder to the outside of the body).

Early Symptoms in the Male

Once gonococci successfully enter the penis, they invade the cells of the urethra, causing inflammation of the urethra. Most infected men notice symptoms 3 to 5 days after the infecting sexual intercourse. Symptoms can appear as early as 1 day, or as late as 2 weeks after infection. At first a thin, clear mucous discharge seeps out of the meatus (opening of the penis). Within a day or two the discharge becomes heavy, thick, and creamy. It is usually white but may be yellow or yellow-green. The discharge is composed of dead urethral cells, bacteria, and white blood cells. The lips of the meatus (skin around the opening of the penis) become swollen, and most men feel pain and a burning sensation in the penis during urination.

Gonorrheal infection can occur in the anus and rectum in persons who engage in anal sex (homosexuals). There may or may not be any mucous discharge or mild irritation.

If a male observes these symptoms, he should immediately go to see a doctor and have a clinical diagnosis made. The doctor can usually decide if gonorrhea is present by just examining the man's genital area. However, a sample of discharge or secretions from within the penis must be tested in the laboratory to confirm a doctor's observation. The simplest test for gonorrhea is a microscopic examination and incubation of a culture plate for 24 to 48 hours. Visible colonies of gonococci on the culture plate media confirm the infection. Such confirmation is referred to as "positive." Thus an immediate checkup of the suspected infection is the easiest way to confirm whether one has gonorrhea.

After about 2 weeks, symptoms of urethritis (inflammation of urethra) begin to disappear on their own. The discharge gradually disappears and urination is no longer painful. However, the bacteria are still present, and the man can still infect his sexual partner. Bacteria now begin to invade the urethra and prostate gland and spread to the vas deferens (the tube from the prostate to the testicles), reaching the epididymis, or the back of one or both of the testicles, causing gonococcal epididymitis. Epididymitis causes pain in the groin, a heavy sensation in the affected testicles and the formation of a small, hard, painful swelling at the bottom of the testicles. If the infection is left untreated, epididymitis may leave scar tissue that closes off the passage of spermatozoa from the affected testicle, causing sterility.

Early gonococcal urethritis is uncomfortable and painful. It causes most men to seek early medical treatment. Modern antibiotic treatment is effective in fighting gonorrhea.

Early Symptoms in the Female

Nine out of ten women infected with gonorrhea may feel or observe no symptoms, and hence may not be aware of the infection (18). This is especially true if the cervical-vaginal area is infected. Many women may not observe or feel the vaginal discharge or irritation as a green or yellow-green pus. Instead they may mistake it for normal vaginal discharge or menstrual flow.

However, women will feel a burning pain during urination if the urethra or meatus is red and swollen from infection. These symptoms are the same as in the male. Thus a woman will have recognizable gonorrheal symptoms when the urethra is infected.

If the infection and symptoms are untreated in the early stage of infection (up to 10 weeks), the infection will spread to the uterus and into the Fallopian tubes. Infected tubes are referred to as salpingitis. Inflammation or subsequent scarring may block the Fallopian tubes, causing sterility.

An infected pregnant woman may infect her baby's eyes as the baby passes through the mother's infected cervix or vagina. This natal infection of the eyes (gonococcal ophthalmalia) can cause blindness. It is common medical practice to put drops of 1 percent silver nitrate solution in the eyes of all newborn infants as a preventive measure. Another preventive measure is to have all pregnant women tested for gonorrhea several times during their pregnancy.

Women need to rely on men to inform them of gonorrheal infection. For many women, the first sign of their own infection is gonorrhea in a male sexual partner. Any man who has gonorrhea should immediately inform his sexual partners of what is usually their common infection. This detective reporting would do much to prevent the needless 60,000 to 100,000 young American females who each year become sterile from untreated gonorrheal infection (22).

SYPHILIS

Syphilis is the most serious and the second most prevalent venereal disease in North America. Although gonorrhea infects more persons, syphilis kills more people. Syphilis is suspected of killing 1000 or more adults each month as a consequence of its long-range crippling, chronic, degenerative effects (2:11).

Syphilis is very different from gonorrhea. Whereas gonorrhea is normally a local surface infection, syphilis is always a systematic infection, spreading throughout the body. It is caused by a spirochete (*Treponema pallidum*). The spirochete is extremely fragile and can survive for only a few minutes when exposed to air. A person contracts the spirochete from an open wound (lesion) onto moist warm skin, thus allowing it to survive long enough to burrow through the skin surface into the blood establishing a colony (infection), and eventually spreading throughout the body. Like gonorrhea, it is spread through physical contact during intercourse or kissing. Washing the skin with soap and water kills T. pallidum immediately. Wearing a condom helps but does not always protect a man against syphilis, since the organisms can enter at the junction of the penis and the rest of the body, which the condom does not cover (3:29). Spirochete in an infected pregnant woman can cross through the placenta and infect the fetus. If the fetus and the pregnant woman are left untreated, the infant may be stillborn, or seriously disfigured and diseased.

Without medical treatment, the initial infection progresses through distinct stages, each with characteristic signs and symptoms.

Primary Syphilis

Infection begins when the spirochete enters a tiny break in the skin. The infected person may show no sign of the disease for 10 to 28 days. During this time, the spirochete multiplies in the body.

The first stage and symptom to appear is a chancre (pronounced skanker) (see Figure 15.5). This is a sore that appears at the exact spot where infection took place. The sore is a dull red bump about the size of a pea and is painless. The chancre is swarming with spiro-

chetes; hence it is highly infectious and can pass the infection on to sexual partners.

The chancre is usually located on or near the sex organs, but it can be on the lip, fingers, or any part of the body. In females it is often within the vagina and usually goes unnoticed. The chancre usually disappears with or without treatment in 3 to 6 weeks. It is about this time that the chancre disappears (3rd to 4th week) and blood tests for syphilis can accurately confirm the infection.

The first stage of syphilis, if untreated, gradually progresses into the secondary stage. About 6 weeks after the appearance of the primary chancre, a generalized skin rash develops (see Figure 15.6). The rash as a symptom varies greatly—some persons may have a rash on the

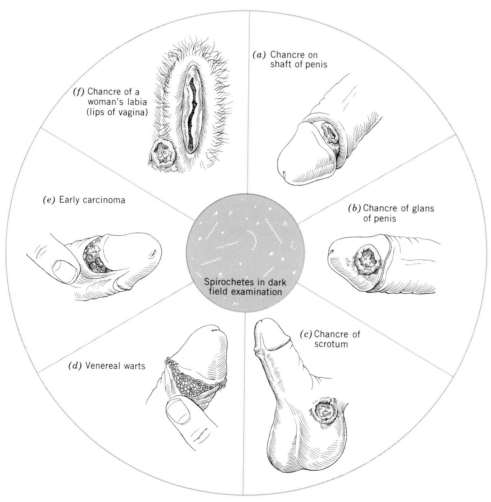

Figure 15.5

Illustrations of symptoms of venereal diseases in male and female genitalia. (Adapted from Frank H. Netter, *Cica Collection of Medical Illustrations*, Vol. 4, *Endocrine System*, © Copyright 1965, CIBA Pharmaceutical Company, Division of CIBA-GEIBY Corporation.)

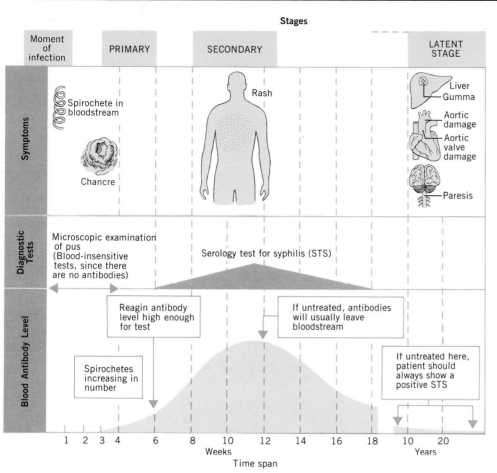

Figure 15.6

Comparative summary of the course of syphilis from the moment of infection, including the development of antibodies and the effectiveness of blood tests.

shoulders, upper arms, chest, back, and abdomen, while others may have only part of the body covered with a rash. The rash bumps are greyish-blue on black skin, and rose-pink on white skin. Rash sores at this time are highly infectious. The rash spots become brownish-colored and fade away. Other symptoms may include sore throat, headache, slight fever, red eyes, pain in the joints, and patches of hair falling out. These symptoms may last from several days to several months and fade away. Since these symptoms mimic those of other diseases, syphilis can easily be mistaken for another disease. It is, therefore, important to have one's physician confirm syphilis. It is at this stage that syphilis is most contagious and a blood test at this stage would be positive.

Most infected persons in this country are treated before or during this stage of syphilis. If untreated for about 2 years, the disease progresses to the third or latent stage.

Latent syphilis is simply hidden syphilis. There are no outward clinical signs or symptoms. A blood test is helpful in diagnosing the disease. The infected male and female person is no longer contagious at this stage, but the untreated pregnant female can pass on the infection to her unborn child (congenital syphilis). Although there are no observable symptoms, the disease is spreading throughout the body, gradually degenerating the brain, spinal cord, hearing, sight, heart, bones, and liver. After 10 to 20 years, the disease can cause heart disease, blindness, mental deterioration, and even death.

The treatment for syphilis is the same as for gonorrhea: antibiotics. The VDRL (Veneral Disease Research Laboratory) test is an accurate, inexpensive, and easy-to-perform blood (serology) test for syphilis. It is accurate only when done during the time that a person has secondary infection (after the 4th week of infection). (See Figure 15.6.)

Patients who are being treated for syphillis should not have sexual intercourse for 1 month after receiving treatment.

To reduce the spread of the disease, prenatal and premarital tests are required by law in 45 states.

VAGINITIS

Vaginitis is an inflammation of the vagina. Vaginitis may be caused by the organism *Trichomonas*, the yeastlike fungus candida albicans and herpes simplex virus. Vaginitis is the most common disease of the female genital system. Although not very dangerous, vaginitis is very uncomfortable. The various kinds of vaginitis have similar symptoms, and it is usually possible to tell them apart by examining a drop of vaginal secretion under a microscope. The doctor should do so before prescribing medication; otherwise the treatment may be ineffective.

Trichomonas vaginitis is an inflammation of the vagina caused by a pear-shaped protozoan. However, symptoms in the female can include intense itching and burning of the vagina, and small rashlike spots in its lining. Most infected women become very uncomfortable because of an abundance of white or yellow discharge that has an unpleasant odor. It irritates the vagina and vulva causing them to become red, itch, and even painful.

Trichomonas infection in the male is usually without symptoms, since the organisms do not survive in the male sexual organs. Both an infected woman and her sexual partner should be treated at the same time with the drug metronidazole (Flagyl). A treated woman should not have sexual intercourse for 1 week after being treated with metronidazole.

Candida albicans vaginitis is caused by a yeastlike organism. This organism is a normal inhabitant of the mouth, skin, digestive tract, and vagina. Pregnancy, diabetes, birth control pills, antibiotic treatment, many hours spent in a wet swimsuit, and lowered body resistance to disease make a woman more susceptible than a man to this infection.

Most women carry candida albicans in their vagina at some time in their lives, although active vaginitis does not always occur. The vagina can become infected by the candida traveling from the anus along the surface of the menstrual pad, or when the woman wipes herself after moving her bowels, or by an infected male penis during sexual intercourse.

Symptoms include intense itching, dryness, redness of the vagina, and painful intercourse. The vaginal discharge is not heavy—it is thick, white, and curdy.

Prevention includes keeping the vaginal area dry; using proper toilet habits; and correcting conditions, such as poor nutrition, that increase susceptibility. The most effective treatment is the antibiotic hystatin (mycostatin) in the form of vaginal tablets.

HERPES VIRUS GENITALIS

This infection is more common in women than in men. Herpes simplex viruses are carried by most people at all times, although usually in a state of latency (dormancy). Most persons are exposed to herpes virus during childhood without much complication. Once the symptoms subside, the viruses continue to live in the cells of the body without causing symptoms for the rest of the person's life. Both males and females may become infected through sexual intercourse. Sores may occur in the genital area as blisters, or as red sores, causing considerable pain and discomfort during coitus.

There is no antibiotic treatment available to kill the virus. The best way to prevent infection is to practice good hygienic habits and ingest a balance of nutrients.

PUBIC LICE (CRABS)

These are small, yellowish-gray insects $1/16$ of an inch long that live as external parasites on the body. They live on pubic hair but will also live in hair on the chest, underarms, beards, and eyebrows. Pubic lice feed on human blood, causing an intense itching and discoloration of the skin. The itching is a kind of allergic reaction to the bite of the louse. Female lice attach eggs, called nits, to the body hair. These eggs hatch in 6 to 8 days.

Pubic lice are usually transmitted from person to person by sexual intercourse or by contacting infected bedding, toilet seats, or clothing. Pubic lice and their eggs are not affected by normal soap, but they can be killed easily by a nonprescription drug—gamma benzene hexachloride, or a lotion shampoo—Kwellada in the United States and Kevell in Canada. After several treatment applications, the lice separate from the body and die. They cannot live longer than 24 hours away from the human body although the eggs will continue to hatch for about 10 more days. The infected person should have a complete change of clean clothing and bedding after treatment.

URINARY TRACT INFECTIONS

The most common urinary tract (kidney, bladder, urethra) infection is cystitis, or infection of the bladder. It occurs mostly in women.

Cystitis is usually caused by the bacteria *Escherichia coli* (E. coli). This organism is present in the large intestine of all healthy men and women. The reason for the infection is not certain.

Symptoms include burning pain on urination and a frequent desire to urinate. The urine is hazy and sometimes reddish in color. If left untreated, cystitis can spread to the kidneys, causing severe complication.

After diagnosis is made on a sample of blood and the bacteria is identified, most doctors will begin treatment with sulfa drugs or antibiotics. Black men and women should refuse to accept sulfa drug therapy unless a test for G6PD deficiency has been performed (3). In such people, sulfa drugs can cause a serious form of hemolytic anemia, a disease in which red blood cells burst and die. Sulfa-induced hemolytic anemia can be fatal (3:39).

WAYS TO REDUCE THE RISK OF VD

1. Choose your sex partner with care. Avoid a partner who is promiscuous or sexually active with many other persons. Limit your contacts to one individual on the assumption that this individual is also limiting his or her contacts.
2. Although not 100 percent safe, a condom will greatly reduce the chances of infection.
3. Insist on good personal hygiene. Wash the genital area thoroughly with soap and water immediately after intercourse and make sure your partner does the same.
4. Urinate as soon as possible after sexual intercourse. Doing so can wash some of the microorganisms out of the urinary tract before they advance further. This measure is more effective for males than for females.
5. Routinely check for VD infection if you are sexually active.
6. Seek medical help immediately when experiencing VD symptoms.
7. If you have infected a partner, or your partner has infected you, you have a moral obligation to let your partner know that you were infected, that your partner may be infected, and that your partner should check for a VD infection.
8. Women should wipe the anus from front to back. Doing so reduces the risk of bacteria from the large intestine entering the urinary tract and bladder and causing urinary tract infections.
9. Do not sit around in a wet swim suit, especially on hot, humid days, as this encourages the growth of yeastlike organisms.
10. Wear cotton underwear and change it daily.
11. Eat a well-balanced nutrient diet. It will help reduce susceptibility to infection.

WHERE TO GO FOR HELP

1. *Allergies*
   (a) Look up an allergist in your local telephone book.
   (b) Write to: Gerald Freeman Inc.
       Public Relations
       850 Third Avenue
       New York, N.Y. 10022
2. *Arthritis*
   (a) Local public health department.
   (b) Local chapter of The Arthritis Foundation.
   (c) Write to: The Arthritis Foundation
       3400 Peachtree Road, N.E.
       Atlanta, Ga. 30326
3. *Diabetes*
   (a) Local chapter of the Diabetic Association.
   (b) Local public health department.
   (c) Local Medical Association.
   (d) Local campus health center.
4. *Respiratory Infections*
   (a) Local public health department.
5. *Venereal Disease*
   (a) Local public health department.
   (b) Local campus health center.
   (c) National VD hotline toll-free number: 800-523-1885.
   (d) Write to: The American Social Health Association
       1740 Broadway
       New York, N.Y. 10019
   (e) Social Issues Research Council
       19075 Ventura Boulevard, Suite 220
       Encino, CA. 91316

Further Readings

Arthritis: The Basic Facts, Atlanta, Ga.: The Arthritis Foundation, latest edition.
Bender, Stephen J., *Venereal Diseases,* Dubuque, Iowa: W. C. Brown, 1971.
Cherniak, Donna, and Allan Feingold, *V.D. Handbook,* Montreal, Canada: Montreal Health Press, June 1975.
Crook, William G., *Are You Allergic?: A Guide to Normal Living for Allergic Adults and Children,* Jackson, Tenn.: Professional Books, 1974.

PART E

LIFE CYCLE CONCERNS

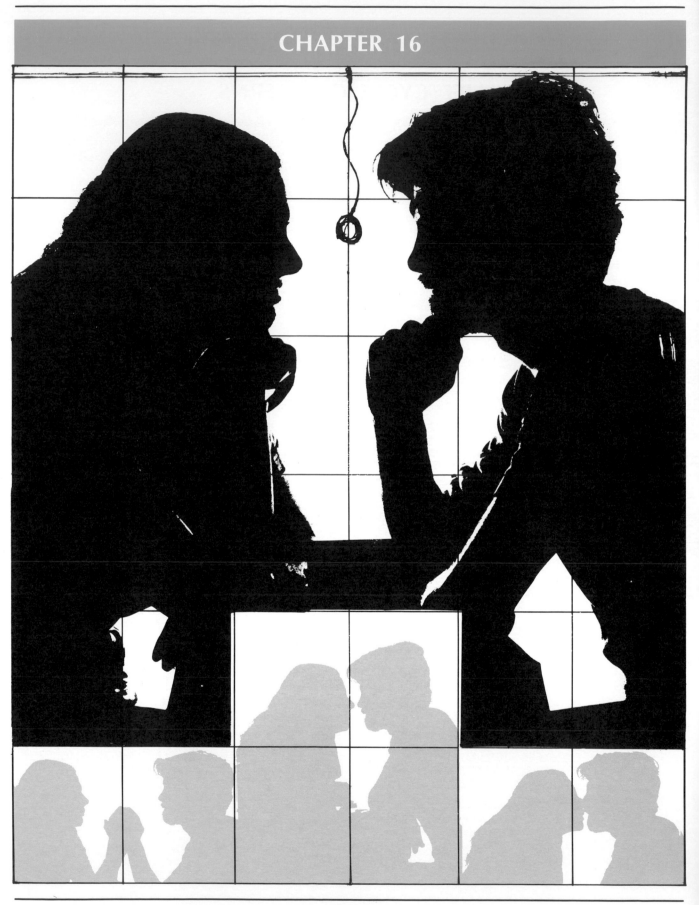

People of all ages have the same love, sex, companionship, and interpersonal needs as their parents, grandparents, and other people have. Although some persons may argue that new attitudes have emerged about sex and marriage, the basic human needs of companionship, love, and emotional fulfillment have not changed. What has happened is that technology has accentuated loneliness and evolved many different ways of fulfilling these vital human needs. Unfortunately, technology has not lifted or updated our social-economic restrictions of the past. Consequently, adults of all ages, including college students, are often unable to feel adequately fulfilled in sex and love. A recent national survey (1) found that people of all ages were more concerned about a strong commitment to a relationship, a search against loneliness, rather than just sex for pleasure.

Sexual intercourse is a natural body function of living, much like eating, drinking, breathing, thinking, exercising, and feeling. Because of this, sex pervades every facet of life. Recent research points out that an active sex life is essential for good health (7:199–201). Coitus provides a valuable combination of physical stimulation and relaxation (7:201).

During sexual activity blood pressure and pulse rate rise, as much as they do when we take a walk or climb a flight of stairs—then promptly return to quiet resting levels. It is this sequence of stimulation and relaxation that is generally considered conducive to good health. In addition, sexual relationships also fulfill emotional and social needs.

Many doctors (7:201) agree that by improving our mood and relieving psychic tensions, sex makes us less vulnerable to the numerous aches, pains, and more serious health impairments, such as emotional distress and depression. Statisticians suspect that continuous sexual activity throughout married life is responsible for married men and women living significantly longer than those who are single, widowed, or divorced. On the other hand, it should be obvious that abstention from sexual activity is not necessarily a cause of poor health.

Commitments relevant to young people include (1) accepting masculine/feminine sex roles, (2) giving love, (3) developing interpersonal socially responsible relationships, (4) accepting the ideas of marriage and family living, and (5) clarifying personal values and ethics as a guide to sexual behavior and family living.

Young people are at a stage of life when they are expected to assume certain sex roles, identities, and commitments and, at the same time, continue to develop as persons while attending college. In spite of such expectations creating real emotional strain on young people, most of them eventually clarify their sexual roles and identities and establish numerous commitments.

This chapter deals with the many aspects of marriage and human sexuality: love and family living and alternative sexual behaviors, sexual responses, and sexual dysfunctions.

The two inventories that follow should be used as a guide to helping you assess how you and your loved one or date feel about sex, dating, companionship, and marriage.

☞ SEXUALITY SCALE

PURPOSE   To help you assess your attitude toward marriage, sex, dating, and other sexual-social relationships.

DIRECTIONS   Nineteen sexual-social relationships have been selected and identified as concepts. Each concept has the same three adjectives which help you to describe the strength of your feelings.

        Select the side of the scale that best describes how you feel about a concept.

        If your feelings about a concept are very strong, check (✔) the space on the extreme left or right side of the scale, for example,

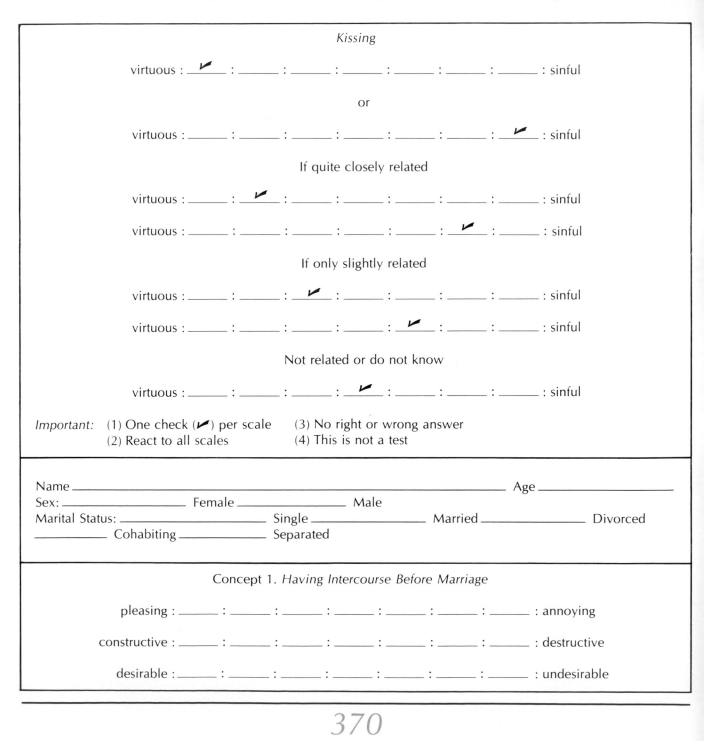

Kissing

virtuous : __✔__ : _____ : _____ : _____ : _____ : _____ : _____ : sinful

or

virtuous : _____ : _____ : _____ : _____ : _____ : __✔__ : _____ : sinful

If quite closely related

virtuous : _____ : __✔__ : _____ : _____ : _____ : _____ : _____ : sinful

virtuous : _____ : _____ : _____ : _____ : _____ : __✔__ : _____ : sinful

If only slightly related

virtuous : _____ : _____ : __✔__ : _____ : _____ : _____ : _____ : sinful

virtuous : _____ : _____ : _____ : _____ : __✔__ : _____ : _____ : sinful

Not related or do not know

virtuous : _____ : _____ : _____ : __✔__ : _____ : _____ : _____ : sinful

Important: (1) One check (✔) per scale   (3) No right or wrong answer
        (2) React to all scales   (4) This is not a test

Name _____ Age _____
Sex: _____ Female _____ Male
Marital Status: _____ Single _____ Married _____ Divorced
_____ Cohabiting _____ Separated

Concept 1. *Having Intercourse Before Marriage*

pleasing : _____ : _____ : _____ : _____ : _____ : _____ : _____ : annoying

constructive : _____ : _____ : _____ : _____ : _____ : _____ : _____ : destructive

desirable : _____ : _____ : _____ : _____ : _____ : _____ : _____ : undesirable

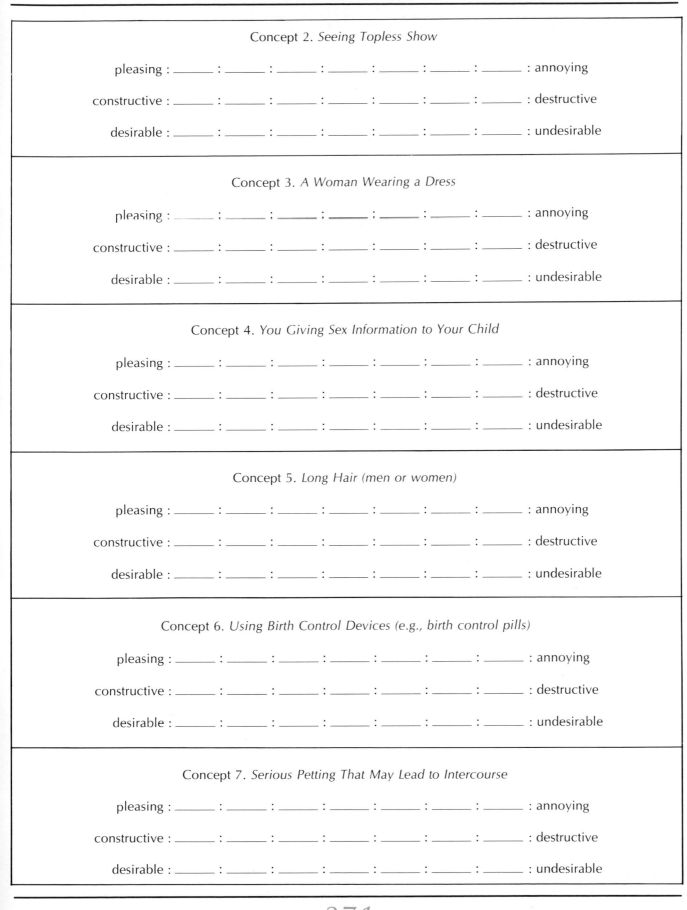

Concept 2. *Seeing Topless Show*

pleasing : _____ : _____ : _____ : _____ : _____ : _____ : _____ : annoying

constructive : _____ : _____ : _____ : _____ : _____ : _____ : _____ : destructive

desirable : _____ : _____ : _____ : _____ : _____ : _____ : _____ : undesirable

Concept 3. *A Woman Wearing a Dress*

pleasing : _____ : _____ : _____ : _____ : _____ : _____ : _____ : annoying

constructive : _____ : _____ : _____ : _____ : _____ : _____ : _____ : destructive

desirable : _____ : _____ : _____ : _____ : _____ : _____ : _____ : undesirable

Concept 4. *You Giving Sex Information to Your Child*

pleasing : _____ : _____ : _____ : _____ : _____ : _____ : _____ : annoying

constructive : _____ : _____ : _____ : _____ : _____ : _____ : _____ : destructive

desirable : _____ : _____ : _____ : _____ : _____ : _____ : _____ : undesirable

Concept 5. *Long Hair (men or women)*

pleasing : _____ : _____ : _____ : _____ : _____ : _____ : _____ : annoying

constructive : _____ : _____ : _____ : _____ : _____ : _____ : _____ : destructive

desirable : _____ : _____ : _____ : _____ : _____ : _____ : _____ : undesirable

Concept 6. *Using Birth Control Devices (e.g., birth control pills)*

pleasing : _____ : _____ : _____ : _____ : _____ : _____ : _____ : annoying

constructive : _____ : _____ : _____ : _____ : _____ : _____ : _____ : destructive

desirable : _____ : _____ : _____ : _____ : _____ : _____ : _____ : undesirable

Concept 7. *Serious Petting That May Lead to Intercourse*

pleasing : _____ : _____ : _____ : _____ : _____ : _____ : _____ : annoying

constructive : _____ : _____ : _____ : _____ : _____ : _____ : _____ : destructive

desirable : _____ : _____ : _____ : _____ : _____ : _____ : _____ : undesirable

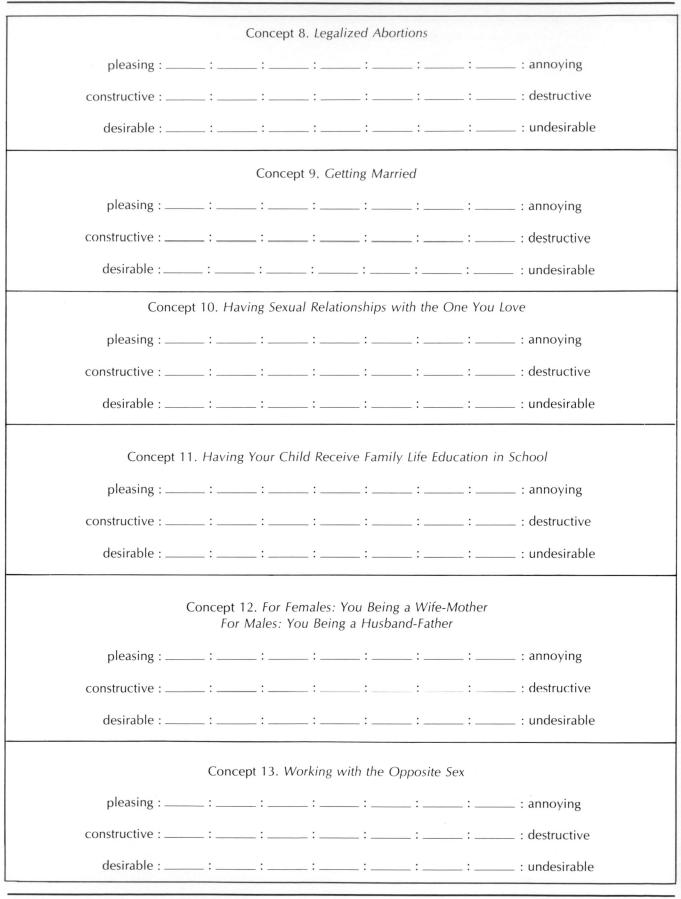

Concept 8. *Legalized Abortions*

pleasing : _____ : _____ : _____ : _____ : _____ : _____ : annoying

constructive : _____ : _____ : _____ : _____ : _____ : _____ : destructive

desirable : _____ : _____ : _____ : _____ : _____ : _____ : undesirable

Concept 9. *Getting Married*

pleasing : _____ : _____ : _____ : _____ : _____ : _____ : annoying

constructive : _____ : _____ : _____ : _____ : _____ : _____ : destructive

desirable : _____ : _____ : _____ : _____ : _____ : _____ : undesirable

Concept 10. *Having Sexual Relationships with the One You Love*

pleasing : _____ : _____ : _____ : _____ : _____ : _____ : annoying

constructive : _____ : _____ : _____ : _____ : _____ : _____ : destructive

desirable : _____ : _____ : _____ : _____ : _____ : _____ : undesirable

Concept 11. *Having Your Child Receive Family Life Education in School*

pleasing : _____ : _____ : _____ : _____ : _____ : _____ : annoying

constructive : _____ : _____ : _____ : _____ : _____ : _____ : destructive

desirable : _____ : _____ : _____ : _____ : _____ : _____ : undesirable

Concept 12. *For Females: You Being a Wife-Mother*
For Males: You Being a Husband-Father

pleasing : _____ : _____ : _____ : _____ : _____ : _____ : annoying

constructive : _____ : _____ : _____ : _____ : _____ : _____ : destructive

desirable : _____ : _____ : _____ : _____ : _____ : _____ : undesirable

Concept 13. *Working with the Opposite Sex*

pleasing : _____ : _____ : _____ : _____ : _____ : _____ : annoying

constructive : _____ : _____ : _____ : _____ : _____ : _____ : destructive

desirable : _____ : _____ : _____ : _____ : _____ : _____ : undesirable

Concept 14. *Having Sexual Intercourse with Another While Married*

pleasing : _____ : _____ : _____ : _____ : _____ : _____ : _____ : annoying

constructive : _____ : _____ : _____ : _____ : _____ : _____ : _____ : destructive

desirable : _____ : _____ : _____ : _____ : _____ : _____ : _____ : undesirable

Concept 15. *Working with a Homosexual*

pleasing : _____ : _____ : _____ : _____ : _____ : _____ : _____ : annoying

constructive : _____ : _____ : _____ : _____ : _____ : _____ : _____ : destructive

desirable : _____ : _____ : _____ : _____ : _____ : _____ : _____ : undesirable

Concept 16. *Endorsing Population Control by Having Two Children Only*

pleasing : _____ : _____ : _____ : _____ : _____ : _____ : _____ : annoying

constructive : _____ : _____ : _____ : _____ : _____ : _____ : _____ : destructive

desirable : _____ : _____ : _____ : _____ : _____ : _____ : _____ : undesirable

Concept 17. *Being Engaged Before Getting Married*

pleasing : _____ : _____ : _____ : _____ : _____ : _____ : _____ : annoying

constructive : _____ : _____ : _____ : _____ : _____ : _____ : _____ : destructive

desirable : _____ : _____ : _____ : _____ : _____ : _____ : _____ : undesirable

Concept 18. *Living with Another Person Before Getting Married (trial marriage)*

pleasing : _____ : _____ : _____ : _____ : _____ : _____ : _____ : annoying

constructive : _____ : _____ : _____ : _____ : _____ : _____ : _____ : destructive

desirable : _____ : _____ : _____ : _____ : _____ : _____ : _____ : undesirable

Concept 19. *Living a Single's Life*

pleasing : _____ : _____ : _____ : _____ : _____ : _____ : _____ : annoying

constructive : _____ : _____ : _____ : _____ : _____ : _____ : _____ : destructive

desirable : _____ : _____ : _____ : _____ : _____ : _____ : _____ : undesirable

INTERPRETATION

The purpose of this scale is to help you understand your feelings about marriage, sex, and sexually related behaviors, and to help you identify the strength of your feelings. No right or wrong answers are intended.

Your reactions to sexually related topics and issues are often masked by group pressure to conform to social customs. People are often inhibited in expressing their opinions about a delicate subject like sex. Such inhibition often leads to a lack of communication, and results in misunderstanding and poor human relationships. By completing this scale you should be able to overcome these problems. Hopefully, it will help you to become more aware of your feelings toward marriage and sexual behavior.

There are many ways to use this scale in the classroom. Your instructor may survey your classmate's reactions and then make a class study for each concept. One study may be made for females and one for males. Or these studies may be used to promote classroom or group discussions. A sample study is given here (Figure 16.1).

Another comparison might be made between your feelings about certain issues and those of another person, such as your date or loved one. This scale is very accurate in determining the sensitivity of your feelings toward a sex-related topic or behavior. Therefore, two people may think that they have similar feelings and not realize that they differ, perhaps greatly. Because the scales are repetitive for each concept, you can easily compare your feelings with others.

This scale may also be used in counseling two people who contemplate marriage. It points out differences and similarities of feelings between them, thus suggesting the present degree of compatibility.

How strongly do you feel about each concept? You can tell by where you placed your response. For example, in Figure 16.1, both males and females found getting married slightly pleasing, females felt it very desirable and constructive, while males felt getting married only somewhat desirable and constructive. Placing your response in the most extreme left or right space indicates having an extremely strong feeling toward or about the human sexuality topic.

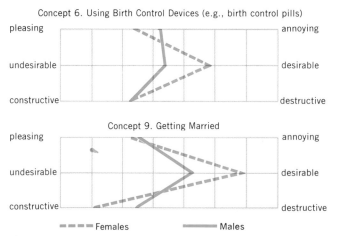

Figure 16.1

Profile analysis of how a class of San Diego State University students felt toward two concepts: using birth control devices and getting married. Students were enrolled in a basic health science class during spring semester, 1970. The solid line represents the average (anonymous) feelings of the males, while the broken line represents the average (anonymous) feelings of the females toward each concept. The profiles illustrate ways of analyzing your responses.

☞ RISKS OF SEX BEFORE MARRIAGE INVENTORY

DIRECTIONS   There may not be any right or wrong consequences. Rate the statements high, average, low, or no risk on the basis of you perceiving the consequences below as a total risk to yourself, to the other person(s), and to society. Total your score.

	(Points)	Degree of Risk			
Consequence		High 5	Average 3	Low 1	None 0
1. Danger of pregnancy					
2. Danger of VD					
3. Forced marriage by parents or pregnancy					
4. Abortion					
5. Guilt of loss of virginity (by engaging in premarital intercourse)					
6. Fear of being a less-desirable marriage partner					
7. Fear of consequences in a future marriage					
8. Female fearing male will lose respect for her					
9. Damage done when guilt feelings are reawakened after marriage					
10. Fear resulting from public or familial disapproval and resultant complications					
11. Social difficulties resulting when relationship is discovered					
12. • Fear of legal difficulties					
13. Delay or prevent couple from marrying					
14. Coitus obligates you to marry partner					
15. Coitus may break up desirable friendship and possible marriage					
16. Likelihood that premarital coitus will lead to later extramarital infidelities					
17. Moral decay of society					
18. Female less capable of responding satisfactorily in marital coitus					
TOTAL					

Source: Adapted from E. M. Schur, *The Family and the Sexual Revolution,* pp. 19–21.

INTERPRETATION

Score Range	Health Complication
90–72	High risk
71–36	Average risk
35–0	Low risk

Young people are often faced with numerous interim problems of living as single persons. One is having sex before marriage. Is it all right to have sex before marriage? This is a difficult question to answer. Perhaps the way to resolve this question is to ask other questions: What do you want to get out of sex before marriage? Are you emotionally stable enough to try it? What would you do in case of pregnancy? Are you using premarital sex as a rebellion against society or your parents? Do you want sex to prove your sex role? Is sex an alternative to reaffirming your self-identity? These and many other questions need to be answered. You should realize that you need to ask yourself these kinds of questions and try to find honest answers.

There are numerous consequences of having sex before marriage. Many of these are covered in the Risks of Sex Before Marriage Inventory. Over a million teenage women become pregnant each year. The death rate from pregnancy complications is 13 percent greater for 15 to 19 years olds, and 60 percent greater for teens 14 and under as compared to women in their early twenties. Since such pregnancies are seldom planned, the babies are often unwanted and may have difficulty developing healthy personalities.

Having sex before marriage is no longer the problem it used to be. Birth control devices now minimize the risk of pregnancy. Perhaps instead of dwelling on sex before marriage, you should contemplate on evolving a life style that helps you to fulfill your human health needs on a long-term basis. Love and affection, intercourse, and emotional and social fulfillments all need to be resolved on a long-range instead of a short-range basis if one is to maintain emotional equilibrium and attain happiness, contentment, and peace of mind.

HUMAN SEXUALITY

Sexuality is how you feel about your own sex role and sexual behavior, and that of others. It reveals how well you accept your sex role, your relationships with others, and your responsibility for having sexual and interpersonal relationships with another, including marriage and having children. Human sexuality is really your attitude toward yourself and others. It is not very different from your attitude toward caring for your body, toward pollution, toward sports, toward physical fitness, toward religion, toward business, toward politics, and toward all other facets of life. Your values and attitudes toward sex should be the same as your attitude toward people—how you deal with them and communicate with them.

Our roles are set by our being male or female. You are a son or daughter, brother or sister, boyfriend or girlfriend, husband or wife, father or mother. (See Figure 16.2.) You are stuck with being either a male or female. Your physical makeup predestines your role in life. Each person must learn to accept his or her role, to he happy with it, and to live with that role. It is essential for one's emotional well-being to identify with a sex role, as well as accept it.

Roles imply relationships. A girl—even if she wishes to be, try as she may—cannot be "one of the boys." She was created to relate to others in ways that only women can relate. Women are taught to be feminine, while boys are expected to be masculine. Their attitudes toward others reflect this makeup.

Roles and relationships are fortified by responsibility. A husband and father has the responsibility to love and cherish his wife and children. Similarly, a wife and mother has certain responsibilities toward her husband and children. Although these responsibilities have undergone changes since 1960, the maintenance chores of life for a family have not changed. No longer is it only the wife's chore to clean house, cook, and wash dishes; husbands often do this as well. (See Figure 16.3.) Many couples make a big issue over these mundane things, but

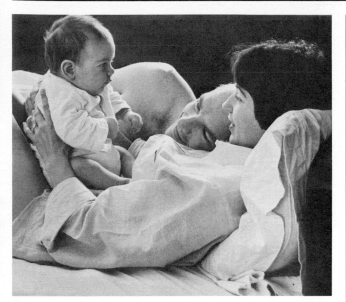

Figure 16.2

A family enjoying their baby. Children require additional sex roles from a husband and wife. What are the sex roles projected in this photo?

the responsibilities for maintaining the well-being of self and family will always be there. Although there has been some shift in responsibilities for maintaining life in a family, the nature of such maintenance has not changed.

In summary, relationships are determined by what we are in relation to what other people are, and our responsibilities are determined by the way we should react toward those with whom we have relationships. Together these aspects of life help structure how we feel and act about ourselves and others. This is what human sexuality is all about. Human sexuality is the same as a healthy attitude toward life.

Sex, as integrated into the total personality, is not simply a physical expression. Because of its interrelation with the emotional, social, and moral spheres, one must find a balance between controlling one's impulses and gratifying them. This requires that a person be "patterned" in his activity by some kind of standards of behavior. This means that one's value system should be founded on respect for other persons. Kirkendall (18) has suggested four prerequisites for good sexual relationships:

1. A genuine friendship between partners.
2. A willingness and ability to discuss and explore sexuality.
3. A knowledge of the physiology and techniques of sex and sexual intercourse.
4. Patience to take reasonable time for working things out together.

One should also be aware that sexual relationships become worthwhile when such a relationship is a warm

social experience, as long as each partner makes the other a better person, neither partner is exploited, and the relationship becomes a positive force in one's life. This recipe for a satisfying sexual relationship is not complete but should give you a basis on which to build.

The Sexuality Scale in this chapter is planned to help you and your friend assess your feelings about marriage, sex, dating, and other sexual-social relationships.

LOVE, INFATUATION, AND SEX

"Love is a many splendored thing!" There is nothing like being in love. This wonderful feeling gives two persons a spiritual strength that, in turn, provides each with a spark for living, a feeling of vitality and power. It's like a flower opening into full bloom and becoming more beautiful. Love gives one a fresh outlook on life, a sense of boundless energy, and a new sense of power. "It gives the stone its brilliance and luster," so to speak.

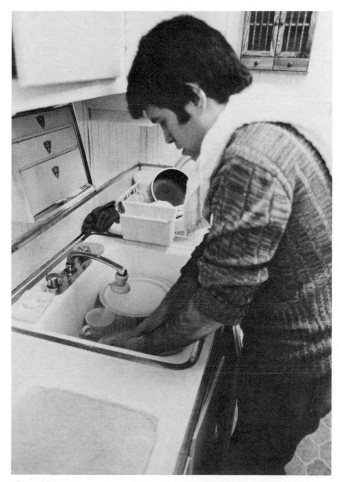

Figure 16.3

A man washing dishes. Washing dishes is more important as a sanitary safeguard and life maintenance chore than as a sex role controversy.

On the other hand, the symptoms of lack of love include: feeling forlorn and sad, feeling inadequate and that no one cares, withdrawal from others, feeling that life has no meaning or purpose, and performing poorly on the job. Those without adequate love often tend to compensate for lack of love through antisocial behavior or getting overinvolved in their job, or hobbies, or projects. Some tend to be aloof and avoid commitments. As a consequence, such persons tend to be low performers.

Once the novelty of the marriage ceremony and the honeymoon wear off, love often loses its newness, spark, and luster and becomes just a comfortable relationship. The result is that those looking for continuous "sparkles and splendor" are disappointed. It is difficult, if not impossible, to keep love on a natural high all the time.

Americans have difficulty recognizing love, much less being sure of it or how to nurture it. Most young people, much like their parents and grandparents, want love (1). Although many also feel a need for sexual pleasure, they feel strongly about having a commitment to another person for love and sex. Thus they perceive marriage as a way of attaining a commitment for love and sex (1).

How do you know that you are really in love? Is it really love or infatuation? Is liking a person the same as being in love with that person? Does getting physically, psychologically, and emotionally excited about a person reflect love?

Obviously, one cannot obtain all the answers from just reading about love, but perhaps sharing a few ideas will help you to clarify your own thoughts above love.

Love is an abstract term that attains meaning through emotional experience. Love is difficult to put into words and describe. Furthermore, there is no mutual agreement on what it is.

There is a time and familiarity difference between love and infatuation. It is infatuation when you are instantly and physically attracted to another person. A kind of animal magnetism takes over, and your "vibes" are impulsive in nature. At this stage of attraction, you do not have a sense of caring for the other person, since you know virtually nothing about him or her. But such an infatuation may grow and develop into love over a period of time if (1) after getting to know more about the other person, you also begin to then (2) care for him/her; and then (3) feel a sense of responsibility for the other person; and (4) have respect for the other person. These are the four elements of love identified by Eric Fromme in *The Art of Loving* (13). Love grows over a period of time, whereas infatuation is an instant physical response of short duration.

Many persons think of physical sex as a consequence of love and a deep emotional-interpersonal relationship. Sex may or may not symbolize love. Many men and women today separate sex from reproduction and sex from love. Sex is often thought of as recreation and pleasure. However, instant sex is about as satisfying as a sneeze. Today young women, more so than men, are still eager for a deep emotionally and mentally stimulating commitment instead of just a physical relationship. Overcoming loneliness through personal commitment is a greater need than sexual gratification. Many young people appear to sense this need, and they look forward to marriage as a way of fulfilling these needs. A recent survey (1) reported in *Time* magazine found that marriage and its commitments have a strong appeal to young people.

MARRIAGE AND MARRIAGE ALTERNATIVE

People get married for different reasons, but it is hoped that the unifying cement in all marriages will be love. Besides love, people also marry for sex, companionship, emotional-social security, wealth, children, and family and social obligations. It is a unity of interacting and intercommunicating of two or more persons enacting the social roles of husband and wife, mother and father, son and daughter, and brother and sister.

Today, traditional marriage is only one of the many alternative styles to fulfilling one's basic human needs. The most common choice of marriage in North America is monogamy, where a husband and wife aspire to enjoy a lifelong one-to-one sexual exclusiveness with each other. (See Figure 16.4.)

Another approach to the traditional monogamous style of marriage is the comarital or swinging kind, where a husband and wife may exchange mates and have very little emotional involvement with their exchange mates. Such extramarital sex is an open physical act and is recreational in nature. The couple have sexual fun and stimulation but nothing else that would jeopardize their marital relationship. Such marital swingers do their swinging in an effort to support and improve their monogamous marriages. They maintain that sex can be detached from the emotional feelings toward a mate and enjoyed apart from those romantic feelings. Thus the sexual-swing act takes up only a few hours in a week or month; everything else in their lives remains intact and conventional. Many couples find this swinging marriage empty and are abandoning this life style.

A contemporary experiment in marriage is group marriage. Small groups of adult males and females, and their children, live together under one roof or in a closely knit settlement, calling themselves a family, tribe, commune, or intentional community. They consider themselves all married to one another. (See Figure 16.5.) Such communes foster a self-sufficient farming and/or handicraft

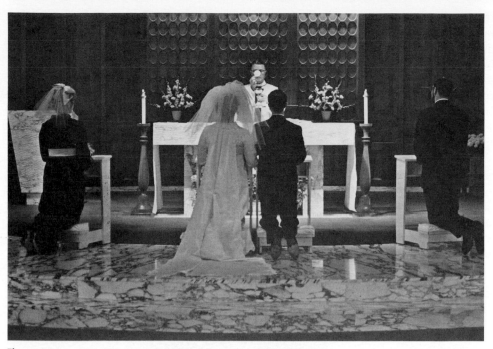

Figure 16.4
A wedding ceremony cements the commitments of both persons to
marriage and each other.

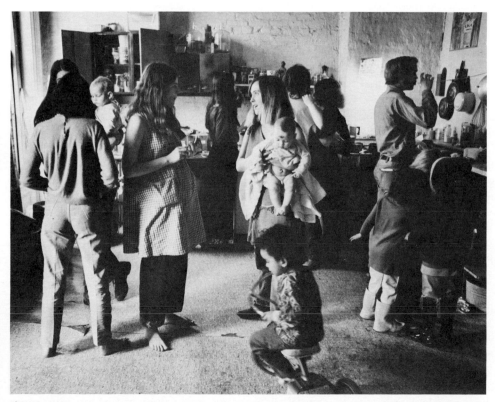

Figure 16.5
A commune is an alternative life style to fulfilling one's needs.

way of life. Many, but not all, of the communes are built around some kind of group sexual sharing.

Although such marriage is a distinct minority today, group marriages provide for collective parenthood and minimize the disruptive effects of divorce on the child's world. Sexual sharing relieves boredom and avoids the problem of infidelity. It avoids the loneliness and confinement of monogamous marriage. These positive aspects of group marriage are offset by numerous negative aspects. Such marriages seldom last longer than two years, since four or more adults have a difficult time living together harmoniously and coordinating the many lives. Leadership is a concern, and this extends into the difficulty of sharing communal work. Eventually, such marriages tend to disintegrate and revert back to the old-fashioned, masculine-feminine work roles. Thus many group marriages often have persons coming and going, very little cohesiveness and interpersonal involvements, and, instead, a continuously changing and unstable encounter group. They are rarely successful or enduring.

Recently, the unwed live-in relationship has become popular as an alternative to marriage. Although such an alternative was considered immoral in the fifties when older couples often secretively lived together in a "common-law" relationship it had increasing appeal in the sixties and seventies to those concerned over property rights and alimony support. This alternative was highlighted in the middle and late seventies by the Lee Marvin v. Michelle Triola Marvin court case (see Figure 16.6). When their live-in relationship broke up after six years, Michelle Triola Marvin sued Oscar-winning actor, Lee Marvin, for half of the property ($3.5 million) acquired during their relationship. Although the court recognized the oral agreement, the judge awarded Michelle Marvin about a $100,000 settlement.

Many young couples view this live-in alternative to marriage as experimental, during which time they "try each other out" and then may decide on marriage. Two persons living together may have a written or orally expressed partnership covering living relationship and the future dissolution of property and money.

Young persons should initially contemplate more about a life-style arrangement that will help them to (1) fulfill their basic human health needs, (2) continue to develop as total persons—that is, strive toward self-fulfillment and self-actualization, (3) test and resolve their compatibilities, and (4) attain satisfaction and happiness through a workable love relationship. Such a life style should eventuate the attainment of a minimum level of individual commitment and emotional maturity and personal adjustment necessary for two people living together and having a family. The couple should identify and refine their developmental levels—social, intellectual, vocational, emotional, and so on—and determine

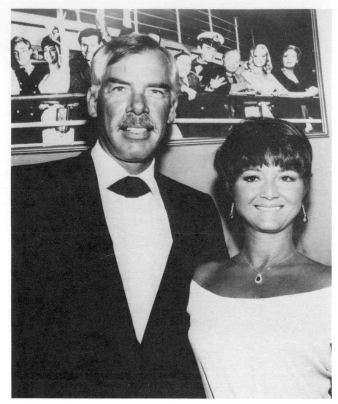

Figure 16.6
The Lee Marvin–Michelle Triola court case drew attention to the unwed. Live-in relationship is an alternative to marriage.

how successfully they are able to mutually fulfill their basic human health needs. They also need to take into consideration that as each person's needs change from time to time, they may become incompatible.

According to Toffler in *Future Shock,* one should expect to marry more than once in a lifetime. For many, relationships may be of short duration and one may end up having several relationships instead of a one-life marriage.

Finally, marriage, whatever style, may not be for everyone, just as motherhood is not for every woman. Many persons can best cope as a single person who relates well to many persons, has varied interests, and is able to fulfill his or her personal health needs without marriage.

Sex for the single person is more liberated and accepted today than in past years. Single persons can have sexual involvements without feeling guilt or the pressures of social restrictions. You can be single in a married society if you have a healthy self-concept, are able to adjust to most of life's situations, and enjoy life in general. Thus being single does not necessarily imply sexual permissiveness. Most single people are able to work out a life style that fulfills their basic human health needs and allows them to function optimally.

WAYS TO ASSESS YOUR MARRIAGE PROSPECT

So you are in love and want to get married. How sure are you that your mate will make a good marriage partner? What are the chances of your marriage working? These and other doubts haunt all those contemplating marriage. There are many things you can do to get reassurances that the person you fell in love with is the right marriage prospect for you. Here are a few suggestions:

1. Date a person often and for at least 6 months. Get to know him or her really well.
2. Date the person under different distress-stress situations, and observe how well he or she adapts and copes with different social situations.
3. Check the hereditary tree of both of you. What good or bad traits will your children inherit?
4. Find out how both of you respond to the marriage and sexuality inventories. Use these as a basis for discussing topics between you and your date. How similar or different are your tastes and interests?
5. Are your marriage and life-style goals similar? Do you want the same things out of life? For example, do you want an engagement, a trial marriage, or neither? Do both of you want children?
6. Are both of you on the same developmental level in the following areas?
   (a) College degree versus grade 9 education.
   (b) Skilled or professional versus nonskilled.
   (c) Literary versus artistic activity.
   (d) Self-improvement versus recreational.
7. Do you have major complementary or compatible interests (even if these are different)? For example, you both exercise but you run and your partner swims; both of you are vegetarians; both of you are religious; both of you like music but you like disco and your partner likes jazz.
8. Are both of you able to communicate with each other? Can you talk about sensitive and personal topics like sexual intercourse, bad breath, body defects, etc.?
9. Do both of you accept responsibility for maintenance of apartment or home? This includes cooking, shopping, cleaning, and record-keeping.
10. How well do you get along with his or her family and friends and vice versa?
11. Are you able to fulfill each other's human needs? Do both of you make each other a better person?
12. Are you able to make a strong loyal commitment to your partner and to your relationship?
13. Do both of you have a steady, adequate income? (Lack of money is the number one cause of broken homes.) Is one of you a spendthrift?
14. Are both of you from the same social class and religious backgrounds?
15. Are both of you emotionally stable and mature? Can you trust each other? Are both of you ready for marriage? Does one of you have a drug, drinking, or smoking problem? How familiar are both of you with the topics in the next section?

You increase the chances that your love relationship and marriage will work if you and your marriage partner contemplate each of these 15 points. If you have a strong difference of opinion, or respond to three or more of these points, then the chances of your relationship's lasting and working are not very good. Physical chemistry (love) between two people may not be enough to make marriage a success.

THINGS TO KNOW OR DO BEFORE MARRIAGE

Most young persons look forward to marriage. Many divorcees and widows remarry. Thus men and women contemplating marriage should know as much as possible about all aspects of marriage.

You may already be familiar with much of this information. Being knowledgeable about this information ensures greater success of your marriage than if you did not have this information. How many of these topics have you honestly discussed with your partner?

1. Anatomy-physiology of male and female reproductive systems.
2. Venereal diseases.
3. Menstruation and sexual activity.
4. Family planning, including birth control and spacing of births.
5. Pregnancy and prenatal care (including nutrition).
6. The process of childbirth and how you want your baby to be born.
7. Diseases and pregnancy.
8. Heredity and genetic counseling, including pharmacological influence of cigarette smoking, alcohol, coffee, sugar, and drugs.
9. The hygiene of pregnancy.
10. Preparation for parenthood (infant-child care and rearing children).
11. Children's diseases and their prevention.
12. Immunizations in infancy and childhood.
13. Child health and juvenile delinquency.

14. Physical well-being.
15. Medical and hospital care for the family.
16. Home nursing and emergency care.
17. Accidents in the home.
18. Family nutrition and weight control.
19. Emotional (mental) well-being (emotional stability and personal adjustment and ability to communicate).
20. Maladjustment problems of marriage and marriage counseling.
21. Present and future goals of you and your partner, including desirable life style.
22. Developmental levels of you and your partner, and potentials for individual growth and self-actualization.
23. Areas of compatibility and incompatibility.
24. Blood test for syphilis.
25. Marriage license—where.
26. Wedding plans.
27. Engagement.
28. Where to go for marriage first aid, sex and marriage counseling.
29. Financial basis for marriage and family living.
30. Fidelity.

ALTERNATIVE SEXUAL BEHAVIORS

Marriage is the most socially accepted way of fulfilling one's sexual needs. Having sexual intercourse with a person of the opposite sex is referred to as heterosexuality. Our society legally condemns other sexual behaviors, such as public nudity, child molestation, and incest. Most states also have laws prohibiting intercourse before marriage (premarital sex) and extramarital sex (adultery), or having a casual "affair" outside of marriage. Rape is both illegal and a crime. It is discussed in Chapter 12.

Other ways of fulfilling one's sexual needs include masturbation, homosexuality, transvestism, transexualism, prostitution, and voyeurism. This section explores these alternative sexual behaviors.

Masturbation

Masturbation is the self-stimulation of the sex organs and/or other parts of the body for sexual pleasure. It is the most common form of sexual activity. Nearly all men and about two-thirds of all women have masturbated, as well as enjoyed sexual intercourse with a partner regularly. Others have recourse to masturbation when no partner is available or use masturbation to replace sexual intercourse during late pregnancy.

There are many untruths about masturbation. It does not cause blindness, lead to homosexuality, cause inad-

equate sexual adjustment or sterility, cause acne or skin disorders, or cause baldness. But, like overeating and drinking alcoholic beverages, masturbation may become a poor substitute for people, social companionship, and heterosexual behavior.

Masturbation for women may be a therapeutic way to improve a sexual life with a partner. Evidence (17) suggests that women having difficulty experiencing orgasm may learn to do so through masturbation. Once a woman learns how to become sexually aroused, she can help her partner in mutual love play (foreplay before coitus) to stimulate her to experience orgasm during coitus.

Orgasm and ejaculation during sleep, or "wet dreams," are fairly common experiences among adolescent males, which tend to disappear later in life; whereas in females orgasm is an uncommon experience in adolescence, but gradually increases up to age forty.

Homosexuality

Homosexuality is the most common sexual deviation. About 10 percent of the American men and women are exclusively or sometimes homosexual (4). They have physical contact and sexual arousal with a person of the same sex. Although homosexual behavior is more accepted by the public now than it was in the past, it remains a controversial issue in this country. Homosexuals have come out of the "closet" and no longer keep their behavior a secret. They have formed "Gay Liberation" organizations to champion for equal rights legislation in cities and states.

There seems to be no one cause of homosexuality in any one individual, but there are a number of predisposing factors. Society's own restrictions on heterosexual behavior push some individuals toward homosexuality. Some persons are predisposed to homosexuality when their marriage fails, or they cannot adequately fulfill their needs through marriage. Others may experiment with homosexual activity during adolescence and accept it as a way of fulfilling sexual needs. Evidence (4) does point to early family influences as a strong contributor to homosexuality. For example, overprotective mothers can develop homosexual tendencies in their sons if the fathers do not provide some input. In similar circumstances, little girls often develop homosexual tendencies (lesbianism) when their fathers lavish them with puritanical attention while masking sexual interest in them. These examples support the theory that parental upbringing can create a social environment wherein the child is unable to make a strong commitment to a sex role.

Gay men and lesbian women look and behave like heterosexual members of society, except in the sexual aspect of their lives.

Relatives, marriage partners, and close friends of gay and lesbian people may find they need help in coping with their own feelings about homosexuality. There are organizations in the United States and Canada that can put them in touch with people in a similar position and help them accept their gay relatives or friends (see end of chapter).

Transvestism

Transvestism is the practice of dressing in the clothes of the opposite sex. Most transvestites or female impersonators are males who feel they are females. They are not homosexual. They usually fulfill a sexual need by wearing women's underclothing, while others masquerade completely dressed in women's clothing.

Transsexualism

A transsexual is one who's anatomy and sexual role identification are incompatible. A male transsexual, for example, feels he is a woman emotionally and was meant to be a woman physically. Male transsexuals are not satisfied by merely dressing as women—they feel an emotional need to physically respond as women. They often seek sex-conversion operations, which include hormone therapy and plastic surgery to reconstruct the external sexual organs so that a female anatomy will be present. These transsexuals are capable of vaginal intercourse following surgery, but they are not capable of giving birth to a child.

Voyeurism

Voyeurism is characterized by the "peeping Tom," who derives sexual satisfaction from watching others who are nude or engaging in sexual activities. Usually these people are harmless and never do anything more than look.

Prostitution

The world's oldest profession, prostitution, is participation in sexual activities for financial reward. Although the majority of prostitutes are women, some men (gigolos) engage in this activity. Although illegal in all states except Nevada, it is widely practiced.

Women become prostitutes for different reasons. Many do so because it is a way to make fast money. Others are talked into doing it by boyfriends or "pimps," while others participate in this activity because they like the frequent and varied sexual experiences. Others do it as a rebellion against their parents and society. Many prostitutes are hooked on drugs and use prostitution as a way to support their drug habits. Most prostitutes have inadequacies in their personality or problems in their life.

Most prostitutes do not find sexual satisfaction with their clients, since they seldom become emotionally involved. For a male client, this lack of emotional involvement may be a very unfulfilling experience.

Many women become prostitutes for a limited period (as when money is scarce or after running away from home) and eventually resume a more conventional way of life.

REPRODUCTIVE SYSTEMS

Having adequate knowledge of the male and female reproductive systems should help people feel more comfortable about their own bodies and body processes. They can have greater appreciation of menstruation, pregnancy, childbirth, and the proper use of birth control techniques. It also helps them to respond more adequately as sexual partners. This section provides the basic information about the male and female reproductive systems.

The Male System

The male reproductive organs consist of the testes, penis, and other structures (see Figure 16.7). The testes which hang outside the body in the scrotal sac, have two main functions: the production of male hormones and the manufacture of sperm. A normal man's testes produce about 500 million mature sperm each day, and this process continues well into old age.

Once spermatozoa have been synthesized, they are stored in the epididymis prior to traveling through the coiled vas deferens in preparation for ejaculation. Ejaculation is the sudden expulsion of semen through the urethra of the penis; this physical reaction is accompanied by a highly distinct, pleasurable sensation and relief of tension known as orgasm. If ejaculation does not occur, spermatozoa disintegrate and are reabsorbed by the testes.

As ejaculation is about to occur, the urethra is lubricated by the secretion of the Cowper's gland. This secretion neutralizes any acidity remaining in the urethra from urine and it also lubricates the urethra. This secretion is most often the preejaculation that may be noticed by males, and it may contain some spermatozoa. As the spermatozoa are physically propelled through the vas deferens, the fluids from the seminal vesicles and the prostrate gland mix with the spermatozoa. Spermatozoa are suspended in a thick whitish fluid called semen.

The penis is the male's primary sexual organ. It is a spongy structure containing numerous arteries. Normally, these blood vessels are constricted and restrict blood flow to the relaxed and flacid penis. However, when the man is sexually excited, the blood vessels

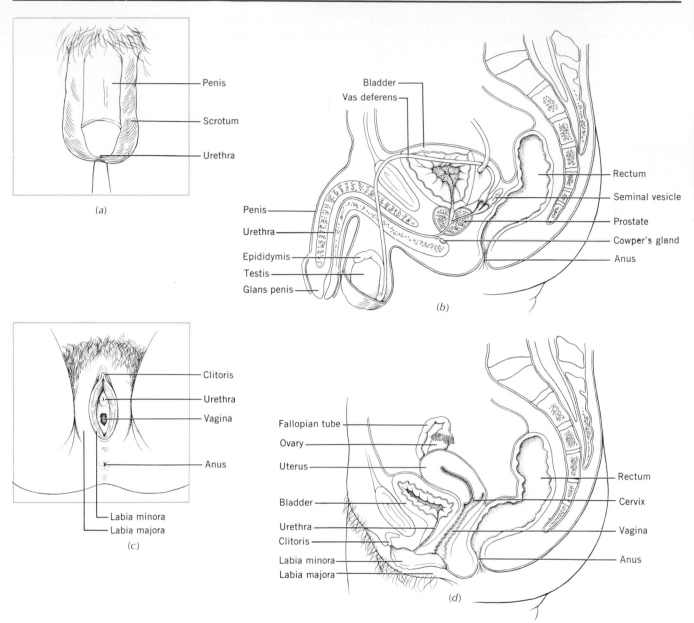

Figure 16.7

Anatomy of male and female reproductive systems. (a) External view of male genitals. (b) Cross section of male organs. (c) External view of female genitals. (d) Cross section of female organs.

dilate to allow blood to engorge the muscle tissues, thereby causing the penis to become erect. Erection allows the male to penetrate the female's vagina so that spermatozoa can be deposited there at the point of ejaculation.

The Female System

Whereas the male genitals are outside the body, all the female reproductive structures are internal: the ovaries, fallopian tubes, uterus, and vagina (see Figure 16.3). The woman's system is designed to produce sex hormones, release mature eggs (ova) about once every 28 days, and provide a place for fertilization and prenatal development to take place.

The ovaries are the primary sex glands of women. They synthesize the hormones (estrogen and progesterone) that regulate the menstrual cycle, prepare and maintain the uterus for potential occupancy, and produce secondary sexual characteristics (breast development and pubic hair). Each ovary is about the size and shape of an unshelled almond and contains thousands of ova in various stages of development. The release of an egg from one of the ovaries is called *ovulation*. The egg travels through the fallopian tube to the uterus (about the size of a fist), and fertilization (uniting with a sperm), if it occurs, happens in the tube. An unfertilized egg simply disintegrates as it passes through the uterus.

The uterus, a pear-shaped organ with elastic walls, has only one function: to house a fertilized egg until it has developed into a baby. The uterus is not a sex gland and does not take part in a woman's sexual responses. Removing it (hysterectomy) does not make a woman fat, bring on menopause, or reduce sex drive. Removing the uterus does, of course, stop menstruation, the monthly shedding of the inner lining of the uterus. Menstruation occurs when the egg is not fertilized; this shedding is referred to as menstrual flow, or period, and lasts an average of 3 to 6 days. The basic physiological and hormonal events in the menstrual cycle are described in Figure 16.8.

Each woman has her own characteristic menstrual cycle, and it may or may not be regular. Most women are aware of bodily changes immediately preceding their period. Some may feel slightly swollen or bloated, their breasts become sore or full, and they may have backache, leg pains, or feelings of depression or lethargy. Such tension is often caused by pooling of blood in the abdomen and can in many cases be relieved through exercising the abdominal muscles. Many women also experience abdominal cramps and other discomforts during their period, and whole body exercise is often helpful with these problems. A few women experience severe discomfort during menstruation; this condition is called *dysmenorrhea*. Menstruation in no way limits a woman's normal activities, including sexual intercourse.

The uterus is joined to the vagina by an opening called the cervix. The vagina is a muscular tube four or five inches long. Its primary purpose is to receive the penis during sexual intercourse, as well as become the birth canal. Sexual excitement causes the vagina to secrete a fluid that acts as a lubricant and aids in the penetration of the penis, making the sex act or coitus easier and more comfortable to perform.

The external lips surrounding the vagina are called the labia majora and libia minora. Together with the mons pubis and the clitoris, these structures constitute the vulva, or outer genital area. The clitoris is the female counterpart of the penis. Ordinarily less than an inch in length, it may enlarge considerably when sexually stimulated—either physically or mentally. It contains an abundance of nerve endings and is the most sexually excitable area of the woman's body.

There are two major dramatic changes that take place in a woman's reproductive life: the onset of menstruation (usually in the early teens) and menopause (usually in the middle forties). During menopause the ovaries cease to release eggs and menstruation ends. Menopause marks the end of a woman's ability to produce children, but it certainly does not end her sexual drive, desires, or abilities.

SEXUAL RESPONSE

Preparation for Coitus

Previous experiences condition one to anticipate the sexual act. For example, a song, an erotic picture, a style of dress, or an exotic perfume can all create a psychic interest and arouse emotional and physical responses as preparation for the sex act—coitus. Such arousal may be initiated by lovemaking or foreplay. Gentle touching and stroking of the body's erogenous zones help to arouse the person sexually. Such body zones include the clitoris, labia, anal area, the hips, armpits, lips, breasts and nipples, neck and ear areas of a woman, and the lips, neck, ears, hips, armpits, nipples, testicles, scrotum, and penis of a man. Foreplay also includes general hugging and caressing and kissing. One needs to be in a relaxed and receptive mood, trust the partner, and be prepared to give and receive pleasure if one is to be sexually responsive and enjoy the sexual act.

Human beings have an enormous potential for sexual pleasure. Unfortunately, the first sexual experience is usually not the most fulfilling, satisfying, or successful. A man may be so sexually excited that he ejaculates early or prematurely, often before he has inserted his penis into the vagina. For a woman, the first experience may be physically painful, dull, or messy and unpleasant. A couple needs to learn how to have coitus in a mutually satisfying and pleasurable way. Mutual satisfaction requires that intercourse become more than just a physical act—that it also include emotional, social, and psychic responses where love and commitment are expressed. Thus a couple needs to learn how to make love.

It helps when both partners are emotionally well adjusted and have a healthy sexuality. Emotionally stable people have a greater potential to relate to and communicate with each other.

A couple can also enhance their potential for sexual pleasure by understanding what happens to their bodies during sexual intercourse. Masters and Johnson studied (21) couples responding sexually during intercourse. They discovered that sexual response is so predictable and orderly in both sexes that it may be divided into four phases:

1. *Excitement phase*. One responds to some sort of sexual stimulation. The entire body reacts to

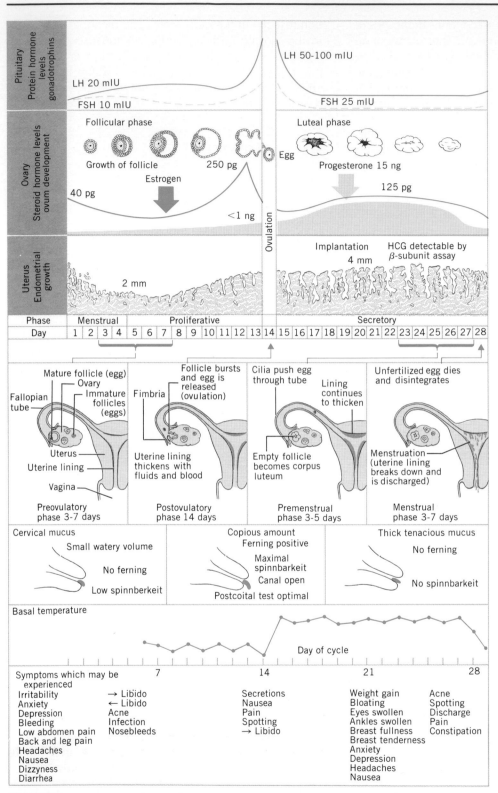

Figure 16.8

Phases of the menstrual cycle, depicting changes in the pituitary gland hormones (LH and FSH), ovary, uterus, cervical mucus, temperature changes, and possible symptoms. Changes in the uterus and ovary are also summarized by four X-sectional views of the reproductive system.

stimulation by general muscular tension, an increase in the heart rate and blood pressure, and vasocongestion or blood accumulation in certain blood vessels. The blood vessels of the penis become engorged with blood causing the penis to become erect while the testes elevate. Women's bodies respond to sexual stimulation with vaginal lubrication, and the clitoris, vaginal lips, nipples, and breasts gradually getting larger. The vagina lengthens and the uterus may elevate.

2. *Plateau phase.* Excitement continues and intensifies into the second stage. Penis size increases in both length and diameter because of vasoengorgement. The outer third of the vagina becomes so congested with blood that it swells and constricts, grasping the penis to increase stimulation for both partners. A sex-flush, or superficial skin vasocongestive reaction, may cause a temporary rash to spread from the breasts to the lower abdomen. The female breasts become enlarged and the nipples erect. As sexual tensions increase and orgasm becomes imminent, respiration, heartbeat, and blood pressure also increase. The heart rate may rise to 180 beats per minute.

3. *Orgasmic phase.* Men ejaculate or discharge semen while women do not. Both males and females sense physiological contractions. Long pelvic muscular contractions, lasting several seconds, may be followed by a series of shorter contractions less than a second apart. Both sexes undergo other muscular contractions as well as continuing increases in respiration, pulse, heart rate, and perspiration. Female orgasm may consist of rapid excitement and plateau stages, followed by a prolonged orgasm with the vagina contracting.

4. *Resolution phase.* After orgasm, the body returns to a normal preexcitement state in 5 to 15 minutes. Vasocongestion disappears and the muscles relax in both sexes. The penis becomes flaccid and returns to about half its erect size, while the testes descend into the relaxed scrotum. Breathing and heart rate return to normal.

Most males need a rest period before being able to get another erection and have coitus. On the other hand, females, after having had orgasm, can experience a series of multiple orgasms.

If an orgasm has not occurred, the return to normal may not take place for a half-hour to a full day.

Many women have enjoyable intercourse but fail to experience orgasm.

Sexual Dysfunctions

A man and woman about to have sexual intercourse for the first time may become concerned about their ability to perform and please each other. This and other psychological concerns of impotence and frigidity are referred to as sexual dysfunction. A male, for example, may not be able to get an erection, or he may lose his erection while attempting to enter the vagina. Or, a woman's vagina may not lubricate, or the vaginal lubricant may dry up during coitus. Some men and women may reach a plateau stage but not be able to have orgasm. Or the sex act itself may not be long enough for one of the partners.

The two most frequent sexual dysfunctions occurring in males are impotence and premature ejaculation. *Impotence* is the inability of a male to attain or maintain an erection long enough to have sexual intercourse. Emotional difficulties are the most frequent cause of impotence. Often a man who fails to have a satisfying erection will worry over his failure and be nervous when he attempts intercourse. This nervousness in turn produces the failure he feared and a vicious cycle has begun. Counseling and education in sexuality can help a man escape from this problem. Maintaining optimal physical fitness and eating a balance of nutrients are the best aphrodisiacs. As long as the penis is stimulated, the man has sexual thoughts, or there are erotic odors or bodily caresses, he will maintain his erection. Drugs and alcohol will depress the body and may contribute to impotence.

Penis size is a cause for concern among many men. The research of Masters and Johnson points out that there is little cause for such concern. They found that smaller organs tend to expand more than larger ones during erection, so that size differences diminish. Furthermore, the female vagina is an elastic organ that adapts to any penis size, so that penis size has little to do with sexual pleasure.

Premature ejaculation is the loss of control of ejaculation; that is, the male ejaculates before the female has had sufficient time to feel intravaginal satisfaction. This dysfunction is usually the result of psychological tension or concern. A male needs to learn to relax during coitus and how to physically and psychically delay — control his sexual responses during the plateau phase. Fortunately, the "squeeze technique" (squeezing the penis when ejaculation is near) is a very effective treatment for premature ejaculation. Refer to Masters and Johnson's description of this sexual therapy in their book *Human Sexual Inadequacy.*

The most prevalent causes of sexual dysfunction in females are the inability to experience orgasm, frigidity, dyspareunia, and vaginismus. Inability to achieve orgasm while enjoying coitus may be due to unawareness of how to attain it through body arousal. Often psychological blocks caused by fear of pregnancy, embarrassment of one's body, or trying too hard to have orgasm may contribute to the problem. Inability to have orgasm may be due to women having sex for the first time with an inexperienced partner, or in an inappropriate setting—such as the back seat of a car. As with a man, a woman's mental attitude toward her partner and sexual intercourse, and her attitude toward life in general, will have a significant impact on her ability to experience orgasm. Other reasons for not being able to experience orgasm may include anatomical defects, hormonal imbalance, and drugs and alcohol ingestion. More often than not, the couple simply fail to communicate about what excites a woman and what turns her off.

Frigidity is lack of interest in sex on the part of the woman. Often a personality problem or emotional conflict, unrelated to the sexual act itself, or a poor attitude toward sex may contribute to or cause frigidity.

Dyspaveunia is a painful intercourse. It may have psychological roots if a woman does not want to have intercourse with or resents her partner. Often there may be insufficient vaginal lubrication. Painful intercourse may also result from jellies, foams, sprays, and creams causing irritation.

Vaginismus is an involuntary tightening of the muscles of the vagina, which makes it difficult for the penis to enter or, if it does, causes considerable pain. This condition is primarily psychological in origin.

Sexual dysfunction is not unusual. Everyone experiences a temporary dysfunction sooner or later. There are many ways to overcome sexual dysfunctions. The next section offers numerous suggestions.

WAYS TO IMPROVE YOUR SEX LIFE

Couples often find that their relationship becomes stale, unexciting, worn out, and sexually unfulfilling. Their sex life needs an uplift and a recharge. Based on an article in *Sexology* (23), here are some ways to improve your sex life:

1. Do not overemphasize on mutual orgasm. It is not necessary for both partners to have an orgasm at the same time. Instead, it is more important that both are satisfied most of the time. There is nothing wrong with each partner having a climax at a different time.

2. Use your imagination and experiment with sex. There is no mutually desired sexual activity that is better than another. Varying sexual activity is sometimes essential to enliven a couple's married life. Trying something new brings the couple closer together.

3. Find the kind of birth control that suits both of you best.

4. Try to stay in good physical condition. Sexual ability is inhibited by overdrinking alcoholic beverages, overeating, fatigue, poor figure, obesity, bad breath, and smoking. All of these contribute to poor physical fitness and sexual inactivity. However, it is true also that lack of or lowered cardiovascular fitness contributes to preejaculation, lack of physical control, and poor sexual experiences. Good physical fitness enhances one' sex life and outlook on life.

5. Do not neglect personal hygiene. A dirty body turns off a partner's sex drive. Cleanliness is essential to personal attractiveness for both men and women. Constant deodorizing and perfuming masks the real problem—body odors result from lack of regular cleanliness. A shower or bath will do wonders to give one a fresh, clean feeling and appearance. If a woman has a persistent odor, this could mean that she has a yeast or trichomonas infection. She should consult a doctor instead of deodorizing it away.

6. Do not hesitate to seek help for problems. Consult a specialist (or a doctor) about a physical or emotional problem. Such problems can create psychosomatic hangups and stifle one's ability to enjoy sex.

7. Talk over your doubts and desires with your mate. It is very difficult to talk about a sex problem with one's partner; instead, one beats around the bush. Every woman must realize that her partner needs to feel that his sexual performance is a good one, and every man should know that his partner is very sensitive to the thought that she might not be "good in bed." Both partners need to be thoughtful and tactful about not just sex, but in all interpersonal daily affairs. Displaying good manners, and showing consideration and respect for the other person go a long way toward establishing communication between two married people.

8. Let your mate know you find him or her attractive. Give credit where it is due and compliment the other person. Do so every day. There is always something good that you can say about your mate. Compliment your partner on how fresh and clean her or his hair looks after she or he washes it, how good she or he looks after losing a few pounds, how good she or he looks in a new outfit, and so on. You should do everything you can to erase anxiety and self-consciousness. Reassurance that "I like you," "You're OK," and "You look beautiful or handsome" will go a long way to improving sexual performance. Poor body image, or a feeling that one is physically ugly, is often a root cause of sexual inhibition

and dissatisfaction.

9. Respect your mate's dislikes and desires. Do not pressure your mate into sexual behavior when he or she feels uncomfortable with it. Do those things that your partner likes—please your partner but be willing to experiment.

10. Remember that sex is basically adult play. Most sexual activity is recreational in nature. It dispels loneliness and our deepest emotional needs. Affection and sex are often ways of expressing not only how we feel, but expressing these feelings in ways that cannot be expressed in any other way. Keep in mind that sex is a tremendous source of warmth, comfort, and energy. Sex is often a time when one can talk about problems and life, as well as forget the worries and cares of the world.

11. Encourage your partner to become a self-actualizing person, to develop talents and abilities, and to express these in public. Doing so makes one feel confident and self-assured, and it lights the "spiritual" fire of life. Do not be possessive and selfish—let go and be encouraging.

12. Remember that a marriage is a continuous and developmental process. This means that it will be constantly changing as the partners change. Be ready to change within your relationship for the betterment of your partner and your life together.

13. Be prepared to develop yourself so as to complement the development of your partner. If your partner is progressing in his or her job, try to do likewise. The same holds true in the social, intellectual, academic, emotional, religious, moral, and spiritual aspects of life. Self-development should help you to grow as a person first, and then it should complement the relationship with your partner. It is important that both persons in a relationship grow in the same direction even though the nature and character of their growth may be different. For example, the woman should develop academically, while the husband develops skills on the job.

14. Learn to communicate with your partner about what turns you on and off. Keep in mind that you can communicate verbally, as well as physically. A woman can gently guide a man's hand to an erotic zone for stimulation, as well as move his hand away from a zone that has become overstimulated. Good communication cements a couple, makes them feel more intimate, and psychically prepares them for more sexual experience.

WHERE TO GO FOR MORE INFORMATION

The references at the end of this chapter are a good beginning. If you need more information about marriage and sex, there are various places you can go for help. Most college campuses and communities have the following resources (refer to local telephone directory where appropriate):

1. Your college or local library—textbooks on various family life, sex, and marriage topics.
2. Planned Parenthood Services.
3. Campus counseling center.
4. Campus health services center.
5. Family and marriage counselors as practiced by licensed and trained sociologists, psychologists, and psychiatrists.
6. Sex counselors, using the Masters and Johnson technique.
7. Local family counseling services.
8. Local public health department (state).
9. Gay Community Center (local).
10. Write for free or inexpensive information to the following organizations:

   (a) Sex Education and Education Council of the U.S. (SIECUS)
   1855 Willow Road
   New York, N.Y. 10023
   (b) Tampax Incorporated
   161 East 42nd Street
   New York, N.Y. 10017
   (c) Association for Voluntary Sterilization, Inc.
   14 West 40th Street
   New York, N.Y. 10018
   (d) Maternity Center Association
   48 East 92nd Street
   New York, N.Y. 10028
   (e) Planned Parenthood Services
   515 Madison Avenue
   New York, N.Y. 10022
   (f) American Genetic Association
   1507 N. Street N.W.
   Washington, D.C. 5
   (g) American Social Health Association
   1790 Broadway
   New York, N.Y.
   (h) American Medical Association
   535 North Dearborn Street
   Chicago, Ill. 60610
   (i) South California Psychotherapy Association
   8730 Wilshire Blvd.
   Beverly Hills, CA 90211
   (j) Parents and Friends of Gays
   Box 24528
   Los Angeles, CA 90024

(k) The National Gay Task Force
Suite 1601
80 Fifth Avenue
New York, N.Y. 10011

For the name of a qualified sex counselor in your area write to:

(l) American Association of Marriage and Family Counselors
225 Yale Avenue
Claremont, CA 91711

(m) American Association of Pastoral Counselors
201 East 19th Street
New York, N.Y. 10003

Further Readings

Calderone, Mary S., *Sexuality and Human Values,* New York: Human Science Press, 1967.

Casler, Lawrence, *Is Marriage Necessary,* New York: Human Science Press, 1974.

Fromme, Eric, *The Art of Loving,* New York: Harper & Row, 1974.

Kirkendall, Lester A., *Marriage and Family Relations,* Dubuque, Iowa: Wm. C. Brown, 1968.

Masters, William H., and Johnson, Virginia, *Human Sexual Inadequacy,* Boston: Little, Brown, 1970.

O'Neill, George, O'Neill, Nena, *Open Marriage.* New York: Avon Books, 1972.

Woods, Marjorie Binford, *Your Wedding: How to Plan and Enjoy It,* New York: Pyramid Brooks, 1960.

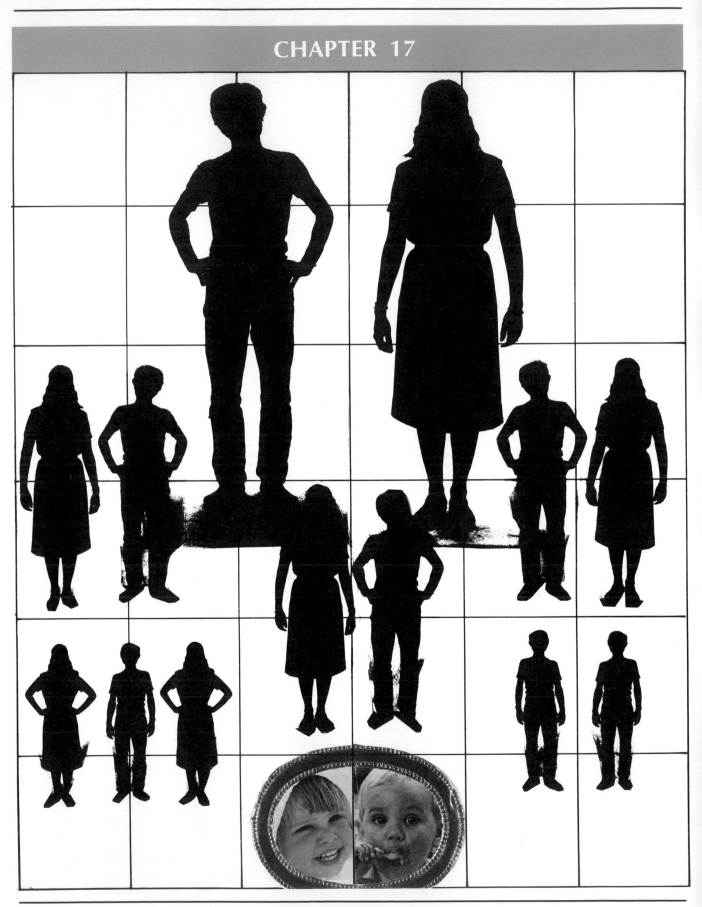

CHAPTER 17

PREGNANCY, CHILDBIRTH, BIRTH CONTROL AND HEREDITY

Biologically, we are all programmed to reproduce our species. We are equipped with systems efficiently designed to bring together sperm and egg in order to create a new human being. It is thus vitally important that each of us understand this fundamental biological part of ourselves. Such understanding is essential for accepting our sexual nature, using sex as a constructive force, and assuming responsibility for the consequences of the sex act — be it pregnancy and a baby, or simply caring for the other person.

In this chapter we will be covering the basic facts of human reproduction — conception, pregnancy, and birth — and the methods used to prevent reproduction (birth control and abortion). We will also be examining hereditary and environmental factors that can affect the health of a fetus and the newborn.

Assess your genetic endownment and your predisposition to genetic diseases and disorders by reacting to the Heredity Checklist that follows.

HEREDITY CHECKLIST												
	Mother	Father	Mother's Mother	Mother's Father	Father's Mother	Father's Father	Sister(s)	Brother(s)	Aunt(s)	Uncle(s)	Cousins
A. *Appearance*											
1. Albinism (white skin)											
2. Dwarfism											
3. Extra fingers (polydactyly)											
4. Webbed toes											
5. Cleft lip (harelip)											
6. Other body deformity											

	Mother	Father	Mother's Mother	Mother's Father	Father's Mother	Father's Father	Sister(s)	Brother(s)	Aunt(s)	Uncle(s)	Cousins
B. *Eyes*											
7. Nearsighted											
8. Farsighted											
9. Color blindness to green-red (Daltonism in males)											
C. *Skin*											
10. Allergy to poison oak ivy											
11. Psoriasis											
12. Eczema											
13. Acne (blackheads)											
D. *Allergy*											
14. Hay fever, asthma, and hives											
15. Milk											
16. Alcohol											
17. Cigarettes											
18. Eggs											
19. Certain fruits											
20. Penicillin											
21. Isoniazid											
22. Anesthetics											
23. Aspirins											
24. Vitamin pills											
25. Smog and car exhaust											
26. Other drugs											
27. Other foods											

	Mother	Father	Mother's Mother	Mother's Father	Father's Mother	Father's Father	Sister(s)	Brother(s)	Aunt(s)	Uncle(s)	Cousins
E. *Cardiovascular System*											
28. Sickle cell anemia											
29. Hemophilia (bleeding)											
30. High blood pressure											
31. Stroke (any part of body)											
32. Heart attack											
33. Varicose veins											
34. Anemia											
F. *Metabolic*											
35. Diabetes											
36. Overweight or obesity											
37. Phenylketonuria											
38. Thyroid or goiter trouble											
39. Other											
G. *Nervous System*											
40. Nervous breakdown											
41. Epilepsy											
42. Tay-Sachs disease											
43. Emotional disturbances											
44. Schizophrenia											
45. Mental retardation											
46. Mongolism (Down's syndrome)											
47. Migraine headache											

	Mother	Father	Mother's Mother	Mother's Father	Father's Mother	Father's Father	Sister(s)	Brother(s)	Aunt(s)	Uncle(s)	Cousins
H. *Cancer*											
48. Moles or warts on skin											
49. Cancer (any part of body)											
50. Leukemia											
51. Hodgkin's disease											
I. *Respiratory*											
52. Emphysema											
53. Frequent colds and flu											
54. Throat infections											
J. *Other*											
55. Muscle diseases											
56. Gout (a kind of arthritis)											
57. Arthritis (rheumatism)											
58. Kidney disease											
K. *Longevity* (age at which relatives died, other than from accidents)											
59. Under 30 years											
60. 31–50											
61. 51–70											
62. 71–80											
63. 81–90											
64. 91–100											
65. 100+											

INTERPRETATION

This is a checklist. It is not a test or a diagnostic instrument. It covers those diseases, disorders, and items related to health that have a reasonably high likelihood of occurring in the general population. Many diseases and disorders are obviously not included in this list.

By reacting earnestly and honestly to this checklist, you will become more aware of the importance of heredity to your health potentials. The items also provide an incomplete list of traits people may inherit (from allergies to longevity).

Diseases seem to run in families. If your mother or father or sister or brother has a disease or disorder, there is a good chance that you might develop it. If you or your mate has a disease or disorder, the chances of your children developing it increase. However, keep in mind that although many disorders, such as hypertension and heart disease, run in families, there is no general agreement about whether or not a tendency toward a disorder is inherited or is the product of a shared environment also (similar eating habits and lack of activity).

As a follow-up to reacting to this checklist, you should verify the incidence of hereditary disorders in your family. Have your relatives confirm your inventory.

PREGNANCY

The biological purpose of sexual intercourse is to unite the sperm from the male with the ovum of the female (see Figure 17.1). The male's ejaculation of semen deposits about half a billion sperm cells into the vagina. However, only about 4000 spermatozoa are able to survive and make their way up through the uterus to the fallopian tube in search of an ovum. Several spermatozoa may penetrate an ovum but only one actually fertilizes it. Since spermatozoa can survive 48 to 60 hours, conception can result only if intercourse occurs within a 3-day period of 2½ days before the release of the egg to a half-day after the release.

Once fertilization takes place, a new organism has begun. The single cell of fertilized egg soon begins to divide and becomes a cluster of cells floating through the fallopian tube and into the uterus. This cluster attaches to the uterine wall and soon differentiates into an embryo, supporting sac (amnion), placenta, and umbilical cord. For the organism, this is the first stage of life — prenatal development. For the mother, it is the beginning of 9 months of pregnancy. The stages of pregnancy and the baby's development are shown in Figure 17.2.

How does a woman know when she is pregnant? Usually, she first suspects something when her menstrual period is late. Pregnancy can be confirmed by laboratory or home tests, or by direct physical examination. Laboratory tests are designed to detect a hormone called human chorionic gonadotropin (HCG) in the woman's urine. The hormone HCG is produced in increasing amounts by the placenta of the developing embryo. By the sixth week of pregnancy, enough HCG is being produced to be detected.

A woman can buy a pregnancy test [(e.g., Early Preg-

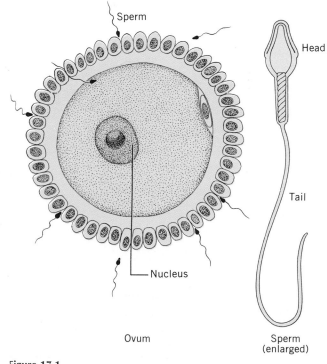

Figure 17.1
When an ovum is penetrated and fertilized by a sperm, which is many times smaller, the result is a single cell that contains all the information for the development of a human being.

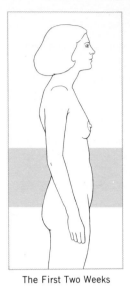

The First Two Weeks

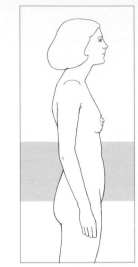

The First and Second Months

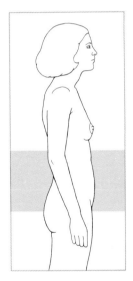

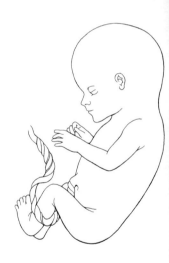

The Third and Fourth Months

Figure 17.2
The nine months of pregnancy, depicting the various stages of the embryo and the fetus and the changes in physical appearance of a pregnant woman.

nancy Test (EPT)] and check for pregnancy at home (28). To perform the EPT, a woman adds three drops of the first urine voided in the morning, along with a vial of purified water, to the chemicals in a test tube. The results are ready to analyze 2 to 4 hours later. If a ring forms at the bottom of the test tube, HCG is present. If the test is negative, it does not necessarily mean the woman is not pregnant because it may still be too early in the preg-

nancy for the hormone to appear. A woman who gets negative results should wait 10 days and try the test again just to be sure. A woman can also go to her doctor, a clinic, or Planned Parenthood and have a quick 2-minute test performed for pregnancy. Pregnancy can also be determined by a brief physical examination in which the doctor checks for color changes in the cervix and enlargement of the uterus.

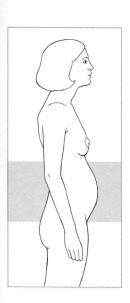

The Fifth and Sixth Months

If a woman thinks she may be pregnant, she should verify this suspicion as soon as possible so she can proceed to make a decision as to what to do about pregnancy. If she chooses to abort the pregnancy, it should be done as early as possible to avoid medical and financial complications.

CHILDBIRTH

The culmination of the 9 months of pregnancy is the birth of a child. It is normal to fear the unknown and many pregnant women fear the pain of the birth process. This fear causes the woman to build up a stage of ten-

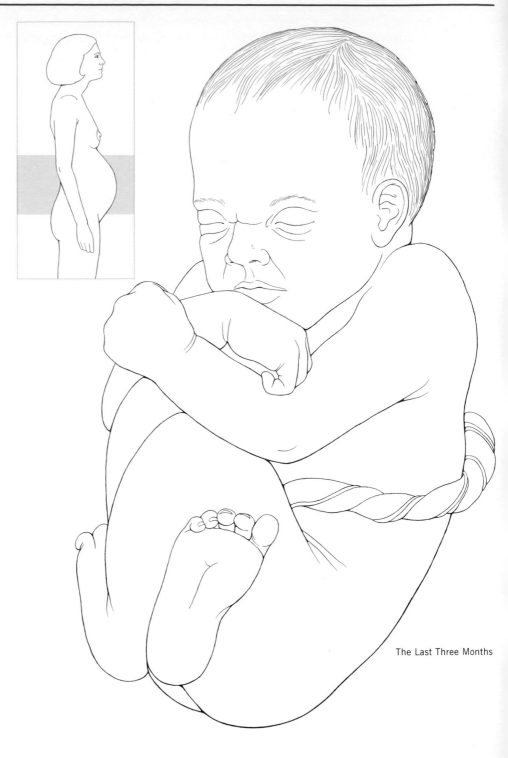

The Last Three Months

sion, which in turn contributes to a painful delivery. How can an expectant mother escape from this fear and tension? There are several approaches to helping pregnant women experience a relaxed and joyful delivery relatively free of pain.

Methods of *natural childbirth* are designed to reduce the mother's fears and emotional stress during delivery. This method involves educating the mother about the entire process of childbirth and preparing her for labor by giving her special exercises to strengthen the abdominal muscles. Emphasis is also placed on learning relaxation and proper breathing. In natural childbirth sedatives are usually avoided, and the father takes part in the process and is present during delivery. One approach to natural childbirth, called the *Lamaze* method, involves conditioning the pregnant woman to associate relaxation, rather than pain, with the contractions of labor. She is given breathing and relaxation exercises and special training in the stages of childbirth.

Which method of childbirth do you want for your child? The birth experience must be good for the mother, father, and baby. In the past, obstetricians would give the mother a pain killer in the hip area called a "saddle block." Many women still choose saddle blocks and other types of sedation or anesthesia to get them through the pain of labor. Most drugs used to sedate the mother find their way through the placenta to the fetus. Just how great an effect such medication has on the baby is uncertain, but the safest way for a baby to be born is without the mother taking drugs or medication.

The stages of labor and birth are shown in Figure 17.3. The baby moves into position for leaving the womb, and the cervix gradually dilates (enlarges). The fetal membranes (bag of waters) break, and the infant begins to move through the cervix headfirst (in most cases). An *episiotomy* (cutting of the vaginal opening to enlarge it) is sometimes performed at this stage. After the baby has totally emerged, the placenta (afterbirth) follows.

Treatment of the infant at the moment of birth has become somewhat controversial. The delivery room in a normal hospital is usually well lit and noisy. The baby is immediately checked for various normal body functions and problems. A French physician, Frederick Leboyer, has suggested that this whole process should be altered to ease the baby's transition into its new world. The newborn emerges from the darkness and silence of the womb. In the Leboyer approach, the delivery room is darkened and no one speaks above a whisper. The newborn infant is immediately placed stomach down on the mother's warm abdomen to retain the prebirth curved

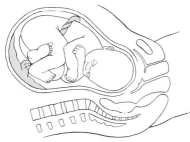

(a) Lightening.

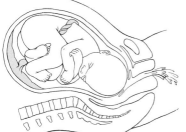

(b) Contractions and breaking of the bag of waters.

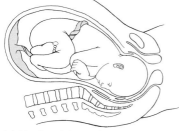

(c) Dilation of the cervix.

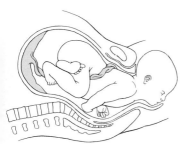

(d) Episiotomy at this stage if needed.

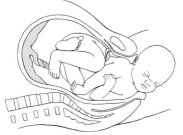

(e) Delivering the head.

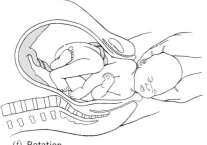

(f) Rotation.

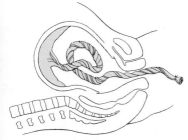

(g) The afterbirth (placenta).

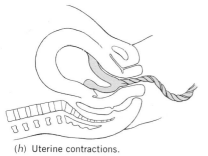

(h) Uterine contractions.

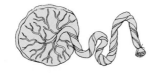

(i) Expulsion of the placenta.

Figure 17.3

Stages of labor and birth. (Original artwork Courtesy of Carnation Company, Los Angeles, Calif. © Carnation Co., 1972.)

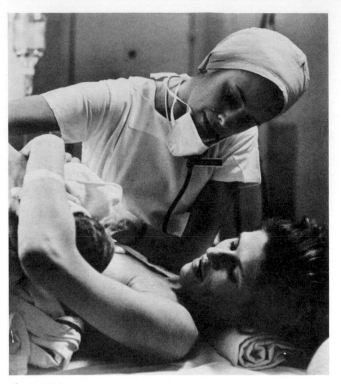

Figure 17.4

A mother cuddling her newborn baby in the delivery room. Does the mother receive emotional satisfaction from this act?

position of the spine. After the umbilical cord is cut, the baby is bathed in warm water, similar to the environment it has just left. Proponents of this technique feel that the newborn has less fear of its new world, is more calm, and becomes a better adjusted child as a result of this less traumatic birth experience.

If the mother is unable to undergo labor, the doctor delivers the baby by an operative procedure called Caesarean section (see Figure 17.5).

ENVIRONMENTAL FACTORS

The health of the developing embryo can be affected by a number of environmental factors that are within the parents' control (refer to Figure 17.6). Both mother and father need to be aware of these factors in order to optimize the development of their unborn child. It is advisable, for example, that both parents maintain physical fitness, eat a balanced diet, and be immunized against infections, such as rubella (German measles), that can possibly be passed on to the child. Furthermore, prospective parents should always have a blood test to check for venereal diseases and to determine blood type and Rh factor. If the man and woman have incompatible

Rh factors, doctors can be prepared to perform a blood transfusion on the fetus.

In addition to her physical condition, many of the mother's behaviors can affect the developing child. For example, it has been found that the mother's use of many drugs, including caffeine, aspirin, nicotine, and alcohol, as well as tranquilizers and over-the-counter preparations, especially during the second and third months of pregnancy, can adversely affect the fetus. The use of such drugs contributes to miscarriages, stillbirths, premature births, low birth weight, and even mental retardation and birth defects (see Figure 17.6). The mother's diet and nutritional state are also important to the baby's healthy development. Malnutrition in the mother has been found to be related to a number of problems in the newborn. Other factors potentially harmful to the developing child include exposure to X rays and other radiation and emotional stress on the part of the mother.

Thus, to reduce the negative effects of environmental factors, prospective parents must (1) educate themselves in the processes of prenatal development and childbirth; (2) be responsible enough to drop harmful habits (such as smoking and drinking); and (3) eat nutrient balanced diets; and (4) be aware of the financial expenses involved in bringing a healthy child in the world and prepare to meet such obligations.

HEREDITY

Heredity, much like nutrition and aspects of the environment, structures the foundation of what we are and can become. Not only do the genes you inherited determine how much health you will have, how long you will live, but also the kind of ailments, disorders, and diseases you might get (see Figures 17.7 and 17.11). One needs to be very cautious in concluding that observable defects are genetically caused, since the environment also plays a part in causing a trait or defect to develop. Thus a fault in a gene, or a fault in the environment, may each independently give rise to the same fault in development (9:246). If a gene is defective, the trait that results is hereditary. If the environment is defective, the trait that results is not hereditary; yet outwardly it may appear identical to the hereditary trait. For example, one should not assume, when a mentally defective child is born, that the family tree is tainted with a defective gene. It may be that this defect is hereditary, but it is just as likely that it is not. Perhaps the mother was infected with German measles during the first 2 months of pregnancy, or exposed to X rays or deficient in some nutrients, or she suffered from oxygen deficiency at a critical time when the brain of the embryo was developing.

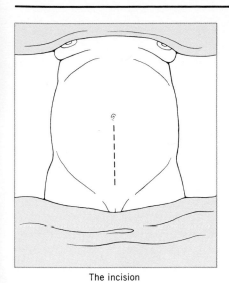
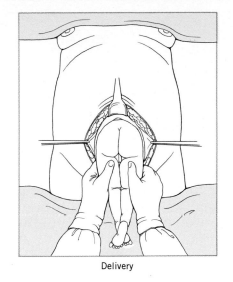

The incision | Delivery

Figure 17.5
Birth by Caesarean section. The physician makes a small abdominal cut, large enough to deliver the baby.

DRUGS	EFFECTS ON FETUS
Caffeine (in coffee) Tannic acid (in tea)	Stimulates fetal nervous system
Sleeping pills	Depressant
Tranquilizers	Possible malformations; but some now designed specifically for safe use by pregnant women
LSD and other psychedelics	Increased risk of miscarriage; possible chromosome damage
Cocaine; amphetamines	Acts as stimulant on fetus
Heroin; morphine	Possible fetal addiction: can mean blood transfusion needed at birth
Aspirin	Large amount can cause miscarriage or hemorrhage in newborn
Phenacetin	Possible damage to fetal kidneys
Antibiotics (a) Streptomycin, geneamycin (b) Sulphonamides (long-term) (c) Tetracycline	(a) Associated with deafness in infants (b) Can cause jaundice (c) Possible deformities: stains teeth
Antihistamines	Possible malformations; some now designed specifically for safe use by pregnant women
Cortisone	Fetal and placental abnormalities —possible stillbirth, cleft lip
Progesterone (for hormone def — iciency and possible miscarriage)	Genital abnormalities in female infants
Catathyroid	Possible goiter
Marijuana	As yet no proof of ill effects
Cigarette smoking (tobacco)	Pre-maturity
Alcohol	Mental retardation; fetal addiction, fetal alcohol syndrome
Malnutrition	Mental retardation; dental caries

Figure 17.6
The effects of some drugs on the fetus. (Adapted from the Diagram Group, *Woman's Body*, New York: Paddington Press, 1977, pp. D62–64.)

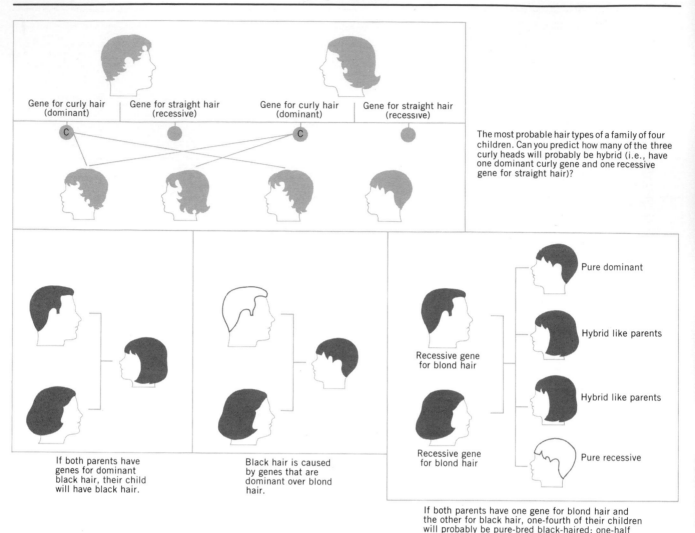

The most probable hair types of a family of four children. Can you predict how many of the three curly heads will probably be hybrid (i.e., have one dominant curly gene and one recessive gene for straight hair)?

Gene for curly hair (dominant)

Gene for straight hair (recessive)

Gene for curly hair (dominant)

Gene for straight hair (recessive)

If both parents have genes for dominant black hair, their child will have black hair.

Black hair is caused by genes that are dominant over blond hair.

Recessive gene for blond hair

Recessive gene for blond hair

Pure dominant

Hybrid like parents

Hybrid like parents

Pure recessive

If both parents have one gene for blond hair and the other for black hair, one-fourth of their children will probably be pure-bred black-haired; one-half hybrid black-haired; and one-quarter blond.

Figure 17.7

Examples of how we inherit hair. Good and bad traits are inherited in similar ways.

Hereditary ailments are more common that anyone has suspected. Medical investigators have now identified nearly 2000 genetic ailments caused wholly or partly by defective genes or chromosomes (4). It is estimated that 25 percent of the nation's medical problems are genetic. These diseases affect 12 million Americans: 1 person in 18 (4). They account for a third of the admissions to hospital pediatric wards, and 40 percent of infant deaths in the United States. (4). Such ailments inconvenience those having them, stifle or undermine the ability of those having them to function optimally and, in many instances, cause great anguish and suffering to the victim and his or her family.

Hereditary disorders range from causing serious health problems to those causing minor problems. For example, premature white hair, early baldness, myopia, and color blindness are not considered serious health problems, while phenylketonuria (PKU) can cripple a baby with severe mental retardation.

A few hereditary diseases are concentrated in certain races or ethnic groups. Sickle-cell anemia, a painful blood disorder, is common among blacks. Tay-Sachs disease, an enzyme deficiency that kills its young victims, is widespread among Jews who came from Eastern or Central Europe. Cystic fibrosis, a fatal glandular disease affecting mostly children and young adults, is confined to Caucasians.

Genetic predisposition is strongly implicated in many

What is Tay-Sachs Disease? Defect occurs when there is lack of a specific enzyme (Hexosaminidase A) in the blood, causing fatty substances to accumulate in brain cells, causing a loss of motor abilities and loss of locomotor function, causing mental retardation and eventually early infant death.

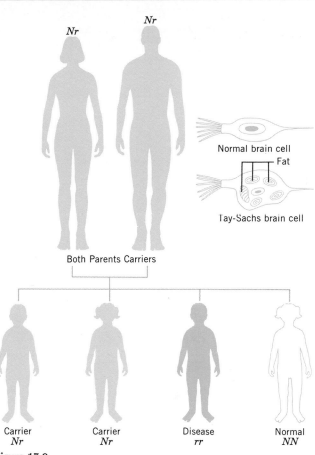

How Dominant Inheritance Works

One affected parent has a single faulty gene *(D)* which dominates its normal counterpart *(n)*

Each child's chances of inheriting either the *D* or the *n* from the affected parent are 50 percent

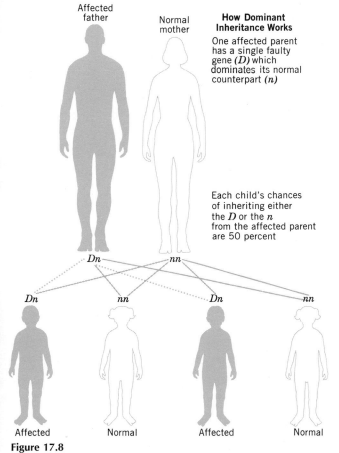

Figure 17.8

An example of how we inherit good and bad dominant traits. In this example, a father has a dominant gene (*D*) for a disorder (affected), while the mother has nondominant (normal) genes. Over 940 human disorders may be inherited this way, such as chronic glaucoma (blindness), Huntington's disease (nervous system degeneration), hypercholesterolemia (high blood cholesterol), and polydactyly (extra fingers or toes). (From *Genetic Counseling* (pamphlet), New York: Permission granted by the National Foundation—March of Dimes, the copyright holder of the original publication.)

Figure 17.9

An example of how recessive inheritance works. Chances of inheriting Tay-Sachs disease.

A child who inherits two recessive Tay-Sachs genes, one from each parent, will have the disease.

But a child who has only one recessive gene, from only one parent, is a carrier. A carrier is completely normal, and is as healthy as anyone else, except for two things—

1. Specific blood tests show only half as much of one particular enzyme (a chemical substance in the blood) as a noncarrier's.
2. A carrier must be aware of his or her carrier state, in case marriage is considered to an individual who is also a carrier.

If two carriers marry, there is a 25 percent risk with each pregnancy that their child will have the disease. There is another 25 percent chance that the child will be totally free of the disease. And there is a 50 percent risk that each child will be a carrier like the parents. (From, *Tay-Sachs Disease* (pamphlet), New York: Permission from The National Foundation/March of Dimes, as the copyright holder of the original publication.)

What is sickle cell disease?
It is a hereditary blood disease in which the red blood cells
sometimes assume a strange shape — like a sickle.

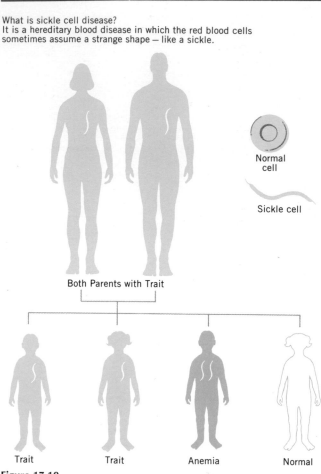

Figure 17.10

Chances of inheriting sickle cell anemia disease when both parents are carriers of this trait. Chances are that two of four children will have the traits of their carrier parents; and be well; one child in four will have sickle cell anemia; and one child in four will have no form of the disease at all. People whose ancestors came from Africa and the Mediterranean are more likely to have this disease. (From *Facts About Sickle Cell Anemia* (pamphlet), New York. Permission granted by the National Foundation-March of Dimes as the copyright holder of the original publication.)

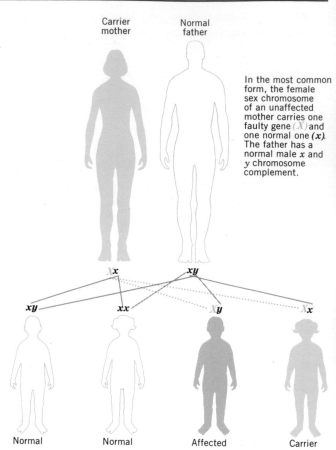

In the most common form, the female sex chromosome of an unaffected mother carries one faulty gene (X) and one normal one (x). The father has a normal male x and y chromosome complement.

Figure 17.11

An example of how X-linked inheritance works. Over 150 disorders may be transmitted by a gene or genes on the X chromosome (e.g., hemophilia or blood clotting defect, agammaglobulinemia or lack of immunity to infections, and muscular dystrophy or progressive wasting of muscles).

The odds for each *male* child are 50/50:
1. 50 percent risk of inheriting the faulty **X** and the disorder.
2. 50 percent chance of inheriting normal x and y chromosomes.
For each *female* child, the odds are
1. 50 percent risk of inheriting one faulty **X**, to be a carrier like mother.
2. 50 percent chance of inheriting no faulty gene.
(From *Genetic Counseling* (pamphlet), New York. Permission granted by the National Foundation—March of Dimes as the copyright holder of the original publication.)

common afflictions such as heart disease, schizophrenia, manic depression, ulcers, diabetes, and lung cancer.

The personal and social costs of genetic diseases reach tragic dimensions. The tragedy of having a genetically defective child affects both the parents and the child emotionally and economically. A mongoloid child, for example, is vulnerable to diseases, including leukemia, even though antibiotics and modern heart surgery now allow many mongoloids to live into adulthood. By the time they reach forty, most mongoloids become susceptible to diseases normally associated with old age. Considering such problems, it is understandable that many parents choose to abort mongoloid fetuses. Furthermore, many scientists agree that this kind of abortion assists nature, for nature is a great abortionist. It weeds out most chromosomal defects through spontaneous abortion. Mongoloids are the distressing exceptions that slip through nature's genetic screen.

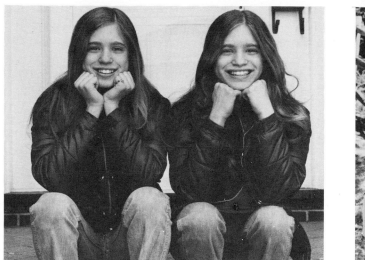
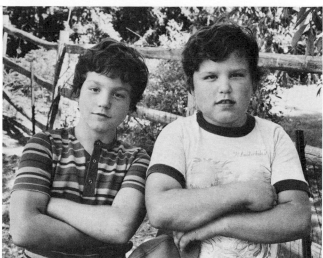

Figure 17.12

Identical twins look alike because they are genetically alike and come from the same egg. Fraternal twins look different, may be male or female, and come from two separate eggs.

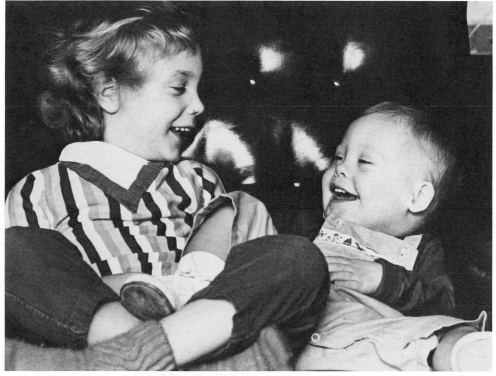

Figure 17.13

A child with Down's syndrome. Can you identify the child with this syndrome?

GENETIC COUNSELING

Fortunately, recent strides in medical genetics can reduce some of the sorrow, suffering, and social cost of abnormal children. About 70 genetic abnormalities can now be diagnosed during pregnancy (4). Parents who want only normal and healthy children can choose abortion for severely affected fetuses. Recently developed tests make it possible to detect some kinds of defective genes, and people who carry such genes can be advised as to their chances of having afflicted children. Today, 40 diseases can be treated and alleviated, mainly by diet and drugs (4). What genetic diseases or disorders might your son or daughter inherit? To find out, react to the Heredity Checklist at the beginning of this chapter.

Once a woman is pregnant, the embryo-fetus can be tested for some of the genetic disorders before birth. In a procedure known as amniocentesis, a needle is inserted through a pregnant woman's abdomen into her uterus to withdraw a small amount of the amniotic fluid that surrounds and protects the fetus (see Figure 17.14). The fluid contains cells shed by the developing fetus, and these cells disclose the unborn child's genetic makeup. Highly trained technicians analyze the cells both for chromosomal defects and for biochemical abnormalities. Using this information, a doctor can tell the parents whether the baby is likely to be normal and healthy. In addition to amniocentesis, certain malformations can be detected by the new technique of ultrahigh-frequency sound reflection (30:477–478).

Genetic counselors can also project risk factors for people. For example, the older a woman is when pregnant, the greater her chances of bearing a genetically defective baby. For example, the risk of bearing a child with Down's syndrome rises dramatically with maternal age. At 25, a mother's risk of giving birth to a mongoloid child is only 1 in about 1500; at 35, the risk rises to about 1 in 290; and at 45, it leaps to 1 in 45 (4) (see Table 17.1).

Who is in need of genetic counseling? Those who want to have children and who are carriers of defective genes, or who exhibit harmful genetic traits or disorders, and women over age 30. It is especially important for parents who already have an infant with a genetic disorder or who have disorders in their families. While having a defective gene usually poses no health problem for you, the carrier, there is always the chance of serious genetic diseases in any child of two carriers of the same harmful trait. When both partners are carriers, the chance of having a genetically defective child greatly increases. Genetic counseling provides information as to

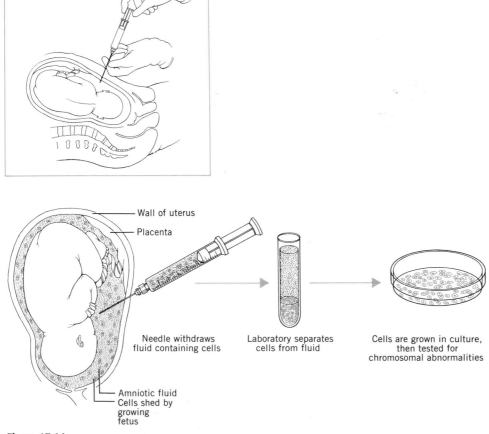

Figure 17.14

The process of amniocentesis. The upper drawing depicts the physician inserting the needle into the amniotic sac. The lower illustration depicts the step-by-step process.

Table 17.1

Risks of Down's Syndrome in Relation to Maternal Age

Mother's Age	Risk of Down's Syndrome in Baby
Under 20	1/2325
20–24	1/1612
25–29	1/1201
30–34	1/869
35–39	1/285
40–44	1/100
45 and over	1/45

Source: E. A. Murphy and G. A. Chase, *Principles of Genetic Counseling.* Copyright © 1975 by Year Book Medical Publishers, Inc., Chicago. Used by permission.

the advisability of their deciding to have children. At present, carrier tests are available for a large number of genetic diseases. At other times, the counselor may predict the possibility of defects after conception, as well as before birth. Often, a genetic disorder may not appear in the affected person until years later, as with glaucoma and Huntingtons's disease (diagnosis possible after age 25).

Medical genetics is fragmented, poorly understood, and is resisted socially. It is difficult for all physicians and other professional persons to be experts in all genetic disorders. One way to overcome these problems is to be aware that one can contact The National Foundation/March of Dimes. This organization lists counseling centers throughout the United States and has information on genetic diseases. Your doctor can call the National Genetics Foundation for information. You can ob-

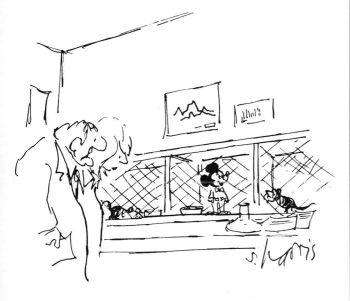

"SOMEHOW I WAS HOPING GENETIC ENGINEERING WOULD TAKE A DIFFERENT TURN."

tain information by contacting a medical school, a teaching hospital, the Public Health Department, your campus health center, and/or a geneticist on your campus.

WAYS TO HAVE A HEALTHY BABY

Whether a baby is born healthy or with birth defects, whether it will be miscarried or stillborn or full term, or whether it will be underweight or chubby—all these conditions are determined by environmental and genetic factors. Knowing these factors can help prospective parents to prepare, even before pregnancy, to have a healthy child.

Birth defects occur with disturbing frequency. Of liveborn infants, 2 percent suffer from major defects, and at least 20 percent of all pregnancies terminate in spontaneous abortions, usually the result of gross fetal abnormalities (13). Poor nutrition and drug use by the prospective mothers are probably responsible for a great majority of birth defects and miscarriages (natural abortions).

You should plan for a healthy baby. Here are some suggestions:

A. Before Pregnancy

1. Identify your own susceptibility to healthy and health-defective hereditary traits. Are you a carrier of certain disorders? Consider marrying a person who is not a carrier of genetic diseases or disorders, as well as adopting children.
2. Avoid exposure to X rays and radiation.
3. Avoid taking drugs, alcohol, smoking, etc. These can undermine the health of the sperm and egg (27:39).
4. Eat a well-balanced nutrient diet. A Harvard School of Public Health study (39:63) found that mothers on superior diets had fewer complications during pregnancy. Well-nourished pregnancy mothers have children with fewer dental caries (39:118–120). Malnourishment in the mother is related to defective development of the fetus (30:197;39:65–68).
5. Get regular exercise and maintain a high level of physical fitness.
6. Get immunizations for recommended viral infections, especially rubella (German measles), whooping cough, measles, mumps, polio, diphtheria, and smallpox. Since these viruses can pass through the placenta from an infected mother, the embryo or fetus may be injured and congenital disorders may occur.

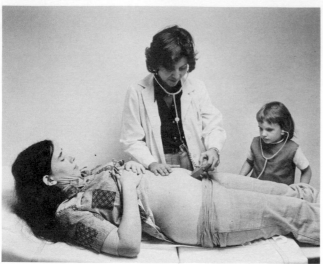

Figure 17.15
A pregnant woman having a medical examination with her daughter looking on. Is this a good way to educate your daughter?

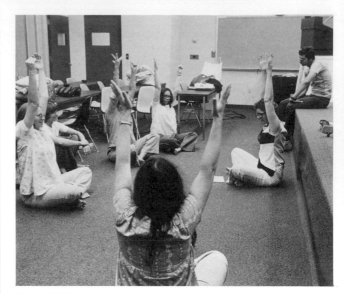

Figure 17.16
Exercises can help a pregnant woman to maintain physical fitness and also strengthen muscles used in delivering a baby.

B. During Pregnancy

1. Follow all suggestions for health care before pregnancy.

2. Avoid exposure to infections in pets, such as cats, which may have toxoplasmosis[1] infection (1). A woman having toxoplasmosis during pregnancy usually recovers quickly, but her unborn baby may have active infection all during the months of pregnancy. Such babies may be born with major defects, including mental retardation, hydrocephalus, epilepsy, eye damage, hearing loss, and premature birth.

3. Avoid all drugs or chemicals (aspirins, sleeping pills, laxatives, reducing pills, hair sprays, insecticides, heroin, marijuana, soft drinks, excess sugar, etc.). A woman who sniffs cocaine or shoots heroin also addicts her unborn baby to these drugs.

4. Don't drink coffee. Heavy coffee drinking (7 or more cups) increases the chances of miscarriage and stillbirth (27).

5. Do not smoke cigarettes. The carbon monoxide in the smoke cuts down the availability of oxygen that the mother's blood brings to the embryo and fetus. Nicotine is suspected of retarding fetal growth and contributing to underweight babies. Smoking mothers have more frequent premature babies. A smoking pregnant woman chokes her unborn baby.

6. Do not drink alcoholic beverages. Women who drink tend to bear a higher than expected number of abnormal and mentally defective children (39:163). Pregnant women who drink make their fetuses addicted to alcohol and greatly increase the risk of fetal alcohol syndrome (27).

7. Try to become pregnant when the sperm and ovum are both fresh by having intercourse within a day of ovulation. An overripe sperm and egg are suspected of increasing the risk of a defective baby.

8. Have a positive emotional outlook on life. An emotionally depressed woman should not become pregnant, as she may lack the coping skills and self-discipline to ensure a healthy baby.

9. Plan to have children when a woman is between 18 and 30 years of age. Women having babies before age 18, and those over 35, increase the risk of defects in their babies.

10. Space your children out 2 to 3 years apart so that each child can receive adequate nutrition and care before and after pregnancy.

11. Plan to have a few children. The more children a mother has, beginning with the third, the fewer the chances that each will be born healthy and normal.

12. Have good medical care insurance during pregnancy and after birth.

---

[1] A serious disease caused by the Toxoplasma. In young people it may cause inflammation of the brain.

13. Get the necessary blood tests during pregnancy (VD, Rh factor).
14. Prospective fathers and mothers should enroll in education classes for childbirth or rearing children.

BIRTH CONTROL

Couples who engage in sexual intercourse have the basic responsibility of planning for the consequences of their act. If they wish to have children, they will want to time their intercourse to the woman's most fertile period, and they will plan for caring for the child once it is born. But, if they do not wish to have children, they will have to take steps to prevent the sperm and egg from meeting. This process can be blocked in several ways: by preventing the spermatozoa from entering the vagina or fallopian tubes, by stopping the release of eggs from the ovaries, or by limiting intercourse to those times when a mature egg is not available. These are all forms of *contraception*, or blocking of fertilization. Contraception is only one form of birth control; others include abortion and abstinence.

The ideal contraceptive is one that a couple finds to be (1) effective in preventing pregnancy, (2) easy and comfortable to use, and (3) hygienically safe, with few, if any, side effects. Before having sexual intercourse, couples should discuss the use of contraceptives and what they will do should pregnancy occur. Which contraceptive method is best for a particular couple? The answer depends on their life style, finances, religious background, psychological makeup, and many other factors. Let us look at the various methods available.

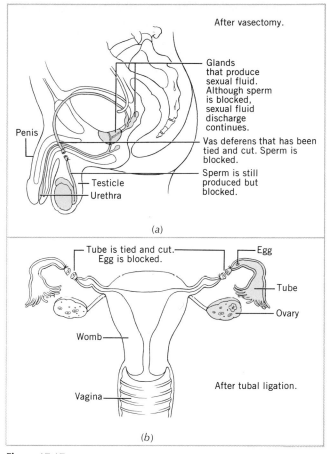

Figure 17.17
Sterilization procedures. Vasectomy in a male as a form of birth control. An incision is made (a) through the scrotum and the vas deferens is cut and tied. (b) Tubal ligation in a female consists of cutting the fallopian tube and then tying both ends.

MALE APPROACHES TO CONTRACEPTION

Although some women prefer that the man assume responsibility for taking measures to prevent pregnancy, there are relatively few options available to the male. *Withdrawal* (coitus interruptus) is seldom reliable, since this practice takes a great deal of control and timing to avoid ejaculation in the vagina. Many men find such control difficult to master. Furthermore, some semen is released prior to ejaculation, and spermatozoa may still make their way up into the uterus and fallopian tubes. Finally, many men and women find withdrawal to be emotionally and psychologically unfulfilling.

A more reliable and time-honored male birth control method is the *condom*, or rubber. If used properly, it is one of the best methods of contraception. It is particularly useful for occasional or unanticipated intercourse,

and it provides some protection against venereal disease. Condoms should not be stored in wallets, nor should they be allowed to age. The most reliable of male approaches is, of course, sterilization. In this process, the man undergoes a minor surgical operation, called a *vasectomy*. An incision is made on the scrotum, cutting the vas deferens, and thus preventing spermatozoa from being discharged (see Figure 17.17a). The testes continue to produce spermatozoa, which simply dissolve and are absorbed by the body. There is no change in the man's ability to have and enjoy sex. He can have erections, orgasms, and ejaculations of seminal fluid as often as before the operation, but the fluid is sperm-free. With the fear of pregnancy removed, both partners are able to enjoy a freer and more relaxed sexual experience.

Several researchers are currently exploring the idea of a male contraceptive pill, and several such pills have been tested. However, the approach has yet to be perfected and it is unlikely that we will see a male birth control pill on the market for some years. Until that day does arrive, it is likely that women will continue to bear the major responsibility for birth control.

FEMALE APPROACHES TO CONTRACEPTION

Today the choice of contraceptive is more important for the woman than for the man, since most of the methods available have been developed for women. The kind of contraceptive most acceptable to a woman depends on her emotional and psychological makeup, her knowledge of contraceptives, her religious and cultural background, her physical health, and how and when she has intercourse.

By using a contraceptive method, a women can assume direct control of her sex life and of her ability to have children. She can use contraception to eliminate the fear and anxiety of unwanted pregnancy and she can plan and space out her children. With this control comes the opportunity and freedom to enjoy sex as recreation and to use sex as a positive force in her life. She can

choose from a wide variety of methods, ranging from the pill and IUD to creams and foams, each with its particular advantages and drawbacks (see Table 17.2). Let us examine briefly each of the major approaches presently available, in the order of increasing effectiveness.

Rhythm Method

The natural, or rhythm method, is "natural" in that it does not involve drugs, artificial hormones, surgical procedures, mechanical devices, or foreign objects inserted in the body. Also known as the "safe period" and "periodic continent" method, this approach involves avoiding sexual intercourse during the fertile period of a woman's menstrual cycle. The fertile period usually falls about 14 days before the beginning of the next menstrual flow (refer to Figure 17.18). Since sperm can survive in a woman's body for 2 to 4 days, and an ovum survives 12 to 24 hours after ovulation, a woman using the rhythm method must abstain from intercourse from 2 to 4 days before ovulation to 1 day after.

The key obstacle in using the rhythm method is difficulty in identifying the day of ovulation, since few women have precise or regular cycles and most women

Table 17.2

Methods of Fertility Control: Factors Affecting Their Utilization

	Foam	Condom	Oral Contraceptive	IUD	Vacuum Abortion	Diaphragm
Cost	$25/yr	$25/yr	$60/yr	$60/yr	$150 each	$60/yr
Effectiveness (theoretical)	97%	97%	99.66%	97–99%	100%	97%
Morbidity						
Major	a	a	1%	1%	1%	a
Minor			40%	40%	8%	
Mortality (per 1,000,000 users/yr)	a	a	0.3–3	1.5	1.9	a
Reversibility	100%	100%	+100%	±100%	0	100%
Skill Required[b]	1	1	1	2	$^2/_3$	2
Anesthesia type	0	0	0	0/Local	Local	0
Time away from work	0	0	Office visit	Office visit	½ Day	Office visit
Hospital or office time	0	0	5–15 min.	5–15 min.	10–15 min	15 min
Recovery time	0	0	0	0	1 hour	0
Facility	—Across the counter—		Office	Office	Office/Outpatient	Office/Across the counter

cannot sense or feel ovulation taking place. One way a woman can try to determine her fertile period is to chart her daily basal body temperature — the temperature goes up a little during ovulation. Even following this precaution, the method is still "chancey" at best. A major advantage of the rhythm method is that it allows the woman to become more familiar with the functioning of her body and, when she does choose to have a child, she will have a good idea of the time when she will be most likely to conceive.

Jellies, Creams, and Foams

When inserted into the vagina before intercourse, spermicidal jellies, creams, and foams prevent pregnancy by blocking the cervix so that sperm cannot enter the uterus and by acting to kill the spermatozoa. The main advantage of these chemicals is that they are inexpensive and easy to use. However, the failure rate is high with this method, probably because the preparations are often used incorrectly. Another drawback to spermicides is that they can cause irritation to delicate tissues in some men and women, and they can leak out of the vagina after intercourse, causing physical discomfort and much psychological concern.

Diaphragms and Creams

The diaphragm is a soft rubber cup sealed over a circular steel spring about 3 inches in diameter. It prevents conception by blocking sperm from entering the cervix. It is most effective when used with a spermicidal cream or jelly. Because diaphragms come in various sizes and because women vary slightly in the length and size of the vagina, a woman must be examined and fitted for a diaphragm by a physician. In order to make sure the diaphragm fits properly over the cervix, the woman should receive instructions on how to insert it. (Refer to Figure 17.19.)

The diaphragm must be smeared with a spermicidal chemical before being inserted. Insertion can be done anytime up to 6 hours before intercourse. With the diaphragm in place, a woman can perform any normal physical activity without discomfort, and the device cannot be felt by either partner during intercourse. The diaphragm should not be removed for at least 5 or 6 hours after intercourse, and additional spermicide should be used before repeated sexual activity.

Use of the diaphragm is especially popular with women who are concerned about taking the pill for long periods of time. It is a relatively effective method when

Methods of Fertility Control: Factors Affecting Their Utilization (continued)

	Late Abortion	Hysterectomy	Laparoscopic	Tubal Ligation Minilap	Culpotomy	Vasectomy
Cost	$600 each	$2000	$800	$1000	$1000	$150
Effectiveness (theoretical)	100%	100%	99+%	99+%	99+%	99+%
Morbidity						
Major	3%	14%	0.6%	0.4%	2–4%	1%
Minor	26%	51%	1.7%	1%	3–13%	5%
Mortality (per 1,000,000 users/yr	17.3	100	1–5	?	?	0
Reversibility	0	0	0–50%	0–75%	0–75%	5–90%
Skill required[b]	4	4	5	4	4	3
Anesthesia type	Local	General	Local/General	Local/General	Local/General	Local
Time away from work	3 days	42 days	2–7 days	2–4 weeks	2–4 weeks	½–5 days
Hospital or office time	12–36 hrs	6 days	½ day	1–2 days	1–2 days	15–20 min
Recovery time	24 hrs	14–42 days	0–5 days	2 weeks	2 weeks	1–5 days
Facility	Hospital	Operating room	Operating room/ Surgicenter	Operating room	Operating room	Office

[a] Pregnancy related only.
[b] On Scale of 1-5: 1 = lay; 2 = short course; 3 = medical; 4 = surgical/gynecology; 5 = surgical/endoscopy.

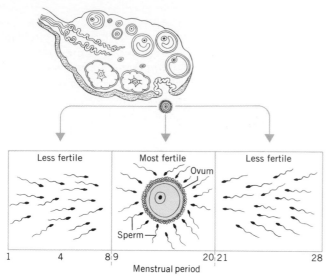

Figure 17.18

THE RHYTHM METHOD of birth control is based on the fact that every menstruating woman has a fertile period in her menstrual cycle. There is great variation among women, and even in the same woman from month to month, but generally a woman is fertile for two or three days sometimes between the 9th and 20th day of her cycle, counting from the first day of menstruation. Conception can be prevented by abstaining from coitus during this period. The method is not reliable. (From *Sexology*, August 1969, p. 45. Reprinted with permission of Mediomatic, Inc.)

Table 17.3

How to Figure the "Safe" and "Unsafe" Days

Length of Shortest Period	First Unsafe Day After Start of Any Period	Length of Longest Period	Last Unsafe Day After Start of Any Period
21 days	3rd day	21 days	10th day
22 days	4th day	22 days	11th day
23 days	5th day	23 days	12th day
24 days	6th day	24 days	13th day
25 days	7th day	25 days	14th day
26 days	8th day	26 days	15th day
27 days	9th day	27 days	16th day
28 days	10th day	28 days	17th day
29 days	11th day	29 days	18th day
30 days	12th day	30 days	19th day
31 days	13th day	31 days	20th day
32 days	14th day	32 days	21st day
33 days	15th day	33 days	22nd day
34 days	16th day	34 days	23rd day
35 days	17th day	35 days	24th day
36 days	18th day	36 days	25th day
37 days	19th day	37 days	26th day
38 days	20th day	38 days	27th day

Note: This is the standard chart for the rhythm method as prescribed by physicians. To use this chart, a woman should keep a record of her menstrual cycles for a year, counting the day on which menstruation begins as the first day of each period. Knowing the number of days in her shortest and longest cycles, she can find her first and last unsafe days from the chart.

used correctly. One drawback is that taking "time out" to insert the diaphragm during a passionate moment can be rather awkward. Furthermore, a woman must take good care of the diaphragm, keeping it clean and checking it occasionally for holes, tears, or cracks.

Intrauterine Devices (IUDs)

An intrauterine device (IUD) is a small object placed into the uterus through the cervical canal (refer to Figure 17.20). As long as the IUD stays in place, it somehow prevents pregnancy by disturbing the normal environment of the uterus. The precise way in which the IUD accomplishes its contraceptive effects is poorly understood.

IUDs come in various shapes, sizes, and materials. The IUD is not for every woman. Most physicians find it easier to insert and fit the IUD in women who have given birth to at least one baby. An IUD should not be used by women who have had an infection in the uterus, fallopian tubes, or ovaries, who have a tipped uterus, who are pregnant, or who have given birth or had an abortion within the previous 8 weeks.

The IUD is inexpensive, and once inserted is effective as long as it remains in place. When the woman desires, the IUD can be removed easily. In some women, the presence of the IUD irritates the uterine muscles, which contract to push the object out of the uterus. About 10 to 12 percent of women who receive an IUD expel the device within the first year of use. Further drawbacks of the IUD include possible irregular bleeding between periods, severe cramps in some women due to contractions, and such potential complications as pelvic inflammation and perforation of the uterus.

Other contraceptive techniques are recommended by physicians in this country and Canada.

Birth Control Pills

The Pill, or oral contraceptive, was the first contraceptive method to be 100 percent effective, easy to use, reversible, and completely controlled by the woman. It is now the most popular form of birth control in the United States, with some 10 million women using it. The most common type of oral contraceptive is the *combination pill*. It contains two artificial hormones, estrogen and progestin (a synthetic progesterone derivative), which take over the menstrual cycle from the normal endocrine

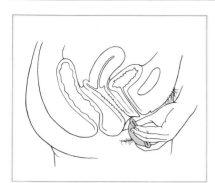

(a) Insertion.

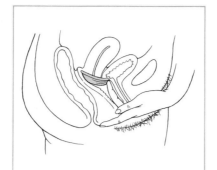

(b) Placement.

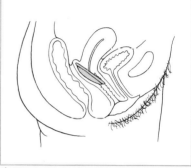

(c) Reaffirming the placement.
The woman knows the diaphragm is in place when she actually feels with her fingers that it fully covers the cervix.

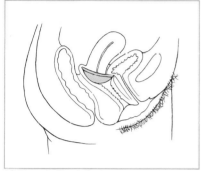

(d) Properly fitted diaphragm.

(e) Diaphragm too small.

(f) Diaphragm too large.

Figure 17.19
Techniques that increase the effectiveness of using the diaphragm. (Adapted from *Sexology*, October 1979, p. 67. Printed with permission of Mediomatic, Inc.).

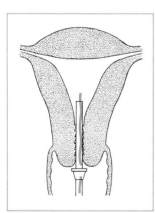
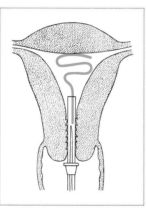
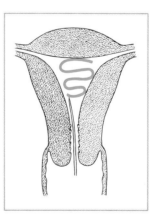

Figure 17.20
Technique used by physician to insert IUD in the uterus.

mechanisms. In so doing, they inhibit ovulation and change the characteristics of the uterus so that it is not receptive to a fertilized egg. The woman takes one pill each day for 21 days, starting on the fifth day after menstruation begins and ending on the 25th day. There is a gap of 7 days during which no hormone is taken and menstruation occurs. Then the pill taking begins again.

Many side effects have been linked to birth control pills, and the main culprit appears to be the estrogen component of the Pill. Among the side effects that some women experience are nausea, stomach cramps, fluid retention, weight gain, increase in size and tenderness of breasts, and periodic depression. Estrogen also increases the chances of elevated blood pressure, increased blood cholesterol, sugar and fat levels, abnormal insulin responses, and blood-clotting diseases in some women. It has also been suggested that birth control pills increase the risk of heart disease and certain types of cancer (37). Thus, although the Pill is the most effective contraceptive available, it does have certain health risks. It is for this reason that the Pill is a prescription drug. It is not for all women.

Any woman on the Pill should see her doctor or gynecologist for regular physical examinations. She should advise her doctor of any physical condition she may have, or her relatives may have had, that would make her use of the Pill undesirable. Such conditions include heart disease, stroke, sickle-cell anemia, endocrine disorders such as thyroid problems and diabetes, liver or kidney diseases, high blood pressure, varicose veins, migraine headaches, depression, asthma, epilepsy, and other ailments (19:19). The hormones in the Pill can aggravate many of these conditions. Furthermore, women who smoke are being advised not to use birth control pills or else to stop smoking while on the Pill. It seems that women who smoke and take birth control pills have a greatly increased risk of heart attack. However, most of these risks are reversible and expill users have risks similar to women who have never used the Pill.

Many doctors advise that women who are on the Pill for several years take periodic "vacations" from the Pill—a few months off every few years to see if the body returns to normal hormonal functioning. Physicians are also now advising that women in their late thirties and their forties, or women who have been on the pill for 10 years or more, switch to another birth control method, as health risks increase with age and long usage.

In addition to the physical drawbacks, the only other major disadvantage to the Pill is that the woman must remember to take it every day. If she misses 2 or 3 days, the contraceptive effect may be lost for the entire month. Taken regularly, however, the Pill is more effective than any other method short of sterilization. Women on the "pill" should supplement their diet with vitamins and minerals (see Chapter 6).

Newer Approaches

Research continues in an effort to find new methods of birth control that are both effective and safe. One unusual drug has been developed for women who have had sexual intercourse without taking any precautions but who do not want to become pregnant. Dubbed the "morning after pill," this artificial estrogen called DES (diethylstilbestrol) is taken every 12 hours for 5 days, beginning as soon after intercourse as possible. If started within 24 hours of sexual activity, the DES pill is almost 100 percent effective in preventing pregnancy.

Women using the "morning after pill" often suffer severe nausea and vomiting, as well as undesirable changes in body chemistry. A further problem with DES is that long-term studies indicate use of the pill by pregnant women can cause vaginal cancer in a female child who reaches puberty (19). If a woman uses DES and becomes pregnant, she should seriously discuss the possibility of abortion with her physician. A woman should ask her doctor to clarify the pill prescribed and what the side effects might be before using the pill.

Among other approaches to birth control currently being tested is a contraceptive nose spray that prevents pregnancy much the same way as the Pill does, and long-acting injections that can be administered once a month.

Sterilization

A woman can be sterilized by removing the ovaries, removing the uterus, or interrupting the fallopian tubes. Removal of the uterus (hysterectomy) is sometimes done because of a disease and, when such is the case, the woman becomes sterile. The most common method of sterilization is *tubal ligation,* or "tying the tubes" (see Figure 17.17b). A part of each fallopian tube is cut out, and the cut ends of the tube are tied and closed. In this way eggs are prevented from making their way to the uterus.

Many couples are turning to sterilization, and it is now the single most popular birth control method for couples who have been married 10 years or more (38). Couples who have had all the children they want find that male or female sterilization is the best solution to their birth control problem.

Abortion

Abortion is the removal of the embryo or premature fetus from a pregnant woman's uterus at an early point in pregnancy. Considerable moral and legal controversy surround the issue of abortion in this country, but the practice is a legal one.

Abortion, like the sex act itself, is a private and personal matter. This form of birth control is often the last resort for a woman who becomes pregnant and who does not want the child or who feels she will be unable to care for it properly.

There are two kinds of abortion—natural and induced. Natural abortion, or miscarriage, occurs as a spontaneous expulsion of the embryo or fetus and usually happens during the first 3 months of pregnancy. Happening in 10 to 15 percent of pregnancies, miscarriage usually occurs because of genetic abnormality or malformation of the embryo or maternal disease. A miscarriage is nature's way of ensuring that a healthy baby will be born.

Induced abortion involves use of artificial means to expel or abort the embryo or fetus during the first few months of pregnancy. There are several different medical methods of abortion, the choice depending on the length of pregnancy (see Figure 17.21).

Vacuum aspiration involves inserting a small tube through the cervix into the uterus and sucking the embryonic tissue from the uterine wall. This method works best for a woman in the first 3 months of pregnancy. Vacuum aspiration is quick, inexpensive, and usually free of complications.

For a woman who is 3 months pregnant, the method of choice is usually dilatation and curetage (D & C). The cervical opening is dilated to allow for the entry of a large instrument called a curette, or scraper. The doctor gently scrapes the fetal tissue from the wall of the uterus. The D & C is more difficult to perform, takes longer, is more painful, and is more dangerous than suction abortion.

Saline abortion is another method used when the woman is more than 3 months pregnant. Using a long hypodermic needle, the surgeon penetrates the uterine wall and the amniotic sac. He injects a strong saline solution, which usually causes expulsion of the fetus within 6 to 12 hours.

Some women try to induce abortion on their own without seeing a physician. The methods they use are highly dangerous, unsuccessful, and often fatal. Any woman considering an abortion should see her physician or other health professional.

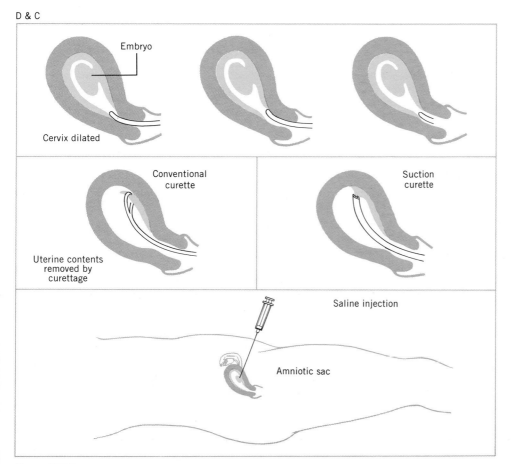

D & C

Embryo

Cervix dilated

Conventional curette

Uterine contents removed by curettage

Suction curette

Saline injection

Amniotic sac

Figure 17.21
Techniques of abortion.

WHERE TO GO FOR MORE INFORMATION

1. Your family physician.
2. Your campus health services center.
3. Your local department of public health.
4. Your local office of Planned Parenthood, or write:
   Planned Parenthood Federation of America
   810 Seventh Avenue
   New York, N.Y. 10019
5. Write to:
   Birth Control Institute, Inc.
   1242 W. Lincoln Avenue, Suite 1
   Anaheim, Calif. 92805

6. Write to:
   National Organization for Non-Parents
   3 North Liberty Street
   Baltimore, Md. 21201
7. Write to:
   The National Foundation/March of Dimes
   Box 2000
   White Plains, N.Y. 10602
   (Ask for International Directory of Genetic Services.)
8. Write to:
   Zero Population Growth
   1346 Connecticut Avenue, N.W.
   Washington, D.C. 20036

Further Readings

———, ''Am I Parent Material?'' (pamphlet), Baltimore: National Organization for Nonparents.

———, *Birth Control Handbook,* Montreal: Montreal Health Press, Inc., 1973.

Bylinsky, Gene, ''What science can do about hereditary diseases,'' *Fortune Magazine,* September 1974, pp. 111–118.

Gerard, Alice, *Please Breast Feed Your Baby,* New York: Signet Books, 1970.

Guttmacher, Alan F., *Pregnancy and Birth: A Book for Expectant Parents,* New York: Signet Books, 1962.

Hause, Aline, ''What contraceptive type are you?'', *Ms Magazine,* March 1973, pp. 7–14.

Holmes, Lewis, ''How fathers can cause the Down's Syndrome,'' *Natural Science* Oct. 1978.

LaMaze, Fernard, *Painless Childbirth,* New York: Pocket Books, 1977.

Leboyer, Frederick, *Birth Without Violence,* New York: Knopf, 1975.

McCary, James Leslie, *Human Sexuality,* New York: Van Nostrand, 1967.

Nofziger, Margaret, *A Cooperative Method of Natural Birth Control,* Summertown, Tenn.: The Book Publishing Company, 1978.

The National Foundation, ''Genetic Counseling'' (pamphlet), New York, The National Foundation/March of Dimes.

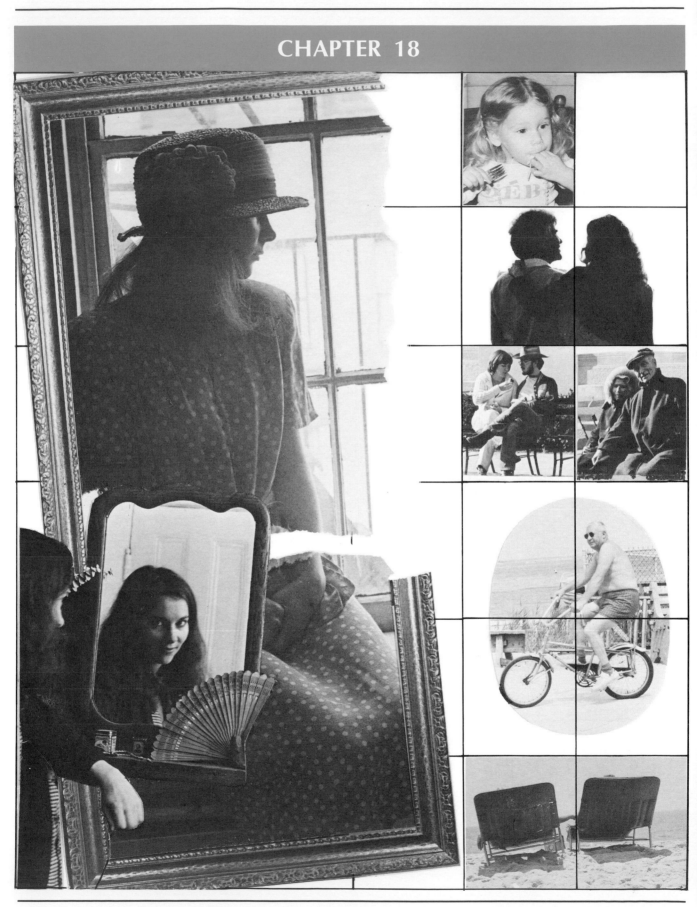

The preceding chapters did more than present information on how to maintain well-being. They also suggested how you can keep fit and postpone the aging process. You can look your present age when you are 40 years old; you can look 35 when you are 60 years old, and 45 when you are 75 years old. Looking and feeling physiologically younger than your actual chronological age should be perceived as successfully postponing the aging process.

The elderly in any society are living proof that they have lived a right and proper style of life. Only outstanding persons reach or surpass 80 years of age. Octogenarians must have deliberately maintained optimal well-being throughout most of their lives because living into old age usually does not happen by chance or accident. Instead, one needs to deliberately mold, plan for, and control each day. What you do today contributes to keeping you healthy at a later time. Aging is not an exclusive characteristic of the elderly or those over 50. Many adolescents and young people today are old and do not know it. Young adults can and do prematurely age physiologically, emotionally, socially, and spiritually. You speed up the aging process when you lack values by which to live; when you lack the will or spirit to live; when you do not have good health habits; when you are depressed and lonely; when you have lost your youthful figure to overweight and obesity; when you get tired easily; when you suffer from arthritis, cancer, heart disease, hypertension, and other disorders; and when you are unable to function in work and society. Skin wrinkles, gray hair, and a rough skin complexion do not necessarily depict the elderly. Today, many young persons are unaware that they may be incubating or already have these symptoms of aging. They just do not look, act, or feel young.

A few young people might argue that we will all die from heart disease or cancer sooner or later, and therefore, the odds are against living past age 70. Besides: "Who wants to live a long time anway?" These are poor arguments, for most persons die because they lack the will to live. No one ever dies from old age (7:206). Most persons die prematurely because of diseases or disorders initiated early in life. They shortchange themselves and do not get the most out of life.

Getting sick during early adulthood in Roman times symbolized that one had not yet learned how to live properly. All young Romans were expected to master the art of successful living before the age of 30. We would be wise to adopt a similar attitude toward health, life, and longevity.

What kind of a life style will postpone aging, help keep you young, and allow you to surpass 80 years of age? This chapter discusses the aging process, problems of the elderly, and identifies life-style factors enhancing both longevity, as well as the quality of living. This chapter will discuss the secrets of longevity, and, it is hoped, make you aware that you cannot ignore the study of aging.

React to the How Long You Will Live Predictor. It will make you aware of the factors affecting longevity, as well as assess your potentials for longevity.

☞ HOW LONG YOU WILL LIVE PREDICTOR[1]

Directions are included in a progressive manner in each section.

Start with a prediction of expected longevity, based on life insurance tables, then add or subtract years to this prediction, ending up with years of life remaining. This is your predicted longevity.

Be sure to react to all the sections and make selections that most closely fits your life.

A. *Year of Birth*

Period	Men	Women
1880–1900	35 − 40	35 − 42
1900–1904	46 + 2 mos.	48 + 8 mos.
1905–1908	48 + 8	51 + 5
1909–1912	50 + 7	54 + 4
1913–1916	51 + 8	55 + 5
1917–1920	52 + 6	56 + 5
1921–1924	58 + 2	61 + 2
1925–1928	58 + 5	61 + 10
1929–1932	58 + 10	63 + 2
1933–1936	60 + 6	65 + 5
1937–1940	62	66
1941–1944	64 + 6	68
1945–1948	65	70 + 4
1949–1952	65 + 11	71 + 6
1953–1956	67	74
1957–1961	67 + 6	74 + 2
1963	67 + 8	74 + 4

Write down your basic life expectancy: _____ years _____ months

B. *Place of Birth*

New England	Add 6 months
Middle Atlantic	Subtract 1 month
South Atlantic	Subtract 1 year
North Central	Add 7 months
South Central	Subtract 7 months
Mountain and West	Add 6 months

New total _____ years _____ months

C. *Present Age*

Age	Add	Age	Add	Age	Add
1–4 Years	1 Year Each	31–35	3 Years Each	61–65	8 Years Each
5–10	2 Years Each	36–40	3½	66–70	9½
11–15	2	41–45	4	71–75	11½
16–20	2	46–50	4½	76–80	12
21–25	2½	51–55	5½	81–85	6½
26–30	3	56–60	6½	86+	4½

New total _____ years _____ months

[1] Permission to reprint this predictor has been received from Dr. Ralph Grawunder, Professor of Health Science, San Diego State University, San Diego, Calif.

D. *Marital Status*

If you are happily married, add 5 years.
If you are over 25 and not married, or unhappily married, deduct 1 year for every unwedded or unhappy decade.

New total _____ years _____ months

E. *Occupation*

Student	Add 3 years
Clergyman	Add 4 years
Teacher	Add 3 years
Nurse	Add 3 years
Lawyer	Add 3 years
Clerical	Add 2 years
Doctor	Add 1 or 2 years
Farmer	Add 2 years
Miner or quarryman	Subtract 10 years
Construction worker	Subtract 5 years

New total _____ years _____ months

F. *Where You Live*

Small town	Add 3–5 years
City	Subtract 2 years

New total _____ years _____ months

G. *Economic Status*

If wealthy or poor for greater part of life, deduct 3 years.

New total _____ years _____ months

H. *Transportation*

Drive or ride less than 10,000 miles annually mostly in full-sized automobile or public transportation	Add 2 years
10,000–15,000 miles as above	Add 1 year
Drive or ride in compact car up to 15,000 miles yearly	Subtract 1 year
15,000 + miles in compact car	Subtract 2 years
Ride motorcycle in traffic regularly	Subtract 4 years

New total _____ years _____ months

I. *Family Background*

If two or more grandparents or parents died before age 65 of causes other than accident or infectious disease subtract 2 years.

New total _____ years _____ months

J. *Physical Fitness*

If you do not exercise or play an active sport

Subtract 3 years

If you exercise lightly (calisthenics, golf, or tennis) 1 or 2 days per week or if you exercise moderately (light exercise 3 or 4 days per week)

Neither add nor subtract

If you exercise heavily (30 minutes or more of jogging, cycling, swimming, or equivalent) and if you are capable of running or running and walking two miles in 17 minutes (men), 20 minutes (women)

Add 2 years

New total _____ years _____ months

K. *Medical Condition*

Blood pressure—subtract ½ year for each 10 mm above 130 resting systolic. Add 1 year for 105–120.

New total _____ years _____ months

Cholesterol:

200–250 mg% (choose this if you do not know)   Subtract 1 year
251–300 mg%   Subtract 2 years
301–400 mg%   Subtract 4 years
401+ mg%   Subtract 6 years
125–175 mg%   Add 2 years

New total _____ years _____ months

Presence of diseases such as diabetes, asthma, kidney disease, or abnormal electrocardiogram alter one's expectancy of remaining years of life but the degree of severity and success of medical treatments are variables that are impossible to assess even in a crude predictive exercise like this.

Illness frequency—subtract 1 year for every day per month on average of incapacitation.

New total _____ years _____ months

L. *Medical Checkups*

Yearly checkups   Add 1 year
No checkup in last 2 years   Subtract 1 year
Never had checkup   Subtract 2 years

New total _____ years _____ months

M. *Your Shape*

Deduct 1 year for every 5 pounds you are overweight. For each inch your girth measurement exceeds your chest measurement, deduct 2 years.

New total _____ years _____ months

N. *Diet*

Never eat breakfast and/or irregular diet	Subtract ½ year
Ingest pastry, ice cream, sweets often	Subtract 3 years
Eat beef meat, hot dogs, bologna often	Subtract 5 years
Eat diet rich in vegetable fiber	Add 2 years

New total _____ years _____ months

O. *Alcohol*

Heavy drinker	Subtract 5 years
Very heavy drinker	Subtract 10 years
Nondrinker	Add 1 year

New total _____ years _____ months

P. *Smoking*

½ to 1 pack per day	Subtract 3 years
1 to 1½ packs per day	Subtract 5 years
1½ to 2 packs per day	Subtract 10 years
Pipe or cigar	Subtract 2 years

New total _____ years _____ months

Q. *Other Drugs* (prescription and nonprescription medical and recreational)

Frequency

10 doses (separate takings or less per year)	Add 1 year
24–100 doses per year	Subtract 1 year
More than 100 doses per year	Subtract 2 years

Variety

Three or more different drugs taken each week on average	Subtract 2 years

New total _____ years _____ months

R. *Sleep*

Less than 6 hours sleep a day or more than 9 hours sleep a day or irregular sleep	Subtract 1 year

New total _____ years _____ months

S. *Relaxation*

Daily relaxation (pleasure reading, TV, music, hobby, meditation, etc.) of one or more hours	Add 1 year

New total _____ years _____ months

T. *Worry*

For each half-hour of worry per day on the average   Subtract 6 months

New total   _____ years _____ months

U. *Contentment*

Feel content 90 percent or more of the time   Add 1 year
Feel content about half the time   Subtract 1 year
Seldom or never feel content   Subtract 2 years

New total   _____ years _____ months

V. *Disposition*

Good-natured and placid   Add 1–3 years
Tense and nervous   Subtract 1–3 years

New total   _____ years _____ months

INTERPRETATION

Your interaction with the instrument made you aware of the many variables that may extend or restrict longevity. Read the remainder of this chapter to get information about the many factors affecting longevity.

FACTORS PROMOTING LONGEVITY

Man today is as interested in postponing, preventing, or retarding the progress of aging and even overcoming death as were the ancients. Reports of the search for the Fountain of Youth, the elusive elixirs, and the philosopher's stone; or the efforts of the ancient alchemists, surgical removal of the colon, hormone injections, gonadal transplants, and the very origin of medicine bear testimony to this curiosity and eagerness (11).

Recently, scientists and gerontologists have renewed this interest by studying the life styles of people in three areas of the world where people are alleged to live longer and remain more vigorous in old age than in most other societies: the Andean village of Vilcabamba in Ecuador; the land of Hunza in the Karakoram Range in Pakistani-controlled Kashmir; and Abkhazia in the Georgian Soviet Socialist Republic in Southern Soviet Union.

As a result of these (7;21) and other studies (5;9–14, 22, 24), the following life-style factors have been identified as contributing to a long and vigorous life:

1. Optimal well-being and fitness (few illnesses and diseases).
2. Positive, emotional, and optimistic outlook on life.
3. Regular, vigorous physical exercise or activity.
4. The desire to live a long time and to be healthy.
5. Positive psychological makeup (motivated self-care) and intelligence.
6. The ability to adjust and cope.
7. Clean, sanitary physical environment.
8. Ample socioeconomic rewards (e.g., enough materialistic goods to live; few stressful changes in life style, such as the loss of job and friends).
9. Life-style satisfactions and fulfillments.
10. Social respect for elders (personal worth in com-

munity; elders occupy high social status in community).

11. Continued close, active family unit.
12. Continued involvement in the community.
13. Marriage and prolonged sexual activity.
14. No abuse of alcohol, smoking, or drugs.
15. Heredity (have long-lived parents and relatives).
16. Low calorie diet (2000 calories).
17. Low salt, animal fat, and low refined sugar diet, but high in fruits and vegetables (vitamins and minerals).
18. Appropriate body weight (lean body mass).
19. Purpose in life.
20. Enjoy leisure, recreation, and play.
21. Minimum stress from work, friends, and life style.
22. Doing challenging and satisfying work.
23. Continuing to do useful and meaningful work throughout life (no retirement).
24. Sex-linked (women outlive men by 5 to 10 years).
25. High-fiber diet (roughage as provided by cereal bran and vegetables).

Longevity is clearly a multifactorial matter. Those having studied longevity are convinced of the importance of genetic factors, perhaps the most important of all these factors. It is generally accepted that the offspring of long-lived parents live longer than others (8:238). Factors associated with nutrition are also of primary importance although the role of specific dietary factors in promoting longevity remains unsettled. Eating a low-calorie diet, however, and one low in sugar and animal fats early in life, appears to extend life considerably. A third important contributor to long life is physical activity. In the three areas of Vilcabamba, Hunza, and Abkhazia, physical fitness was an inevitable consequence of the active life led by the inhabitants. The benefits of continuous exercise and physical activity are summarized in Chapter 5. Psychological factors (stress and outlook on life) also play a part in determining how long a person will live. Contributing, productive, and self-esteemed persons are happier and live longer than those who are unproductive and unhappy. People in these three areas have no fixed retirement age, and the elderly make themselves useful doing many necessary tasks around the farm or the home. Unlike the situation in the United States and Canada, there is no retirement, and increased age is accompanied by increased social status. People who continue to play an active social and economic role in society live longer.

It should be obvious by now that those attaining old age evolve life styles that include most of these positive factors. Young people (college students) would be wise to structure their life style so that it includes most of

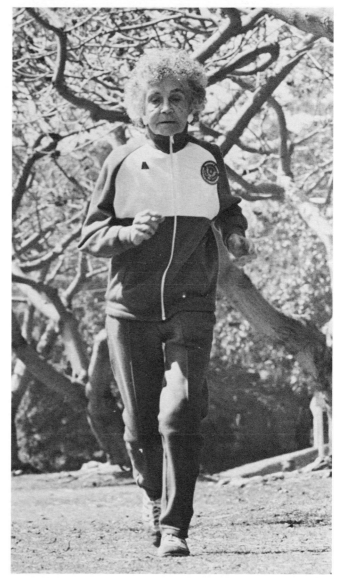

Figure 18.1

Eighty-eight year old Eula Weaver of Los Angeles runs a mile a day, goes to the gym three times a week, and peddles a stationary bicycle 10 miles before dinner. When she was stricken a decade ago, her doctor gave her a choice: become an invalid or get out and get going. Exercise is wonderful therapy as we get older. Everyone, and especially older persons, need exercise. Will you be as spry at age 88 as Eula Weaver?

these predictors of long life. In essence, they detail the fulfillment of one's basic health needs (Maslow's hierarchy of human needs). The key here is for young people to evolve such a life style early in life. Evolving a sound way of life is probably more important than getting a college degree and job skills.

Most of us have many preconceptions about growing older and what to expect when we do reach old age. For example, many people believe that humans are living longer today than we ever have. That is not true (5:10). What is true is that, for many today, there is a fixed maximum lifespan of about 100 years (4:18), but it is the likelihoood of reaching that age that has increased dramatically in developed countries since 1900 (5). (See Figure 18.2.) The maximum lifespan for our species is not increasing, but what has happened is that we are now more likely to reach that fixed, immutable end point (see Figure 18.3). Even if we could resolve or eliminate the major causes of death today (heart disease, cerebrovascular, various cancers, motor vehicle accidents, influenza and pneumonia, diabetes, and tuberculosis), babies born today would have a life expectancy of about 96.5 years, and those 65 years old today could hope to live until they are about 101 years old (5). The chances of living beyond age 100 are affected by the increased vulnerability of older people to disease (see Figure 18.4). That this is probably so is attributed to losses or changes occurring in our immunological defense system as we get older. Our vulnerability increases as we become less capable of coping with diseases like cancer or heart disease. Then too, Hayflick (4) discovered that normal human cells grown in laboratory glassware will divide some 50 times and then die. In other words, there seems to be a limit as to how long the average person will live. Thus, based on today's knowledge of medicine and technology, a life span of 100 to 130 years represents a very probable maximum limit for humans. The fact that a few people may live to be 110 or 115 merely shows that the figures used are averages. There will always be some lucky people who will beat the averages, as well as some unlucky individuals who will die earlier than the average.

In spite of the evidence that the length of life may be programmed, everyone should evolve a life style that ensures reaching old age. It is important to live out the human cycle and make the most of the only opportunity one ever has of living. We must work at "staying alive," for this in itself can become a functional purpose.

All individuals age in all three dimensions: biologically, psychologically, and socially (28:8). Aging may be different in the same individual. People also age at different rates.

BIOLOGICAL ASPECTS (OF AGING)

As we grow older, there appear to be losses in functional capacity at the cellular level, the tissue level, the organ level, and the human body in general. As the saying goes "we tend to die a little each day." The functional capacity of the individual is gradually lost through aging and other circumstances of living.

There is also ample evidence (6) that aging probably begins about 12 years of age, when the thymus gland atrophies. People are perceived to be healthiest at ages

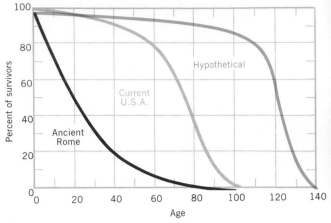

Figure 18.2
The intrinsic life span of the human species has remained unchanged since the Biblical "three score and ten," but a far greater proportion of people now live out that full life span. Roy Walford of University of California, Los Angeles, who designed this chart, thinks that the new discoveries about aging herald the day when this intrinsic life span can be stretched by pushing diseases of old age into the final stage of a longer life. Source: Fortune Art Department/George Nicholson. Originally photographed by Alfren.

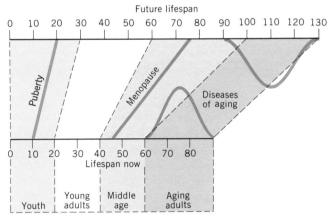
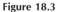

Figure 18.3
Life's milestones might be moved back by age-retarding agents. This version of the future ages of man, drawn up by Roy L. Walford, assumes that treatment would begin early, as is now the practice with laboratory animals. Puberty would be postponed until the twenties and menopause pushed back toward the seventies. The diseases of old age would be delayed and exposure to them would cover fewer years than now. Source: Fortune Art Department/George Nicholson. Originally photographed by Alfren.

10 to 12 (2;6). Thus, since the thymus gland is part of the immune system, and since its function is suspected to be closely allied to the hypothalmus in the brain, and the endocrine system in pacing the aging process, the adolescent body has already begun to gradually age. Man reaches his peak strength at about age 19 (10). The aging process accelerates after age 30 when osteoporosis[1]

[1] A loss in bony substances producing brittleness and softness of the bones.

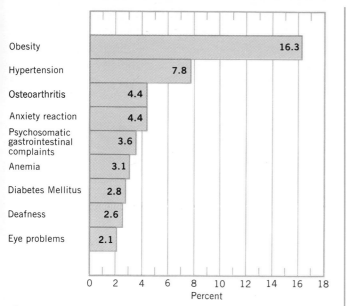

Figure 18.4

Disorders of middle age that college students should guard against. These disorders can become aggreviating and debilitating as one gets older and indicate that the aging process is well on its way. Reproduced by courtesy of Pitman Medical Ltd., from "Pre-Symptomatic Detection and early diagnosis," Sharpe and Keen, 1968.

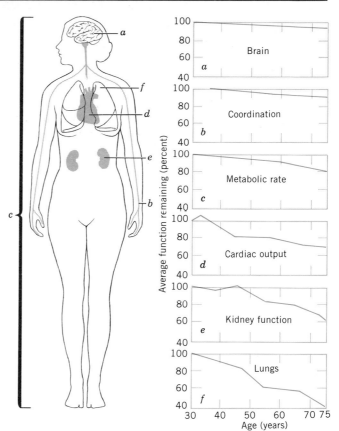

Figure 18.5

Graphs showing the loss of body function with advancing age. Loss of function does not occur at the same rate in all organs and body systems. Level of function at age 30 represents 100 percent. Brain weight has diminished to 92 percent of its age-30 value by age 75. Coordination (nerve-muscle conduction velocity) has diminished to about 90 percent of age-30 value. Basal metabolic rate has diminished to 84 percent, cardiac output to 70 percent, filtration rate of the kidneys to 69 percent, and maximum breathing capacity to 43 percent. Adapted from "Getting Old," by Alexander Leaf. Copyright © 1973 by Scientific American Inc., all rights reserved.

gradually sets in, and when brain cells are suspected to die at the rate of about 100,000 per day (5). As aging progresses and accelerates with advancing age, there is a decline in the levels of the key brain chemical—the neurotransmitter dopamine. These and other physiological detriments are shown in Figure 18.5 Interestingly enough, the body's organs do not deteriorate dramatically with age. The healthy heart does not age significantly. Likewise, the old liver, if given the time, seems to be just as good as a young one in disposing of alcohol and chemicals. Although body organs are able to maintain most of these physiological functions, these functions appear to be impaired or disrupted by overeating, a nutrient-deficient diet, excess body weight, inactivity, drug and alcohol abuse, cigarette smoking, and distress. These habits appear to accelerate the normal aging process. Those initiating these deleterious habits during adolescence and early adulthood begin to vacillate slowly toward physical degeneration. Young adulthood is a prime time to assess personal habits, behaviors that may accelerate aging and predispose the body to degenerative diseases and disorders.

Numerous theories have been proposed to explain cellular aging. A few of them include the following (7:78–87;28:222–224).

1. *Collagen theory.* The formation of cross-links between collagen (fibrous, protein-forming connective tissue) molecules and fibrous proteins that support bone, tendons, cartilage, and connective tissue lessens. Over the years, these cross-linked collagen molecules shrink and strangle many healthy cells. Reactive free radicals formed from radiation, fat, alcohol, nicotine, ozone, and other chemicals are responsible for part of the cross-links (refer to loss of nucleic acids).

2. *Stress theory.* Constant stress gradually wears out the cells and drives them to the point where they become completely worn out, and where cell division stops early. Excess stress in the cells makes them age faster than normally. Faulty nutrition, lack of exercise, smoking, air pollution, mental stress, and an excessive amount of alcohol are major stress factors.

3. *Metabolic products theory.* Metabolic products, which are not excreted fast enough, tend to build up and poison the body.

4. *Immunologic theory.* The breakdown of the immune system (e.g., relationships between the pituitary, thyroid, and thymus glands, and the production of the hormone thymosin makes one more and more vulnerable to the diseases of aging.

5. *Programmed or genetic theory.* The biological clock keeps track of cell division and initiates the aging sequence when certain limits are reached. It has been estimated that the human cells have the capacity to divide about 50 times.

6. *Mutation theory.* Errors introduced in the transmission of information from the DNA molecule to the formation of vital proteins (enzymes) in the cell can stifle new cells from carrying out chemical reactions essential to cell life; then the cell dies. Thus the capacity for regeneration of tissues (skin and bone) slows down. Cells also decrease in performance due to damaged DNA.

7. *Loss of nucleic acids.* After many cell divisions, there is a remarkable loss of DNA and RNA (7:33). Eventually, the damage becomes so serious that the performance of the DNA becomes completely unsatisfactory and ceases to function. Old DNAs are suspected of being unable to produce normally functioning cell enzymes. The most serious damage to cells occurs when the DNA is damaged by agents called "free radicals" (7:67–74).

Free radicals are fragments of molecules that have become unattached. These free floating molecules are very eager to recombine and react with anything nearby. Unless free radicals are neutralized and converted into less reactive and harmless forms, they can produce considerable damage to the fats in the membranes of cells, to enzymes and proteins, and even to genetic material. When a polyunsaturate or a protein is damaged in such a reaction, a telltale pigment is left in the tissue, this pigment, Lipo fuscin (and ceroid) is suspected of causing cellular aging (26).

Free radicals are formed mainly from the oxidation of products of fats, caffeine, alcohol, sugar, sodium nitrate, radiation, tobacco substances, smog, lead and mercury (26). Formation of these radicals may be prevented by a diet rich in all essential nutrients, and especially antioxidant vitamins E and C, the mineral selenium, and sulfur amino acids like methionine and cysteine (26).

In addition to these, other theories have also been proposed (4:12). The real magical causes(s) of aging has yet to be scientifically verified. Be that as it may, definite biological changes take place gradually.

Many scientists predict that living to age 100 is within the reach of all of us today. Others, such as Bylinsky (2), Kugler (7), Prehoda (17), and Tappel (26), perceive humans living to 200 years and beyond if we unlock the mystery of cell metabolism. They feel that life can be greatly extended if we can select a diet that is rich in antioxidants (vitamins A, C, and E, and trace minerals, such as selenium). Antioxidants slow down the oxidation of fats in the cell, aid in combating carcinogens, and in general, slow down the aging process. Vitamin C, for example, is essential for the synthesis of collagen in the bodies of human beings. Collagen is a fibrous protein that forms connective tissue and is largely responsible for the strength of bones, teeth, skin, tendons, blood vessel walls, and other parts of the body. When these collagen protein molecules cross-link for long periods of time, they bind together. This chemical sewing together causes the body structure to become rigid and lose elasticity. Furthermore, the constantly increasing number of these large molecules throughout the body interferes with the biochemical processes in the cells.

Cell function is gradually lost in most body systems. This is summarized in Figure 18.4. The older kidney has fewer nephrons; muscles lose strength; brain cells continue to die gradually; and the old brain has fewer neurons. The skin grows thinner; wrinkles accumulate; and pigmentation is more widespread (26). Bones become more brittle; the hair thins out and grays; and the eyes appear grayer and cataracts may develop as one gets older. This may be more of a nutritional than an actual physiological deterioration. As muscle size and strength diminish with age, there is an increase of interstitial fat and lipids within muscle fibers. The older person may not weigh more, but the body fat to body weight ratio increases (25).

The body senses lose their sensitivity (25). The eye lens thickens, and the eye muscles do not accommodate as well with aging. Hence an older person needs more light than a younger person to be able to read and see. Ability to hear high tones and to hear in general declines with age. Many olfactory (smell) receptors in the nose die. Two-thirds of the taste buds in the mouth die by the time an individual is 70 (27). The skin receptors for touch and pain are also lost. There is a decline in the sense of balance, reaction time, and coordination, thereby making the older person more susceptible to falls and accidents.

There is a reduction in breathing efficiency. With a diminished metabolic rate, the energy level requirements drop, and the older person needs fewer food calories compared to young adults.

The digestive system in many—but not all—persons may undergo many changes (25). Smaller amounts of digestive juices are secreted. There may be altered gastric pH level, a reduction in peristalsis, and fewer absorptive cells; and intestinal blood flow may be reduced. Persons over the age of 50 may eat balanced diets, but their digestive system may be unable to absorb nutrients and they may experience vitamin and mineral deficiencies. They may suffer digestive disorders and delay in elimination. Such elimination delays often result in constipation although this is probably due to a low-fiber diet and inactivity more so than because of physiological changes (10:105;11).

Peripheral resistance increases and blood flow slows down (25). Arteries may lose their elasticity, and blood pressure usually increases with age. However, many cardiovascular changes may be a consequence of poor diet and inactivity rather than the aging process itself.

Numerous sexual changes occur gradually as the individual ages. Gonadal hormones decrease over time in both men and women. Women lose their fertility much sooner than men. In menopausal and postmenopausal women, there is a gradual atrophy of ovarian, uterine, and vaginal tissues, and a decreased level of vaginal lubrication (26). Testosterone levels decline in men although such hormonal decline starts much later in men than women. Sex hormones are secreted but in lesser amounts in old age. There is a decrease in viable sperms; the prostate may become enlarged; the force of ejaculation is reduced; and although an older male takes longer to reach an erection, he is able to maintain the erection longer than a young male (26). To sum it up, older men and women can and do have sexual desires and do have a capacity for sexual relations. Masters and Johnson found that the capacity to have satisfying sexual relations continues well into the 80s and beyond for healthy partners (5). Previous sexual experiences (enjoyment, frequency, pleasure) in early adulthood are important predictors for sexual activity in the last half of life (25). With loss of a spouse, sexual activity is often hampered by lack of an intimate partner.

Psychological factors usually are the main block of sexual activity at any age. "People stop having sex for the same reason they stop riding a bicycle." Someone tells them it is inappropriate at their age (1:72). This is a ridiculous viewpoint, for older people have great need for warm human contact, love and affection, physical contact, intimate social involvement, and recreation.

Older people are much more sensitive to drugs than young people. Toxic substances may accumulate, since detoxification and excretion of drugs is often slower in older individuals (26). Since body fat in older persons increases even though body weight may not, and since many drugs, such as barbiturates, are stored in adipose tissues, the total metabolism and elimination of drugs from the older person's body may be delayed. Thus drugs may be more active in older people even at reduced dosage levels (26).

Physiological changes accompanying the aging process may not be the result of aging alone. Incipient disease processes, undiagnosable and unrecognized in their early state, could also contribute to the losses in body function (27:263). DeVries reviewed the effects of exercise on aging, and concluded that physiological declines more often that not result from disuse and lack of activity rather than the aging process (27:272). Furthermore, both middle-aged and older healthy men and women are trainable and able to improve their physical fitness equivalent to that of the young. The effects of exercise training are definitely therapeutic and cathartic, and important health benefits can result, such as decreased percentage of body fat, lowered blood pressure, relief from arthritis, and a better ability to achieve neuromuscular relaxation. When older people exercise, they not only regain some of their physiological capacity, they also feel better.

SOCIOLOGICAL ASPECT (FOR AGING)

The discussion on physiological and psychological aspects of aging are closely related to the sociological aspect of aging. Personal loss of physical vigor and appearance, and greater susceptibility to diseases, undermine the self-esteem of the older person. Psychological feelings like insecurity and self-worth are further compounded by a series of sociocultural events, as when the individual reaches forced retirement, and loses a spouse, friends, income, or residence. These events collectively compound the psychological stresses of the elderly. These life style change events often tend to isolate the older person from his former professional associates, from his friends, and from his community. Physical debility makes one more dependent on public buses, relatives, and friends for transportation. When the elderly become both environmentally isolated and personally immobilized, their social roles change. Thus, after age 65, many individuals undergo a transformation of self-identity. They must reluctantly give up their life's work and in its place are expected to substitute less important social activities, including card playing, bingo, and other games that contribute little in the way of a positive self-image. Although acquisition of a new role and adjustment to other elderly persons and to society in general is to be expected, it is often not too rewarding, satisfying, or acceptable to the older person. It is something to put up with! Such social conditions can generate feelings of being dispensable, unneeded, incompetent, and result in a general loss of self-esteem. Retirement further isolates them from direct personal day-to-day contact with their professional or vocational friends and community activities (see Figure 18.6). More important, it isolates them more and more from the real social world—from children, adolescents, young adults, and middle-aged adults. They tend to substitute television for society. They end up living in a sterile social arena. Cutoff from the essential and meaningful social contacts of the past, the elderly have limited opportunities for getting psychologically and spiritually recharged from social involvements.

Life and work itself take on meaning when one accomplishes and functions, and these efforts are appreciated and recognized by society. With retirement, such social rewards can quickly disappear. Verbal compliments, pay raises, and other recognition become fewer and fewer for older persons. There are contrasting patterns of how various segments of American society deal with this. For example, some Mexican-Americans are likely to attach a stigma to old age, while some blacks

tend to respond with a feeling of pride at having survived to such an age (28:72). Consequently, the elderly may feel less motivation to continue to live. Retirement, once perceived as a utopia and a reward for having worked hard all your life, has now become slow suicide in North America. Many people who live a long time have continued involvements with their families, friends, and society in general. Although they may be forced to retire from work, they remain active as people and do not retire from living itself.

PSYCHOLOGICAL ASPECTS (OF AGING)

Older people are just as capable of learning and memorizing as the young (28:8). A person's intelligence changes very little over the years. As long as older people are reasonably healthy, intellectual abilities and skills do not decline (28:120). Instead, such abilities and skills usually become obsolete. The real problem of older people is that they are frequently functioning at a level they attained in their younger days, but which is no longer appropriate for successful performance in contemporary society. Older persons need compensatory education to update old learnings (see Figure 18.9).

Depression appears to be one of the major psychological problems of the aged. At both the biochemical and social levels, the elderly may be predisposed to depression (27:180). The social environmental effects of significant life losses—loved ones, income, employment—

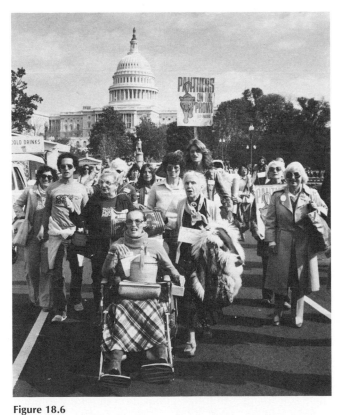

Figure 18.6
Senior citizens can do useful community work. The Grey Panthers is an activist group that has a lot of support from young persons.

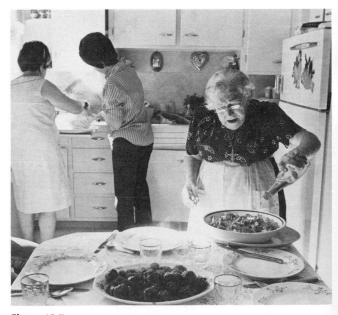

Figure 18.7
An elderly woman helping to prepare a meal. Being involved in useful work is an essential human need, especially for older persons.

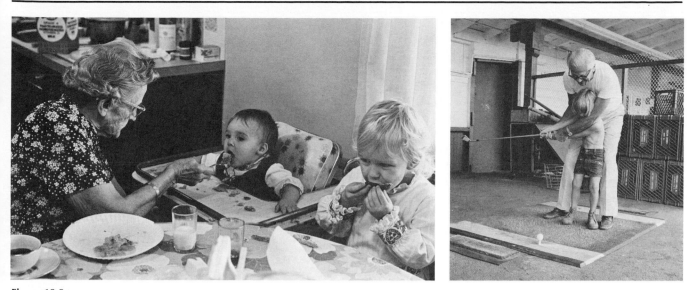

Figure 18.8
Grandparents are a vital educational link in molding the health habits and values of children.

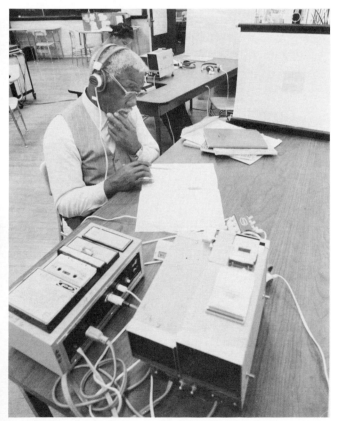

Figure 18.9
A senior citizen learning new job skills.

cause older individuals to feel depressed. Losses in physical capacity and energy level also undoubtedly play a role.

Older people are much more perceptive and realistic about their own ability to function, and their station in life, than are the young (28:197). Senior citizens experience many life changes that tend to occur in close frequency after age 60. For example, retirement may lead to loss of role, status, self-esteem, and income; isolation through disability; loss of friends and spouse; loss of physical vigor; and so on. Collectively, these create psychological stress that often becomes overwhelming.

Thus physical and psychological impairments may cause older people to be restless, irritable, and even hostile. They often experience changes in sleep patterns, in which the frequency and duration of wakeful periods are greatly increased.

Physical survival by itself has little value. One also needs a meaningful, spiritual, and satisfying psychological life.

CONCLUSION

Everyone will get old—only some of us age quicker than others. Aging is a natural process of life and we must face this realistic fact. Aging should be a rewarding time of life when one can appreciate the many accomplishments and happenings of the past. One needs to accept and act out the role of a senior citizen and enjoy doing so.

Aging results in a constant loss of cells. Numerous theories have been proposed to explain the cause of aging. You do not have to wait for the cause(s) to be verified in order to slow down or postpone the aging process. You can control stressful factors that drive cells to divide too early or form cross-linkages.

You should not rely on heredity for long life. It is not your sole assurance for longevity, since getting old is the result of the interplay of biological, social, psychological, and behavioral forces. Imagine that you had grandparents who lived to their eighties. Nevertheless, your personal life style might lead you to be 30 percent overweight, to smoke, and to drink alcohol heavily. These ecological factors could eliminate the genetic advantage of having long-lived grandparents.

As a young person, you can do many things to slow down and postpone the aging process. Aging is no more than the changing of body structure and function over a period of time. Perhaps the major factors that you can definitely and immediately control in this process are physical activity, obesity and overweight, overeating, poor nutrition, mental attitude, cigarette smoking, drugs, the establishment of close ties with your family and community, and the ability to cope with the stresses of living. Physical deterioration is speeded up by the interplay of these conditions at all ages, but the earlier in life that they occur, the more serious their consequences, because aging progresses on a logarithmic progression (12). For example, Kugler in his book, Slowing Down the Aging Process (7:91–92), has projected the years lost to various stressful causes. These are summarized in Figure 18.10 and Table 18.1. The total number of years lost for all causes ranges from 42 to 68 years.

If we add the loss of years due to all causes (42 to 68) to the present average life expectancy (71 years), we come up with the maximum possible life span of 113–139 years for humans who lead an orthobiotic life style (71 years + 42 years lost = 113; 71 years + 68 years lost = 139). Although these are rough estimates, they do give you an idea of how long you could live, if you lived a clean, health-oriented life style. On the other hand, Bjorksten (7:79) has shown that prevention of only 10 percent of all causes of aging could lead to an average life span of about 170 years.

The basic rules of good health and good living are the skills needed for long life. You should develop longevity skills early in life, for this is your only insurance for living

Table 18.1

Loss of Years due to All Causes

Cause (lifetime effects)	Decrease in Life Span (years)
Smoking	8.3
Air pollution	5–8
Malnutrition	6–10
Stress (psychological and physiological)	5–9
Alcohol	6–10
Inactivity	6–9
All other causes	10–15
Total of all causes	42–68

Source: Projections adapted from Hans J. Kugler, *Slowing Down the Aging Process,* New York: Pyramid Book, 1976, pp. 91–92.

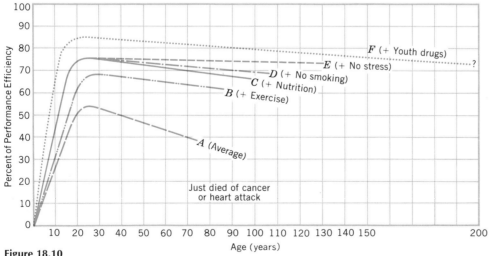

Figure 18.10

Possible extension of life through orthoboisis. Curve *A* typifies an average person who does not know or practice good nutrition, does not have a well-planned and continuous exercise program, smokes more than 20 cigarettes per day, lives in an air-polluted community, does not get enough, rest, has psychological stress, and does not take any drug compounds to slow down the aging process. This person lives to about 72 years of age. The curve *B* person exercises and can extend life to 85 years. The curve *C* person exercises, has good nutrition and can live to 95. The curve *D* person does everything the curve *C* person does and does not smoke, and extends life to 105. The curve *E* person does what the curve *D* person does, but has very little stress, lives in a nonpolluted community, and extends life to 120 years. The curve *F* person extends life by also taking youth extension drugs.

a long time (see Figure 18.5). Most of your life is still in the future, and you can expect to get the most out of life when your life style keeps you young physically, emotionally, socially, and spiritually throughout your life.

Although functional decline and reaching the retirement age accelerates functional decline, most elderly people have learned to age with grace and dignity. What is significant is not that aging does take place, but that the majority of older persons accommodate well to these changes. Approximately 86 percent of the 22 million people over 65 remain in their communities and demonstrate more than adequate coping behavior in meeting the challenge of everyday living (27). Many social contributions to art, music, literature, and science are made by people in their 70s and 80s (see Figure 18.11). It is not socioeconomical to retire people from work or soci-

ety; a good society needs the gifts of all of its senior citizens and should not "lead them out to pasture."

Chronological age is a poor index for physiological age. Many young people have physiologically old bodies. Thus one needs to add both life to years, as well as years to life. To extend life without maintaining vigor is to invite trouble.

WAYS TO MAINTAIN YOUTH AND POSTPONE AGING

The following rules of good health and good living will help you to fulfill your basic human needs.

1. Participate in vigorous physical activities four or more times a week. Walk if you cannot run!

(a)

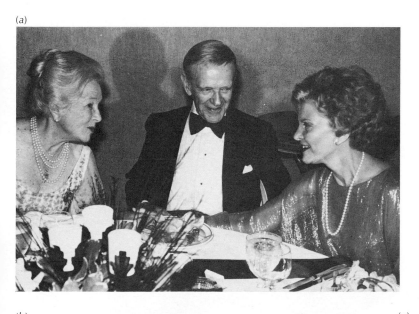

Figure 18.11

(a) Fred Astaire, America's most celebrated star, has channelled his dancing talent into movie and television acting. He has kept busy working while reaching his 80th birthday in 1979. Astaire was honored by former first lady Betty Ford (right) and moviestar Helen Hayes (left) at a dinner on October 7, 1978. (b) Senior citizen George Burns and Art Carney in a gambling scene from the movie *Going in Style*. (c) Doing meaningful work throughout life helps one to live past age 65. Married for 64 years, historians Will and Ariel Durant, now in their nineties, have spent a lifetime studying and writing about people and events of more than 2000 years. Both co-authored 11 volumes of the *Story of Civilization,* since their retirement.

(b)

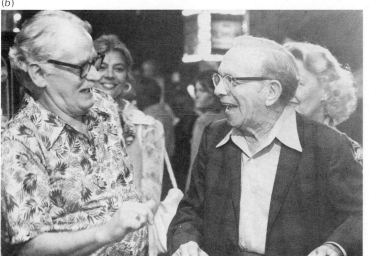

(c)

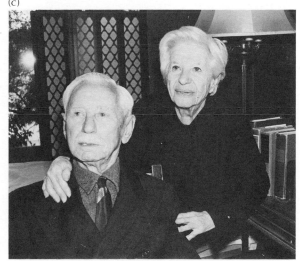

2. Eat a well-balanced nutrient diet. This also implies that you periodically (every 3 or 6 months) assess your diet for nutrient balance and good eating habits.

3. Refrain from overeating excess calories.

4. Stay slim and thin and maintain low body fat.

5. Refrain from ingesting too much salt, animal meats and fat, refined white sugar, and refined white flour products.

6. Eat a high-fiber diet.

7. Develop varied vocational, recreational, and other life skills to be able to accomplish many things in your lifetime, so that you can receive social recognition and feel a sense of satisfaction, fulfillment, and personal worth. It is important to do useful and worthwhile things throughout your lifetime.

8. Have a purpose(s) in life. Goals give us direction and purpose.

9. Evolve a desire to live a long time.

10. Have an optimistic outlook on life.

11. Learn to cope with the stresses of living.

12. Cultivate a close, active family.

13. Stay married and enjoy prolonged sexual activity.

14. Cultivate many, dear friends and socialize with them each day.

15. Continue to be involved in the community and thereby receive social recognition and social status.

16. Minimize emotional, physical, social, and environmental stresses.

17. Do not retire from a job, marriage, friends, or the community. Continue to be actively interacting in all of these dimensions of life. Never retire from hobbies, physical activity, friends, recreation, and your community.

18. Have periodic medical-physical checkups and periodically assess your personal well-being.

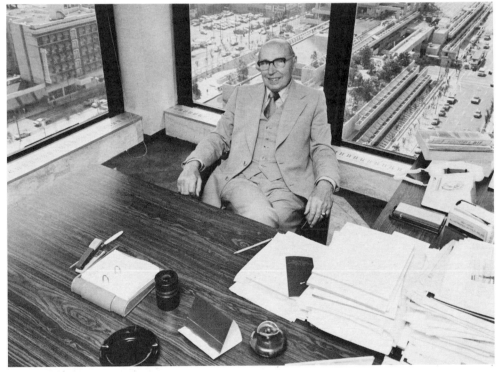

Figure 18.12
Dr. Gordon Shrum of Vancouver, British Columbia, Canada, at age 82, is a good example of how a successful and meaningful life style enables one to stay healthy, youthful, and productive, throughout one's lifetime. Since forced retirement at age 65, as a physicist and outstanding university administrator, he has done more in his 17 years of retirement than the vast majority of people do in their entire lifetime. Among his many accomplishments since retirement are the following: (1) head of the energy board for the province of British Columbia, (2) director of construction of the massive Peace River power project, (3) director of the building of Simon Fraser University in an amazing 18 months; and (4) director of building the Centennial Museum-Planetarium in Vancouver, Canada. To quote Dr. Shrum, "Life is made of experiences and the more experiences you have, the more you live."

BEHAVIOR MODIFICATION TECHNIQUES

Refer to the previous chapters for ways to modify or change life-destructive habits.

Where To Go For More Information

1. Refer to your local telephone book for:
   (a) Gray Panthers
   (b) American Association of Retired Persons (AARP)
   (c) National Retired Teachers Association (NRTA)
   (d) National Council of Senior Citizens (NCSC)
   (e) Seniors in Action

Further Readings

Bylinsky, Gene, "Science Is on the Trail of the Fountain of Youth," *Fortune*, July 1976.

Leaf, Alexander, "Everyday Is a Gift when You Are Over 100." *National Geographic*, January 1973, pp. 93–118.

Prehoda, Robert W., "Our Children May Live to Be 200 Years Old," *The Futurist*, February 1969.

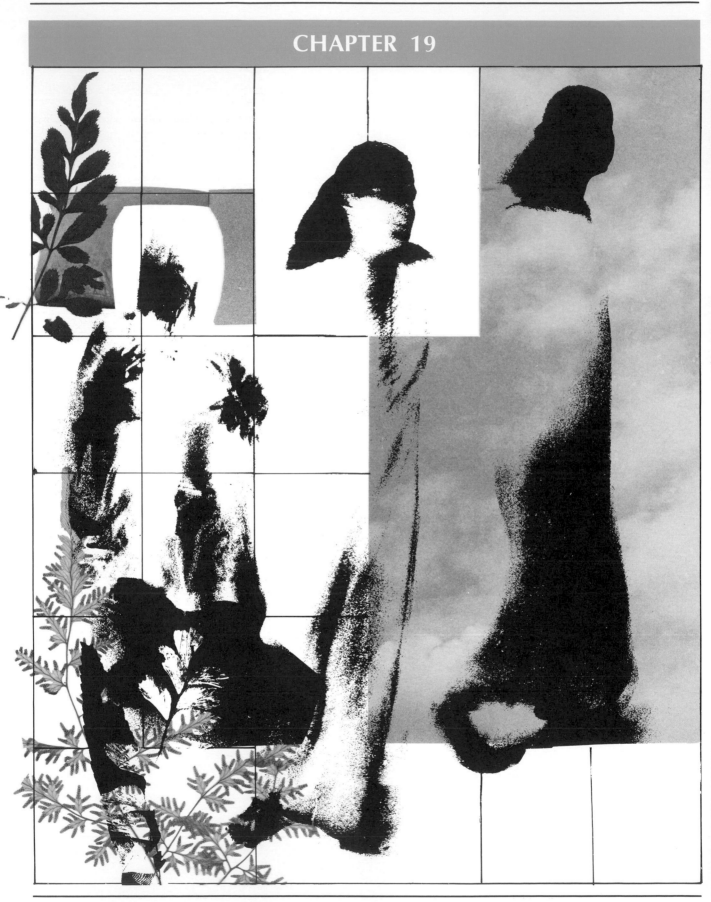

One of the most stressful situations of life is the death of a family member or a close friend. Death is stressful because it often happens when we least expect it, when we are unprepared for it, and/or because we do not usually see people dying in real life. Since most people die in a hospital, death has become secretive, removed from the reality of life, impersonal, and mechanical.

Everyone must face the possibility of death, for it is inevitable. What is death? How is it different from dying? How should one die? How can the process of dying be made easier for the terminally ill and the family and close relatives? Should the plug be pulled for a person who is terminally and chronically ill? Is there a best place to die? How can the dying person make dying a growth experience? What should you say to a dying person? These and other questions will be answered in this chapter.

Respond to the Death-Dying Questionnaire that follows. It will help to make you become more aware of the process of dying and death itself. The questions also will help you to explore the values of life and the process of dying.

☞ DEATH-DYING QUESTIONNAIRE[1]

DIRECTIONS   Select an answer that is most appropriate to you. There are no right/ wrong answers.

1. How often do you think about your own death?
   (a) Very frequently (at least once a week)
   (b) Frequently (once a month)
   (c) Occasionally
   (d) Rarely (no more than once a year)
   (e) Very rarely or never
2. What does death mean to you?
   (a) The end: the final process of life
   (b) The beginning of a life after death, a transition, a new beginning
   (c) A joining of the spirit with a universal cosmic consciousness
   (d) A kind of endless sleep; rest and peace
   (e) Termination of this life but with survival of the spirit
   (f) Do not know
   (g) Other
3. What is your present orientation to your own death?
   (a) Death-seeker
   (b) Death-hastener
   (c) Death-accepter
   (d) Death-welcomer
   (e) Death-postponer
   (f) Death-fearer

4. To what extent are you interested in having your image survive after your own death through your children, books, good works, etc.?
   (a) Very interested
   (b) Moderately interested
   (c) Somewhat interested
   (d) Not very interested
   (e) Totally disinterested

5. If you had a choice, what kind of death would you prefer?
   (a) Tragic, violent death
   (b) Sudden but not violent death
   (c) Quiet, dignified death
   (d) Death in line of duty
   (e) Death after a great achievement
   (f) Suicide
   (g) Homicidal victim
   (h) There is no appropriate death
   (i) Other

6. If you were told that you had a terminal disease and had a limited time to live, how would you want to spend your time until you died?
   (a) I would make a marked change in my life style, satisfying hedonistic needs (travel, sex, drugs, and other experiences)
   (b) I would become more withdrawn: reading, contemplating, or praying
   (c) I would shift from my own needs to a concern for others (family and friends)
   (d) I would attempt to complete projects, tie up loose ends
   (e) I would make little or no change in my life style
   (f) I would try to do one very important thing
   (g) I might consider committing suicide
   (h) I would do none of these things

7. What efforts do you believe ought to be made to keep a seriously ill person alive?
   (a) All possible effort: transplantations, kidney dialysis, medication, etc.
   (b) Efforts that are reasonable for that person's age, physical and mental condition, and amount of pain
   (c) After reasonable care has been given, a person ought to be permitted to die a natural death
   (d) A senile person should not be kept alive by elaborate means

8. If it were entirely up to you, how would you like to have your body disposed of after you have died?
   (a) Burial
   (b) Cremation
   (c) Donation to medical school or science
   (d) I am indifferent

9. How important do you believe mourning and grief rituals (such as wakes and funerals) are for the survivors?
   (a) Extremely important
   (b) Somewhat important
   (c) Undecided or do not know
   (d) Not very important
   (e) Not important at all

---

[1] Adapted with permission from ———, "You and Death," *Psychology Today*, August 1970, pp. 66–72.

DYING AND DEATH

Death is the opposite of optimal well-being. This was illustrated and discussed in the first chapter of this book (see Table 19.1). Death is the end of the life cycle itself. However, the prelude to death itself is dying. That is, most persons die gradually over an extended period of time. The previous chapter on getting older alluded to the aging process and to the fact that we tend to die a little each day. Without being aware of it, most persons die gradually, then the process is accelerated over a period of from several days to several years, until one day the vital life-support organs, such as the heart, lungs, liver and/or kidneys, give out and the body dies in a few days or hours.

Most persons understand the more obvious signs of dying as characterized by prolonged illness and/or terminal disease. This can occur at any age, as with a teenager who suffers from leukemia, or a man who, at 40, suffers from rheumatic heart disease. The dying person gradually loses physical mobility, is unable to perform or function socially, and becomes more and more dependent on others for personal health care. This phase may last from a few days to several years. There is a gradual loss of body system/organ efficiency. How quickly we die is determined by our lifetime orthobiosis — it is accelerated by deleterious and self-destructive life styles of our youth and middle age.

Many young persons die needlessly and prematurely from accidents and suicides, thereby not experiencing the gradual physiological dying process. As Kubler-Ross points out in her book *Death: The Final Stage of Growth*, such persons rob themselves of a peak developmental experience in life — dying.

DEATH DENIAL

Americans do not accept the death and dying phases of life realistically. One reason for this is that our society hides death in many ways. In spite of the fact that death occurs all the time, we seldom, if ever, see dying or dead persons. Most persons die in a hospital, where they are magically whisked away before anyone gets upset. Dead persons are dressed up to appear lifelike and placed in velvet-lined caskets. Many young people go through life

Table 19.1

Relationship of Phases of Death to Levels of Wellness in the Continuum of Life

Phase	Wellness Characteristics	Levels of Wellness
Youth retained	Perform at highest or best levels in social endeavors, no debility or illnesses, peak vitality, and vim and vigor	Optimal well-being
Normal aging	Loss of some physiological functions (body immunity drops; decreased digestive enzymes; loss of hearing, sight, etc.) emotional, social, and spiritual deterioration	Average wellness
Aging accelerated	Some illness on occasion, some disability on occasion, malnutrition, often eat lots of junk foods, do not exercise regularly, may smoke or drink, live in air-polluted community, poor emotional or spiritual being, inability to function optimally, vegetate in everyday life, and lack purpose in life	Minor illness
Dying	Prolonged illness, terminal disease, immobility, nonfunctioning in society, depend on care by others	Major illness
Death	Vital organs (heart, lungs) stop functioning, spiritual death, brain death, no EKG for 24 hours	Death

without attending a funeral. Children are also sheltered from death and the dying, thereby being deprived of the death experience. Such sheltering creates a sense of fear and nonacceptance of death.

In addition to hiding death, our culture unconsciously rejects and denies death in everyday life. For example, women deny the aging process when they fight to retain a girlish figure, when they use cosmetics to look young and attractive, and when they have face-lift surgery to hide wrinkles. Experiencing partial failure in tasks, jobs, and marriage symbolizes the inability to "hack it" in a success-oriented society. Likewise, when one puts on body weight or gets obese and shows wrinkles with age, he or she is dubbed as getting old and close to the time of dying. Such attitudes deny that death is inevitable and make it very difficult for most Americans to cope with the death of a loved one or a dear friend, much less their own death.

STAGES OF DYING

Dying is a process of change in the life of the person. Although one cannot choose the age or time for dying, most people sense when they are about to die. Such psychological reactions to impending death have been researched by Elizabeth Kubler-Ross (2) in interviews with hundreds of terminally ill patients. She has classified such reactions into five stages of death (2:10).

Stage one: *Denial and Isolation:* "No, not me! It can't be!" The dying person is in a temporary state of shock in which he denies the fact and isolates himself from further confrontation with it. By denying the possibility or reality of dying, the denial acts as a buffer against shock and gives the person time to get himself together emotionally and mobilize other defenses.

Stage two: *Anger:* "Why me?" This is what people think when they realize the truth. The dying person is angry that it is he and not someone else. He vents his anger at doctors, nurses, family, and even God. Such projected anger makes it increasingly difficult for the hospital staff to care for the person, even though the expressed anger is not really aimed at them.

Stage three: *Bargaining:* "Yes me . . . but, please God, may I have one more chance to live again! I promise to be good (or do something)!" The dying person bargains with God as a means of marshalling hope for recovery and as a way of postponing death. The dying person accepts the fact of death but strikes bargains for more time.

Stage four: *Depression:* "Yes me!" The dying person mourns past losses, things not done, and wrongs comitted. The person is bothered by the loss of personal strength and looks. He is also bothered by losing possessions, friends, and loved ones. One enters a "preparatory grief" period as a way of getting ready for the arrival of death. The dying person grows quiet and refuses to see visitors. Refusal to see visitors is a sign that the dying person has finished his unfinished business with you. He can now go peacefully.

Stage five: *Acceptance:* "My time is very close now, and it's all right." A dying person progressing through the earlier stages will accept death. He or she slowly drifts away from all but one or two people. He or she will feel tired and weak, want to be left alone, and doze off often. The hours of sleep becomes longer and longer. It is a time without feelings, pain, or discomfort. The family must "let go." The person is at the end of a struggle. Death is close at hand.

These stages provide a useful guide to understanding the different phases that dying persons may go through. These stages are not absolute, that is, not everyone goes through each stage in a predictable manner. Dying persons sometimes go back and forth from one stage to another.

WHEN IS A PERSON DEAD?

A person is dead when the vital organs of life stop functioning. This basically means:

1. *Functional death*—the absence of heartbeat and spontaneous breathing. Most persons are pronounced as medically dead when the heart stops beating.
2. *Brain death*—there are no electroencephalographic (EEG) reactions to detect electrical impulse activity in the brain. No one has survived without an EKG reaction for 24 hours.
3. *Cellular death*—somatic cells may continue to live for some time after the heart and brain stop functioning. Cellular death results in rigor mortis (stiffening of the body's muscles).
4. *Spiritual death*—loss of meaningful awareness of others and self, although the heart and lungs function. A person may be spiritually dead while life-support systems of a hospital keep him in a vegetative state.

EUTHANASIA

Thousands of people who were at one time very ill or disabled are alive and well enough to function in our society. Many would have died had not medical technology provided them with a heart pacemaker, an artificial limb, or a surgical operation to restore their eyesight and hearing. These are positive advances in reclaiming people and helping them maintain meaningful lives.

Doctors and hospitals do not always help people to lead useful lives. Several years ago the story of 21-year-old Karen-Anne Quinlan was in the newspaper headlines. While in a state of coma, she was kept alive by a breathing machine. When there was no improvement in her condition after many months, her parents requested that the "plug be pulled," allowing Karen-Anne to die. This raised several medicolegal questions: Should a person be kept alive by a machine if there is no hope of recovery? Are such mercy killings legal and ethically proper? Does a physician have the right to "play God" with a patient's life? Although the answers to these questions are not satisfactorily answered or resolved as yet, these questions do help us to think about how one might or should die.

Pulling the plug is referred to as a mercy killing, or "passive" euthanasia (eu = good, and thanotos = death). It is the painless allowing of death that many people feel should be available to the terminally and chronically ill. The terminally ill person may not be emotionally and spiritually ready to die, nor willing to die, but others decide when he or she will die. This approach to death may be considered when there is no hope for the terminally ill patient, all medical lifesaving and restorative efforts have been exhausted, the patient is in a coma for at least 24 hours, the patient must have continuous life-support and extending machines, and/or the cost of keeping the terminally ill person is so financially overwhelming that neither the immediate family, friends, medical doctors, and hospitals can endure the financial burden (10;12). There is very little rationale for prolonging or deferring the physiological act of dying.

PHYSICIANS AND THE DYING PERSON

Unfortunately, doctors and other medical professionals are not trained to help people die with dignity or to allow dying persons to accept sickness and death as part of the human experience of living. Since ours is an achievement-oriented society where success and winning are accentuated, doctors do not consider losing patients as indicators of medical success regardless of how they die. Death to many physicians is the ultimate defeat, a sign of failure. Consequently, many physicians are ill at ease with dying and death.

Most physicians would rather not deal with terminally ill patients, much less help them to die with dignity (12:46). Thus the terminal patient may desperately want rest, peace, and dignity; yet he may receive only infusions, transfusions, a heart machine, a kidney dialysis machine, and a team of experts all struggling to prolong the life of a patient by monitoring his heart rate, his pulmonary functions and his secretions, but not dealing with him as a feeling and still living person.

STAGES OF GRIEF

Relatives and close friends grieve for those dying and those who are dead. Grief is the emotional (psychological) pain or suffering accompanying death or separation of a loved one. Mourning is the expression of grief. Mourning expresses and releases one's emotions. People mourn by talking, crying, writing poetry, painting, walking alone, preparing a meal, and other ways, in addition to taking part in a ritualistic funeral. Mourning is like a cleansing of the whole body. On the other hand, unresolved grief that is full of pent-up emotions about death can become emotionally debilitating. It can stiffle one's ability to perform or to function effectively.

A person losing a loved one through death or separation usually goes through three states of grief (13):

Stage one: *Shock* —disbelief, numbness, loneliness, weeping, and agitation. It occurs before and after death, and usually lasts from 1 to 3 days.

Stage two: *Painful* —longing for the dead: sadness, despair, insomnia, irritability, restlessness. This stage peaks between the second and fourth weeks and usually subsides after 3 months.

Stage three: *Postvention* —acceptance and adjustment to live without the significant other person within a year after death.

The ultimate goal of grief or mourning is to be able to remember without emotional pain and to be able to reinvest emotional surpluses. In death and grief, we do not need as much protection from painful experiences as we need the boldness to face them. We do not need as much tranquilization from pain as we need the strength to conquer it.

Mourning cannot be hurried. One has to work things out and eventually an emotional balance returns to the grieving person. Appropriate mourning will allow one to form new relationships eventually. There are many ways to facilitate grieving. The most culturally accepted way is through mourning at rituals and funerals.

WAYS TO GRIEVE AND GROW

One has to accept change—that a loved one has died and is gone. More important, one has to carry on with life after the death of a loved one. A funeral is designed to facilitate such changes.

Kubler-Ross suggests that participation of the grieving

persons in a funeral can help to accomplish the following (2:87–96):

1. Facilitates grief work. Grief work begins with the acceptance of death. Acceptance of death must be intellectual and emotional.
2. Saying the last goodbyes to dead person.
3. Making death real through actively participating in the preparation of a funeral.
4. Beginning to live again by making a commitment to continue living.
5. Growing through this experience.
6. Becoming a more complete and beautiful person. Such complete persons have an appreciation, a sensitivity, and an understanding of life that fills them with compassion, gentleness, and a deep loving concern. They know defeat, suffering, struggle, loss, and have learned to cope with these realities of life. They become realistic about life but can at the same time temper it with ideals.
7. Accepting own personal death.

A funeral can be a catharsis for those in grief. A mourning person should participate in the planning of a funeral, in the rituals of a funeral, and in the burial or cremation of the dead person. Doing so shortens the grief period, works out the pain and sorrow, and makes it easier to come to grips with death and change. Those working through a funeral unload tremendous surges of emotion. Shock, denial, and the hostility of death are left behind. But this happens most often when the grieving person is allowed to be actively involved in the planning of the funeral. Having a funeral director do most of the funeral planning takes away the catharsis advantages from the mourning.

Funerals provide for mourning to be shared by friends, relatives, and the entire community. Most acquaintances of the dead person want to be involved in the funeral. Sharing one's grief with others in the community is psychoemotionally necessary for the mourning persons. It is more comforting and helpful to share your sorrow and hurt with others than by yourself. Friends become a source of comfort. More important, the friends and com-

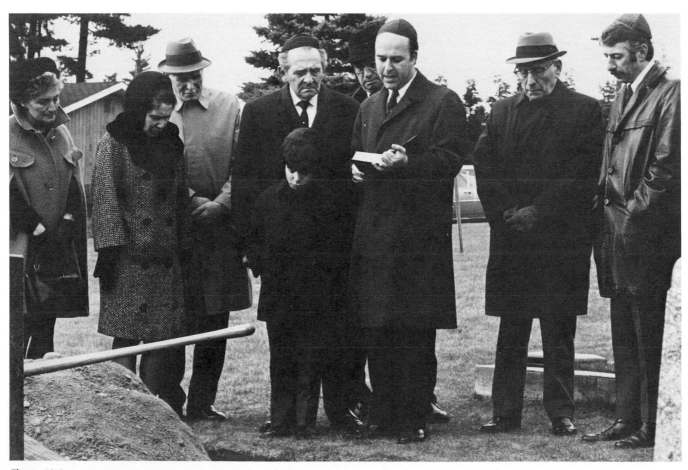

Figure 19.1
Attending a funeral can be a way to give and to grow as a person.

munity provide an emotional-social acceptance of a commitment to carry on with life after the funeral.

Mourning does not stop at the end of a funeral. Mourners closest to the dead person will continue to mourn for many months after the funeral.

WAYS TO MOURN

Mourning helps ease the pain of loss of a loved one. It allows the fullest possible outpouring of grief. Mourning at a funeral provides the opportunity for the family, friends, and community to reknit after the loss of one of their members, so that they may continue to be able to love and to work (2:3).

Ways to mourn include the following:

1. Become involved in making funeral plans.
2. Allow children and the entire community to share grief.
3. Eulogize the dead person—make the mourner aware of what he has lost.
4. Bury the dead by actually doing some of the shoveling.
5. Have a lunch or meal for all those returning from a funeral. A meal is a visible sign of communal solidarity reassuring the mourner that he is not

alone and that others are ready to help him. A meal also restates the theme of life for the mourner—that life must go on.

WHERE TO DIE

Eighty percent of all deaths now take place in hospitals (10:97). Others take place in nursing homes and at home. Hospitals are probably the worst place for people to die (12:97). Hospitals create a dishonest and artificial climate for death. Too many people die in the isolation of a hospital room, under medication and sedation, and often with a battery of life-support systems. Such medical care does little to offer human warmth, the emotional comfort of social contact, and the opportunity for the dying to be understood and loved (10:37). Hospitals strip away all that is personally meaningful to the dying person. The dying person gets very little reassurance to continue living. Instead, dying in the familiar surroundings of one's home, with those you love and who love you, can take away much of the fear and discomfort of death.

An alternative to dying in the home or in the hospital is a hospice (11). It is a home for dying patients where no heroic life-saving techniques are used, and the only medications given are those to relieve pain. A happy, honest and pleasant social atmosphere prevails. Family and friends can visit the dying person as often as they wish. Many communities have initiated hospices or are about to do so.

PROCESS OF DYING

We die a little each day in numerous ways. Most people die because of a lack of will to live and not from a chronic disease. Before losing the will to live, a person loses friends or withdraws from friends and from actively participating in the community—hence, social death. Social death is accompanied by emotional death and intellectual death. Intellectual death occurs when people stop learning, stop taking risks in discovering new alternative life styles, and stop creating. People die a little when they vegetate or are low performers in everyday life. People die spiritually when they do not have a purpose in life and when life has no meaning. The ability to function completely—physically, emotionally, socially, spiritually, gradually diminishes until the person needs to be cared for instead of caring for self. This debilitated state of staying alive is often a preliminary to death. Such slow dying in one or all of these ways can occur early in one's life and gradually gets worse. The somatic cells lose the vigor and vitality to perform optimally. The im-

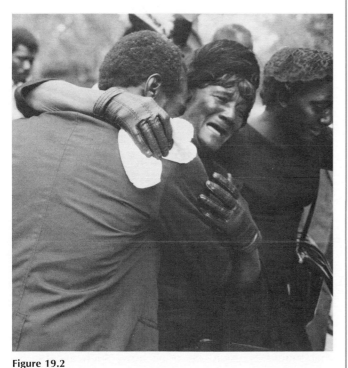

Figure 19.2

Mourning, as by crying at a funeral, is an expression of grief and helps to ease the pain or loss of a loved one.

mune system loses its ability to physiologically fight infections and disease. There is a gradual loss of quality of life.

WAYS TO PREPARE FOR DYING

You can do many things throughout your life to prepare yourself to accept dying and death. One of the most important is to live a useful and meaningful life. Persons who do live useful and meaningful lives acquire goals and purposes through love and marriage, work or profession, hobbies and recreation, and community involvements. It is the attainment of their goals that gives them a sense of satisfaction and fulfillment. A rich and meaningful life also provides experiences that force one to replace old ways of living with new ways. Not only does one feel fulfilled in later life, but one develops the courage to face the unknown and unfamiliar, including dying and death. Setting goals and having a purpose in life in the prime of health contributes to a fuller acceptance and understanding of death (2:73).

One can add richness and meaning to life by cultivating friends of all ages and cultivating lasting relationships with relatives. Visit your parents, grandparents, uncles, and aunts. Spend time with them. They have been where you are going and have experienced what you are going to experience. They can share with you their wisdom of life only if you socialize with them. Enjoying their companionship is also part of the reality of life, for by interacting with friends and relatives of all ages, one is able to gain a more wholistic insight into life and death. Socializing with relatives cements the bonds of life that allow us to develop an appreciation of the true meaning of life and death.

Perhaps the most important preparation for dying is not to deny dying and death experiences. As a young adult, you should visit the terminally ill in hospitals or at their homes and attend religious funerals of dead friends, neighbors, and relatives. Observe dying pets, wild animals, birds, and insects. Experiencing broken bones, minor surgery, and near-fatal accidents should make you feel lucky to be alive. Collectively, such life-time experiences should remind us that our time is very limited, that life is very precious, and that we had better make the most of the one life we now have.

Another way to prepare yourself for dying is to share the dying period of someone who understands the meaning of death. Talking to the dying person gives that person a chance to appraise their readiness to die and at the same time share their philosophy of life and death with you. It will give you a chance to develop greater insight into life and death. Individuals who have been fortunate to share in the death of someone who under-

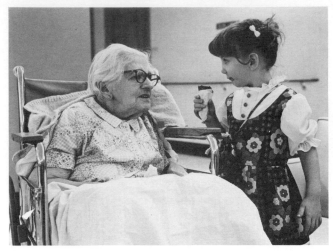

Figure 19.3
A granddaughter visiting with her ailing grandmother. Does the girl relate sickness to dying and death? How will such an experience prepare a young child to face future death?

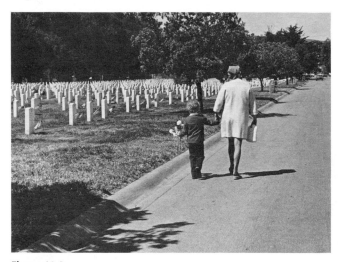

Figure 19.3
A mother and son visit a cemetery to commemorate the death of a loved one.

stands its meaning seem better able to live and grow because of this sharing experience. They have more empathy, compassion, and are more humane than others without a death experience.

Other ways of preparing for dying and death are summarized in Table 19.2

According to Kubler-Ross, those denying death or not facing up to it tend to live empty, self-destructive and purposeless lives. They live as if they will live forever, making it easy for them to postpone doing those things that should or could be done now. Such an attitude results in living one's life in preparation for tomorrow, or in remembrance of yesterday—meanwhile, each day is

Table 19.2

List of Experiences to Help Cushion Future Dying and Death

1. Attend funerals.
2. Visit a mortuary and find out what a mortician does to a corpse.
3. Read a book on death and dying.
4. Visit a nursing home for the aged. Make a friend in the nursing home and do something for him or her.
5. Visit a hospice in your community.
6. Make out a dying and death will.
7. Take a course on dying and death. The highest spiritual values of life originate from the thought and study of death (2:21).
8. Cultivate deep and loving relationships with family and friends of all ages.
9. Visit a terminally sick friend or relative.
10. Decide on whether you would or should be hooked up to a life-saving extension machine, and include this decision in your dying will.
11. Plan to reassess your life now (bad and good habits, goals) and impregnate it with quality of living. Reassess your goals and the priorities for attaining these goals.
12. Evolve a plan to improve yourself as a person by developing your talents and abilities.
13. Accept dying as a highly creative force.
14. Think of death in later life as a final growth experience.
15. Learn to listen to your own body's warnings when it is hurting and not able to perform. These warnings were summarized at the end of Chapter 1.
16. Discuss death and dying frankly with others.
17. Welcome the opportunity to become close to someone who is presently facing terminal illness with inner peace and dignity.
18. Prepare a living will. Such a will is prepared when the person is in good health; whereas a dying will is prepared when a person is terminally ill.

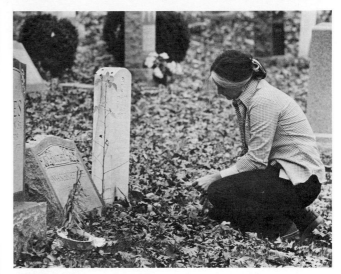

Figure 19.4

Visiting a cemetery can help a person to mourn and accept the loss of a loved one. It can also help to prepare one to face death in the future.

The most important and desirable response to dying and death at any age is to try to grow when you become a terminally ill person. This is best done by reaching out to others, as when the dying person shares his intimate feelings of joy, sorrow, anger, and hate. He reaches out when he gives and takes in social relationships, continuing to honor his social, family, and community commitments. As he struggles with the reality of death, he also struggles with growing as a person, searching and clarifying the meaning and significance as a person. Dying persons also need to maintain strong bonds with others in order to maintain their self-images, their dignity, and their sense of self-worth. Terminally ill persons have a great need to communicate their feelings to others in efforts to reassure themselves that they are valuable persons. Receiving adequate responses creates within them a readiness for death.

WAYS OF HELPING A DYING PERSON

The dying person should be perceived as having the same needs as a nondying person. Help the dying person fulfill his or her needs. Consider their needs as a normal phase of living, subject to personal growth, self-esteem, obligations, and commitments. Help them to accept the reality of death and to become psychologically ready to die.

1. Center your questions and help around:
   (a) What do you want (or need)?
   (b) Is there someplace you would like to go?

lost. Those who have not really lived are not ready to face the mask of death. They have left issues unsettled, dreams unfulfilled, hopes shattered, have let love pass them by, have not spent enough time with relatives, and so on. According to Kubler-Ross (2:xi), these are the persons whose consciences will not allow them to die peacefully. They will fear dying and death.

In contrast, when one is aware that each day may be your last, you take time to grow and to develop as a person, to reach out to human beings, to create, and to perform. Life takes on immediate direction and meaning. You find your true self-identity in a hurry. You find the strength and courage to face the possibility of change, as well as the possibility of death when it comes.

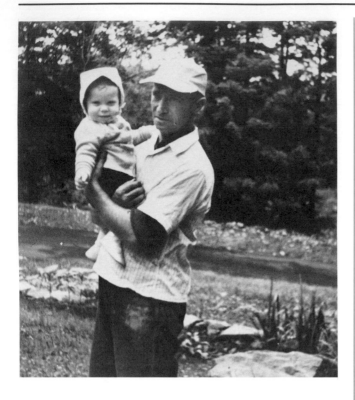

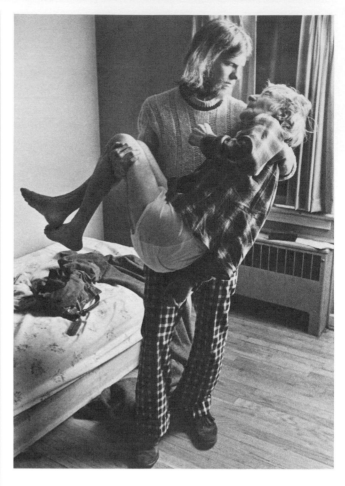

Figure 19.5
Roles in life reverse themselves. Grandfather caring for his year-old grandson and, 25 years later, the grandson caring for his dying grandpa.

(c) Would you like to give someone a gift?

(d) Would you like to visit a son, daughter, grandchild, or friend?

(e) Are there things you wish to do or accomplish?

(f) Would you like to go to church or have your clergyman visit with you for prayers and blessings?

(g) Are there any business or financial matters that need to be taken care of?

(h) Would you prefer to stay at home or with me, or in a hospice?

2. Be a pleasant and helpful companion.

3. Help the dying person live each day as joyfully and peacefully as possible.

4. Help the family of the dying person deal with dying, loss of a loved one, and with death. The dying person is often more concerned about how the family members will adjust to his death than about his death.

5. Help the dying person to decide about how he or she wants to die.

6. Listen to the dying person talk.

7. Do not:

(a) Give false hope for speedy recovery to a terminally ill person.

(b) Play games. Dying persons want to know the truth about their illness and chances for recovery.

(c) Allow doctors and nurses to cover up the truth about the dying person's condition.

(d) Say ''You'll be all right—you'll get over it!''. This often has the opposite effect.

WAYS OF HELPING SOMEONE WHO HAS LOST A LOVED ONE

1. Listen to the mourning person talk.

2. Be ready with an understanding smile.

3. Be silent instead of making idle chatter. Do not try to divert the person in mourning by talking about something else. Allow the person to grieve.

4. Show empathy by helping the person do something.

5. Cry, if you feel like it, with your friend. Tears help express grief in a healthy way—they relieve tension and guilt.

6. Communicate—don't isolate yourself from the mourning person. A person in mourning and grief needs consolation. Aloneness is best replaced by companionship.

7. Socialize with the mourning person by going out to social and cultural affairs.

8. Instill in the mourning person the hope and the will to continue to live.

9. Do not say "buckle-up" or "you'll get over it." This idle talk serves no useful purpose.

10. Reassure—do not argue.

11. Help the grieving person face the fact of death or the loss and accept a new altered life style.

A LIVING WILL

Everyone should have a will made out. A written will tells others what to do with possessions and the dead person's body after death. It can also tell the doctor, hospital, and others how and where you wish to die. You should draft such a will now and modify it later on in life. Here are a few suggestions for a living will.

Part A. Instruction For Final Care (An Example)

(This part of the will to be drafted with you and your family physician.)

I, _____, do not wish to live in a
       (Name)

vegetative state, unable to function mentally or intellectually, nor receive therapy so risky, arduous, or experimental so as to have physicians overtreat me. I accept relevant therapy as long as my physiological body organs and systems and mental and intellectual capacities allow me to eventually function in a coherent self-maintenance fashion in my own home and in society.

Furthermore, I wish to be fully informed and apprised of all circumstances regarding the nature of my illness, disorder, or debility, the nature of treatment and the probabilities for extending my life if therapy and treatment are offered.

_____
(Signature)

WITNESSED: _____

WITNESSED: _____

DATE: _____

Copies of this request to be given to:

_____

_____

_____

Part B. To Attending Physicians and Hospitals: Instructions For Final Care While Dying (An example)

(This part of the draft should be completed with your family, with your family physician, and with your lawyer.)

1. In event of unconsciousness from a homicide or an automobile accident, length of time to remain:
   (a) In hospital in coma—not longer than 2 weeks.
   (b) If at home, only one practical nurse to attend.
   (c) No tube feeding or intravenous fluids at home.

2. In event of coma, all life-support equipment to be turned off when EEG is flat and nonresponsive for 24 hours.

3. In event of stroke or cerebral accident (other than subarachnoid hemorrhage), no treatment of any kind until it is clear that you are going to be able to think effectively. No stomach tube and no intravenous fluids.

4. In event of subarachnoid hemorrhage, physician to use own judgment in the acute stage. If there is considerable brain damage, send me home with a practical nurse.

5. In event of becoming mentally incapacitated, but remaining in good physical condition, do not spend money on private care. Institutionalize in a state hospital or a hospice.

6. In event of *cancer or emphysema:*
   (a) No respiratory or heart-lung machine.
   (b) (other) _____

7. In event of heart attack:
   (a) No intravenous feeding.
   (b) No dialysis or heart machine.
   (c) *(other)* _____

8. In event of other debilitation resulting from advanced aging process or inability to function or perform life maintenance and self-care tasks: (other).

9. If additional complications happen, then all of the above are subject to be reassessed by my own mental-value capacities, providing I am so capable.

10. Perform autopsy as needed but without harassment to family and close friends.
11. Anatomical or organ gifts: organs may be removed for transplantation but only after adherence to the 24-hour EKG time limit.
12. Disposal of corpse: burial, cremation, cryogenesis, or bequeath to a medical school
13. Disbursements of possessions:
    (a) Real estate—commercial investments.
    (b) Place of residence—home.
    (c) Dissolution of partnerships.
    (d) Personal possessions.
    (e) Continuing royalties, securities, trust deeds, etc.
    (f) Cash in bank.
    (g) Establishment of a trust fund.
14. Inform the following persons of my death:
    (a) Specific funeral home, crematory, or cryogenic center.
    (b) Lawyer: to carry out this will.
    (c) Accountant: to update the bank account, stocks, bonds, possessions, etc., and to help fill out tax forms.
    (d) Insurance person or company: to help pay hospital-medical bills and other debts.
    (e) Social security office: (to help pay hospital bills if dead person is over 65).
    (f) Family and dear friends.

WHERE TO GO FOR HELP

1. Your church clergy or minister.
2. Your family members.
3. Your close friends and acquaintances.
4. Your family physician.

FOR MORE INFORMATION—WRITE OR CONTACT THE FOLLOWING:

1. Make Today Count (local community chapter)
2. (Dr. Warren T. Reich)
   Kennedy Center for Bioethics
   Georgetown University
   Washington, D.C.
3. Continental Association of Funeral & Memorial Societies
   59 E. VanBuren Street
   Chicago, Ill. 60605
4. Memorial Society Association of Canada
   207 W. Hastings
   Vancouver, B.C., Canada
5. National Hospice Organization
   765 Prospect Street
   New Haven, Conn. 06511
6. (Concern for Dying)
   Euthanasia Society (living will)
   250 W. 57th Street
   New York, N.Y. 10019
7. National Kidney Foundation (organ donorship)
   2 Park Avenue
   New York, N.Y. 10016

Further Readings

Kubler-Ross, Elizabeth, *Death: The Final Stage of Growth*, Englewood Cliffs, N.J.: Prentice-Hall, 1975.

Stoddard, Sandol, *The Hospice Movement*, New York: The Hospice Movement, 1978.

PART F

ENVIRONMENT AND HEALTH

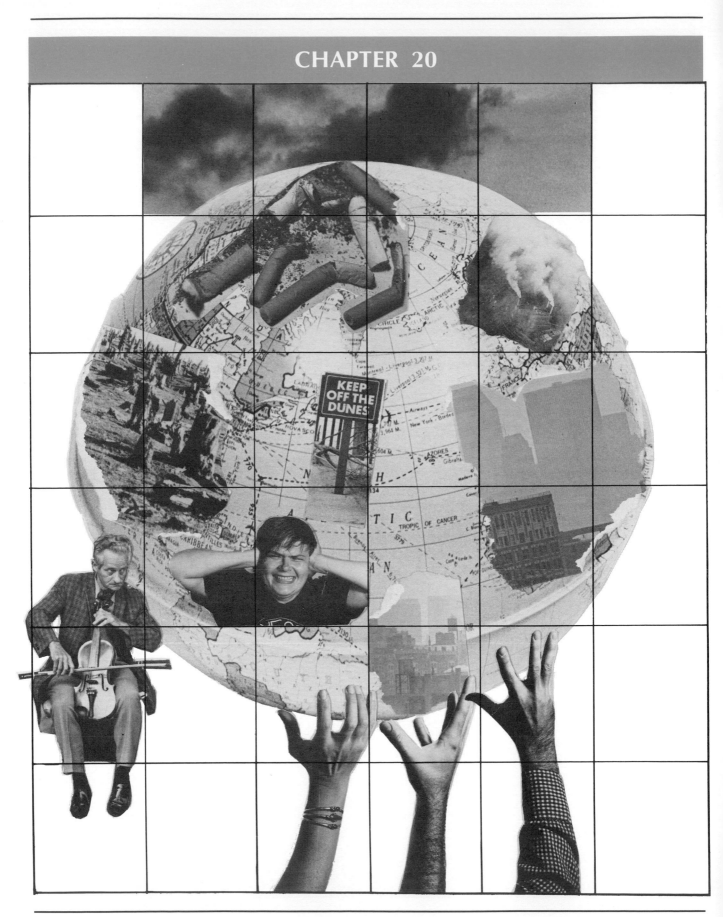

Our environment is made up of social and physical dimensions. It is made up of everything that surrounds us and with which we interact. People make up the social dimension, and this includes the working or job-people environment. Work, friends, relatives, and the comradery of fellow workers structure social well-being, (this was discussed in Chapter 4).

Our physical environment is composed of water, air, soil, food, and living and nonliving things. For thousands of years, man has used air, water, and soil as "natural sumps or sinks" to dump our wastes. Since 1940, man has accelerated the pollution of the environment, which has raised some major health issues. Is photochemical smog really dangerous to your health? Is the food we eat contaminated with chemicals? Is noise from cars and jets a chemical stressor?

Recently, the energy crisis has focused attention on nuclear power and the dangers of radiation. Is the threat of nuclear power radiation greater than that of dental and medical X rays?

This chapter takes a look at the different ways we pollute our environment and how such pollutions may affect our well-being.

Respond to the two inventories that follow.

☞ YOUR COMMUNITY—A GOOD PLACE TO LIVE INVENTORY

PURPOSE
1. To make you aware of how a community can enhance you.
2. To help you find out whether your community is a good place for *you* to live in.

DIRECTIONS
1. On the left side of the scale are statements describing opportunities or services. The columns on the right side list the frequency, availability, or accessibility of services in your community.

    React to each statement by relating it to yourself. To what degree does it help you to fulfill your health needs, help you to grow as a person, and generally make you a better person?
2. Circle *one* number for each statement that best describes its status in your community.
3. Answer all items.

Community Opportunities Contributing to Good Living	Availability of Opportunities (In Your Community)			
	Most Usually	Often	Sometimes	Almost None
A. **Psychoemotional Security** Does your community help you to:				
1. Feel mentally relaxed where you live?	5	3	1	0
2. Feel content and happy where you live?	10	7	2	0
3. Use your talents and intellect?	15	10	5	0
4. Find relief from tensions?	5	3	1	0
5. Grow as a person?	10	6	2	0
6. Be productive?	5	3	1	0
7. Become involved in improving the community?	15	10	3	0
8. Work with people of all ages?	5	3	1	0
9. Have protection against robbery?	15	10	3	0
10. Have protection against rape?	5	3	1	0
11. Have protection against fires?	5	3	1	0
12. Have protection against drug pushers?	5	3	1	0
13. Have civil defense and disaster care?	5	3	1	0
14. Have marriage counseling services?	5	3	1	0
Subtotal				

	Very Many	Many	Some	None
B. Economic Opportunities				
Does your community provide opportunities for:				
15. A variety of jobs?	5	3	1	0
16. Earning adequate income?	10	7	2	0
17. Affording to buy a home?	20	15	5	0
18. Affording to rent a place?	10	7	3	0
19. Living near supermarkets (groceries and clothes)?	15	10	5	0
20. Using a rapid transit system?	15	10	5	0
21. Attracting big business?	5	3	1	0
Subtotal				
C. Social Opportunities				
22. Meeting people of your age group	20	15	7	0
23. Mixing with people of all age groups and races	10	7	3	0
24. Going to parties and dances	5	3	1	0
25. Becoming involved in local activities and projects	5	3	1	0
26. Having many close friends	5	3	1	0
27. Joining social clubs (music, art, drama, etc.)	5	3	1	0
28. Joint interest groups (4-H Club, bookclub, vocational, etc.)	5	3	1	0
29. Joint service clubs (Lions and Kiwanis)	5	3	1	0
30. Joining professional societies (medical, teacher, cancer, heart, epilepsy, etc.)	5	3	1	0
Subtotal				

Community Opportunities Contributing to Good Living	Availability of Opportunities (In Your Community)			
	Very Many	Many	Some	None
D. Educational Opportunities				
31. Good public school buildings	5	3	1	0
32. Good qualified teachers	10	7	2	0
33. Good junior colleges	5	3	1	0
34. Night adult classes	5	3	1	0
35. Preparation for parenthood classes	5	3	1	0
36. Weight-control or dieting, and physical fitness classes	5	3	1	0
37. Stop smoking classes	5	3	1	0
38. Vocational-technical counseling and training	5	3	1	0
39. Business training schools	5	3	1	0
40. Medical health seminars or forums open to public	5	3	1	0
41. Bookstores	5	3	1	0
42. Educational TV programs	10	7	3	0
43. Legal aid services	5	3	1	0
44. Health behavior counseling	5	3	1	0
Subtotal				
E. Man-Made Environment				
Does your community have:				
45. Good roads?	5	3	1	0
46. Bikeways?	5	3	1	0
47. Camping sites?	5	3	1	0
48. Wooded areas (open spaces)?	5	3	1	0

Community Opportunities Contributing to Good Living	Availability of Opportunities (In Your Community)			
	Very Many	Many	Some	None
49. Playgrounds?	5	3	1	0
50. Gardens, green grass, and parks?	5	3	1	0
51. Walkways?	5	3	1	0
52. Quiet neighborhoods?	5	3	1	0
53. Clean beaches or swimming pools?	5	3	1	0
Subtotal				
	A	B	C	D
	Most of the Time	Often	Sometimes	Never
F. Climatic-Geographic Conditions				
54. Clean fresh air (outdoors)	5	3	1	0
55. Bright sunshine (year round)	10	7	3	0
	None	Sometimes	Many or Often	Very Many
56. Smog (air pollution)	10	3	1	0
57. High-low temperature changes year round	5	3	1	0
58. Rainfall or snowfall	0	6	10	4
59. Tornadoes or hurricanes	10	8	3	0
60. Earthquakes	5	3	1	0
61. Thunder and electrical storms	5	3	1	0
62. Dust storms	5	3	1	0
63. Foggy evenings and days during the year	5	3	1	0
Subtotal				

Community Opportunities Contributing to Good Living	Availability of Opportunities (In Your Community)			
	A	B	C	D
	11+ Miles Away	5–10 Miles Away	Edge of City	In City
G. Airports (distance from)				
64. Residential and commercial areas	40	30	10	0
Subtotal				
	Very Often	Often	Sometimes	Never
H. Environmental Law Enforcement Does your community enforce laws on:				
65. Noise ordinance?	5	3	1	0
66. Litter?	5	3	1	0
67. Sewage dumping?	5	3	1	0
68. Dogs on the beach?	5	3	1	0
69. Industrial wastes dumping?	5	3	1	0
70. Pesticide spraying?	5	3	1	0
71. Airplane air pollution?	5	3	1	0
72. Automobile air pollution?	10	8	3	0
73. Industrial air pollution?	10	7	3	0
74. Disturbance of the peace?	5	3	1	0
Subtotal				
	Twice a Week	Once a Week	Once Every 2–3 Weeks	Seldom or Never
I. Sanitation				
75. Garbage collection	20	12	2	0

		Buried and Soil Covered	Taken to Re-cycling (pyro-lysis) Plant	Burned in Open Dump	Not Collected
76.	Refuse-solid waste disposal	10	7	2	0
		Within 50 Miles	Within 100 Miles	Within 300 Miles	Over 300 Miles
77.	Distance to safe water supply	10	7	2	0
		Very Often	Often	Sometimes	Never
78.	Working in a cigarette smoky office	30	20	5	0
	Subtotal				

		Miles away from Dump Site			
		20+	19–10	9–5	5–10
79.	Living near a chemical, plastic, or petroleum plant. Living near a radium-uranium dump site as in Colorado, Utah, or a chemical dump site as in the Love Canal site of Niagara Falls, N.Y.	0	10	40	50

Community Opportunities Contributing to Good Living		Availability of Opportunities (In Your Community)			
		Very Many	Many	Some	None
J.	Medical Services Does your community have:				
80.	Nursing hospitals for sick care and treatment?	5	3	1	0
81.	Hospital surgery services?	5	3	1	0
82.	Nursing homes for the aged?	5	3	1	0
83.	Psychiatric treatment centers?	5	3	1	0
84.	Day-night walk-in hospitals?	20			0

Community Opportunities Contributing to Good Living	Availability of Opportunities (In Your Community)			
	Very Many	Many	Some	None
85. Drug counseling services?	5	3	1	0
86. Fast ambulance service?	10	7	3	0
87. Dental care services?	5	3	1	0
88. Drug-treatment rehabilitation services?	5	3	1	0
89. Alcohol-treatment rehabilitation services?	10	7	3	0
90. Nursing services?	5	3	1	0
Subtotal				
K. Recreation and Entertainment Opportunities				
91. Professional sports	5	3	1	0
92. Amateur sports competition and leagues	20	15	5	0
93. Dramas, theater plays, and shows	10	7	3	0
94. County or city fairs or festivals	5	3	1	0
95. Public golf courses and tennis courts	5	3	1	0
96. Public gymnasiums (civic centers)	5	3	1	0
97. Live music concerts (symphonies) and live entertainment	10	7	3	0
98. Water sports (boating and swimming)	5	3	1	0
99. Horseback riding, fishing, and hunting	5	3	1	0
100. Art displays and craft shows	5	3	1	0

	Very Many	Many	Some	None
101. Square dancing and public social dances (not in bars)	10	7	3	0
102. Zoo, museums, and art galleries	5	3	1	0
103. Senior citizens' social clubs	15	12	5	0
Subtotal				

SCORING

1. Total the values for each section.
2. Add all the section totals for your community area.

INTERPRETATION

Classify your community score in the side range:

Score Total	Interpretations
850–700	*Very satisfying place to live*
669–520	*Desirable place to live*
519–360	*Acceptable place to live*
359–201	*Tolerable place to live*
200–0	*Stifling place to live*

The nature of this inventory may disturb the pure ecologist, who would probably expect this scale to deal exclusively with the physical dimensions of the environment. Such a position is not a realistic one because a good place to live in is more than just a clean and safe environment. Just as man does not live by bread alone, he cannot enjoy good health by having only a sanitary physical environment.

One should not get the impression that the environment is not important. Indeed, it is essential that the environment provide the necessary reinforcements for better living. What needs to be emphasized is that our environment is multidimensional—physical, social, and cultural in nature. This inventory includes many environmental dimensions that help people fulfill their health needs.

This inventory should show you that a good community provides many alternative opportunities. Unfortunately, many communities today are not providing positive reinforcements for optimal well-being. The recent ecology movement, concern about the increasing crime rate, the energy crisis, and inflation should have made us very conscious of the importance of living in a safe community.

Future humanity will strive to live in communities that provide psychoemotional security, a comfortable climate, disaster-free location, a clean man-made environment, adequate and accessible medical services, enforceable laws, sanitary refuse-garbage disposal, and numerous personal-family growth opportunities: economic, sociocultural, educational, and recreational.

A good place to live has everything people of all ages need to live happy, fulfilling, satisfying, and healthy lives. The community should provide ample opportunities for personal growth, community involvement, and self-motivation for its citizens. A good place to live is a perfect place to raise a family, to happily spend your life, and to finally age with grace. It is a community that has a serene and clean environment, provides numerous opportunities, and, at the same time, is stimulating.

Obviously, a good place to live for one person may be a poor place for another. Personal choice of a desirable community is a value decision. Most of us are busy fulfilling our basic health needs (food, clothing, and shelter), satisfying our social needs, often starving our emotional needs, and stifling our self-actualization. A community should help you fulfill all of these needs. The ideal place to live is where you feel most comfortable and happy.

☞ YOUR RADIATION DOSE INVENTORY

We live in a radioactive world. Radiation is all about us and is part of our natural environment. By filling in the blanks on this form, you will get an idea of your annual exposure to radiation.

	Common Sources of Radiation	Your Annual Dose (mrem's)
WHERE YOU LIVE	**Location** Cosmic radiation at **sea level**	44
	Elevation: Add 1 mrem for each 100 feet of elevation . . . . Elevation of some U.S. cities (in feet): Atlanta 1050; Chicago 595; Dallas 435; Denver 5280; Las Vegas 2000; Minneapolis 815; Pittsburgh 1200; St. Louis 455; Salt Lake City 4400; Spokane 1890. (Coastal cities are assumed to be zero, or sea level.)	
	House Construction (based on ¾ of time indoors) . . . . Brick 45 Stone 50 Wood 35 Concrete 45	
	Ground: (based on ¼ time outdoors): U.S. Average	15
WHAT YOU EAT, DRINK, AND BREATHE	**Food** **Water** **U.S. Average** **Air**	25
	Weapons test fallout	4
HOW YOU LIVE	**X-ray diagnosis** . . . . Number of Chest X-rays _____ × 10 Number of lower Gastrointestinal tract X-rays _____ × 500 U.S. Average Dose: Whole Body _____ × 100	
	Jet plane travel: For each 1500 miles add 1 mrem . . . . **TV viewing:** For each hour per day _____ × .15	

HOW CLOSE YOU LIVE TO A NUCLEAR PLANT	At site boundary: average number of hours per day _____ × 0.2 ....
	One mile away: average number of hours per day _____ × 0.02 ....
	Five miles away: average number of hours per day _____ × 0.002 ....
	Over 5 miles away: .... None ....

| My total annual mrem's dose |

| *Compare your annual dose to the U.S. annual average of 228 mrem's* |

| **One mrem per year is equal to:** Moving to an elevation 100 feet higher, Increasing your diet by 4%, Taking a 5-day vacation in the Sierra Nevada mountains. |

Source: Permission from American Nuclear Society, 1980.

ECOSYSTEMS

The study of relationship patterns between different organisms and their environment is referred to as *ecology*. For example, flowers depend on bees and other insects for pollution, while the insects in return depend on the flowers for food. Green plants harness energy from the sun and photosynthesize starch. Plants, as first-order producers of food, are eaten by herbivores, a second-order food user; which in turn, may be eaten by a third-order food consumer, the carnivores, and so on (see Figure 20.1). The different levels of food consumers illustrate the complex interdependent relationships found in nature. All such relationships are based on the food web or chain (see Figures 20.1 and 20.2), and form stable and healthy ecological communities or ecosystems. The more cross-connecting strands a food web has, the more it is able to compensate for the changes imposed on it. All members of the community are linked by their eater-eaten relationships. As long as these ecosystems are balanced, the wastes of one organism are scavenged by another. One species of organism is held in check by another as a source of food. No pollution occurs in this balanced state of nature.

This balance of nature between living things is often disrupted by man's wastes or excesses. The pesticide DDT is a good example of this. DDT was overused on farms in the early 1950s to kill insects. It was washed off the farms by rain and snow into streams and eventually into lakes and oceans. Small water plants, called plankton, picked up trace amounts of DDT. Small fish, like

sardines, would eat the plankton and DDT, thereby increasing the DDT concentration in their bodies. Tuna would eat many sardines and continue concentrating the DDT in their bodies. At each food or trophic level, there was a DDT buildup (see Figure 20.2). This process is called biomagnification. The concentration of DDT was small at the lowest trophic level and did not affect the low-order organisms.

When the DDT fish were eaten by birds, the DDT accumulated in their fatty tissues and interfered with the birds' calcium metabolism, resulting in very brittle eggshells. The eggshells broke so readily that many young chicks failed to survive the incubation period. With the bird population diminishing, the ecosystem was disrupted by an overpopulation of insects.

Mankind is inadvertently exterminating birds, fish, and animals at the rate of one species or subspecies per year by destroying their natural habitats (36). Over 300 species of animals have vanished since historic times (36); over 300 animal species have been killed off in the past three centuries; today at least 982 mammals, birds, reptiles, amphibians, and fishes are threatened with extinction (36).

Man is disrupting his own habitat in much the same way by producing an excess of wastes. Although large bodies of water, such as lakes and oceans, are natural "waste sinks," they can get overloaded in time, and a degradation takes place. All large bodies of water have the necessary waste decomposers, scavengers, and carbon-nitrogen cycles to recycle the wastes into usable plant growth substances. However, an excess of wastes

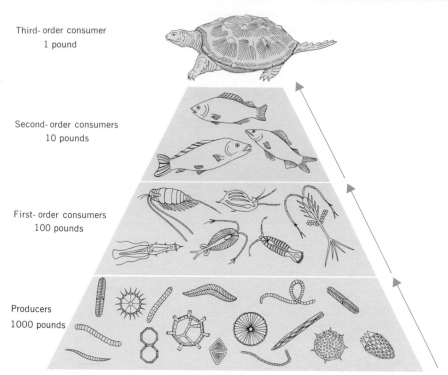

Third-order consumer
1 pound

Second-order consumers
10 pounds

First-order consumers
100 pounds

Producers
1000 pounds

Figure 20.1

A food web that also transfers energy. The dependence of one trophic level on another is depicted. The transfer of food energy from the pond's producers to successively higher orders of its consumers results in about a 90 percent loss at each step. The pond must produce 1000 pounds of plant plankton to feed 100 pounds (first-order consumers) of cope pods, which in turn, is converted into 10 pounds of mud minnows (second-order consumers), which allows the snapping turtle to gain 1 pound.

eventually chokes the large lake, resulting in speeding up the aging of the lake (eutrophication). Lake Erie is an excellent example of this.

Air is another natural "waste sink." When we overload the air with chemical wastes, we end up with photochemical smog (see Figure 20.3). Often nature itself creates pollution. The blue haze in the Appalachian Mountains of Kentucky, Tennessee, and West Virginia is created by pine trees giving off hydrocarbons that are photochemically transformed into a bluish-colored smog.

Soil is also a "natural sink" for wastes. There is ample evidence that man has been unwittingly disrupting his ecosystems for many centuries. As a result of the unsound use of land, such as overgrazing by goats, sheep, and cattle, and by overproduction of crops without fertilizing the soil, the once fertile soils have become arid deserts (see Figure 20.4). The famed Sahara desert at one time was a teeming jungle. Historians believe that

vast herbivorous animals, such as elephants, cattle, and goats, aided by the Romans using trees to build ships, defoliated the Sahara region (12). The soil eroded and topsoil was washed off the heavily wooded slopes, resulting in plant changes, which brought climatic changes and drought. This ecological upheaval has affected man's well-being, as witnessed by the droughts and famines in the African countries of Chad and Upper Volta in 1972. Desertification has become a malignancy undermining the food-producing capacity in many parts of the world today—the Rajasthan Desert of India; the LaRioja, San Luis, and LaPampas regions of Argentina; the Coquimbo Region of Chile; Australia; and parts of New Mexico, Arizona, Oklahoma, and California (12).

Today technological progress in the form of concrete and asphalt freeways is disrupting our natural habitat much like the Romans disrupted the ecosystems of the Sahara region thousands of years ago. Thousands of people and millions of acres of fertile farmland have been

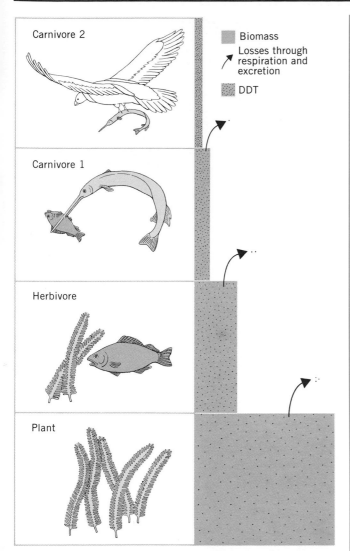

Figure 20.2
The build-up of DDT in higher-order organisms through the aquatic food chain. DDT occurs in low concentrations in sea plants (as indicated by the sparse number of dots (DDT) in the lower space. The concentration of DDT at each trophic level is passed along to the next order in this simple food chain. The concentration of DDT and other toxic substances is highest in the top of the food chain. (With permission from "Toxic Substances and Ecological Cycles" by George M. Woodwell, *Scientific American,* March 1967. Copyright © 1967 by Scientific American, Inc. All rights reserved.)

displaced by expressways (see Figure 20.5). Two-thirds of our fertile urban land has been turned over into roads for automobiles (20).

The most recent evidence of environmental degradation was observed in 1978 when acid rain, made up of nitric and sulfuric acids, fell on heavily industrialized areas of the world (1). The rains ate away at buildings, and killed fish and plant vegetation. Scientists believe

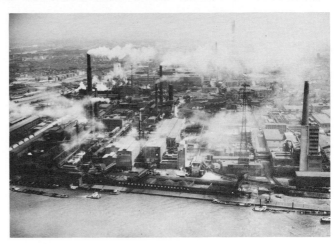

Figure 20.3
Chemical factories in Duisberg, Germany, emitting wastes into the air. Who fines factories in the United States for polluting the air? How much is the fine?

that acid rains result from waste overload from fossil-fuel power plants, smelters, and automobile exhausts (1).

The examples of desertification—disappearing bird and animal species, the desecration of fertile lands, and acid rains—are incomplete evidence of how our ecosystems have been disrupted and our physical environment degraded and made unsafe. Humans are big polluters. The remainder of this chapter briefly reviews the major ways we pollute our environment.

WATER POLLUTION

Without water there is no life. Unfortunately, we misuse much more water than our bodies need to sustain life. Our bodies need less than 2 gallons of drinking water a day although we use an average of 60 gallons a day per person in the home to cook, wash, and flush the toilet. Industries consume almost 70 percent of our water supply, and in return, create an estimated 60 percent of the water pollution.

Water systems are polluted by (1) the discharge of domestic sewage containing mostly human excrement, (2) industrial wastes, (3) agricultural wastes that include animal excrement, fertilizers, and pesticides from cultivated land, and (4) liquid wastes from slaughter houses, dairies, and canning and packing plants. Water polluted in these ways carries pathogenic bacteria and viruses that can cause viral hepatitis, polio typhoid, dysentery, cholera, yellow fever, tapeworm and salmonellosis in the United States and Canada. In addition to the disease threats, chemicals, bacteria, and algae give water a foul

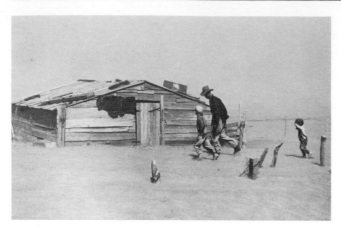
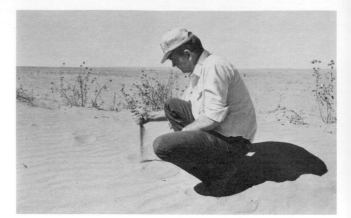

Figure 20.4
Desertification of farm land in Oklahoma in 1936 and the same land in 1979.

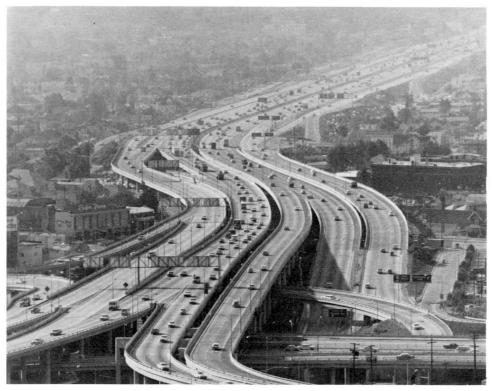

Figure 20.5
Our cities have become blacktop cement jungles. Concrete and asphalt freeways have disrupted a once natural habitat.

odor and discolor it, thereby making it unesthetic in appearance and distasteful to drink.

We obviously need to purify our drinking water to make it safe and palatable for us. Most communities in the United States and Canada have built water treatment plants to purify the drinking water. Such treatment plants use sand and charcoal filters, chemicals, and chlorine or ozone to kill or remove most of the pathogenic bacteria and viruses and make it appealing to drink. One can

travel to any community in the United States and Canada and drink pure water. This is a tribute to the daily vigilance of our public health departments.

Many streams, rivers, and lakes in this country in the 60s were polluted by tons of synthetic-phosphate-hydrocarbon detergents (see Figure 20.6). These substances cannot be decomposed by bacteria (biodegradability). When they were dumped in large quantities, ''soapsuds'' were observed in streams and lakes, causing large masses of "algae blooms." Algae used up much of the oxygen needed by fish and other aquatic organisms, killing the fish, thereby disrupting the lake's ecosystem.

Potential drinking waters in many communities are now being polluted by farmers using nitrate fertilizers (see Figure 20.7). Bacteria react on the nitrates, causing the water to be toxic to human beings. Toxic nitrate compounds interfere with the oxygen-carrying capacity of red blood cells and may cause suffocation in babies and children. Most water purification plants do not remove chemicals (nitrates) or minerals from the water.

Considerable controversy surrounds the dumping of hot water from nuclear power plants. Perhaps the greatest threat is from radioactive material seeping into drinking water.

Water pollution occurs when wastes accumulate in a body of water to the point where the water's natural purification processes cannot break them down into harmless and inoffensive forms. All water systems have the natural ability to self-purify. We disrupt this natural process by dumping domestic, industrial, and agricultural wastes into our waterways.

SEWAGE

Raw domestic, agricultural, and industrial wastes can greatly pollute streams, rivers, and lakes. Sewage, or waste water, is used water that is very rich in organic matter and is teeming with microorganisms. Major industries, such as pulp and paper mills, petroleum refineries, steel mills, and chemical plants, create three times as much waste as is discharged from domestic sources. For example, 200,000 gallons of water are used to synthesize 1 ton of viscose rayon; 770 gallons of water are used to synthesize 1 barrel of petroleum; and 600,000 gallons of water are used to manufacture 1 ton of synthetic rubber. Making matters worse is that most industrial plants are clustered close to each other, thus overburdening local lakes and rivers with industrial wastes.

Sewage is 99.9 percent water and 0.1 percent solids. These solids include fats and oils, dirt, settleable solids, suspended solids, soluble organic and inorganic material, chemicals, and bacteria. Obviously, bacteria can thrive on such wastes and increase in number. The danger of bacterial sewage increases when these are

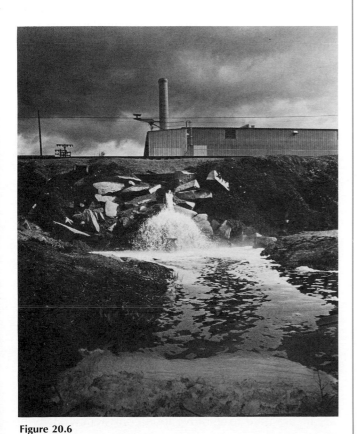

Figure 20.6
Chemical wastes from a factory polluting a stream in California. Who should monitor such pollution? To whom should you report it?

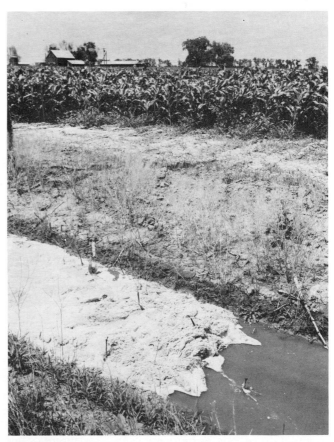

Figure 20.7
Agricultural wastes (chemical fertilizers and pesticides) are often washed off farmland and end up polluting streams.

dumped into rivers and lakes that, in turn, are used as drinking water. As an example, over 13 cities along the Ohio River use the river water for drinking purposes, and in turn, dump their sewage into the river. Fortunately, all of these cities treat their drinking water and also their sewage before dumping it into the river. A sewage treatment plant works much the same as a water treatment plant.

Since sewage is mostly water, and water is expensive and difficult to provide, many cities are now considering reclaiming effluent or waste water that comes from a sewage treatment plant. Waste water in Santee, California, is recycled into recreational ponds, is used to irrigate golf courses, and is even used in the local swimming pool.

Many ancient civilizations dumped their raw sewage into large ponds. Bacteria in the ponds would digest the organic matter and the waste water would become pond water. The small community of Orange Grove, Mississippi, dumps its raw sewage into a lagoon loaded with pesky water hyacinths. These plants suck pollutants out of the water and are nature's sewage treatment system. Water flowing out of the lagoon exceeds state health standards for purity. More communities should consider using water hyacinths to recycle waste water.

FOOD POLLUTION

Over 10 million persons receive medical aid from food spoiling and food poisoning each year (see Table 20.1). Millions more suffer an upset stomach and diarrhea several times a year, but never relate this to poorly prepared meals or contaminated foods. Most such discomforts are due to poor sanitary practices.

The food humans eat is also the same food that over 2 dozen bacteria eat: precooked hams, fish, fowl, milk, custards, potato salads, and eggs. Bacteria produce invisible waste products called *Toxins*. When we eat food, we also ingest the toxin, hence the term *food intoxication*. The more toxins you ingest, the more severe your reactions. Similarly, the more toxins ingested, the quicker the onset of the symptoms. Toxins irritate the nerve endings inside the digestive system, causing stomach-intestinal cramps and pain, diarrhea, fatigue, and nausea. These symptoms are referred to as food poisoning. Between 75 and 95 percent of all food poisoning is transmitted by persons infected with staphylococci who handle food that others eat.

The potential for getting sick from contaminated foods is very great in this country, since 50 percent of our population eat one or more meals in a restaurant or fast food establishment each day, and many more eat frozen and canned foods, and many cold meats.

Table 20.1

Mechanisms of Food Poisoning by the Leading Infectious Microbial Agents

Microbes	Symptoms
Clostridium perfringens	Most common source is re-heated cooked meat; incubation period 8–24 hours. Symptoms include diarrhea and abdominal cramps. Symptoms are usually gone after 8 hours.
Staphylococcus	Most common sources are custard- and cream-filled bakery goods, also ham, tongue, processed meats, cheese, ice cream, potato salad, hollandaise sauce, chicken salad. Incubation period 1–6 hours. Symptoms include severe and sudden abdominal cramps, nausea, vomiting, and diarrhea. Recovery usually follows in 6–8 hours. Organisms gain entrance via food handlers.
Salmonella	Most common sources are poultry, eggs, and products containing dried eggs such as cake mixes. Incubation period 8–24 hours. Symptoms include nausea and vomiting followed by chills and high fever. Symptoms may persist for 2 weeks; the disease can be fatal to infants.

Food intoxication may be prevented by washing hands with soap and water before handling food, keeping hands away from the mouth and nose, promptly refrigerating all perishable foods below 40°F, properly cooking the food so that toxins are destroyed, and keeping infected persons (flus and cold) from handling food others eat (see Figure 20.8).

Another form of food pollution has been created by the food industry. Farmers spray pesticides on vegetables. The pesticide residues often remain on vegetables purchased from supermarkets. A more serious and emergent food problem is the additives that the food industry adds to many foods to retard bacteria and molds from spoiling food. Additives are also used to enhance flavor, while dyes and nitrates improve food color and sugars are used to improve food consistency. Many of these chemicals cause allergic reactions in sensitive persons such as hyperactivity, headaches, anxiety, mood

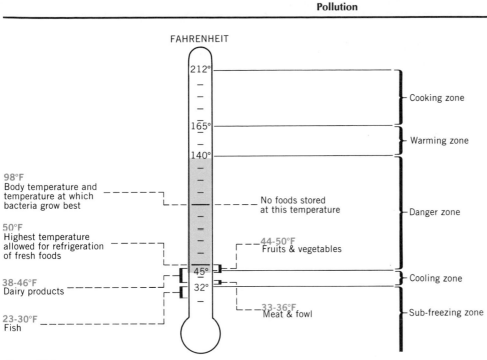

FAHRENHEIT

212° — Cooking zone

165° — Warming zone

140°

98°F
Body temperature and
temperature at which
bacteria grow best

No foods stored
at this temperature

Danger zone

50°F
Highest temperature
allowed for refrigeration
of fresh foods

44-50°F
Fruits & vegetables

45° Cooling zone

38-46°F
Dairy products

32°

Sub-freezing zone

33-36°F
Meat & fowl

23-30°F
Fish

Figure 20.8

Prevention of food-borne illnesses (food poisoning and diarrhea) through the proper temperature control of bacteria. Food must be kept hot above 140° F or cold below 45° F. Bacteria grow best at temperatures between 50° F and 140° F. Freezing food merely slows down the bacterial growth to a minimum. When food is thawed out, bacteria begin to reproduce again.

changes, and depression. The nitrates used to preserve ham, sausage, and weiners are suspected of causing cancer.

To avoid ingested food additives, read the labels, and select and eat fresh foods that you can prepare yourself.

SOLID WASTES

Our most visible and annoying pollution is the piling up of trash, garbage, rubbish, and solid wastes. These include food peelings and meal leftovers, plastic and paper wrappers, beer cans, pop bottles, metals, junked cars, dirt, paper and wood crates, clothing, and just about everything and anything that householders discard. The average American creates about 6 pounds of these wastes each day, more than persons in any other country (16). In the course of a year, a city of 10,000 people creates enough such garbage to cover an acre of ground to the height of 7 feet.

Our traditional approach to getting rid of solid wastes is to put them in the garbage can, have the garbage truck pick up the wastes one or two times a week and dump the wastes at the landfill or open dump. Communities in the past would burn the open dump, creating smoke and

unpleasant odors. A cleaner approach is the landfill dump, which covers the solid wastes with a layer of dirt each day (see Figure 20.9). If left uncovered, garbage becomes a breeding place for pests such as flies, mosquitoes, bacteria, and rodents. The pests can cause diseases (e.g., the rat carries every disease endemic to humans); this threat is aggravated by noxious odors and an unaesthetic appearance. Many cities along the Atlantic coastline dump their garbage 20 to 30 miles out into the ocean, only to have it wash ashore and pollute the beaches and shoreline.

Our methods of collecting household solid wastes and disposing of them have not changed much in the past 100 years. Eighty percent of the total costs is spent on trucks and labor collecting the solid wastes. One way to reduce the expenses of collecting and getting rid of solid wastes is to reclaim or recycle materials. Such demonstration recycling plants have been built in numerous communities. These plants retrieve metals, paper, glass, and clothing, then shred the remaining garbage and trash, kiln heat it to high temperatures, and decompose this shredded material by a process of pyrolysis so that gases and fuel oils are produced. One ton of trash can produce 42 gallons of low sulfur oil, as well as methane gas.

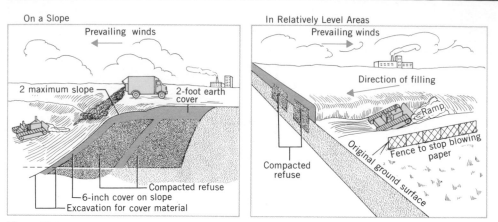

Figure 20.9
Schematic representation of a well-planned sanitary landfill.

TOXIC CHEMICAL WASTES

Many persons are working or living in areas that were once factory dumping sites for such hazardous chemicals as mercury, chlorine, benzene, toluene, and persistent carcinogenic pesticides. These toxic chemicals were dumped as wastes years ago and left to decompose. As these dump sites were forgotten and city land became scarce, cities and industries built on or near these sites. Only recently has the public become aware that residents on or near such sites, as the Love Canal in Niagara

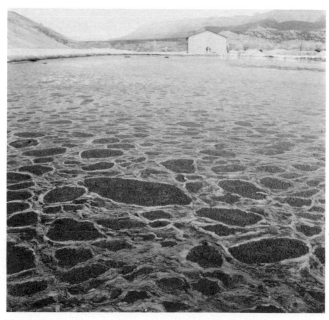

Figure 20.10
Abandoned uranium wastes dumped into a settling pond near Rifle, Colorado. Such wastes release radioactive gases that may accumulate to dangerous levels. Are there any such ponds or abandoned mine wastes near where you live?

Falls and others in Michigan and Louisiana, were having high incidences of headaches, mental and respiratory illnesses, cancer, and birth defects. These sites were assumed to be nonhazardous until now.

A similar occurrence has taken place near abandoned radium and uranium mine milling sites in this country (see Figure 20.10). Inadvertently, many of these dumping sites in Colorado, Utah, Arizona, New Mexico, Pennsylvania, and Wyoming are emitting 24-hour radiation equivalent to getting one or two daily X-rays. Such cumulative radiation exposures over a long period of time are great enough to cause cancer, chromosome damage, and birth defects (27).

The complete picture on the long-range, cumulative chemical and radiation exposure is only surfacing. It will be a few more years before we have the complete picture of the impact all dumping sites have on human well-being. We need to do a better job of disposing of chemical and radiation wastes than we have in the past.

AIR POLLUTION

Air is another of nature's "waste sinks." There is no air pollution as long as wastes (smoke, dust, and chemical gases) are discharged in a slow fashion, and the winds disperse and dilute these wastes. The air is able to cleanse itself. However, air pollution usually occurs when gaseous and particulate wastes accumulate quicker than the air is able to remove them.

Polluted air is distasteful and irritating to inhale and look at, and it is physiologically dangerous to our well-being.

The chief sources of air pollution are waste-burning, manufacturing plants, electric power plants, and motor vehicles (see Figure 20.11). Most of these sources burn fossil fuels or their products—coal, oil, gas, and gaso-

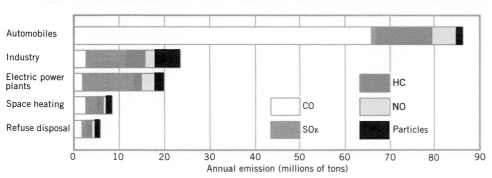

Figure 20.11

Sources of air pollution emissions ranked. Automobiles can cause over 85 percent of the air pollution in big cities. Five points of each bar represent (from left) carbon monoxide (CO), sulfur oxides (SOx), hydrocarbons (HC), nitrogen oxides (NO), and particles.

line. Eighty percent of the photochemical smog in a big city comes from automobile exhausts.

The air we breathe is polluted in two major ways. The first type of air pollution occurs from burning coal. Burning coal gives off sulfur oxides and smoke that hovers close to the ground causing irritation to the respiratory system. Respiratory congestion and death can occur in those persons already weakened by cardiopulmonary diseases, red blood cell deficiencies, malnutrition, allergies, and other respiratory ailments. Such pollution is common in coal-burning, industrial centers of eastern United States.

Photochemical smog, characteristic of Los Angeles and most big cities, is the second type of air pollution. It is caused mostly by automobiles spewing nitrogen oxides and hydrocarbons. In the presence of ultraviolet rays of sunlight and warm temperature, these gases are changed photochemically to produce ozone, peroxyacetyl nitrate (PAN), and other chemical pollutants (see Table 20.2). These pollutants referred to as oxidants by most local public health departments, form a whitish gray haze called photochemical smog. Ozone and PAN

Table 20.2

National Air Quality Standards for Automobile or Related Pollutants

Pollutant	Standard
Carbon monoxide (CO)	9 ppm for 8 hours[a]
	35 ppm for 1 hour
Hydrocarbons (nonmethane)	0.24 ppm for 3 hours
	(6–9 A.M.)
Nitrogen dioxide (N_2O_2)	0.05
	(annual arithmetic
	mean)
Oxidant	0.08 ppm for 1 hour

[a] Not to exceed more than once a year.

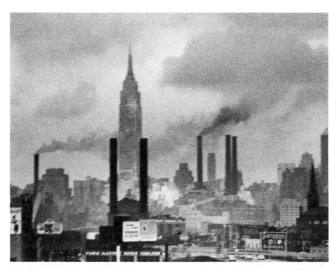

Figure 20.12

Smokestacks in a city spew chemical wastes into the atmosphere. Who is supposed to monitor such pollution in your community?

destroy leaf tissue, cause chlorosis or fading of green color in plants, and stunt plant growth. Smog usually irritates people's skin, eyes, and respiratory mucosa, and constricts the bronchial tubes, causing nasal discharge, coughing, sore throat, fever, headache, nausea, and vomiting. Collectively, these pollutants may also induce biochemical stress in the body and impede metabolic processes as well. Recent research suggests that exposure to high levels of oxidants can impair the efficiency of the central nervous system and may even cause genetic damage. Smog exposure quickly depletes vitamins A, C, E, and selenium, thereby lowering the body's resistance to infectious diseases. Smog exposure also aggravates many preexisting cardiac and respiratory conditions, such as asthma, emphysema, and chronic bronchitis. Perhaps the greatest long-range exposure danger of smog is lung cancer. Smog, like cigarette smoke, aggravates cancer in genetically predisposed individuals. Future research in this area will clarify this cause-effect relationship.

Auto exhausts and manufacturing plants also emit great amounts of carbon monoxide. When inhaled, this odorless gas displaces oxygen in the hemoglobin, thereby reducing the oxygen-carrying function of red blood cells. Hence the oxygen supply to the brain and heart may be greatly reduced, which affects the efficiency of the brain and judgment. Since cigarette smoke contains carbon monoxide as well, a smoker living in an air-polluted area is subjected to even greater quantities of this gas. The inhaled synergistic effect of cigarette smoke and the by-products of photochemical smog increase the risk of cancer and heart attack in genetically predisposed persons. Even nonsmokers are 10 percent more likely to develop lung cancer if they live in smog cities and communities than were they to live in clean air communities.

Trucks and cars are the greatest polluters of air. The reason we have photochemical smog in the big cities is that there are just too many cars being driven too many miles each day in an area that lacks winds to waft and disperse the auto exhausts (see Figure 20.13).

Numerous alternatives to the use of the automobile have been proposed as steam and electric engines, faster and more reliable rapid transit systems, and living closer to where we work. Unsuccessful attempts have been made to control exhaust emissions and reduce speed limits to 55 mph. Very little federal and state progress has been made since the 1973 energy crisis to curb air pollution. Federal laws promulgated in the 1970s to reduce auto emissions by 1976, then extended to 1978, have been rolled back indefinitely and placed in the government "suspense file." Other ways proposed to curb air pollution are to tax people who drive cars instead of using rapid transit, raise the cost of gasoline, tax two-car families, mandate annual car inspections, encourage car pools, prohibit automobiles in congested downtown areas, tax cars with big engines, and give tax write-offs to those using small cars or who do not own cars. What is really needed to reduce photochemical smog is to change our style of living and identify common goals and purposes of life.

WAYS TO REDUCE THE THREAT OF AIR POLLUTION TO YOUR HEALTH

1. Stop cigarette smoking immediately and get others to follow.
2. Identify your health risks to air pollution.
3. Influence industries to cut down spewing air pollutants.
4. Reduce the number of times you drive your car unnecessarily and travel long distances.
5. Influence others to reduce auto travel.
6. Keep informed of air pollution episode days when the oxidant level rises to a dangerous level.
7. Reduce your exposure to pollutants by staying indoors during periods of high risk.
8. Equip your home (at least one room) with an ac-

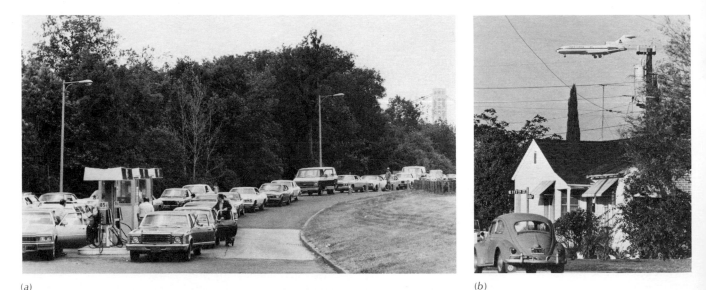

(a)   (b)

Figure 20.13

(a) Automobiles are responsible for most of the air pollution in the cities. Which chemical pollutants disrupt blood circulation? What are some good outcomes of a gasoline shortage? (b) Airplanes and automobiles concentrated into overcrowded cities are a major cause of air pollution.

tivated charcoal air filter, which will eliminate most of the oxidants from the inside air.

9. Use a bicycle, walk, or use rapid transit instead of driving a car.

10. Fight legislatively for clean air as a major public issue.

11. Periodically, check your need for vitamin A, C, and E, and seleniun intake. You may need to supplement them if smog depletes these substances in your body and your daily diet does not fulfill your body's needs. (See Chapter 6 for more information.)

NOISE POLLUTION

Noise pollution is really air pollution, since noise travels in the form of air waves. Loud noise, or mumbo-jumbo and unwanted sound, has almost become a way of life in America. Fraternity houses on many campuses blast rock and roll music in the late afternoon. Rock bands at discotheques and rock concerts blare deafening sounds with electronically amplified instruments in the evenings. Public works crews use jack hammers to repair streets (see Figure 20.14), while big diesel trailer trucks roar noisily down the freeways. Housewives use noisy can openers, washing machines, and hi-fi's at home. It is not surprising to read in Richard Carmon's book, *Our Endangered Hearing* (7), that noises of modern living are causing millions of Americans to lose their hearing.

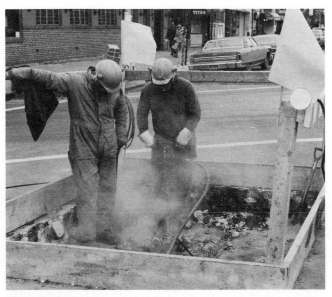

Figure 20.14
Noise created by city maintenance workers using a jackhammer. How are these workers protected from the noise? Are nearby street merchants and pedestrians protected from the noise? Does your community have noise control laws?

About 15 percent of the people in the United States now have significant hearing loss (7). Over 19 million industrial workers have hearing impairments, while an estimated 5 million young people under 18 have impaired hearing. Environmental noise is the culprit of this epidemic. Larger and more powerful machines invade nearly every aspect of life.

Studies on animals and humans show that in addition to causing hearing loss, high noise levels during a typical working day can produce physiological effects, such as increased adrenalin secretion and involuntary muscle spasms causing stomach contractions and constrictions of blood vessels and capillaries (see Figure 20.15). This results in high blood pressure, thereby preventing adequate blood supplied from reaching the inner ear and

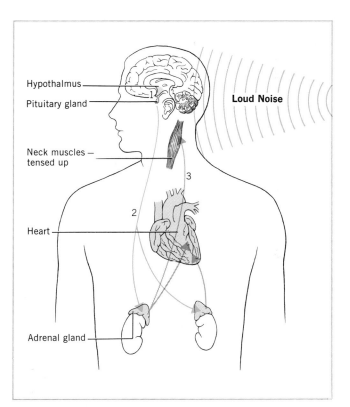

Figure 20.15
Noise is a chemical stressor. A loud jet noise interferes with our communication, irritates the hypothalamus, causing the pituitary gland to release chemical hormones into the blood. The blood transports this hormone to the adrenal gland. The adrenal gland, in turn, releases its own chemical messengers (adrenaline) into the blood. Adrenalin speeds up the heart rate and breathing. Adrenaline also tenses the muscles, as in neck area. A person can become hypertense when exposed to such stresses for much of the day; neck muscles tense up, causing a tension headache. (With permission from Walter D. Sorochan and Stephen Bender, *Teaching Secondary Health Science*, New York: Wiley, 1978, p. 442. Copyright © by John Wiley & Sons Publishers, 1979.)

brain. Many suffer from tension and migraine headaches because noise is definitely a chemical stressor (30). Human bodies react to noise as though it were danger; the body gets ready for the "fight or flight" reaction.

In addition to inducing physiological-chemical changes in the body, prolonged noise exposure disrupts your sense of balance, making you more susceptible to accidents. Noise-induced stress hormones may cross the placental barrier in a pregnant woman and cause irritation to the fetus. Constant fetal exposure to noise may contribute to a hypertense baby.

Noise can also cause discomfort; interfere with your work, sleep, rest, and privacy; and disrupt speech communication. If prolonged, it causes annoyance, irritation, fatigue, anxiety, hypertension, personality changes, and can sever intimate relationships.

Noise, as from an airplane taking off or a party next door, also disrupts one's dream pattern during sleep. By dreaming and escaping into a fairyland for an hour or two, such dream-sleep states replenish the cortisone stress hormones. Upon waking up, one feels rested and fresh. One of the benefits of dreaming is to revive the nervous system. When noise disrupts the mental revival process, you wake up feeling tired and irritable. Such feelings can be prevented by keeping the noise level below 40 decibels when sleeping.

The human body tolerates noise at low levels, becomes uncomfortable and annoyed as the noise level approaches 90 decibels, is irritated from 90 to 120 decibels, and feels pain from 120 to 140 decibels (see Figure 20.16). Prolonged or sudden "bang" noise exposure causes the hair cells in the organ of corti in the cochlea of the inner ear to drop off. Since these hairs do not regrow, this results in permanent hearing loss. Loud rock music is known to be a contributing factor to hearing loss.

The U.S. Occupational Safety and Health Administration (OSHA) has outlined what it considers to be safe time limits for exposure to specific noise levels. One can work safely each day for 8 hours in a 90-decibel or less noise environment, or for 4 hours at 95 decibels, or for 15 minutes or less at 115 decibels. Sounds over 115 decibels should be avoided by everyone.

People exposed to high-noise environments should wear earplugs and/or earmuffs, or consider another job. Noisy engines and noisy machines should be muffled. For example, loud sounding typewriters should be enclosed in a plastic transparent cage so as to cut down office noise. Homeowners should refuse to buy products that do not have a label signifying the amount of noise the products make or not use such products in the first place.

RADIATION

People have recently become most concerned about the safety of nuclear power plants and microwave ovens. Of perhaps greater importance is radiation from medical and dental X-rays.

Most persons are unaware that humans have always lived in a radioactive environment and that man himself is radioactive (21) (see Table 20.3). Most of this radiation in the environment, known as *"natural background radiation,"* comes from the atmosphere as cosmic rays, from radioactive substances in the earth's crust, and from certain natural radioisotopes such as potassium 40 (see Table 20.4 and Figure 20.17). Of the 92 elements found in the earth's crust, the oceans and the atmosphere, 16, or approximately $1/6$, are naturally radioactive. Atoms of the heavy metals uranium and thorium are constantly, though very slowly, breaking down, in the process giv-

Table 20.3

Radiation Exposures in the United States.[a]

	Millirems[b]
Natural Sources	
A. External to the body	
1. From cosmic radiation	50.0
2. From the earth	47.0
3. From building materials	3.0
B. Inside the body	
1. Inhalation of air	5.0
2. Elements found naturally in human tissues	21.0
Total of natural sources	126.0
Man-Made Sources	
A. Medical Procedures	
1. Diagnostic X-rays	50.0
2. Radiotherapy X-ray and radioisotopes	10.0
3. Internal diagnosis and therapy	1.0
Subtotal	61.0
B. Atomic energy industry, laboratories	0.2
C. Luminous watch dials, television tubes, radioactive industrial wastes, etc.	2.0
D. Radioactive fallout	4.0
Subtotal	6.2
Total of man-made sources	67.2
Overall total	193.2

[a] Estimated average exposures to the gonads based on the 1963 report of the Federal Radiation Council.
[b] One thousandth of a rem.

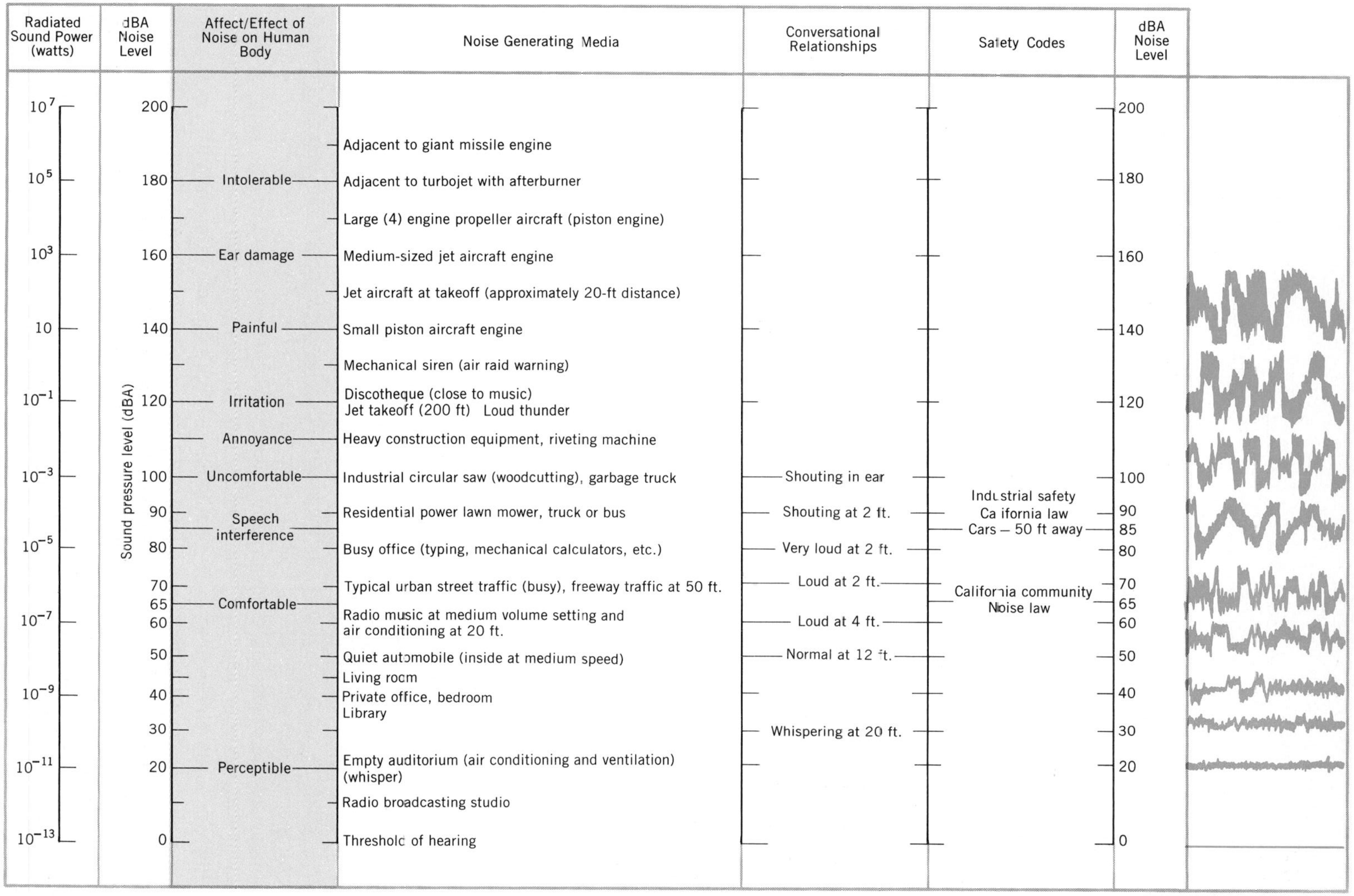

Radiated Sound Power (watts)	dBA Noise Level	Affect/Effect of Noise on Human Body	Noise Generating Media	Conversational Relationships	Safety Codes	dBA Noise Level
10^7	200		Adjacent to giant missile engine			200
10^5	180	Intolerable	Adjacent to turbojet with afterburner			180
			Large (4) engine propeller aircraft (piston engine)			
10^3	160	Ear damage	Medium-sized jet aircraft engine			160
			Jet aircraft at takeoff (approximately 20-ft distance)			
10	140	Painful	Small piston aircraft engine			140
			Mechanical siren (air raid warning)			
10^{-1}	120	Irritation	Discotheque (close to music) Jet takeoff (200 ft) Loud thunder			120
		Annoyance	Heavy construction equipment, riveting machine			
10^{-3}	100	Uncomfortable	Industrial circular saw (woodcutting), garbage truck	Shouting in ear		100
	90	Speech interference	Residential power lawn mower, truck or bus	Shouting at 2 ft.	Industrial safety / California law	90
	85				Cars – 50 ft away	85
10^{-5}	80		Busy office (typing, mechanical calculators, etc.)	Very loud at 2 ft.		80
	70	Comfortable	Typical urban street traffic (busy), freeway traffic at 50 ft.	Loud at 2 ft.	California community Noise law	70
10^{-7}	65		Radio music at medium volume setting and air conditioning at 20 ft.	Loud at 4 ft.		65
	60		Quiet automobile (inside at medium speed)	Normal at 12 ft.		60
	50		Living room			50
10^{-9}	40		Private office, bedroom / Library			40
	30		Empty auditorium (air conditioning and ventilation) (whisper)	Whispering at 20 ft.		30
10^{-11}	20	Perceptible	Radio broadcasting studio			20
10^{-13}	0		Threshold of hearing			0

Sound pressure level (dBA)

Figure 20.16

Relationships of noise levels, noise generating media, and their effects on the human body and conversational relationships. Compiled by the author from numerous sources. This table is merely for comparison, since all noise levels vary with background or noise, distance, acoustics, and so on.

Table 20.4

Sources of Natural Background Irradiation

| Sources of Irradiation | Dose rate (millirems[a] per year) | | |
	Gonad	Bone Marrow	Haversion Canal
External irradiation			
Cosmic rays[b] (including neutrons)	50	50	50
Terrestrial (including air)	50	50	50
Internal irradiation			
Potassium-40	20	15	15
Radium-226 (and decay products)	0.5	5.4	0.6
Radium-228 (and decay products)	0.8	8.6	1.0
Lead-210	0.3	3.6	0.4
Carbon-14	0.7	1.6	1.6
Radon-222 (absorbed in the bloodstream)	3	3	3
	125	137	122

[a] The *rem,* an acronym for *roentgen equivalent man,* is a unit of the absorbed dose of ionizing radiation that accounts for biological effectiveness. A dose in rem is numerically equivalent to a dose in rad. The rem is useful to measure permissible exposure levels and where mixtures of radiation must be considered, as it takes into account the biological damage produced by a given unit of energy. For X- and gamma rays the rem and rad are the same. A *millirem* (mrem) is $1/1000$ of a rem.

A *roentgen* (R) is a unit of exposure to either X- or gamma radiation.

The *curie* is a unit of radioactivity. A material or substance is said to have an activity of 1 curie if it is transformed at the rate of 3.7×10^7 disintegrations per second.

[b] The radioactive activity of cosmic rays increases with altitude; thus Denver, the "mile-high city," is exposed to greater radiation than New York City, at sea level.

ing off alpha rays, beta rays, and gamma rays. These rays, as radioisotopes or radionuclides, are widely distributed in very low amounts in nature—in the food we eat, in the air we breathe, and in the liquids we drink (see Table 20.5).

The human body has sufficient concentrations of radioactive elements that can be measured with modern radiation-detecting instruments. These elements include potassium 40, carbon 14, and radium. This is referred to as the *internal dose.*

We have been exposed to cosmic radiation since conception. Such radiation originates in interstellar space and penetrates our atmosphere. The ozone layer, high in the atmosphere and surrounding our earth, blocks most of the strength of the cosmic and ultraviolet rays so that we receive a very weak dose of it (see Figure 20.15). In fact, such natural radiation is believed to be important in producing the mutations on which evolution is based. We have reason to believe that certain genetic defects, cancers, and stillbirths are associated with the natural background radiation and that additional exposure from man-made sources will increase these defects.

Since 1900 we have been creating new radiations, such as medical and dental X-rays (see Figure 20.18), ra-

dioactive isotopes, industrial X-rays, fallout from exploding atomic and hydrogen bomb blasts, nuclear weapons, nuclear ships and submarines, and radioactive wastes from nuclear power plants. These radiations by themselves account for 41 percent of man's total ionizing radiation "exposure." But the largest source of radiation "damage" exposure to man, 90 percent, comes from the medical and dental uses of X-rays for diagnosis and therapy (21). Man-made radiation from all sources is now being absorbed at nearly twice the rate that natural radiation is. To put it another way, Americans are just about tripling their radiation dosage through exposures to man-made radiations (3:35) (see Tables 20.6 and 20.7).

Radiation risk from nuclear power plants is real. Such plants can release radiation during all stages of power production: in the mining and processing of the fuels (uranium and plutonium), in generating power, and in storing long-lived radioactive wastes. Although safeguards against radiation accident leakages are built into the nuclear energy reactors, they are judged unsafe by large insurance companies and many scientists. Insurance companies have refused to underwrite the potential liability policy for a major nuclear power plant accident.

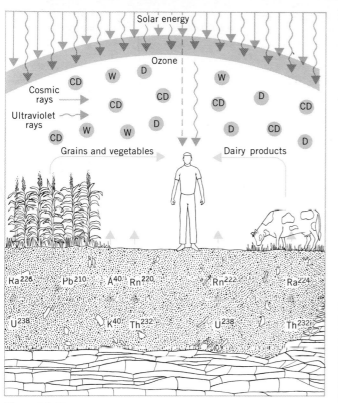

Figure 20.17

Source of natural background radiation coming from the atmosphere and the soil and earth's crust. Most of the cosmic and ultraviolet rays are screened off by the ozone layer and atmospheric gases such as carbon dioxide (CO), water vapors (W), and dust (D). Radioactive substances in the earth's crust and soil include uranium (U^{238}), thorium (Th^{232}), and potassium (K^{40}). These radioactive substances gradually decay into radioisotopes such as K^{40}, argon (A^{40}), radium (Ra^{226}), lead (Pb^{210}), and radon (Rn^{220} and Rn^{222}). Plants absorb the radioisotopes and are reabsorbed by animals (cattle) and humans. We ingest these isotopes directly when we eat grains, leafy green vegetables, and dairy products. This is a simplistic diagram of the radiation sources. (Adapted from James R. Arnold and E. A. Martell, "The Circulation of Radioactive Isotopes," *Scientific American*, September 1959, pp. 85–94.)

Table 20.5
Relative Alpha Activity of Foods

Food Stuff	Relative Activity
Brazil nuts	1400
Cereals	60
Teas	40
Liver and kidney	15
Flours	14
Peanuts and peanut butter	12
Chocolates	8
Biscuits	2
Milks (evaporated)	1–2
Fish	1–2
Cheeses and eggs	0.9
Vegetables	0.7
Meats	0.5
Fruits	0.1

Note: Whenever scientists bring up the question of internal exposure due to natural radioactivity in food they immediately think of Brazil. Not only because of the very high gamma-ray activity of the soil, which exists in certain areas of Brazil as well as India, but also because of the Brazil nut with its extraordinarily high radioactivity—14,000 times that of common fruits. Of course the Brazil nut is exceptional and by no means characteristic of nuts in general. Cereals are also relatively high—perhaps as much as 500–600 times that of fruits, which have the lowest concentrations of natural radioactivity. Table 20.6 points out pretty clearly that it pays to keep away from rich foods for more than *one* reason.

Source: From *Proceedings of the Second United Nations International Conference on the Peaceful Uses of Atomic Energy,* September 1–13, 1958, Geneva, Switzerland, United Nations Publication, Volume 23, Experience in Radiological Protection, p. 153, W. V. Mayneord.

Radiation exposure damages the complex molecules within a body cell, interfering with its chemical machinery and, in extreme cases, killing it. Radiation therapy kills cancer cells in this way. Radiation can easily damage chromosomes and genes, causing actual cell death.

In addition to genetic structural damage, radiation is most harmful to those tissues whose cells undergo division throughout life, or whose cells are periodically replaced. Large doses of all types of radiation kill cells, while with small doses, cell recovery is possible and the cells can continue to function. However, recovery may not be complete, and malignancy changes may occur later. The tissue cells most vulnerable are those that actively regenerate, such as embryonic tissue, fingernails, the inner linings of the mouth, stomach and intestines, blood cells, gonadal germ cells, and the skin.

Harmful effects from radiation can occur by exposure to a single large dose or by cumulative repeated exposure to small doses of radiation. The greatest danger is from relatively small doses of radiation over many years. Early research workers exposed to radiation materials for a long period of time, as were Pièrre and Marie Curie and their daughter Eve, died of cancer (3:32). The short-term effects of acute, high-level radiation exposure have been known since the atomic bomb explosions in Japan in 1945. These include nausea, fatigue, blood disorders, intestinal problems, the temporary loss of hair, skin burns, vomiting, fever, and the appearance of open sores

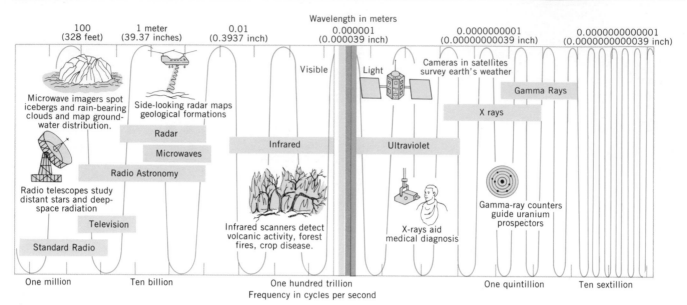

Figure 20.18

The spectrum of radiation or electromagnetic energy and some of its uses. (With permission from "Remote Sensing: New Eyes to See the Old World," *National Geographic,* January 1969, pp. 48–49.)

Table 20.6

The Spectrum of Radiation Exposure — Estimates of Radiation Levels Sometimes Encountered by People

Flight from Los Angeles to Paris (cosmic rays)	4.8	millirems
Chest X-ray (1 film)	22	millirems
Contamination measured one-half mile from Three Mile Island during nuclear accident	83	millirems
Apollo X astronauts on moon flight (cosmic rays)	480	millirems
Dental X-ray (whole mouth)	910	millirems
Dose on Three Mile Island site during accident	1,100	millirems
Breast mammography (1 film)	1,500	millirems
Current yearly occupational-exposure limit	5,000	millirems
Fallout in St. George, Utah, from 1953 atomic-bomb test	6,000	millirems
Barium enema	8,000	millirems
Heart catheterization (before bypass surgery)	45,000	millirems
Pacemaker insertion with fluoroscopy	132,000	millirems
Radiation treatment for Hodgkin's disease	4,500,000	millirems
Radiation treatment for bone cancer	6,000,000	millirems

However, radiation doses are not strictly comparable. Some affect the entire body, while others — such as dental X-rays — are confined to extremely small portions of the body. Therefore, the danger from radiation will vary not only by the amount of exposure, but also by what parts of the body are exposed. A millirem is a standard unit for measuring radiation absorption.

Source: With permission from "Growing Debate over Dangers of Radiation," *U.S. News and World Report,* May 14, 1979, p. 25.

in the mouth and throat. At high-enough doses, death occurs rapidly.

Most of what is known about the dangers of radiation comes from studies of people exposed to extremely high levels, such as the survivors of the atom bombs dropped on Hiroshima and Nagasaki, and patients who were massively dosed with X-rays for ailments now no longer treated in this way. Problems that eventually surfaced,

Table 20.7

Guidelines for Safe Radiation Exposure

NCRP recommended guidelines, 1971.	
Maximum permissible dose	
Equivalent for occupational exposure	5000 mrem[a] in 1 year
Skin	1500 mrem in 1 year
Hands	7500 mrem (2500 per quarter)
Forearms	3000 mrem (1000 per quarter)
Dose limits for the public	
Individual	500
Student	100
Population dose limits	
Genetic	170
Somatic	170

[a] mrem - millirem.

sometimes after 20 to 30 years, included clouding of the lens of the eye, leukemia, thyroid cancer, and changes in the genetic material. Particularly vulnerable are fetuses, primarily during the first 3 months of development, and children under 10. Over 400,000 U.S. military personnel and civilians have been exposed to various levels of radiation while witnessing over 183 nuclear bomb detonations in the Pacific and Southwestern United States test sites from 1945 until 1965. Especially high incidences of leukemia have been observed among those exposed to low levels of radiation. Residents of Arizona, Nevada, and Utah—who witnessed these early atomic tests and were showered with fallout, and workers in nuclear plants and shipyards—may be most vulnerable to leukemia, lymphatic cancers, and their offspring to birth defects.

The interpretation and prediction of long-term effects of low-level radiation is difficult for several reasons. The effects of radiation may go unnoticed and may take several generations to become observable. Thus cancers may not appear for 20 to 30 years after continuous small doses of radiation exposure. Adding to the confusion of predicting long-range effects of radiation is the observation that the effects of radiation may mimic those of other diseases, which may not be radiation-related. Long-range effects of small-dose radiation exposure include increased susceptibility to secondary infections, leukemia, bone and skin cancers, sterility, and accelerated aging. Genetic damage may result in the birth of malformed children in later generations, while fetal exposure to radiation is associated with various cancers during childhood (leukemia). There is no specific treatment for radiation sickness. Radiation exposure can also cause damage to the sperm and/or egg, causing malformed fetuses, which are often naturally aborted.

Recently, controversy began over the safety of microwave ovens. Microwaves have been associated with the production of eye cataracts and with temporary sterility. Microwaves are absorbed by food, producing an instant temperature rise that causes food to cook quickly. These ovens have a nonionizing form of radiation and will not make food or other materials radioactive (see Figure 20.19). However, exposure of such waves to human or animal bodies causes the waves to be converted into instant heat and absorbed into the body. The heat causes molecules to vibrate very rapidly, thereby pulling the molecules apart, bringing chemical changes and eventual cell death.

The effects of radiation exposure are dependent on dose and the period of exposure. It makes considerable difference to the body whether a large dose of radiation is absorbed over the space of a few minutes or a few years. When a large dose is absorbed over a short interval of time, so many of the growing tissues lose the capacity for cell division that death may follow. If the same dose is delivered over a period of years, only a small bit of radiation is absorbed on any given day, and only small proportions of growing cells lose the capacity for division at any one time. The unaffected cells will continually make up for this defect and will replace the affected ones. As the body is continuously repairing the low-exposure radiation damage, no serious symptoms develop.

If a moderate dose is delivered, the body may show visible symptoms of radiation sickness but the body will recover. It will be capable of withstanding another moderate dose, and so on.

The situation is quite different with respect to genetic effects. Even the smallest doses will produce a few mutations in the chromosomes of those cells in the gonads that eventually develop into sex cells or sperms and eggs. The affected gonad cells will continue to produce sex cells with those mutations for the rest of the life of the person. Every tiny bit of radiation adds to the number

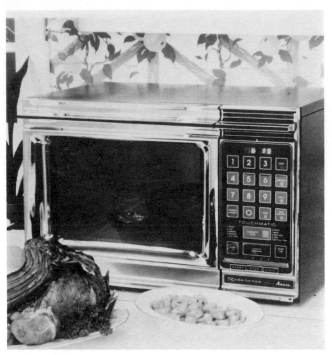

Figure 20.19
Microwave ovens save up to 75 percent of the electricity normally used in cooking foods. Microwaves cause food molecules to vibrate which in turn cooks the food. The waves pass through nonmetallic objects.

of mutated sex cells being constantly produced. Sex cells do not recover. What counts is the total sum or cumulative buildup of radiation and not how much or when one is exposed. In light of this hard fact, it is important for everyone to minimize radiation exposure, especially to sex cells. Reading about radiation has probably made you wonder whether you are exposing yourself to hazardous levels of radiation. Respond to the Radiation Dosage Inventory at the beginning of this chapter.

WAYS TO CUT DOWN EXPOSURE TO X-RAYS AND RADIATION

1. Have an X-ray only when a qualified M.D. specialist requests it.
2. Do not have an X-ray to detect tuberculosis.
3. Tell your M.D. and dentist about previous X-rays and urge them to use these.
4. Pregnant women should avoid X-ray exposure.
5. Use a lead shield to protect your reproductive organs if you must have an X-ray. Such a shield is not a complete safeguard, since radiation waves do not travel in straight lines.

6. Ask your doctor or dentist to explain how it will help in your diagnosis. Can an alternative nonradiating technique be used?

ALTERNATIVE SOURCES OF ENERGY

We are enormous consumers of energy in the Western world. Since the turn of this century, energy in the form of water and steam has been displaced by the gasoline and diesel engines. The latter, in turn, have been displaced by electric engines. We have evolved a life style at home and at work centered around the use of electricity. Our well-being is indirectly related to the use of energy. Our major concern today is to generate electricity in an ecologically clean and humanly safe way. We are presently doing so by burning fossil fuels, which are also major environmental polluters.

Man has used more energy in the past 30 years than in all history. We will need five times more energy by the year 2000 than we now use if we expect to continue to develop technologically at the same rate. The American need for energy surpasses all other countries. With only 6 percent of the world's population, we use 40 percent of the available world's natural resources, and 35 percent of the world's available energy. In 1979, the United States imported approximately one-half of its crude oil needs from foreign countries. Much of this oil is used to generate electricity. Since foreign oil markets are unreliable and cause economic problems, we need to explore alternative sources of power to generate electricity.

There are many ways to generate electricity (see Figure 20.20). The major alternative ways are summarized as follows:

1. *Steam generator plants* are fueled mostly by fossil fuels.
2. *Fossil fuels* to run electricity-producing generators, which generate 80 percent of our power today.
    (a) *Coal burning*—the dirtiest form of fuel; mining it creates waste lands and a real health hazard.
    (b) *Low sulfur oils*—big polluters of air, and limited availability.
    (c) *Natural gas*—the cleanest of fossil fuels, expensive, and limited in quantity.
3. *Hydroelectric plants* (4 percent) are good sources of energy, but most good locations for hydrodams have already been used up.
4. *Geothermal energy* is limited only to certain regions and has not been harnessed.
5. *Wind energy* is unreliable in many parts of the United States.

Energy Sources

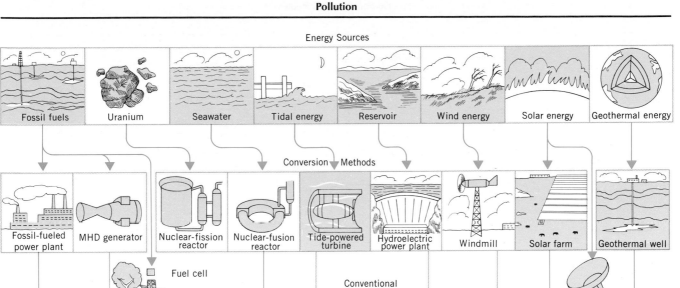

Figure 20.20

Summary of different alternatives for harnessing nature's energy surces. (With permission from Kenneth F. Weaver, "The Search for Tomorrow's Power," *National Geographic*, November 1972, pp. 650–681.)

6. *Nuclear fission plants* (supply 10 percent of our energy needs) use a limited supply of uranium-235, whose atoms are split, producing heat used to convert water into steam that, in turn, drives a turbine to generate electricity (see Figure 20.21). The accumulation of radioactive wastes and the possibility of the plant's blowing up make nuclear power a real life risk. There were 72 such plants operating in 1979 in this country (see Figure 20.22 and 20.23).

7. *The nuclear fusion plant* melts or fuses hydrogen atoms together to produce heat and energy. Hydrogen, in the form of deuterium and tritium, is readily available in inexhaustible quantities in seawater. This is the same kind of energy used by the sun, the stars, and the hydrogen bomb. This reactor is still in the developmental stage.

8. *Nuclear fast-breeder or fission plants* split uranium-238 or thorium-232 to produce 1 pound of plutonium-239 and 4 pounds of uranium-233. It produces more fuel than it uses. This type of nuclear reactor is more difficult to handle and control, and is potentially more dangerous than the conventional reactor. There are no fast-breeder plants operating in this country at the present time.

9. *Solar energy* is clean, readily available, but expensive, and 25 years from being harnessed on a large-scale basis. Solar energy is being harnessed to heat water, which, in turn, heats homes (see Figures 20.24 and 20.25).

10. *Pyrolysis* of waste refuse and garbage is presently very expensive and in a developmental stage. By-products include gas, fuel oil, heat, and recyclable products.

11. *Ocean currents and tide changes* may be harnessed in much the same way as water in a dam to generate electricity. These sources are in the developmental stage and would be nonpolluting.

12. *Ocean temperature-gradient-change power plants*—a temperature difference between warm surface water and near-freezing cold water 4000 feet deep would cause warm water to vaporize ammonia, which would then drive a turbogenerator and produce electricity. This power

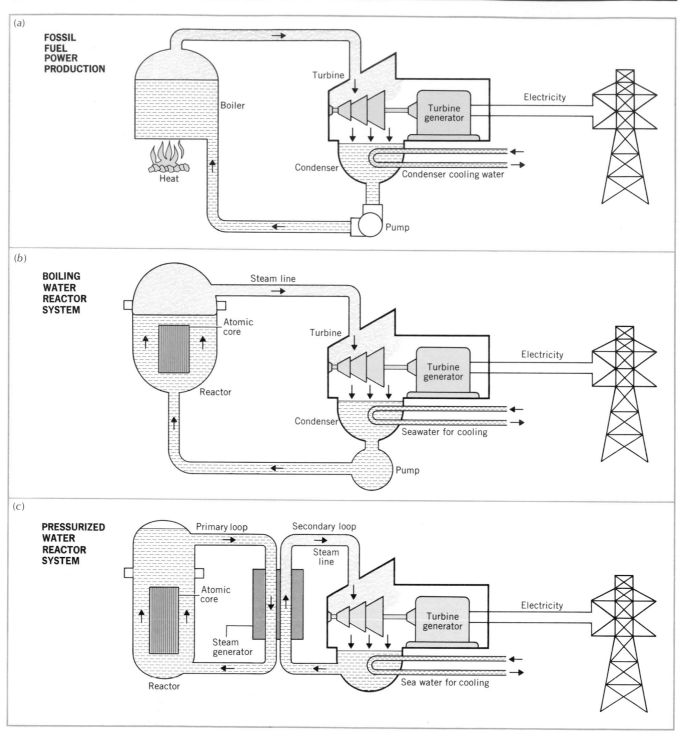

Figure 20.21

Comparison of two major ways of generating electricity. (a) Fossil fuel is used to heat water into steam which, in turn, drives a steam turbine that generates electricity. Nuclear power is substituted for fossil fuel to do the same thing. Two types of nuclear power systems [(b) and (c)] are used today. The system in (c) uses a closed primary radioactive loop to carry heat from the atomic core to the heat exchange unit (steam generator) which, in turn, heats water in the secondary loop to steam that drives the turbine. (Reproduced with permission from *Nuclear Power and the Environment,* (pamphlet), the U.S. Atomic Energy Commission and printed by American Nuclear Society, 1972.)

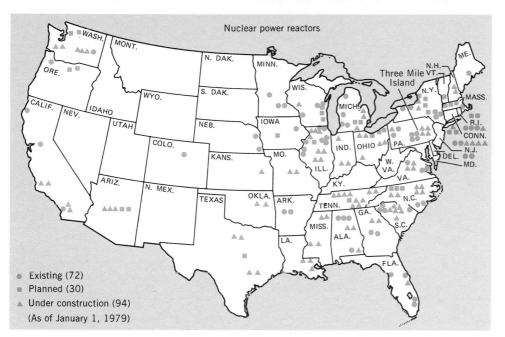

Figure 20.22
Locations of existing, under construction, and planned nuclear power plants in the United States as of January 1, 1979. (With permission from *Time, The Weekly Magazine,* Copyright © Time Inc., 1979.)

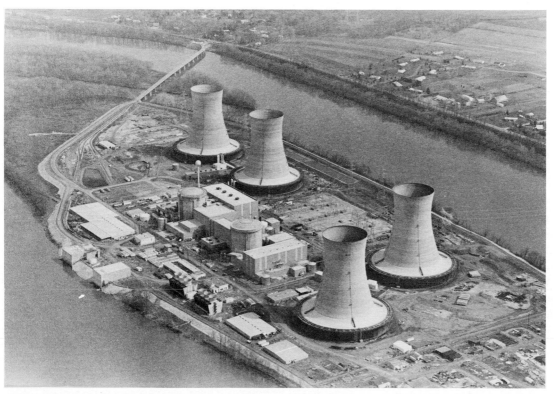

Figure 20.23
Fission reactor and nuclear power plant at Three Mile Island near Harrisburg, Pennsylvania. In 1979 this was the site of the greatest nuclear power plant disaster in this country. Did the incidence of birth defects in this area increase since then?

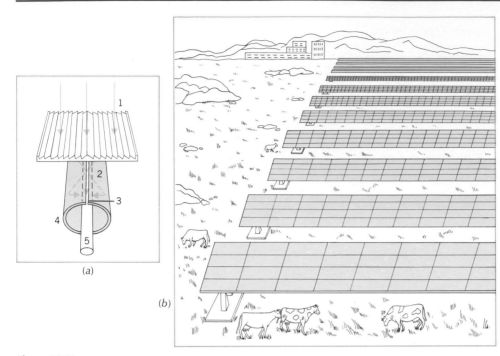

Figure 20.24
A suggestion for harnessing solar energy. (a) To reap the sun's enormous energy, Professor Aden B. Meinel and his wife, Marjorie, would cover areas of the Southwest with louverlike solar collectors. The land beneath them could still be used for grazing cattle or farming. In (b), ridged lenses (1), tilted toward the sun, train rays (2) down through a slot (3) into a glass pipe (4). Its mirrored inside surface reflects the heat onto a coated inner steel tube (5) that circulates gaseous nitrogen. Reaching temperatures of 1000° F., the gas flows to tanks of molten salts capable of storing the heat for nightime use. Steam heated by the salts drives turbines. The Meinels estimate a square mile of solar farm could supply power for a city of 60,000.

plant is in the developmental stage and would be nonpolluting.

13. *Salinity power plants* (see Figure 20.26) move fresh (river) water through a permeable membrane into salty ocean water at a flow pressure about 24 times atmospheric pressure, or equivalent to the water pressure of a dam 780 feet high. Every river outlet is such an untapped source of energy. This is in the developmental stage and would be nonpolluting.

14. *Human and animal power* provided most of the energy prior to 1700.

NUCLEAR PLANT CRISIS

The safety of nuclear power plants came to a head in April 1979, when the worst commercial nuclear accident in United States history occurred at the Three Mile Island power plant near Harrisburg, Pennsylvania. A broken pump in the reactor's secondary loop, coupled with errors in human judgment, led to other complications, eventually causing radioactive steam to escape into the air. The area outside the plant became radioactive. For 13 days, chaos and confusion marked the possibility of nuclear meltdown of the sort fictionalized in the popular film: "The China Syndrome" (see Figure 20.26). The Three Mile Island accident came at a time when the safety of nuclear power plants was being seriously challenged by outspoken critics, and on the eve of the second energy (gasoline) crisis. It demonstrated to the general public that nuclear power plants are not as safe as the Federal Nuclear Regulatory Commission, the utility and power companies, and nuclear scientists have led us to believe. There are many aspects of plant design and operation, and plant and waste security that have not been resolved. Almost all of the nuclear power plants have had physical breakdowns and shutdowns.

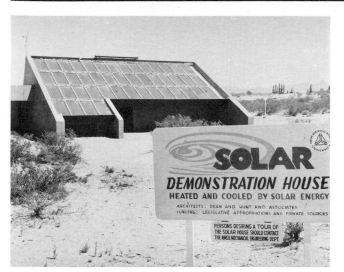

Figure 20.25

A home designed and built to harness solar energy to heat and cool it. In what way is this house designed differently from conventional homes?

Currently, nearly 5000 tons of radioactive wastes from 72 commercial reactors (1979) are temporarily stockpiled in vast underwater tanks at reactor sites and elsewhere, awaiting a permanent graveyard where they can be safely stored for 500 years or more that must pass before they decompose and are no longer toxic (27) (see Figure 20.27). The Three Mile Island accident has brought the controversy over the safety of nuclear power plants to a head. It exemplifies the threat of radioactivity to our well-being and environment. We need more reliable information about the safety of such plants. Summarized below are various considerations about the safety of nuclear power plants:

1. Building site—is it in an earthquake hazard area?
2. Melting point of core uncontrollable.
3. Breakdown in heat exchangers.

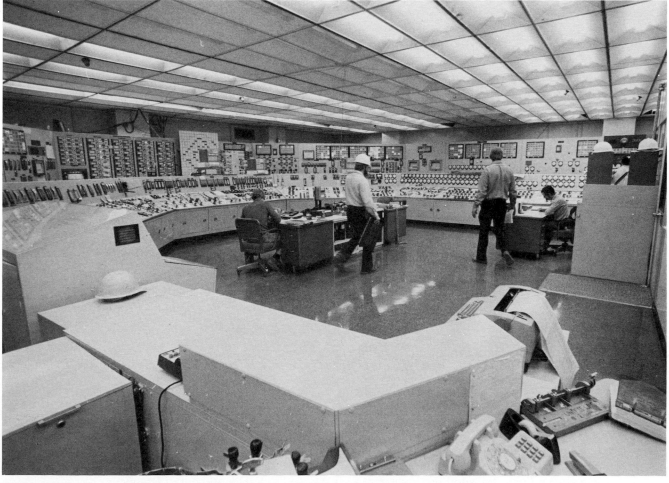

Figure 20.26

The control room at Three Mile Island. A real life crisis here in April, 1979, recalled *The China Syndrome,* a movie about a meltdown crisis in a nuclear power plant.

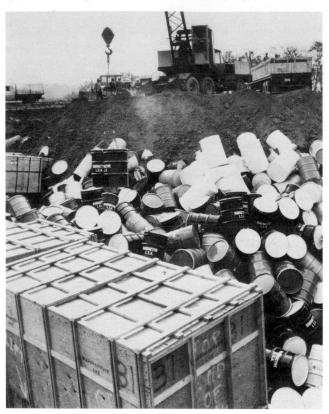

Figure 20.27

A nuclear dump site near Sheffield, Illinois. Steel drums containing low-level nuclear waste are dumped into a block-long, 30-foot-deep trench. How long will such plutonium and uranium wastes be radioactive? How far away from this dumping site must you be in order not to be exposed to radiation?

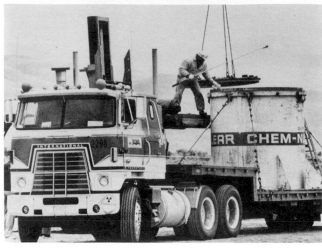

Figure 20.28

Workers at a radioactive waste disposal site in Hanford, Washington, remove lid from cannister holding sealed containers of low-level radioactive waste. The waste was transported to this site from Three Mile Island nuclear power plant in Harrisburg, Pennsylvania. How safe is it to transport radioactive wastes by truck across this country? Who authorizes such transportation of radioactive wastes?

4. Breakdown in primary and secondary hot water or sodium loop exchangers.
5. Dome as questionable safety system.
6. Lack of safe storage site for radioactive products.
7. Lack of validity testing of emergency safety systems in plants.
8. Great duration of half-life of radioactive substances.
9. No real accident radiation insurance available.
10. Nuclear power sites built in populated areas.
11. No public disclosure of results of periodic inspection of current nuclear power plants.
12. No evacuation plans for citizens near nuclear plants in the event of release of radioactivity.
13. Questionable nuclear power plant's emergency core-cooling system.
14. No nuclear radioactive waste-recycling plants to recycle such wastes (wastes are stored).
15. Extreme hazard of transporting radioactive wastes; impossible security.

16. Security of current nuclear power plants very weak.
17. Availability of uranium very limited and in short supply.

WHERE TO GO FOR MORE INFORMATION

1. Local or state Public Health Department
2. Local American Cancer Society chapter
3. Local American Lung Association chapter
4. Campus biology or life science department
5. Your health instructor
6. Local ecology group
7. State Department of Industrial Hygiene
8. Write to (re: pesticides, radiation, and pollution):
   Barry Commoner
   Citizen Soldier
   175 Fifth Avenue
   New York, N.Y. 10010
9. Write to (re: hazards of nuclear power):
   Union of Concerned Scientists
   1208 Massachusetts Avenue
   Cambridge, Mass. 02138
10. Write to (re: energy):
    U.S. Department of Energy
    Washington, D.C. 20585

11. Write to (re: energy publications):
    U.S. Department of Energy
    Technical Information Center
    P.O. Box 62
    Oak Ridge, Tenn. 37830
12. Write to (re: X-rays and radiation):
    Health Research Group
    2000 P Street N.W.
    Washington, D.C. 20036
13. Write to (re: nuclear energy hazards):
    Nuclear Information and Resources Service
    (NIRS)
    1536 Sixteenth Street N.W.
    Washington, D.C. 20036

14. National No Nukes Report
    628 Rubel Avenue
    Louisville, Ky. 40204
15. National Solar Heating & Cooling Information
    Center
    P.O. Box 1607
    Rockville, Md. 20850

Further Readings

Carmon, Richard, *Our Endangered Hearing,* Emmaus, Pa.: Rodale Press, 1977.

U.S. Department of Energy, "Put the Sun to Work Today," Pamphlet No. 0033(8-78).

Nader, Ralph, *The Menace of Atomic Power,* New York: Norton, 1979 (paperback).

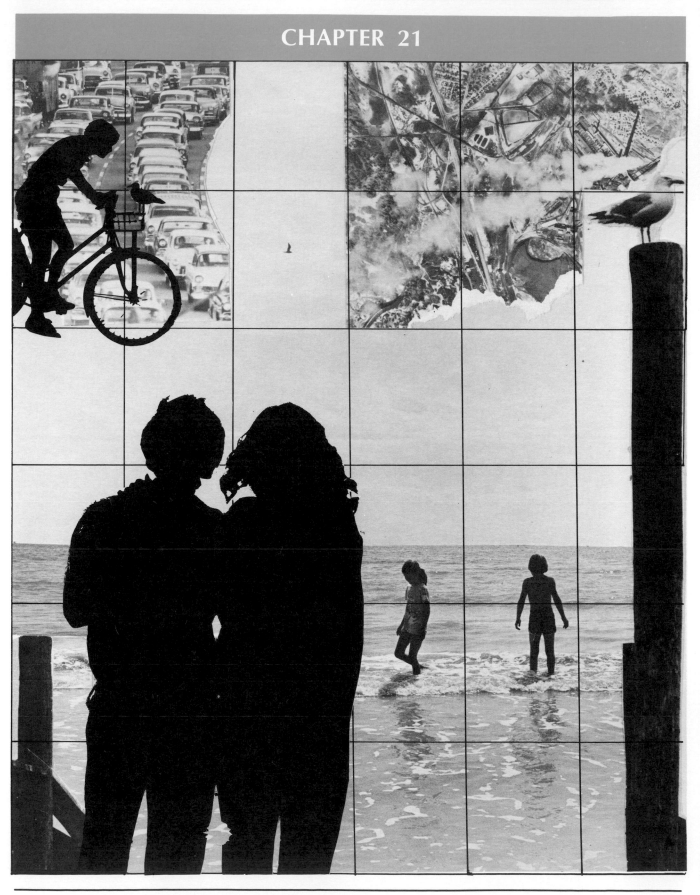

CHAPTER 21

APPROPRIATE TECHNOLOGY

Does eating beef meat contribute to our energy crisis?
Is your life style polluting our environment?
What really caused air pollution in the big cities?
How do fossil fertilizers contribute to the energy problem?
Does industrial progress dehumanize people?
Does technological progress result in more health?

These are just some of the questions that are discussed in this chapter. Using a philosophical approach, the chapter points out how our present technologies have displaced the old ones, thereby causing pollution, dehumanizing people, and indirectly contributing to many of our health problems. Inappropriate technologies have evolved an economical, political, and social way of life that needs to be assessed and modified if we are to attain optimal well-being.

React to the inventory that follows before reading this chapter.

☞ APPROPRIATE TECHNOLOGY INVENTORY

OBJECTIVES   1. To make you aware of the meaning of appropriate technology.
2. To help you determine whether you are using low-labor, inexpensive, energy-saving, and health promotional ways of living.
Are you an appropriate technology person?

DIRECTIONS   Circle the number to the right of each statement that best fits your behavior in this situation.
React to all statements.

	Always	Often	Sometimes	Never
A ☐ *Air Pollution* Do you:				
1. Walk to work, to stores, etc.	5	3	1	0
2. Bicycle to work, to stores, etc.	10	7	2	0
3. Use rapid transit (bus or train)	5	3	1	0

	Always	Often	Sometimes	Never
4. Go to work or shop in a car pool	5	3	1	0
5. Drive a small-engine car	5	3	1	0
6. Use unleaded gasoline	5	3	1	0
7. Live within 1 mile of your place of work or school	10	7	2	0
8. Drive under 55 mph	10	7	2	0
9. Have annual auto inspections	5	3	1	0
10. Get a car engine tuneup every 6 months or as needed	5	3	1	0
11. Avoid smoking cigarettes	10	7	2	0
12. Avoid using recreational campers	5	3	1	0
13. Have one car per family	10	7	2	0
14. Try to run many errands and shop with one trip	10	7	2	0
Subtotal				
B ☐ *Water Pollution*				
Do you:				
15. Use nondetergent soaps	5	3	1	0
16. Recycle waste water (kitchen sink) to water plants and garden	5	3	1	0
17. Shower instead of bathe	10	7	2	0
18. Wash car yourself instead of using car wash	5	3	1	0
Subtotal				
C ☐ *Soil Pollution*				
Do you:				
19. Use Plant humus and animal manure fertilizers instead of commercial nitrogen fertilizers	10	7	2	0
20. Use lady bugs and other natural ways to control insects instead of pesticides	10	7	2	0
21. Pull weeds out of garden and lawn by hand instead of using chemical weed killers	10	7	2	0

	Always	Often	Sometimes	Never
22. Use hand hoes and rakes to till gardens instead of gasoline-engine rotor tillers.	5	3	1	0
Subtotal				
D ☐ *Solid Wastes Disposal*				
Do you:				
23. Use biodegradable paper, cloth, or wooden wrappers, boxes and containers instead of plastic ones	10	7	2	0
24. Separate paper, glass, metals, and wood scraps from garbage (food wastes) and recycle these	10	7	2	0
25. Not litter	5	3	1	0
26. Recycle waste paper instead of burning it	10	7	2	0
Subtotal				
E ☐ *Food*				
Do you:				
27. Grow your own vegetables or fruit	20	15	5	0
28. Eat fresh vegetables or fruit	20	15	5	0
29. Drink water instead of soft drinks or beer	20	15	5	0
30. Cook your own meals at home instead of eating at restaurants and fast-food places	20	15	5	0
31. Have very few, if any, leftovers after a meal	10	7	2	0
32. Eat fish and vegetables instead of beef meat	20	15	5	0
33. Eat fresh vegetables and fruits instead of processed, refined, or canned foods	20	15	5	0
Subtotal				
F ☐ *Energy*				
Do you:				
34. Turn off room lights when not used	5	3	1	0
35. Use a manual can opener instead of electric one	10	7	2	0

	Always	Often	Sometimes	Never
36. Use a manual lawn mower instead of an electric or gaso-line-powered one	10	7	2	0
37. Insulate your house (apartment)	10	7	2	0
38. Buy or use cotton clothes instead of rayon or polyester clothes	5	3	1	0
39. Ship freight packages by train instead of by truck or air	10	7	2	0
40. Press or clean your own clothes instead of using a laundry	10	7	2	0
41. Have only one TV set at home	10	7	2	0
42. Buy recyclable bottled soft drinks or beer instead of canned soft drinks	5	3	1	0
43. Use paper instead of plastic bags	5	3	1	0
44. Avoid using air-conditioners	5	3	1	0
45. Shop for groceries not more than twice a week	5	3	1	0
46. Air dry your clothes on an outdoor clothes line	10	7	2	0
47. Wash dishes by hand instead of using a dishwasher	10	7	2	0
48. Sew (make) your own clothes instead of buying commercial ones	5	3	1	0
49. Use reusable plates and cups instead of paper ones	10	7	2	0
50. Put your sweater on in cold weather instead of turning the heat up	5	3	1	0
51. Buy clothes that last and are fashionable for 2+ years	5	3	1	0
52. Use sunlight (solar energy) to heat your house (and swimming pool water)	10	7	2	0
53. Use your radio only when you can listen to it	5	3	1	0
Subtotal				
G ☐ *Miscellaneous*				
Do you:				
54. Treat yourself for minor injuries, like small cuts and bruises, instead of going to the doctor or hospital	10	7	3	0

	Always	Often	Sometimes	Never
55. Relieve headaches yourself instead of going to the doctor or taking aspirin	10	7	3	0
56. Relieve the inability to sleep yourself instead of taking sleeping pills or going to the doctor	10	7	3	0
57. Self-assess or analyze your eating habits and diet every 6 months	20	15	5	0
58. Self-assess your high risks to health once a year or more often instead of having the doctor do it for you	20	15	5	0
59. Feel happy in your job (work)	30	20	5	0
60. Find your job (work) meaningful	30	20	5	0
Subtotal				

SCORING

Add your scores for each section.

INTERPRETATION

Each section has its own score range, and classifies you as an appropriate, intermediate, or inappropriate technology person. Upon completion of each section, you can study your behaviors or habits that make you an inappropriate technology person and determine how to change your life style in order to become an appropriate technology person.

Section A   Air Pollution

Score Range	Classification
+80	Appropriate, *efficient, thrifty, low polluter, energy saver, promoting optimal well-being*
79–35	Intermediate *(can improve)*
34–0	Inappropriate, *inefficient, extravagant, polluter, high-energy user, not promoting well-being; need to immediately change your behaviors and life style*

Section B   Water Pollution

+20	Appropriate, *efficient, thrifty, low polluter, energy saver, promoting optimal well-being*
19–12	Intermediate *(can improve)*
11–0	Inappropriate, *inefficient, extravagant, polluter, high-energy user, not promoting well-being; need to immediately change your behaviors and life style*

Section C   Soil Pollution

+25   Appropriate, *efficient, thrifty, low polluter, energy saver, promot-*
               ing optimal well-being

24–10   Intermediate *(can improve)*

9–0   Inappropriate, *inefficient, extravagant, polluter, high-energy*
               user, not promoting well-being; need to immediately change
               your behaviors and life style

Section D   Solid Waste Disposal

+25   Appropriate, *efficient, thrifty, low polluter, energy saver, promot-*
               ing optimal well-being

24–8   Intermediate *(can improve)*

7–0   Inappropriate, *inefficient, extravagant, polluter, high-energy*
               user, not promoting well-being; need to immediately change
               your behaviors and life style

Section E   Food

+120   Appropriate, *efficient, thrifty, low polluter, energy saver, promot-*
               ing optimal well-being

119–40   Intermediate *(can improve)*

39–0   Inappropriate, *inefficient, extravagant, polluter, high-energy*
               user, not promoting well-being; need to immediately change
               your behaviors and life style

Section F   Energy

+125   Appropriate, *efficient, thrifty, low polluter, energy saver, promot-*
               ing optimal well-being

124–50   Intermediate *(can improve)*

49–0   Inappropriate, *inefficient, extravagant, polluter, high-energy*
               user, not promoting well-being; need to immediately change
               your behaviors and life style

Section G   Miscellaneous

+105   Appropriate, *efficient, thrifty, low polluter, energy saver, promot-*
               ing optimal well-being

104–40   Intermediate *(can improve)*

39–0   Inappropriate, *inefficient, extravagant, polluter, high-energy*
               user, not promoting well-being; need to immediately change
               your behaviors and life style

This inventory assesses whether your life style is made up of appropriate technology. It should make you aware of the degree to which you are using low-labor, simple, inexpensive, non- or low-pollution, energy-saving, and health promotion ways of living. Remember that your daily habits and ways of living are reflected in how you contribute to environmental degradation, the energy crisis, and well-being. Statements selected were those that you have choice or control over and, therefore, can make subjective and behavioral decisions about.

Most of the statements used in this inventory should be self-explanatory by now or will be explained in this chapter. Statement 32 is an exception and illustrates appropriate technology. Beef meat is one of the most energy-intensive foods because of the fuel and petroleum-based fertilizer needed to produce feed grains for cattle. If everyone in the United States were to substitute a pound of fish once a month for a pound of beef, we would save 100 million barrels of oil annually. Replacing red meat with vegetable proteins and fish not only saves energy, but reduces the risk of heart disease and cancer. An appropriate technology person is one who eats more fish and vegetables than red meat.

If your score classified you as an intermediate or inappropriate technology person, you should review each section and identify those statement behaviors that were inappropriate, and try to change your life style.

Read the remainder of this chapter for more information on appropriate technology.

Our way of life has been built upon a prodigious consumption of energy—energy derived mostly from the burning of fossil fuels. Numerous technologies (2;5;10;12;13;16;17;22) have been created that need energy to produce consumer products and services. We have been obtaining energy and using it to manufacture products without ecological checks or balances to stop the pollution of our environment.

The quest for more energy and the degrading of our environment began with the end of World War II. Overnight, so it seems, the industrial era was transformed into a technological era. Electricity gradually replaced the internal combustion engine as a source of factory energy (see Table 21.1). Consumer commodities were produced on assembly lines and flooded the consumer markets. Human labor was gradually displaced by automation and computers—both of which increased the demand for electricity. This kind of "want" and "keep up with the Joneses" progress was not free and was obtained at the expense of degrading the environment.

Thus most pollution problems festered gradually in the years following World War II. For example, from 1940 to 1970, phosphate pollution of river and lake waters increased sevenfold; nitrogen oxides from automobiles (which trigger the formation of smog) increased 630 percent; tetraethyl lead from gasoline increased in the air by 415 percent; mercury from chloralkali plants increased by 2100 percent; synthetic pesticide pollution increased 270 percent; use of inorganic nitrogen fertilizer (some of which leaches into surface water) on farms increased by 789 percent; and the quantity of nonreturnable beer bottles increased by 595 percent (5:125). These are only a few examples of the consequences of technological progress. The last 50 years have seen a sweeping revolution in science, which in turn has harnessed technology into industry, agriculture, transportation, and communication (5:122–138).

World War II was a decisive turning point in this historical transition. Chemistry and physics knowledge that gathered dust before World War II was pressured into military use. The new production technology, as we know it now, is based on the harnessing of that chemistry and physics knowledge. Under the military demands of World War II, scientific knowledge was rapidly converted into new technologies and productive enterprises. Chemical industries, for example, increased productivity between 1958 and 1968 by 73 percent as compared with only a 39 percent increase for all manufacturing (5:131). Between 1949 and 1968, the population of the United States increased by only 34 percent, while the annual agricultural use of nitrogen fertilizer increased by 648 percent (5:147). Similarly, for the same period, the production of organic chemicals increased 746 percent in an effort to provide raw chemicals for the synthesis of new synthetic fibers, plastics, detergents, pesticides, and drugs (5:167). Chemical products increased the stress on our environment. Just as the industrial revolution had a detrimental effect on the living conditions of city workers, so the chemical feast in the 1950s and 1960s concentrated populations in cities, causing overcrowding, and worsening the pollution problems. Also, just as the Industrial Revolution provoked social deprivation and the loss of values, so the urbanization of the 1950s and 1960s deteriorated social conditions and contributed to confusion about human values and the meaning of life.

Urbanization itself is not to blame for pollution. Nor is the increase in population. Instead, urbanization created a maldistribution of the living and working places in metropolitan areas (5:132). Urbanization compacted the density of cars in metropolitan areas, which immediately compounded the pollution problems. For example, in the years from 1947 to 1968, the total number of vehicles on United States roads increased 166 percent, the total vehicle-miles traveled increased by 174 percent, resulting in an increase in total emissions of nitrogen oxides by about 700 percent and twice as much lead pollution. Overall, smog levels in the cities from 1947 to 1968 has been estimated as increasing by about 1000 percent (5:165). Thus most of the sharp increase in air pollution levels is due not so much to population or affluence as to changes in production technology and the style of living.

Urbanization trends in the United States also reflect the lack of a plan for growth and development. It is really helter-skelter for profit development. Urbanization illustrates inept and disgraceful management of both our environment and social life styles. This country

Table 21.1
How Man's Life Style and Energy Sources Have Changed Through History

Historical Era	Stone	Agriculture	Bronze + Dark	Industrial Revolution	Technology	Post-technology Electro-magnetic
Time	1,000,000–15,000 B.C.	15,000–4000 B.C.	4000 B.C.–1700 A.D.	1700–1930	1930–1960	1960 to present
Time span (years)	4,500,000	11,000	6000	300	30	?
Vocational lifestyle	Hunter	Hunter Farmer	Farmer Craftsman artist	Factory worker Craftsman Farmer	Professional Factory worker	Consumer Professional Factory worker
Housing, life style	Live in caves, packs	Life in huts in tribal village	Houses Walled Cities	City dwellers	City dwellers Track homes	Apartments and condominiums City dwellers Urban sprawl
Major mode of transportation	Foot	Foot	Horse and buggy Sailing ships	Train Steam ships Horse and buggy	Auto Ships Airplanes	Jets and space travel Auto and trucks Ships (diesel)
Source of power (major)	Man	Man Water and wind	Slaves Man Animals Solar Wind	Coal Water (hydro) Fossil oil Machines replacing man	Fossil oil Natural gas Hydro	Electricity Nuclear power Coal Solar Electro-magnetic
Food production	Animals Wild Berries	Domesticated animals Crops	Crops Animals Fowl	Grazing animals Crops Fruits	Animal fertilizer Refrigeration Canning Grazing animals	Fossil fertilizer Frozen foods Fast foods Stock-fed animals
Communication of ideas	Probably sounds	Symbols Talk	Songs Story telling Horse	Wireless Newspapers Radio	Newspapers Radio Telephone	Television Telecommunications Computer
Dominant theme	Hunting survival	Survival Till soil Domesticate animals	Horse and Buggy Commerce Metallurgy	Steam engine Train Radio Movies Newspapers Capitalism	Internal combustion engine Autos Trucks and freeways Chemical technology	Electricity Nuclear technology Mass media (TV) Computers Space flight Leisure time

produces more pollution for the size of its population than any other country in the world (5:133).

Thus there is a similarity between the impact on environment that the influx of people from the country into the cities had during the industrial era as compared to the concentration of populations in large cities since World War II. In both instances, human waste and pollu-tants accumulated at a faster pace than they could be disposed of, or degraded, by nature.

Urbanization has brought about economic growth. Economic growth, in turn, has evolved new demands for consumer products (foods, clothing, shelter, and transportation), new ways of using them (plastic food packaging and frozen foods), and new ways of producing such products. Not only did the technologies change, but they initiated emergent life styles that created continuing demands for products and services. The kinds of goods produced have changed and new production technologies have displaced old ones.

It is important to illustrate this concept—the displacement of old production methods by new technologies. The concept of displacement is to a large measure responsible for pollution. For example (5:142–143), soap powder has been displaced by synthetic detergents; natural fibers (cotton and wool) have been displaced by synthetic ones; steel and lumber have been displaced by aluminum, plastics, and concrete; railroad freight has been displaced by truck freight; returnable bottles have been displaced by nonreturnable ones. On the road, the low-powered nonpolluting automobile engines of the 1920s and 1930s have been displaced by high-powered polluting ones. On the farm, artificial fertilizer has displaced stubble and animal manure fertilizers. Older methods of insect control have been displaced by synthetic insecticides such as DDT, and

herbicide sprays have replaced the cultivator in controlling weeds. The range-feeding of livestock has been displaced by feedlots (see Figures 21.1 and 21.2). In each of these cases, what has changed drastically is the technology of production rather than the economic goods produced (see Table 21.2).

Although the production of goods has changed, this change has not significantly increased the average person's consumption of basic goods. We still eat about the same calories of some foods, use about the same number of clothes, require about as much freight, and so on. However, the food is now grown on less land with much more fertilizer and pesticides than before; clothes, made of synthetic fibers rather than cotton or wool, are laundered with synthetic detergents rather than biodegradable soap; the goods are shipped by truck rather than rail, and so on.

These primary changes have led to other changes. To provide the raw materials needed for the new synthetic fibers, pesticides, detergents, and plastics, the production of synthetic organic chemicals has grown rapidly.

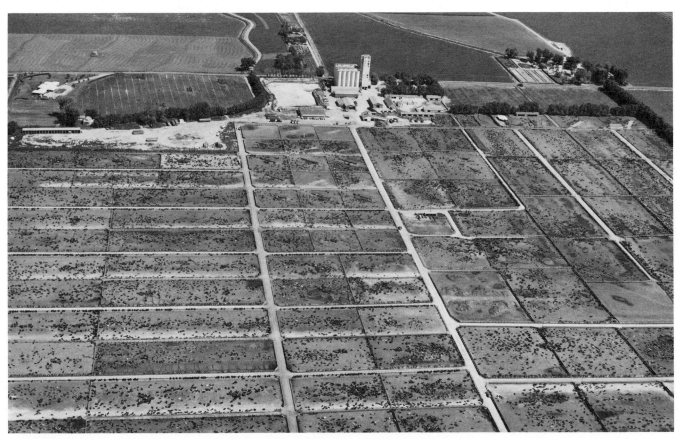

Figure 21.1
Sprawling cattle feedlot in Colorado. Here thousands of steers are fattened by minimizing their activity, force-feeding, and using chemicals in feeds to stimulate a quicker weight gain. Beef meat from such steers contains more fat than found in beef meat of grass-grazing and active steers. Does force-feeding cattle cause beef meat to have chemicals hazardous to your health?

497

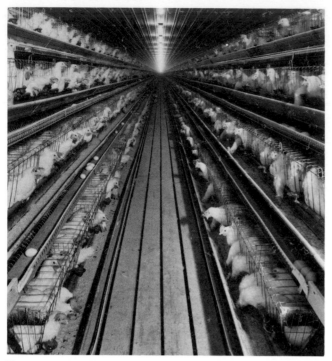

Figure 21.2

Chicken-ranch technology. Chickens are cooped up in cages and fed special chemicals along with chicken feed to force-produce more eggs. Does this farming approach cause eggs (and chicken meat) to have excessive amounts of chemicals?

Such synthetics require large amounts of chlorine. To make chlorine, large amounts of electricity are passed through a salt solution by way of a mercury electrode. Consequently, mercury consumption for this purpose

has increased almost 4000 percent since World War II (5:143). Similarly, chemical products, as well as aluminum, gobble up large amounts of electrical power. This escalation of economic growth is the major cause of environmental degradation.

Economic growth has created an increasing demand for electricity. The annual power consumption in the United States is about 20,540 kilowatt-hours per capita (5:170). Electricity produces goods that, in turn, contribute to human health needs. However, new postwar technologies are more costly than the technologies they have displaced. For example, aluminum, in displacing steel and lumber as a construction material, requires for its production about 15 times more fuel energy than steel and about 150 times more fuel energy than lumber (5:170). (See Figure 21.3.) Thus there is a growing demand for more electricity. The demand for energy has become an octopus.

An interesting but disturbing aspect of technological displacement is that many products, having a very low human value and need, are manufactured in increasingly larger amounts of environmentally harmful wrappings and nondegradable plastic containers. The result is mounting heaps of rubbish.

The environmental crisis entered into this country's political arena in 1970. Numerous pieces of environmental legislation were enacted to clean up the air, water, and soil. The ecology movement reached a national peak in April 1970, when Earthweek focused on environmental awareness. Earthweek died a slow death in the next 2 years, when this country suffered a series of small economic setbacks. Still struggling to clean up the environment, the country was gripped by unexpected energy crises in 1973 and 1979. We started to run short

Table 21.2

Displacement of Inexpensive, Old Production Methods by Expensive Technologies

Inexpensive Products of Old Industry (factories)	Expensive Products of New Technologies
1. Soap powder	Synthetic detergent
2. Natural fabric clothing (cotton and wool)	Synthetic fiber clothing (rayon)
3. Lumber and steel	Aluminum
	Plastics
	Concrete
4. Railroad freight	Truck and airline freight
5. Returnable bottles	Nonreturnable bottles
6. Auto engines small and low-powered	Large, high-powered engines
7. Fertilizer—manure and stubble	Fossil fertilizer
8. Natural biological control of insects	Synthetic insecticides and spraying
9. Open-range grass feeding of cattle	Feedlots
10. Steam and animal power	Fossil power

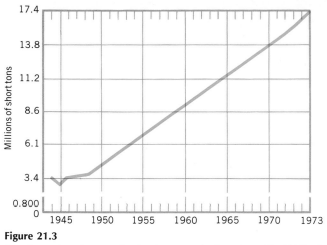

Figure 21.3

The stupendous increase in aluminum production since World War II reflects the worldwide economic expansion that has led to the scarcities of recent years. Almost no aluminum was produced before 1900; today aluminum follows iron as the world's second most used metal. (With permission from David Novick, "Facing Up to a World of Scarcities," *The Futurist,* August 19, p. 220. Copyright © by *The Futurist,* published by the World Future Society, 4916 St. Elmo Avenue, Washington, D.C., 20014.)

of gasoline and crude oil; crude oil production in the United States was unable to meet the domestic energy demands. At this time, despite promises of self-sufficiency in oil production, we were importing almost 50 percent of our annual crude oil needs in 1976 to 1979 as compared to about 25 percent in 1973, while our total consumption of barrels of crude oil per day was the same in 1973 and 1976 (37). About 43 percent of the imported crude oil in 1979 came from the Mideast oil-producing nations (see Figure 21.4). Imported oil siphons off the spendable dollars that this country so desperately needs. Since there is an economic trade-off ("You don't get a free meal"), we export food products to balance our importing-of-oil spending. Consequently,

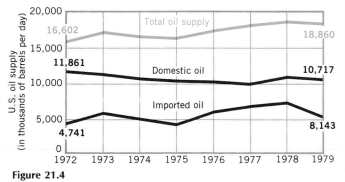

Figure 21.4

Crude oil supply and amount used by the United States in 1972 to 1979. Imported oil as a share of all U.S. supply has risen from 29 percent in 1972 to 43 percent today. (With permission from *U.S. News and World Report,* July 30, 1979, p. 25. Copyright © 1979, U.S. News and World Report, Inc.)

this added cost is passed on to the American consumer, who pays more for a loaf of bread, for vegetables, fruit, and dairy products (32;40). Thus, once more, people are theorizing about who is to blame for the energy crisis.

From the energy crises of the past, we can anticipate future energy crises. The transportation technology exemplifies an energy-economics holocaust. Let us take a look at what technology has done to transportation to disrupt ecology. Trucks have displaced railroads in hauling freight. The energy required to move 1 ton of freight 1 mile by rail now averages about 624 btu, while trucks require about 3460 btu per ton-mile (see Table 21.3). This means that, for the same freight-haulage, trucks burn nearly 6 times as much fuel as railroads and emit about 14 times as much environmental pollution (5:169). At the same time, the amount of power required to produce the cement and steel needed to lay down a mile of four-lane highway (essentially for truck traffic) is 3.6 times the power needed to produce the steel track for comparable rail traffic (5:169). This analysis points out the gross economic mismanagement of our transportation system. We do not need more freeways. We need transportation systems that use less oil and gasoline, that pollute less, and that use up less land space.

An analysis of the mismanagement of our transportation system and other similar technological displacements illustrates several important concepts about our economy, politics, style of living, and pollution. The expansion of energy products in the United States is not an accurate measure of increased economic good, being badly inflated by the growing tendency to displace power-thrifty goods with power-consumption ones (5:197). Our life styles have become extravagant, thoughtless, and unplanned. We could get by without many electric gadgets and high-energy products. Moreover, the real payoff in the use of energy and displaced low-cost materials should be improved social welfare, the attainment of optimal well-being, the control of debilitating diseases, and extended longevity. None of these socially aspiring goals are being fulfilled. Even wealthy industrialists, like the late Howard Hughes, have been unable to enjoy these utopian luxuries of technology.

Thus environmental degradation is caused by politics, economics, and life style. Many new technologies currently dominating production in this country are in conflict with the human-natural environmental ecosystem. Environmental degradation results from the introduction of new transportation, industrial, and agricultural production techniques. These technologies are ecologically faulty because they are designed to solve singular, separate problems and fail to take into account the inevitable side-effects that arise. In natural ecosystems, no part is isolated from the whole ecosystem. Un-

Table 21.3

Energy and Price Data for Intercity Freight Transport: 1970*

Mode	Btu per Route (ton-mile)	Freight Price (cents/ton-mile)	Btu per Route (passenger mile)
1. Pipeline	450	0.27	
2. Bicycle (@ 8 mph)			310
3. Ship (waterway)	440 domestic	0.30	
4. Railroad train	680	1.4	3230 intercity 3500 commuter 2750 rapid transit
5. Passenger bus			1010 intercity 2180 transit (excluding school buses)
6. Highway trucking	2470 intercity	7.5	
7. Private automobile			5400 5210
8. Jet plane	14070	21.9	6440

Source: Data taken from Hirst, Eric, 1973. "Energy intensiveness of passenger and freight transport modes, 1950–1970." Oak Ridge National Laboratory, Oak Ridge, Tennessee, operated by Union Carbide Corporation for the Department of Energy; and update March 14, 1980 by A. B. Rose, of Oak Ridge National Laboratory, Oak Ridge, Tennessee.

fortunately, most of today's wastes of technology are not being recycled into the ecosystems.

Population growth was considered a favorable indicator of social and economic progress up to 1970, but such population growth in this and other countries is making more and more demands for resources on our environment. We are taking fresh water out of the ground roughly twice as fast as natural processes replace it. The demand for electric power in the United States has been doubling every 10 years, and most of our power still comes from heavily polluting fossil fuels. We are building 10 million cars a year, twice as many as we built only 17 years ago. Cars burn gasoline and spew oxides

and lead as chemical pollutants; grind rubber tires to dust; and wear asbestos brakes into an acrid powder, which we inhale. Until 1970 these figures were considered proud evidences of progress. It was falsely assumed that the standard of living would also improve.

Numerous economists and scientists have studied the population explosions and their impact on pollution and the quality of life. Professor Jay W. Forrester of the Massachusetts Institute of Technology met with two dozen of the best political, economic, scientific, medical, and administrative persons in the world in Switzerland in 1970 to discuss the ecological problems of the world (14). The result was the design of an ecological computer program to predict the consequences of continued technological growth and its inherent social way of living. The questions raised were: Is there a limit to how many people we can support? Will we run out of natural resources? Can we produce enough food to feed all the people in this world? Will we create too much pollution while producing food and consumer products? Is there a limit to growth? After several years of computer analysis, they concluded that there is a limit to growth. Their conclusions are summarized in Figure 21.5 Unless we place limits on population growth and technology, the effects of population, food shortages, and depletion of natural resources will cause global diseases, malnutrition, and starvation, a lowering of the quality of well-being, and world wars that collectively threaten the survival of man in the near future. The pollutions discussed in the previous chapter are merely early warning signs that this is already happening. Many scientists do not agree with these doomsday projections, but such

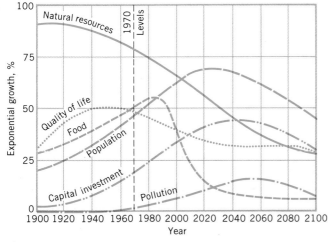

Figure 21.5

Limits to growth. This graphic computer model of Forrester and Meadows is based on a world standard. All variables plotted follow the historical values of five representative world countries from 1900 to 1970. This model assumes no major change in physical, economic, or social relationships in the world. Food and industrial output and population grow exponentially until rapidly depleting resources force a slowdown in industrial growth. Population and pollution continue to increase for some time after industrialization peaks. Decreased food supplies and lack of medical services are perceived as eventually causing population growth to slow down. The projected critical time for "all hell to break loose" is between 1975 and 2000. (*Source: The Limits to Growth: A Report for The Club of Romes' Project on the Predicament of Mankind,* by Donella H. Meadows, Dennis L. Meadows, Jorgen Randerg, William W. and Behrens, III. A Potomac Associate book published by Universe Books, New York, 1972, 1974. Graphics by Potomac Associates and adapted by author.)

projections have forced everyone to take a hard, objective look at our environment, our technologies, and our way of life.

Other scientists and economists, such as futurists Marquis de Condorcet of France and Willis Harman of Standford University, have attempted to identify probable alternative futures of the United States (11). Their collective conclusions suggest that the pollution, food, health, natural resources, economic and quality of life problems and solutions are a "world macroproblem." This means that our current social-economic-political-health problems (e.g., depression and emotional distresses, alienation, drug and alcohol abuse, poverty, health-medical problems, unemployment, inflation, environmental deterioration, crime, and so on) can only be solved on a world (or macro) basis. We need to transform our technological society and its materialistic attitudes and assumptions into a posttechnological society where the life style would be more compatible with fulfilling the basic human needs of all people. In a sense, it means rediscovering many enduring values, attitudes, and stable ways of living of the past.

The world-renowned English economist, Fritz Schumacher (16;17) in his books, *Small is Beautiful* and *A Guide for the Perplexed,* has presented some of the most advanced thinking on such a transformation. He suggests restructuring the world's present technological system into more "appropriate or intermediate technology" and a way of resolving our present social-ecological and economic problems. Schumacher's basic thesis is that the present political, economic, and social systems result from today's technology and cannot be basically altered except by changing the practices of technology and its assumptions and prevailing attitudes. He suggests decentralizing complex, big-energy-using, and automated low-labor-involved technologies into simple, small, high-labor-employed, and low-energy-using technologies (see Figure 21.6). These more *appropriate technologies* would utilize methods and equipment that would be inexpensive, would employ many human beings in meaningful work, would be accessible to everyone, would be suitable for small-scale application, would be discreet in the use of scarce materials, would be compatible with man's need for creativity and work, and would be less polluting (16:34). Appropriate technology implies a redefinition of economic efficiency. An example of *appropriate technology* for use in the third-world countries is the use of a new irrigation pump that is inexpensive and operates with human labor rather than diesel power (21) (see Figure 21.7). The use of human labor reduces the need for fossil fuel, thus easing the farmer's capital outlays, easing his country's need for foreign exchanges, and thereby easing the world's energy problems. Examples of appropriate technologies in

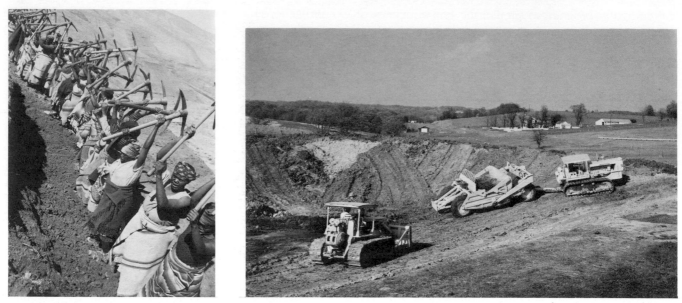

Figure 21.6

An example of simple and appropriate technology (on the left) as contrasted with modern and complex technology (right). Laborers in Basutoland, South Africa, do the same job that a bulldozer and carryall does in this country. Use of labor-intensive rather than capital-intensive methods makes sense in countries with large numbers of unemployed people and little capital or foreign exchange. Can we save money and energy in this country by using less expensive technology?

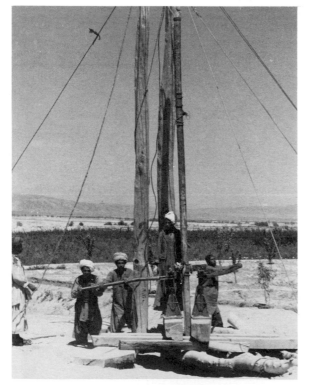

Figure 21.7

Using human power to drill a water well in an arid area near Quetta, in Baluchistan. What are the advantages of using this manual drill over a diesel power drill for the people in this country?

this country include using manual can openers, using recyclable bottles, using solar energy heaters, and using wind-driven electric generators on the roofs of homes to generate domestic electricity. This would allow people to become energy-independent, to find pleasure and meaning in work, and to evolve more purposeful life styles (see Figure 21.8).

Our obsession with technology and pure science has overlooked how to parallel such progress with values and a wise philosophy of life. According to Schumacher (17), ''the result of the lopsided development of the last 300 years is that Western man has become rich in means and poor in ends.'' His will is paralyzed because he has lost the grounds on which to base a hierarchy of values. Man must get to know himself as a social being or continue to suffer a steady decline in health and happiness, no matter how high his standard of living or how successful health services are in prolonging his life. We need metaphysical answers to life if we are to avoid living in a state of continuous anxiety, and if we are to stop providing ever more organized welfare to an emotionally, spiritually, and socially crippled society that lacks social cohesion (17:150–154). We must spread concepts of values and metaphysics (philosophy of the origin, meaning, and purposes of life) so that people will have the wisdom to deploy natural resources and use technology and energy for the benefit of all mankind.

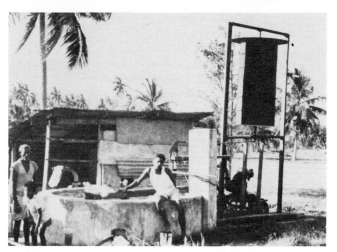

Figure 21.8
A windmill made from a split oil drum pumps water for these villagers in Sri Lanka.

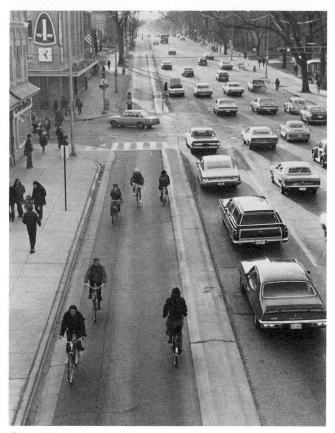

Figure 21.9
Bicycle lanes are given priorities in Madison, Wisconsin. Is this an example of appropriate technology in this country? Are bicycles more efficient than automobiles in terms of energy consumed?

These are ways that Schumacher suggests to resolve our environmental degradation on a long-range basis.

How then do we solve our immediate pollution prolems? The answer is obvious: Technologies need to be selected that minimize the hazards to people, that do not pollute, and that provide meaning to life. Present production technologies need to be redesigned to conform as closely as possible to ecological requirements. The technologies contributing most to pollution are industry, communications, agriculture, and transportation. We need to redesign our technology to include systems that return sewage and garbage directly to the soil, replace many synthetic materials with natural ones, reverse current agricultural policies from land retirement to cultivation, encourage the use of natural fertilizers instead of heavy nitrogen fertilizers, replace synthetic pesticides with biological ones, discourage power-consuming industries, encourage the return to low-cost and efficient land transportation (see Figure 21.9); recycle more refuse (paper, glass, and metals), build ecological solar homes, and institute better land management policies. This is not a comprehensive abatement list, but it suggests ideas for class and home projects. In addition to redesigning our technologies, we cannot overlook the need to reconstruct our life styles. Although redesigning technologies will affect individual life styles, reconstructing individual life styles at the same time eases the pain of change and evolves receptivity to such change. These life style changes should include using a train or bus instead of a car or airplane, growing your own garden, using a mechanical can opener instead of an electric one, and so on. We need to rely more on natural products and human energy and less on expensive electric and fossil energy.

Perhaps more important than these suggestions for dealing with our physical problems is to return to the traditional education of values, skills of socializing, and the identification of meaning and purpose in life. With natural resources shrinking and worldwide unemployment growing rapidly, our society needs to immediately transform its present technology and life style into those that are more compatible with our human needs.

WHERE TO GO FOR MORE INFORMATION

1. The following groups and publications:
   (a) National Center for Appropriate Technology
       Box 3838
       Butte, Mont. 59701

       Started with an initial grant from the Community Services Administration, the National Center for Appropriate Technology is working to develop appropriate technologies in low-income neighborhoods. It provides technical assistance and grants to cummunity action agencies.

(b) Appropriate Technology Project
Volunteers in Asia
Box 4543
Stanford, Calif. 94305

Volunteers in Asia is a small group of young university students who have gone to Asia each year to assist in developmental projects. One of their important contributions is their "Appropriate Technology Sourcebook," which summarizes the many plans available from alternative technology design centers.

(c) Brace Research Institute
P.O. Box 400
MacDonald Campus of McGill University
St. Anne de Bellevue 800
Quebec, Canada

Since 1961 Brace has been working in active collaboration with rural dwellers throughout the world to develop technologies that make the villager feel part of the achievement. Outstanding products include solar stills, wind pumps, solar driers, steam cookers, sulfur block houses, greenhouses, and low-cost steam turbines.

(d) Rain
2270 N.W. Irving
Portland, Oreg. 97210

America's most comprehensive *Journal of Appropriate Technology* reports on who is doing what in recycling, energy, agriculture, architecture, community development, ecotopia, health, and environment.

(e) Intermediate Technology Publications Ltd.
9 Kings Street, Covent Garden
London, WC2E, 8HN, England

Intermediate Technology Publications Ltd. publishes its quarterly journal *"Appropriate Technology"* as well as documents in the fields of agriculture, building, chemistry, rural health cooperative accounting, industry, rural workshops, water, and similar topics.

(f) Walden Foundation
P.O. Box 5
El Rito, N.Mex. 87530

The Walden Foundation's James DeKorne is well known for his "Survival Greenhouse," the bestseller publication which describes an ecosystem approach to home food production. His current system combines hydroponic gardening in a carbon dioxide atmosphere maintained by maximized rabbit production and fish farming. In addition, he has added a Windcharger electric system solar heating and worm composting to supply both food for catfish and an organic hydroponic solution for vegetables in a semiunderground greenhouse.

(g) For more publications and groups, refer to *The Futurist,* April 1977, p. 101

2. Write to:
   (a) National Center for Appropriate Technology, Butte, Mont.
   (b) Office of Appropriate Technology
   1530 Tenth Street
   Sacramento, Calif. 95814
   (c) National Solar Heating/Cooling Information Center
   P.O. Box 1607
   Rockville, Md. 20850
   (d) Your state center for appropriate technology.

Further Readings

Commoner, Barry, *The Closing Circle,* New York: Bantam Books, 1974.

Schumacher, E. F., *Small Is Beautiful: Economics as if People Mattered,* New York: Harper, 1973.

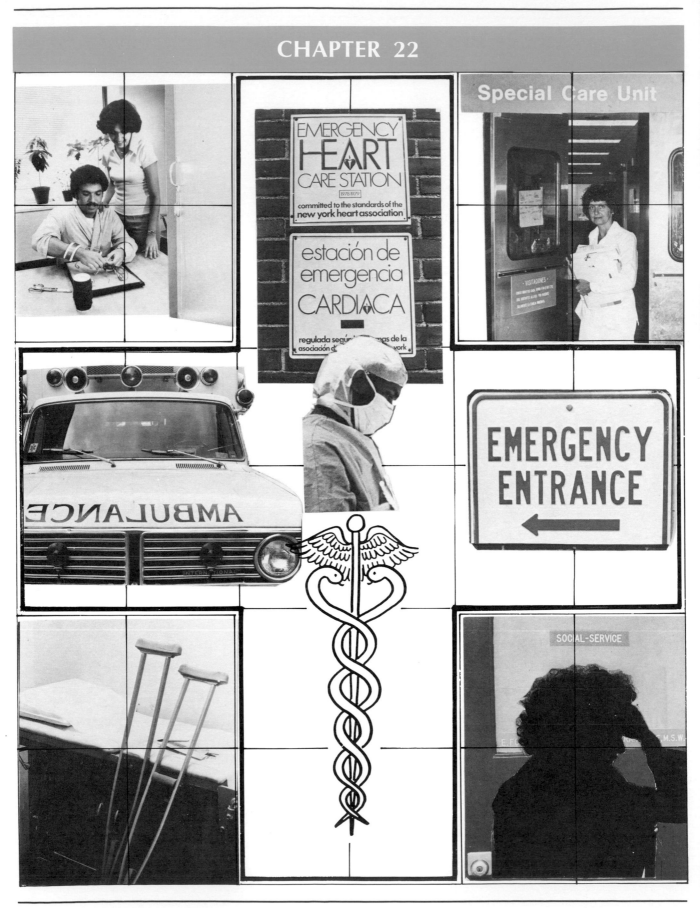

Health care services are one of the four determiners of health. These four factors were mentioned in the introductory chapter and structured the format of this book. Heredity, self-destructive habits and behaviors (overeating, taking pills, smoking, and inactivity), and the environment (food, tobacco, and drugs) have been discussed in great detail up to now. This chapter deals with the fourth determiner of health—that of providing and using health care services.

What kind of health care services do you need to attain and maintain optimal well-being? How are they provided in this country? How can you use the health care delivery system to your best advantage and cut down the spiraling costs of medical and hospital care? What kind of health insurance should you have? This chapter deals with these issues.

Respond to the Health Care Insurance Inventory. It will make you aware of the kind of medical-hospital-dental-care insurance policy you need now and in the future.

☞ HEALTH CARE INSURANCE INVENTORY[1]

DIRECTIONS   1. Pick up your insurance policy first and have it immediately and readily accessible for evaluation *before* you react to this inventory.
2. React to all the statements in each section by circling the number in the vertical column that best describes or typifies the kind of benefit coverage your health insurance policy gives you.
3. React to all the statements in each of the sections.
4. If you cannot find a clause or statement covering the benefit, then you should classify it in the "not-covered" or "do not know" column (in the first or "A" vertical column).

[1] I am grateful to Dr. Aubrey McTaggart, Ph. D., Professor of Health Education, San Diego State University, San Diego, Calif., for his review of, and suggestions to, this inventory.

Benefit	Coverage			
	A	B	C	D
	Duration			
	30 Days or Do Not Know	100 Days	70 Days	70 Days
	Cash Amount			
A. Hospital Service Expense (while in hospital)	$1000 or Less	$5000 or 80% of Costs	+$10,000	Paid in Full
1. Room (3 bed + ward)	0	5	10	20
2. Food and food services	0	5	10	20
3. Anesthesia	0	5	10	20
4. Use of operating room	0	5	10	20
5. Maternity	0	5	10	20
6. Routine nursing care	0	5	10	20
7. Blood transfusions	0	5	10	20
8. Prescription drugs and medicines	0	5	10	20
	Number Visits Limit + Costs			
	10 per Year + $1000 or Less	5 per Year + $5000 or 80% of Costs	No Limit + $10,000	No Limit + Paid in Full
9. X-rays	0	5	10	20
10. Local ambulance service (to and from hospital)	0	5	10	20
11. Physiotherapy	0	5	10	20
12. Diathermy	0	5	10	20
13. Medical baths	0	5	10	20
14. Massage	0	5	10	20
15. Radiotherapy	0	5	10	20
Total	_____ +	_____ +	_____ +	_____

Benefit	Coverage Restrictions			
	A	B	C	D
	Number Limit + Cost Amount			
B. Surgical Expenses (physician fees while in hospital)	10 per Year + $1000 or Less	5 per Year + $5000 or 80%	No Limit + $10,000	No Limit + Paid in Full
16. Operations in general	0	1	3	5
17. Operations for fractures	0	1	3	5
18. Operation for dislocations	0	1	3	5
19. Operation for Caesarean section	0	1	3	5
20. Operation for complications	0	1	3	5
21. Consultations	0	1	3	5
Total	_____ +	_____ +	_____ +	_____
	Cost			
	$1000	$5000 or 80%	$10,000	No Limits
	Number Made			
C. Regular Medical Expenses: Physician fees for Non-surgical Care in your Home or M.D.'s Office (may be covered in A&B Sections)	10 per Year	10–15	No Limits	No Limits
22. Visit by physician to you	0	1	3	5
23. Visit by you to physician	0	1	3	5
24. Diagnostic X-ray in M.D.'s office	0	1	3	5
25. Lab tests in M.D.'s office	0	1	3	5
26. Medical examin in M.D.'s office	0	1	3	5
Total	_____ +	_____ +	_____ +	_____

Benefit	Coverage Restrictions			
	A	B	C	D
	Number Limit + Cost Amount			
	5 per Year	10 per Year	None	None
D. Special Services when prescribed by your M.D., services in addition to previous sections)	$1000 or Less	$5000 or 50%	+$10,000	None
27. Well-baby checkups	0	4	7	10
28. Prenatal care checkups	0	4	7	10
29. Multiphasic screening for well person	0	4	7	10
30. Nutrition counseling	0	4	7	10
31. Weight control services	0	4	7	10
32. Rest cures	0	4	7	10
33. Physical fitness therapy	0	4	7	10
34. Stop-smoking therapy	0	4	7	10
35. Alcohoism treatment and rehabilitation	0	4	7	10
36. Drug use treatment and rehabilitation	0	4	7	10
37. Psychiatric treatment and care	0	4	7	10
38. Burial or cremation	0	4	7	10
39. Hearing aids	0	4	7	10
40. Eye glasses or contact lens	0	4	7	10
41. Allergy shots	0	4	7	10
42. Cosmetic surgery	0	4	7	10
43. Marriage counseling	0	4	7	10
44. Health counseling	0	4	7	10
45. Hysterectomy	0	4	7	10

		$1000 or Less	$5000 or 50%	+$10,000	None
46.	Vasectomy (sterilization)	0	4	7	10
47.	Abortions	0	4	7	10
48.	Heart surgery	0	4	7	10
49.	Terminal cancer	0	4	7	10
50.	Artificial kidney or heart services	0	4	7	10
51.	Treatment of incurable disease or disorder	0	4	7	10
52.	Organ transplant	0	4	7	10
53.	Physiotherapy	0	1	3	5
54.	Therapeutic X-ray plus radium therapy	0	1	3	5
55.	Diagnostic laboratory procedures	0	1	3	5
56.	Diagnostic X-ray	0	1	3	5
57.	Postoperative care (outside hospital)	0	1	3	5
58.	Private duty nursing	0	1	3	5
59.	Prescription drugs outside hospital	0	1	3	5
60.	Treatment for tuberculosis	0	1	3	5
61.	Treatment for other infectious diseases (VD)	0	1	3	5
62.	Specialists fees (pediatricians, gynecologists, chiropractors, osteopaths, podiatrists, dental surgeons, optometrists, physiotherapists, etc.)	0	1	3	5
	Total	_____ +	_____ +	_____ +	_____

Benefits	Coverage Restrictions			
	A	B	C	D
	Number Visits + Cost			
			Unlimited Visits	
E. Dental Services and Expenses (in dentist's office or hospital)	Number Visits + Cost	10 Visits + $100 to $500 Deduct.	20–50% Deduct. Pay up to $5000	No Limits Full Payment
63. Oral examination	0	3	5	10
64. X-ray	0	3	5	10
65. Fillings	0	3	5	10
66. Cleaning	0	3	5	10
67. Extractions	0	3	5	10
68. Inlays	0	3	5	10
69. Bridgework	0	3	5	10
70. Dentures	0	3	5	10
71. Oral surgery	0	3	5	10
72. Root canal therapy	0	3	5	10
73. Orthodontia	0	3	5	10
74. Treatment of gum infection	0	3	5	10
Total	_____ +	_____ +	_____ +	_____

SCORING

Total the point values for all four columns for each section. This is the section total. Add all the totals for all sections. This total is referred to as your health insurance score.

INTERPRETATION

Classify your score in the appropriate score scale:

Score Scale	Interpretation
700–800	Excellent *benefits and coverage*
575–699	Very Good, but a few weaknesses in policy
400–574	Fair, *too many benefits limited or omitted*
0–399	Inadequate *for living in America in next 10 years. Too many services and benefits omitted and too many restrictions.*

Your grand score is an estimated assessment of the comprehensiveness of your health insurance policy.

HEALTH CARE SERVICES

What kind of hospital and medical services do people of all ages in this country need? What kind of health care will raise the quality of well-being and extend life? What kind of health care do you need at various stages of life? It seems logical to answer these questions by saying that such services should be offered on the basis of this country's health problems. The major health problems of this country, like those of most of the world's industrialized nations, are affected by a wide range of life styles and health hazards, including careless driving, poor nutritional habits, smoking, alcohol and drug abuse, inactivity, and the mental-physical stresses of urban living (11;26;27;29;35;46). Based on an analysis of mortality and morbidity rates of premature death (occurring before age 70), the principal causes of death in this country are automobile accidents, heart disease, cirrhosis, respiratory diseases, cancer, and suicide (see Figure 22.1). Since people become sick before they die, sick people are usually hospitalized and, since hospitalization accounts for almost half of all medical-hospital expenses (see Figure 22.2 and Table 22.1), it is also important to identify illnesses and diseases that require long-term hospitalization. These illnesses include heart disease, cancer, illness from accidents or violent acts, and emotional disorders (29;46).

The answers to the introductory questions are obvious. We need hospital and medical services for health promotion that provide treatment and care to the chronically ill and disabled. We also need health care that is inexpensive and that we can afford. Many persons neglect to get medical care because it is beyond their ability to pay for it. Perhaps we can reduce health care costs by learning to care for ourselves instead of always running to the doctor. Being knowledgeable about how physicians and hospitals work and provide health care services will help us to decide when to see a doctor and when to take care of our illness!

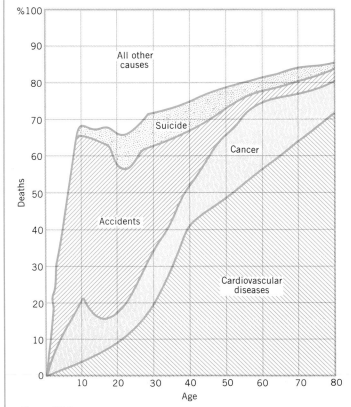

Figure 22.1

Causes of death in the United States today. Two-thirds of all deaths are due to cardiovascular disease, cancer, accidents, suicide, and cirrhosis.

Table 22.1

National Health Expenditures and Percent Distribution, According to the Type of Expenditure for the U.S. Selected Fiscal Year 1977

Expenditures	Percent	1977 Expenditure
1. Hospital care	40.3	$ 65.6 (Billion)
2. Physician services	19.8	32.2
3. Dentist services	6.2	10.0
4. Nursing home care	7.7	12.6
5. Other professional services	2.0	3.2
6. Drugs and drug sundries	7.7	12.5
7. Eyeglasses and appliances	1.3	2.1
8. Expenses — prepayment	4.7	7.6
9. Public health activities	2.3	3.7
10. Other health services	2.6	4.3
11. Research	2.3	3.7
12. Construction	3.1	5.0
Total	100	$162.6

Source: Health: United States: 1978, Washington, U.S. Public Health Service, Washington, D.C., December 1978, p. 385.

HEALTH CARE DELIVERY IN THE UNITED STATES

The traditional medical approach to providing health care in this country has been to have doctors practice medicine privately, or in a clinic, and to treat you for an illness whenever you got sick (20;35;46). A cursory annual physical exam was also given on request. Doctors would charge you a fee for providing this service. Many, but not all, families subscribed to some form of hospital-medical insurance, such as Blue Cross or Blue Shield. Since most doctors are usually affiliated with a hospital, they would hospitalize patients as needed. The idea of using the same doctor for all members of the family in the 1960s was assumed to allow the doctor to become more acquainted with each family member, thereby providing more personalized and adequate medical-health care. But with many families, or their members, moving each year and becoming affluent, the idea of having a family doctor has become somewhat impractical. Family affluence, coupled with rising medical costs and indifferent medical services, has resulted in general dissatisfaction with medical care and increasing distrust of physicians and other health providers (26;35;105).

This federal government's reaction to the public's dissatisfaction in the 1960s was to spend money without interfering in any way with the structure of the health care system (35:6). Public administrators spent vast amounts of money in increasing, or in developing, new programs on the theory that benefits would trickle down to those who needed help. Unfortunately, those needing health care the most — the poor, elderly, and disabled — were unable to get adequate health care because they had no money or they had inadequate hospital-medical insurance. The public's attitude of taking good health for granted and then depending on someone else to look after their ill health compounded this indigence dilemma. To overcome these limitations, comprehensive health planning, requiring citizen involvement in the planning of community health care delivery, was evolved in the mid-1960s. Although still in use today, this approach has had a limited impact on improving health care or keeping its costs under control in this country.

As it became obvious that federal efforts were not providing better health care delivery, nor controlling expenses, the approach in the 1970s shifted to additional regulations. One approach was to reorganize the delivery of health care for the needy and aged. Medicare and Medicaid were introduced in 1965, amidst much confusion, by the federal and state governments. Still in existence today, Medicare is a health plan that did improve the well-being of the elderly and the poor. The plan is voluntary with the government sharing most of the costs of a patient's doctor and other medical expenses. For example, a separate program, Medical, was evolved in California to pay for some of the health care costs of the poor. Medicare and Medicaid both resulted in an enormous enlargement of the nursing-home industry because they provided benefit dollars for post-hospital and long-term health care (35:56). Needless to say, both programs allowed hospital-medical care costs to escalate. Neither of the programs provided health care for the well and those working.

Runaway medical costs tempted the federal government to impose continuous rules and regulations. For example, by 1976, Comprehensive Health Care, including Medicare and Medicaid, became a proliferation of piecemeal regulatory processes that became expensive, poorly designed and administered, complicated, and encouraged fee-for-service medical practice. Adding to the problem of runaway health delivery costs and poor care delivery was the medical profession's encouragement of the public in general to overuse the medical care system (25:1). The cumulative result has been spiraling hospital and medical care costs (see Figures 22.2 and 22.3).

Our health care system of the past is an episodic and crisis-oriented system that encourages physicians to treat diseases through surgery and drugs (31:7). Under the traditional system, doctors and hospitals were paid (many still are) on a fee-for-service or piecework basis. The more illnesses they treated, and the more services they rendered, the more their incomes rose. It meant that

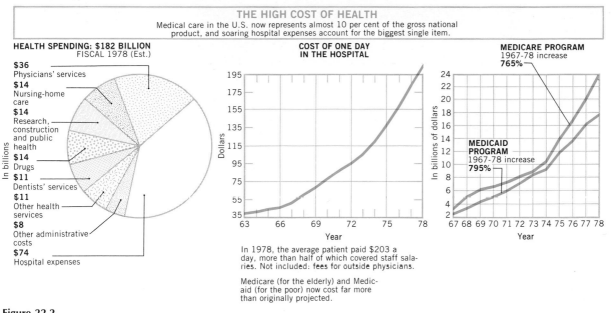

THE HIGH COST OF HEALTH
Medical care in the U.S. now represents almost 10 per cent of the gross national product, and soaring hospital expenses account for the biggest single item.

HEALTH SPENDING: $182 BILLION
FISCAL 1978 (Est.)

$36 Physicians' services
$14 Nursing-home care
$14 Research, construction and public health
$14 Drugs
$11 Dentists' services
$11 Other health services
$8 Other administrative costs
$74 Hospital expenses

COST OF ONE DAY IN THE HOSPITAL

In 1978, the average patient paid $203 a day, more than half of which covered staff salaries. Not included: fees for outside physicians.

Medicare (for the elderly) and Medicaid (for the poor) now cost far more than originally projected.

MEDICARE PROGRAM
1967-78 increase
765%

MEDICAID PROGRAM
1967-78 increase
795%

Figure 22.2
Graphic illustration of the high costs of health care in the United States. (With permission from Health Care Financing Administration, Medicaid Bureau 1967 to 1970 data for Medicaid include other similar Federal-state programs.)

there was no economic incentive for them to concentrate on keeping people healthy. A fixed-price contract for comprehensive health care reverses this illogical incentive. The concept of fixed-price contracts was revived in the late 1970s.

Referred to as the HMOs, or Health-Maintenance (preventive) Organization, it allows the physician's income to grow not with the number of days a person is sick, but with the number of days the patient is well. Therefore, HMOs have a strong interest in preventing illness, or failing that, in treating it in its earliest stages, in promoting a thorough recovery, and in preventing any reoccurrence. Like doctors in ancient China, they are paid to keep their clients healthy. HMOs are growing rapidly in this country.

A major obstacle to providing adequate health care for everyone is the high cost of the delivery system itself. Although we have the best health care facilities and technological-medical services in the world, they have become too expensive for the average person on modest income to be able to use. Private medical-hospital insurance up to now has provided inadequate coverage. This shortcoming prodded the federal government in 1979 to unsuccessfully legislate for national health insurance so that everyone can have access to adequate health care.

Up to and through the 1960s, there was a trend away from the general practice (GP) type of doctor and toward specialization. Although many doctors are continuing to specialize, the trend toward specialization has been reversing with an advent of family practitioners and a move toward self-care and wholistic medicine. Although controversial in some aspects, wholistic medicine attempts to promote optimal health practices and keep the whole body in ecological balance with the physical and social environments, thereby lowering medical-hospital costs by eliminating the need for the same.

We have been pouring money into the traditional health care system with the assumption that the public will receive more and better health care. This has not been the case. It is now recognized by public health officials in this and other countries (20;26;27;29;35;46) that pouring more and more funds into costly curative measures will not improve health in general. Instead, changes in the social and political structures, and changes in personal behavioral patterns that promote optimal well-being will do far more than doctors and drugs can do to minimize the burden of disease and the tragedy of premature death. Thus, while the medical profession needs to change its focus from treatment to prevention, we need to change some of our self-destructive habits and behaviors and maximize optimal well-being.

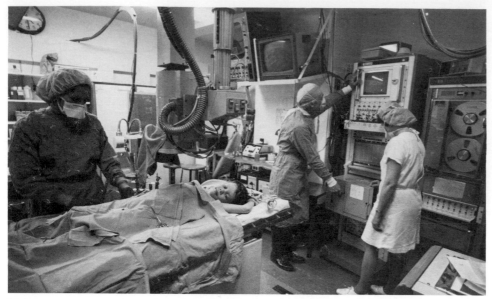

(a)

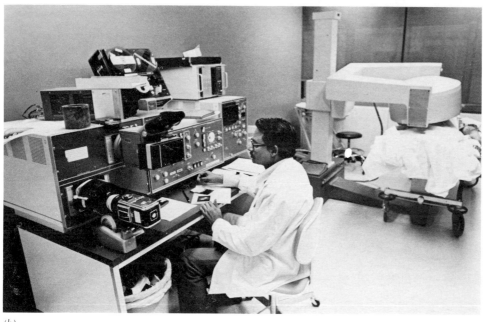

(b)

Figure 22.3 (a) Patient undergoing tests in pediatric cardiology unit at a metropolitan hospital. Is all this medical gadgetry necessary? (b) An example of sophisticated and expensive medical laboratory diagnostic equipment at Mt. Sinai Hospital in New York. Does this kind of equipment result in better health care of well persons? Has it extended life expectancy in this country since 1950?

CRITERIA OF A GOOD HEALTH CARE DELIVERY SYSTEM

A good health care delivery system is one that does more than just treat the ill and those with disease. It has a preventive segment (like health education) that encour-

ages you, the consumer, not to get sick; at the same time, it encourages the providers (hospitals, physicians, drug companies, and others) to deliver adequate and cost-controlled (inexpensive) preventive-treatment care. The delivery program should encourage you to become the steward or manager of your own health. It does not spend enormous sums of money to treat people who should not have been sick; nor does it misplace money and effort on the medical system. A good health care delivery system allows everyone to use a system that is inexpensive and treatment cost-effective, comprehensive in nature, is prevention-oriented and promotes optimal well-being, orthobiosis, and long life. In short, it provides for your care when you cannot do so.

WAYS TO USE THE HEALTH CARE DELIVERY SYSTEM EFFECTIVELY

How can you cut down your hospital-medical costs and, at the same time, effectively use the system and maintain optimal well-being? There are four good ways to do this (see Figure 22.4).

1. The first thing you can do is *to evolve a positive life style or orthobiosis that reduces high risks of illness and premature death* so you will not have to use hospitals and doctors. In the long run, this cuts medical expenses regardless of who pays for them, and second, it also reduces your hospital-medical insurance premiums. More importantly, you will stay healthy and live longer. Improving your level of wellness lies mainly in improving your environment, moderating self-imposed risks, and adding to your understanding of human well-being. Start practicing preventive well-being, thereby reducing the need for health care. It is hoped that the preceding chapters have helped you to do this.

2. A second way to keep hospital-medical costs down and to use the health care delivery system effectively is to *practice self-care.* Self-care or home care is assuming responsibility for taking care of yourself when you are sick, in a sense doctoring yourself. You can, for example, help your body to fight a cold in its own natural way by giving your body rest, fluids, and vitamins such as A and C and by letting the natural body defenses fight the viral cold for you instead of taking antibiotics. You can also take a first aid, emergency care, or self-care course to develop skills in administering emergency and home self-care. Much immediate care for illness and accidents is really common sense and you can and should develop and practice self-care skills. Many illnesses require home care from you and not the doctor.

3. You can reduce hospital-medical costs and use such services more effectively by going to see a doctor when you cannot help yourself. Ways to do this are explored in later sections of this chapter.

4. You can effectively utilize the health care delivery system by *having adequate medical-hospital-dental-laboratory insurance,* such as through the HMO, Blue Cross, or Blue Shield. Many people cannot get proper health care because they do not have the money to pay for their needed health care. They cannot enter the health care delivery system. A good insurance policy charges you a predetermined annual premium and assumes the financial burden for hospital and medical expenses. For most persons, this is financially essential, since they do not have a large savings account, or they are unable to pay off large hospital-medical expenses in case of acute or long-term illness, accident, or any emergency. About 20 million people in the United States are unable to afford medical insurance and so many of these people do not get medical-hospital aid and care. The section on medical-hospital insurance

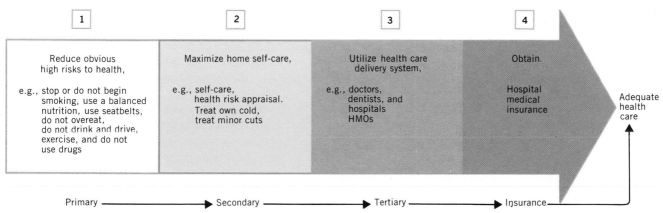

Figure 22.4
Four ways to get adequate health care and, at the same time, keep hospital-medical costs down. The most important baseline approach is to reduce the high risks to health: (1) in your lifestyle, then buttress this with personal home self-care. (2) These first two are preventive in nature and do not need medical intervention. If you do get sick, then use the health care delivery system. (3) By having adequate health care insurance (4).

provides information about proposed national health insurance and cancer insurance, and discusses what an adequate insurance policy should cover.

HOME SELF-CARE

Your body has alarm and defense systems to keep you well (see Chapter 1). Illness makes itself known to you through changes in your bodily feelings, sensations, and reactions referred to by doctors as signs and symptoms. Some symptoms are very familiar, as coughing, fever, pain, nausea, itchy skin, vomiting, headache, and diarrhea. Others may be strange and not as related to the alarm system, such as blindness, a sharp pain in the abdomen, and localized paralysis. An easily recognized collection of symptoms—running nose, slight fever, and sore throat—are analyzed as the common cold. The common cold could be your body telling you that you are overworking, that you have run down your body defenses, or that you have been exposed to hazardous substances in the environment and that it is time to give your body some much-needed rest. A symptom is a signal that there is something wrong with your body's machinery or its processes. It is a red light alerting you to the first breakdown and that you had better pay attention now before there are more breakdowns. You interpret these alarms or symptoms by the way you feel—good, comfortable, and at ease; or sick uncomfortable, tense, and tired. Body defenses become somewhat lowered when these alarm symptoms go off. Self-care deals with recognizing these alarm symptoms and doing something about them at home.

Self-care means giving people enough basic health information so that they can treat themselves and others in the cases where a visit to the doctor is not needed or would not do much good. It is assuming responsibility for personal well-being instead of relying on others to take care of you (see Figure 22.5). Self-care is an important and effective way to cut down hospital-medical costs, since 70 to 80 percent of most first-time complaint visits to a physician may be treated with a home remedy (14;40;41;42;47), while 50 percent or more of patient's visits to doctors are for complaints without any clear biological basis (26).

WAYS TO PRACTICE SELF-CARE

1. You can get information on self-care and emergency care and develop life-saving skills by taking a first aid or self-care class. The preceding chapters should be helpful in the prevention of illnesses and diseases.

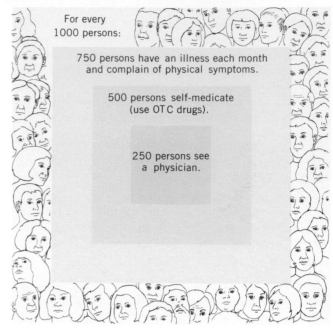

For every 1000 persons:

750 persons have an illness each month and complain of physical symptoms.

500 persons self-medicate (use OTC drugs).

250 persons see a physician.

Figure 22.5
Half of the people who feel sick care for themselves instead of seeing a physician.

2. In addition to health information, self-care can also include self-assessment or identifying your high risks to well-being and reducing them. (Self-care has been suggested as a secondary separate approach to that of reducing high risks to health. The two could easily be combined.) The numerous self-assessment inventories and checklists throughout this text were included to help you assess your predispositions to various illnesses and diseases. By cutting down the high risks to illness and disease, and responding to the early-warning alarm symptoms of your body, you are preventing illnesses and diseases. This means fewer doctor and hospital bills now and in the future. Self-assessments should be done at least once a year and should be shared with your physician.

3. Self-care also means giving yourself an annual home health checkup. Such a checkup is comparable to the annual physical examination that doctors did in the 1950s and 1960s. You can check for vital signs of well-being by doing all of the following once a year, or as often as you feel you need to (14;18;21;28;42;45;47;49;50).

(a) Pulse—count your pulse rate to assess your cardiovascular system. Exercise, trauma, stress, drugs, illness, fever, allergy, and eating will send the pulse rate up. (See Chapter 2 for interpretation.)

(b) Respiration — count the number of times you breathe per minute. A normal adult rate is 14 to 20 breaths per minute. The more physically fit you are, the slower the respiration rate. Like the pulse rate, respiration increases with stress, exercise, fever, etc.

(c) Temperature — a normal temperature of 98.6°F can vary by time of the day and body function. A thermometer reading of over 100°F is likely to indicate illness.

(d) Blood pressure — take the blood pressure with a sphygmomanometer and stethoscope. (See Chapter 2 for interpretation of blood pressure.)

(e) Skin — check your skin for redness, tenderness, moles, warts, and lumps that do not go away within 2 to 4 weeks. Women should self-examine their breasts each month, while men should examine their testes every 6 months.

(f) Eyes — observe for redness of the white of the eye, eye soreness, and styes, and test your eyes for visual acuity.

(g) Urine — observe color changes in your urine. Yellow straw-colored urine may reflect an excess of protein foods, while red-colored urine may indicate an infection or bleeding in the kidney or bladder.

(h) Lymphatic system — palpate the lymph nodes of the throat-neck area and in the armpits. Any lumps or tender spots may indicate an infection.

(i) Insomnia — inability to sleep may reflect overstress, overwork, lack of physical exercise, ingesting drugs, and drinking coffee or cola soft drinks before going to bed — all implying a deleterious life style.

(j) Bleeding — reoccurring or uncontrolled bleeding over a period of a week or longer suggests a health problem that needs medical attention.

(k) Body weight and body-fat change in body weight (gain or loss) — usually indicates that there may be a health problem. Keep a monthly diary of your weight. (See Chapter 7.)

(l) Physical fitness — assess your physical fitness at least once a month. (See Chapter 5.)

(m) Rectal examination — check for bleeding. Men over 40 should palpate the prostate gland for suspected cancer. (See Chapter 15.)

(n) Nutrition analysis — analyze your diet at least once a year. (See Chapter 6.)

(o) Emotional well-being — assess your level and state of happiness, contentment, and fulfillment. (See Chapter 3.)

(p) Social well-being — assess your interactions with others and how your friends are affecting your well-being (See Chapter 4.)

(q) Immunization status — review the immunization you have had. Do you need new ones or booster shots?

By giving yourself an annual comprehensive home checkup, you will save money, save time, and assume responsibility for your own well-being. Many health tests and immunizations may be obtained through Public Health Departments at city or county expense. Use the results of your checkup to guide you in maintaining and conserving your well-being.

"WHEN" YOU NEED MEDICAL HELP

A. You need to see a doctor within a few days when you (42;47):

1. Have a fever of 100°F for more than 3 days or if the fever is over 101°F.
2. Cough up blood.
3. Pass red-colored urine.
4. Observe blood in the stools (red or dark stools).
5. Experience excessive bleeding in the vagina or rectum.
6. Have frequent nosebleeds.
7. Have continuous or recurring headaches.
8. Have a lump in the breast or lymph glands in the neck area that does not regress in 2 to 4 weeks.
9. Have unexplained weight loss.
10. Reoccurring or continuous skin-eye-ear-genital problems.
11. Have persistent dizziness or fainting spells.
12. Have shortness of breath.
13. Feel tired most of the time (exhaustion or fatigue).
14. Have an upset stomach or diarrhea that persists for more than 2 days.
15. Have a serious injury and cannot put weight on an ankle or injured knee in the first 24 hours, or when there is very little significant improvement in 3 to 4 days.
16. Have been stung by an insect (bee or spider) or jellyfish that results in a rash, breathing difficulties, nausea, cramps, vomiting, fainting, an extreme pain, and swelling.
17. Have painful urination and the discomfort has not subsided after 3 days.

B. You need to see a doctor immediately when you:

1. Cannot stop bleeding by direct pressure.
2. Receive a heavy blow to the head.
3. Have a puncture wound that is deep.
4. Get poisoned from an overdose of drugs or mix drugs with alcohol (beer or wine). Head for the hospital emergency room immediately.

GETTING MEDICAL AID

Where can you go to get medical help when your health problem is more than you can handle? Do you need a specialist or a general practitioner? Should you go to a hospital, a doctor, or an HMO?

The kind of medical help you get will be determined by the kind of hospital-medical-dental insurance you have or do not have, the nature of your illness, and the availability of medical care. As a college student, you should have insurance to defray unexpected costs in case you get sick or injured. If you are not covered by your parent's or spouse's policy, then you should subscribe to a similar insurance policy at the campus or student health center. Most hospitals and medical centers require you to be interviewed or examined by a general practitioner or nurse practitioner and then referred to a specialist if needed. See Figure 22.6 to identify the kind of specialist you may need to see. Additional information and help can be obtained from your local public health department; voluntary health agencies such as the Heart and Cancer societies; local free clinics; the local Red Cross chapter; the local medical society; and various health workshops and conventions.

A new national trend is to get hospital-medical services by joining a Health Maintenance Organization (HMO). Instead of going to a private or family doctor, the federal government is encouraging both providers (physicians) and consumers of health services to join HMOs.

The time to choose your personal physician is before you become ill. If you postpone choosing your doctor until you are ill, you may make your choice under the stress of a sense of urgency that may affect your judgment. Furthermore, a doctor who sees you for the first time, when an illness is already in progress, knows nothing about your usual health condition, and this may place both you and the doctor at a disadvantage. Your initial visit to your doctor should be when you are healthy, and he can observe through a general checkup how your body functions when you are well. It is also during this initial visit that you, as a consumer of health services, have an opportunity to evaluate the doctor for his practice style, the kind of office he runs, the staff he

has hired to help him, his personality, and his bedside manner. If you like your doctor, his health philosophy, and approach, can talk to him and he to you, get along well with him, find he will be there when you need him, and your illnesses respond to his therapy, then you have found a good doctor. But, if you find you and your doctor to be incompatible after the first visit, then you should resume searching for another doctor.

The traditional family doctor and general practitioner are now referred to as family practitioners. They receive special patient-care training and experience to deal with most of the health problems people have. They must pass a certification reexamination every 3 years. This means that family practitioners need to take continuing medical education in order to continue providing competent medical services and health care.

An alternative to choosing a doctor in private practice is to choose a group of doctors practicing medicine in a group multispecialty medical clinic or a Health Maintenance Organization (HMO) (42:92–106). Such clinics and HMOs usually have 10 or more doctors specializing in various branches of medicine and have supporting paramedical staffs (nurses, nurse practitioners, laboratory assistants, medical librarians, and record keepers) and medical laboratories, as well as affiliations with nearby hospitals, thereby offering complete medical services to their clients. Upon entering the clinic, you are examined and then assigned to a physician. As a patient, you can be referred to medical specialists within the clinic or HMO as needed. You can identify with a doctor in the clinic or HMO and be covered by his associates when he is away on vacations, evenings, or weekends. Group clinics and HMOs are usually open in the evenings and on weekends, whereas family practitioners in solo or private practice are not. Group medical clinics and HMOs have other advantages over doctors practicing solo medicine; they screen their doctors for competence before hiring them; they can consult or refer with each other; they can lower medical costs by making more efficient use of paraprofessionals such as nurse practitioners and physician assistants; they tend to be better informed on the latest medical-drug advances; and they tend to do a better job of keeping records through a central office. Since most of our health care needs throughout life are of a minor nature, such as health promotion, health maintenance, and disease prevention, we do not really need to see a doctor very often. Instead, the doctor's paramedical staff, such as the nurse practitioner, can cater effectively to most of your health needs. This not only allows the doctor to use his expertise to care for persons having serious health problems but also it greatly cuts costs down without lowering the quality of health care.

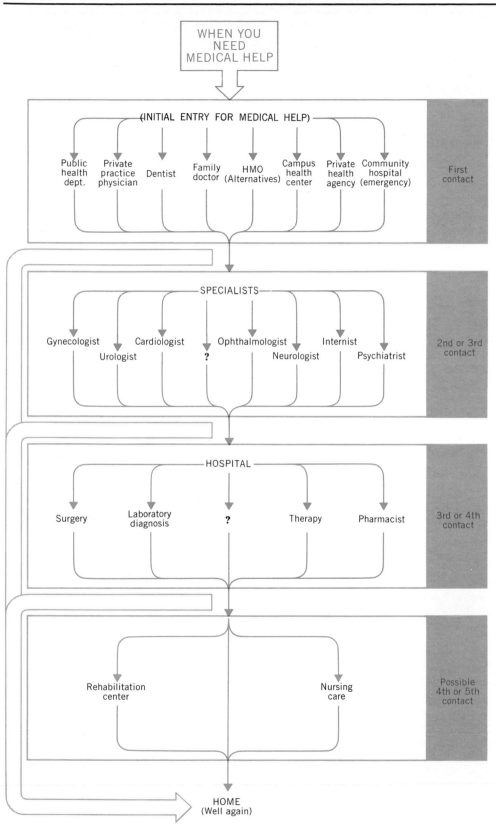

WHEN YOU
NEED
MEDICAL HELP

(INITIAL ENTRY FOR MEDICAL HELP)

| Public health dept. | Private practice physician | Dentist | Family doctor | HMO (Alternatives) | Campus health center | Private health agency | Community hospital (emergency) |

First contact

SPECIALISTS

Gynecologist | Urologist | Cardiologist | ? | Ophthalmologist | Neurologist | Internist | Psychiatrist

2nd or 3rd contact

HOSPITAL

Surgery | Laboratory diagnosis | ? | Therapy | Pharmacist

3rd or 4th contact

Rehabilitation center | Nursing care

Possible 4th or 5th contact

HOME
(Well again)

Figure 22.6
Procedure for using the health care delivery system.

HEALTH MAINTENANCE ORGANIZATIONS (HMOS)

HMOs are an emerging alternative to the traditional practice of medicine by private physicians and hospitals. Instead of paying as you get sick and using services whenever you get sick, HMOs offer medical-hospital insurance at a very low rate. This kind of plan pays for all of your expenses whenever you get sick, as well as your costs for staying well. It encourages physicians to practice medicine as a group on a self-sustaining basis. HMOs were approved by Congress in 1973 to encourage providers and consumers to organize for comprehensive medical services on a voluntary basis. The costs of all health care are mutualized or shared among all the subscribers so that a total health care budget is funded for the HMO. The budget is then paid by contract to the physicians, nurses, technicians, and others in the HMO facility, who, in turn, agree to deliver their respective services for an agreed-upon-in advance cost. All subscribers (patients) are assured of convenient access to all health services on an around-the-clock, 365-days-a-year basis.

The best-known example of an HMO is the Kaiser Foundation Health Plan (23;24), whose roots go back to 1933 when a small group of doctors were retained to care for workers on a construction project in the Mojave Desert. The plan gradually expanded to cover Kaiser employees and the public in other parts of the United States. In 1979, there were over 200 HMOs providing medical-health care to over 7½ million Americans (41).

With prepayment each subscriber contributes to a fund in advance. Caring for illness takes money out of that fund so that each case prevented or hospitalization avoided allows more money to remain in the funds for the doctors and the patients to share. The HMO physician earns more money by promoting health, whereas the traditional fee-for-service physician earns money when the patient is sick. The HMO system is much like the practice of medicine in ancient China where the physician got paid to keep the patient well. It is less expensive to prevent illness and disease than to treat it.

A typical HMO assembles several health services under one roof as contrasted to the fragmented services of traditional medicine. Besides primary-care physicians (general practitioners, pediatricians) there are other specialists available, such as radiologists, surgeons, obstetricians, gynecologists, neurologists, health educators, and others. The HMO team of doctors, nurses, health educators, laboratory technicians, and administrative staff work together in a single building. Thus you as a patient make one trip to a health center for all services.

The HMOs have other advantages over other health care delivery and insurance plans. They reduce medical costs from 20 to 40 percent (23;10;40); they save money by providing economic incentives for everyone not to use the hospital. A major benefit is the removal of the financial threat of catastrophic and long-term illness which often occurs with cancer, heart disease, and accidents. Because HMO members have already paid in advance, they are more likely to seek medical attention for illness in its early stages and be more aware of and receptive to modifying or changing high-risk-of-disease behaviors and habits. Unneeded surgery and and medication is greatly reduced. Medical, nursing, treatment, emergency care, and preventive services are available at all times. Such comprehensive availability in itself encourages subscribers to provide better health care for themselves, to monitor for diseases in their early stages, and to maintain optimal well-being. A major advantage is that one has comprehensive health insurance coverage at an affordable cost. This allows one to fix a health care insurance budget in advance. Health maintenance organizations encourage you to evolve a life style that excludes inactivity; overeating; eating refined sugar, salt, and white flour products; obesity; ingesting fatty foods; and not getting immunizations.

There are some drawbacks to joining an HMO. You must use the doctors and hospitals specified by your HMO. Should you seek medical care or advice from anyone else, you will have to pay for it yourself. You may have to wait to see a doctor. You may find it difficult to join an HMO, for most persons up to now were able to join through their employers. However, as more HMOs are being evolved, and as they become more competitive, these and other disadvantages will be overcome.

The HMOs are forcing physicians to shift from practicing traditional medicine (treatment and crisis oriented) to practicing preventive medicine.

If the HMO idea sounds good to you, the easiest way to join one is through your employer or union group. Your employer will pay part of or all of the premium. You might also be able to locate an HMO in your community that allows individual or nonemployer memberships. To locate an HMO nearest you, refer to the end of this chapter.

NATIONAL HEALTH INSURANCE

Although a few HMOs are keeping hospital-medical costs down, such costs have escalated dramatically in the past 15 years. The majority of the people in this country do not belong to HMOs. Since the federal government today pays indirectly for most of the hospital-medical costs, it seems reasonable to have national health insurance built into the HMO plan. In 1979, over

18 million Americans had no health insurance coverage, 19 million had insurance that did not cover ordinary hospital and physician services, and another 46 million had inadequate insurance against large medical bills (2). To make sure that everyone gets adequate health care insurance, national health insurance plans were proposed by President Carter and Senator Edward Kennedy in 1979 (1;3;16;17;19;25). Their rival proposals are summarized in Table 22.2.

Unlike Carter, Kennedy wants stiff new controls on both the insurance business and doctor's fees. Both plans would merge Medicare and Medicaid into a new federal "health care program," similar in concept to that of Canada and England.

OTHER HEALTH CARE INSURANCE INCLUDING CANCER

Private insurance companies, such as Blue Cross and Blue Shield provide various health care insurance plans. Like the HMOs, they usually have restrictive or contingency clauses limiting the amount of coverage. For ex-

Table 22.2

Comparison of Two Proposed (May 1979) National Health Insurance Plans

	Kennedy-Waxman Plan	Carter Plan
1. Coverage	Full hospital, physician, laboratory, X ray, drugs, ambulance service, nursing home costs paid after plan is 5 years old Limited psychiatric costs	You pay first $2500. Government pays hospital, physician, laboratory, and X rays
2. Package	Total	Piecemeal
3. Cost (federal)	$28.6 billion in 1983 (federal) 11.4 " " " (private) $40. billion total	$30 billion in 1983 (federal and private) + additional sums later on
4. Who is covered?	Everyone, all ages, rich, poor, and disabled	Only those able to pay initial costs below $2500 per year
5. Who pays premium?	The government and employers pay 65 percent Employees pay 35 percent Unemployed covered by funds from a pool of Government-employer premiums After a 5-year phase-in, you would pay nothing	You pay first $2500; the government pays rest Premium-employer pays 75 percent You pay 25 percent Unemployed and poor to be subsidized by state and federal taxes
6. How much premium per year?	Single person — $ 800 Family — $1950	Single person: $114 Family: $185
7. Who insures?	Private insurance firms	Private insurance firms
8. Preventive medicine emphasis	Yes, e.g., premium rebates to nonsmokers	Yes
9. Regulate spending	Strict cost-control over doctor, hospital, and insurance spending Hospitals operate on annual budget	Establish ceiling on physician fees; limit purchase of new equipment and hospital construction
10. HMO supported	Yes	Yes
11. Medicare and Medicaid	Yes	Yes

ample, an insurance policy may pay only up to 120 to 180 days of hospital care, exclude psychiatric care, maternity benefits, and preventive costs, or have a maximum ceiling cost for medical expenses incurred for emergency or accident care. Nonmedical expenses, such as medical treatment and the care of terminal cancer, may not be covered. Yet one in four Americans can expect to be striken by this disease, and two of every three households will be affected by it. Cancer expenses can range from $5000 to $50,000 (51). Since most private insurance companies, including Blue Cross and Blue Shield, reimburse only 30 to 60 percent of the actual medical treatment costs for cancer, the average cancer victim and his family can end up with exorbitant medical bills that can bankrupt family members. To overcome such catastrophies, over 14 million Americans in 1979 subscribed to supplemental insurance that covered cancer (51) (HMOs may or may not cover cancer). Private insurance companies, such as the American Life Assurance Company of Columbus, Lloyds of London, Mutual of Omaha, Bankers Life and Casualty, Continental Life, and The Kemper Group are among 300 companies now selling cancer insurance. You may wish to investigate such supplemental insurance if you have a high predisposition to cancer. You should also inquire about heart disease insurance.

PURCHASING HEALTH CARE INSURANCE

By now, you probably have some idea of what a hospital-medical-dental or an HMO insurance policy should cover. Whether you have one or are interested in getting one, respond to the inventory at the beginning of this chapter. It will help to make you aware of the hospital-medical-dental benefits that should be covered in a policy, as well as assess your present policy. If you feel uncomfortable or uncertain about the kind of coverage your policy provides, then you should discuss these feelings with your individual or group agent, a health science instructor, the insurance clerk in a hospital, or practice facility. Evaluate each section to identify your weak and strong benefits.

You should be aware that there are many aspects of an insurance policy that were not included in this inventory. These are usually listed in "fine or small print" in your policy as the following restrictions, limitations, or omissions:

1. Dependents not covered.
2. Age restrictions—newborns and senior citizens may not be eligible for benefits.
3. Age restriction on issuance of policy.
4. Income restricting on issuance of policy.

5. Coverage of treatment of preexisting conditions (such as terminal cancer, diabetes, allergy, etc.).
6. The free choice of doctor and hospital may be restricted.
7. Renewing clauses as to who has the right to review the policy.
8. Compensation against loss of personal income when the head of household is sick (also referred to as disability allowances).
9. Injury in situations or activities that will not be covered (such as earthquakes, floods, riots, snow or mud slides, auto racing, rodeo horse riding, sports events, deep sea diving, hunting, handling explosives, etc.)
10. Locations that may make the policy void, such as when you get sick in another state or country.
11. Dismemberment benefits or lump sums payable for accidental loss of life, sight, or limbs.
12. Established residency of 30 days or more in a state.
13. Need for a medical examination before qualifying for a policy. This may be required to verify or discover restriction 5 on existing impairments and later used to disqualify you.
14. Grace period before the policy is in force (often a waiting period of 30 days).

Most of us subscribe to other insurance policies such as automobile travel insurance. The benefits in these policies are sold as a package deal and, in most cases, duplicate what you often have as hospital, surgical, regular, or special services. This is unnecessary and uneconomical coverage. You should talk to your auto insurance agent about deleting these services from the company's policy.

The five sections in the inventory are considered to be the most important and essential health protection you need from day to day. The greatest expenses an average American can expect, in times of illness, accident, or disaster are, in order of expenses: (1) hospital, (2) surgical or physician fees while in hospital, (3) regular medical expenses and physician fees outside the hospital, (4) special services prescribed by your physician not covered in item (3), and (5) dental services.

Hospital expenses are at least twice as costly as surgical or physician fees. The point values assigned to Section A in the Inventory reflect this difference.

Many of the services and benefits listed in Section D (special services) may be included in your policy under hospital services, or surgical or physician expenses. This may be a very satisfactory procedure. However, these were listed separately to avoid duplication and to focus special attention on a few services essential to fulfill or resolve your present and future needs. Such needs are really an extension of preventive medicine and should be thought of as maintenance of health or as aids to, or modification of your harmful behaviors or life style. These include such services as multiphasic screening and /or health risk appraisal for well persons to keep them well, nutrition counseling, weight control counseling, physical fitness therapy, stop-smoking therapy, alcoholism and drug treatment and rehabilitation, and health and marriage counseling.

Policy provision for funeral or cremation for family members should be a definite consideration and inclusion in future health insurance policies. Often funeral directors play on the distress of the entire family at a time when bereavement makes the family members most susceptible to an excessively expensive funeral package. Somehow the play on sentiment attempts to create the illusion that the more expensive the casket and funeral arrangements, the more dignified is the death and the easier it is to overcome loss of the dead person. It is unfortunate that the funeral establishment continues to take advantage of people who are encumbered financially.

The last section covering dental services and expenses is long overdue as an essential insurance policy. High fees discourage the practice of oral hygiene by all of us. Because of these and other reasons, dental coverage was included in the inventory. Many persons in this country now have a limited form of dental insurance. Hopefully, such coverage will be part of a comprehensive hospital-medical-dental health package in the future.

A good health insurance policy is essential as a way of caring for one's health. It is a way of helping you to maximize your potentials for optimal well-being and enjoy a longer and more productive life.

Such aspirations for a health cornucopia are possible only when one receives medical-hospital-dental health aid when he or she needs it! Sickness and accident strike randomly and often when we are least prepared financially to afford therapy and care services. The principle of health insurance was evolved to meet such uncertainty and unpreparedness.

Since the cost and type of sickness and accident vary in degree and duration for each person, the cost, type, and amount of treatment will also vary. The idea of insurance is that everybody prepays a small amount, called a premium, into a common pool out of which are paid the large unpredictable expenses of the few who are sick at any given time.

CRITERIA FOR CHOOSING A DOCTOR

A. The following are suggestions for finding a doctor:

1. Ask for recommendations from friends, neighbors, and others such as the local voluntary agencies (cancer and heart disease societies).

2. Validate these recommendations by calling your local county medical society, or go to your local library or hospital and look up the doctor in the *American Medical Directory*. This directory will give you information about the doctor's age, professional education, and affiliations with professional organizations.

B. The following questionnaire helps to rate the doctor of your choice before you visit him or his clinic:

1. Is he licensed to practice medicine in the state in which he resides? (A licensed MD meets the minimum state qualifications by passing a basic medical examination.) The doctor's license should hang in a conspicuous place in his office.

2. Is he board certified? (A board-certified doctor receives 2 to 7 years of additional training and experience beyond his 4 years of medical school and has passed a medical examination.)

3. Is he a fellow? (A fellow is a specialist who is highly esteemed by his peers.)

4. Is he a family practitioner? (Most of your health care needs can be taken care of by a family practitioner and his paramedical staff.)

5. Does he have a teaching appointment at a medical school or hospital? Such an appointment implies competency and expertise.

6. What kind of hospital does your prospective doctor work in? (A small hospital having fewer than 200 beds may not have specialized equipment, intensive coronary care units, etc. that a larger hospital has. Larger hospitals usually have stricter controls and better supervision. Keep in mind that a surgeon affiliated with one hospital will have more time to give you than one who performs surgery in three or more hospitals.)

7. Does he practice by himself or with other physicians in a multispecialty group or HMO setting?

8. Is he a family practitioner or a specialist?

9. Does he participate in continuing medical education programs? (Many states now re-

quire a minimum of 75+ hours of medical education over a 3-year period.)

10. Does he practice preventive medicine or health promotion, or is he treatment and crisis medicine oriented?

11. Does he or his clinic have office hours that allow for evening or weekend appointments?

12. Does he accept Medicare and Medicaid patients?

13. Does he participate socially and culturally in your community affairs? Does he have a commitment to you and your community in nonmedical ways?

C. Things to observe and questions to ask of your doctor on your first visit to reaffirm your choice:

1. Did the doctor (or his staff) do a complete medical history, having you fill out a health-life style questionnaire about your past health and that of your family (or ask you specific questions)?

2. Did the doctor (or his staff) do a careful, complete physical examination? Did he check all parts of your body?

3. If you are a woman, did he (or his staff) do breast and pelvic examinations and a Pap smear test?

4. Did he (or his staff) do a rectal exam?

5. Does he measure and explain your blood pressure?

6. Did he (or his staff) do or ask you to do a 1-week diet eating analysis? Does he ask whether you use table salt? Ingest refined sugar foods? Eat too many fat foods?

7. Does he (or his staff) ask whether you exercise and how often?

8. Does he (or his staff) evaluate your emotional well-being?

9. Does he (or his staff) evaluate your social-cultural well-being?

10. Does he (or his staff) ask about your smoking and alcoholic beverage habits?

11. Does he (or his staff) do any patient education, such as explaining your problem or referring you to literature or recommended books?

12. Does he (or his staff) spend enough time with you to give you a chance to explain your problem? (As a rule of thumb, a doctor should spend a minimum of 15 minutes with each patient.)

13. Does he (or his staff) encourage you in self-care and self-health maintenance, such as

improving your diet and exercising regularly?

14. If he wants you to have special blood-urine lab tests, does he (or his staff) explain why, what they will be, and any side effects?

15. If he prescribes a medication, does he (or his staff) tell you what it is, make you aware of possible side effects, and warn you about synergistic effects? Should you take the prescription until it is empty or only long enough to alleviate the symptoms?

16. Does he (or his staff) make notes in a health record folder about your examination and visit? Does he refer to it in future visits?

17. Does he talk to you in a manner you can understand?

18. Are you able to ask questions and get satisfactory answers?

19. Does he (or his staff) inform you in advance what your total health expenses will be?

20. Does he (and his staff) have a pleasing manner, a wholesome personality, and a neat, clean appearance?

21. Does he (and his staff) exemplify optimal health by not smoking cigarettes, not allowing smoking in the office and clinic (no ashtrays), and not being overweight?

22. How often does he want you to have a medical-maintenance-health risk appraisal? If he is interested in promoting your health, he will suggest frequent and regular medical checkups.

23. Ask him when he would solicit a second medical opinion about your health problem?

24. Ask him when he would refer you to a medical specialist?

25. Does he (or his staff) evaluate your family or home life?

26. Does he (or his staff) evaluate your sex life?

WHERE TO GO FOR INFORMATION

1. To locate private medical multispecialty group clinics in your area, contact:
The American Group Practice Association
P.O. Box 948
Alexandria, Va. 22313

2. To locate HMOs in your area, contact one of the following:
(a) The Group Health Association of America
1717 Massachusetts Ave., N.W.
Washington, D.C. 20036

(b) c/o Dr. Frank Seubold
HMO Program
Room 7-39
Parklawn Building
5600 Fishers Lane
Rockville, Md. 20852

3. For information about dental-care prepared plans, contact:
Digest of Prepaid Dental Case Plans
U.S. Department of Health, Education, and Welfare
Public Health Service
NIH
Division of Dental Health
Bethesda, Md. 20014

4. For information on hospitals, write:
JCAH
837 North Michigan Ave.
Chicago, Ill. 60611

Further Readings

Ferguson, Tom, ed., *Medical Self-Care Magazine,* Inverness, Cal., 1977 (current issues).

Illich, Ivan, *Limits to Medicine (or Medical Nemesis),* Toronto, Canada: McClelland and Stewart, 1976.

McKeown, Thomas, "Determinants of Health," *Human Nature,* April 1978, pp. 60–67.

Sehnert, Keith W., and Howard Eisenberg, *How to Be Your Own Doctor—Sometimes,* New York: Grosset, 1975.

APPENDIX A   TABLES

Table A.1
Essential Amino Acid Values in Typical American Foods

Food Item	Measure	Weight g	Calories	Protein g	TRP	LEU	LYS	MET	PHA	ISL	VAL	THR	Men (160 lb)	Women (124 lb)
BREADS, CEREALS, GRAINS, AND GRAIN PRODUCTS														
Bread														
Cracked wheat	1 slice	23	61	2	24	134	54	30*	98	86	92	58	4	5
Cracked wheat, toasted	1 slice	19	60	2	24	134	54	30*	98	86	92	58	4	5
French, enr flour	1 slice	20	58	1.8	22	139	41	23*	99	83	77	52	4	5
Italian, enr flour	1 slice	20	58	1.8	22	139	41	23*	99	83	77	52	3	4
Pumpernickel	1 slice	32	79	2.9	32	194	119	46*	136	125	151	107	6	8
Raisin	1 slice	23	60	1.5	18	100	40	22*	74	64	69	30	3	4
Raisin, toasted	1 slice	19	60	1.5	18	100	40	22*	74	64	69	30	3	4
Rye	1 slice	23	56	2.1	23	141	67	32*	101	90	109	67	4	6
Rye, toasted	1 slice	20	56	2.1	23	141	67	32*	101	90	109	67	4	6
White, enr	1 slice	23	62	2.0	24	159	60	29*	108	96	92	62	4	6
White, toasted	1 slice	23	62	2.0	24	159	60	29*	108	96	92	62	4	5
Whole wheat	1 slice	23	55	2.1	29	166	71	37*	117	106	113	72	5	7
Whole wheat, toasted	1 slice	19	55	2.4	29	166	71	37*	117	104	113	72	5	7
Bread stuffing, uncooked	1 cup	190	704	24	292	1916	646	330*	1330	1146	1086	732	46	58
Bread crumbs, dry	1 cup	88	345	11.0	133	871	294	150*	605	522	494	333	21	27
Buns, soft, enr flour (hamburger, hotdog)	1 avg	30	89	2.5	31	200	82	38*	134	124	121	82	5	7
Cornflakes	1 cup	25	93	1.98	14	272	40	35*	92	80	100	72	5	6
Corn grits, cooked	1 cup	242	123	2.9	17	377	84	55*	131	134	147	116	8	10
Cornmeal, cooked	1 cup	240	115	2.64	14	313	71	46*	108	111	122	96	6	8
Cracker														
Graham	1 med	7	28	0.56	10	54	22	12*	39	35	37	23	2	2
Standard, round, snack	1 med	3	17	0.24	3	22	7	4*	16	13	12	8	1	1
Soda	1 square	6	26	0.55	6	44	14	8*	32	26	22	16	1	1
Danish pastry	1 sm	35	148	2.6	33	205	77	42*	144	128	125	84	6	8
Farina, instant cooked	1 cup	38	131	4.1	—*	262	76	46	198	186	167	106	—	—
Flour														
Buckwheat, light	1 cup	110	382	7.0	119	437	416	134*	296	267	394	282	19	24
Potato	1 cup	110	386	8.8	97	442	468	115*	389	389	468	345	16	20
Rye, medium	1 cup	110	385	13.0	138	840	514	200*	197	1201	652	464	28	36
Soy, full flat	1 cup	110	418	45.0	605	3428	2784	605*	2179	2380	2339	1734	84	108
Wheat, enr, all-purpose	1 cup	110	394	12.0	139	893	267	151*	638	534	499	336	21	27
Whole wheat	1 cup	120	410	15.0	192	1072	432	240*	784	688	739	464	33	43
Macaroni, enr, salt-cooked	1 cup	140	155	5.3	58	317	154	72*	250	240	274	187	10	13
Muffin														
Plain, enr flour	1 med	48	139	3.7	49	312	157	68*	202	199	202	136	9	12
Blueberry	1 med	40	112	2.9	38	243	122	53*	157	155	157	106	7	9
Noodles, enr, salt-cooked	1 cup	160	200	6.6	73	436	218	112*	317	323	389	277	16	20
Oatmeal or rolled oats, cooked	1 cup	236	130	4.7	76	501	221	86*	275	275	319	205	12	15

Column group header: Essential Amino Acids, mg (TRP, LEU, LYS, MET, PHA, ISL, VAL, THR); Percent of Limiting Amino Acid Supplied† (Men, Women).

* Limiting amino acid.

† Percentages are based on Recommended Dietary Allowances for limiting amino acid of each particular food.

Table A.1 Continued
Essential Amino Acid Values in Typical American Foods

Food Item	Measure	Weight g	Calories	Protein g	Essential Amino Acids, mg TRP	LEU	LYS	MET	PHA	ISL	VAL	THR	Percent of Limiting Amino Acid Supplied† Men (160 lb)	Women (124 lb)
Pancake, buckwheat	1 med	45	90	3.1	46	258	189	68*	153	168	192	131	9	12
Rice														
Brown, cooked	1 cup	150	178	3.8	41	327	148	68*	190	179	266	148	9	12
Brown, raw	1 cup	190	744	14.3	159	1233	558	260*	717	675	1004	558	36	47
Instant	1 cup	148	161	3.3	36	284	129	59*	165	155	231	129	8	11
Parboiled, cooked, long grain	1 cup	150	155	3.2	35	275	125	58*	160	150	224	125	8	10
White, cooked	1 cup	150	158	3	33	258	117	54*	150	141	210	117	8	10
White, raw	1 cup	191	675	13	140	1107	503	230*	643	604	900	503	32	41
Rice flakes	1 cup	30	111	1.77	15	—*	19	—*	96	—*	—*	—*	—	—
Roll														
Sweet	1 avg	50	158	4.25	54	349	155	71*	232	218	215	145	10	13
Dinner, enr flour	1 med	38	113	3.12	38	249	102	47*	166	153	149	102	7	8
Popcorn, with oil and salt	1 cup	14	66	1.4	9	182	40	26*	63	65	72	56	4	5
Tortilla, yellow corn	6-in.-diam cake	30	63	1.5	8	242	38	28*	64	88	78	60	4	5
Waffle	1 avg	75	206	6.98	94	598	331	144*	379	391	404	272	20	26
Wheat														
Bran	1 oz	29	62	4.6	74	273	190	56*	167	185	213	130	8	10
Flakes	1 cup	36	125	4.4	49	363	147	52*	195	202	233	145	7	9
Germ	1 tbsp	6	24	1.8	16	110	99	26*	58	76	88	86	4	5
DAIRY PRODUCTS														
Cheese														
Brick	1 svg	28	103	6.2	87	608	453	161*	335	415	446	229	22	29
Camembert, domestic	1 svg	28	84	4.9	69	475	358	127*	265	328	353	181	18	23
Cheddar, American	1 piece	17	68	4.3	60	417	310	111*	230	285	306	157	15	20
Cheddar, American, grated	1 tbsp	7	28	1.75	25	176	131	47*	97	121	129	67	7	8
Cottage, creamed	1 cup	225	235	31.0	336	3294	2562	854*	1647	1769	1769	1434	119	153
Cottage, uncreamed	1 cup	260	223	44.2	469	4608	3584	1195*	2304	2475	2475	2005	166	209
Edam	1 oz	28	87	7.7	108	755	562	200*	416	516	555	285	28	36
Gruyere	1 oz	28	115	8.1	105	778	591	211*	429	543	575	300	29	38
Limberger	1 oz	28	69	5.9	83	578	431	153*	319	395	425	218	21	27
Parmesan	1 oz	28	110	10.0	140	980	730	260*	540	670	720	370	36	47
Pasteurized, processed, American	1 oz	28	103	6.5	91	631	475	169*	351	436	468	240	23	30
Pasteurized, processed, pimento (American)	1 oz	28	103	6.5	91	631	475	169*	351	436	468	240	23	30
Roquefort	1 oz	28	103	6	81	601	453	161*	329	415	441	227	22	29
Swiss, domestic	1 oz	28	99	7.8	123	884	665	235*	485	609	650	336	33	42
Cream														
Half and half	1 tbsp	15	20	0.48	7	50	39	12*	24	32	35	23	2	2
Half and half	1 cup	240	322	7.68	106	752	592	182*	364	486	524	350	25	33
Heavy or whipping	1 cup	238	861	5.24	71	512	401	123*	246	329	357	238	17	22
Sour	1 oz	30	57	0.8	12	83	65	20*	40	53	58	39	3	4
Egg														
Boiled, poached, or raw	1 med	50	79	6.5	102	559	406	197*	369	420	470	318	27	35
Fried	1 med	50	108	6.2	99	546	397	192*	360	409	459	310	27	34
Scrambled or omelet	1 med	64	116	7.6	112	644	476	215*	407	472	527	355	30	39
White	1 med	31	16	3.4	51	296	204	133*	214	218	262	150	18	24
Yolk	1 med	17	58	2.72	39	235	185	70*	123	171	190	140	10	13

* Limiting amino acid.
† Percentages are based on Recommended Dietary Allowances for limiting amino acid of each particular food.

Table A.1 Continued
Essential Amino Acid Values in Typical American Foods

Food Item	Measure	Weight g	Calories	Protein g	TRP	LEU	LYS	MET	PHA	ISL	VAL	THR	Men (160 lb)	Women (124 lb)
Milk, cow's														
Buttermilk	1 cup	246	90	8.9	90	809	678	188*	433	514	613	384	26	34
Skim, dry, instant	1 cup	64	228	23	320	2260	1780	570*	1095	1461	1575	1073	79	102
Skim, fortified	1 cup	246	89	8.9	137	970	764	235*	470	627	676	451	33	42
Whole, fortified	1 cup	244	159	8.54	118	832	655	202*	403	538	580	386	28	36
Milk, goat, fresh	1 cup	244	163	7.7	94	663	741	156*	289	203	328	515	22	28
Milk, human, fresh	1 oz	30	23	0.3	5	27	19	6*	13	16	18	13	1	1
Yogurt, part skim	1 cup	250	125	4.3	93	842	706	196*	450	536	638	400	27	35
DESSERTS AND SWEETS														
Banana bread	1 slice	49	134	2.4	33	178	92	45*	123	117	119	81	6	8
Doughnut														
Cake	1 avg	33	129	1.52	20	126	55	27*	85	79	78	53	4	5
Raised or yeast	1 avg	33	136	2.1	26	169	74	35*	114	107	106	72	5	6
Raised, jelly-filled	1 avg	65	226	3.4	44	276	120	58*	186	174	172	116	8	10
FISH AND SEAFOODS														
Anchovy														
Canned	3 fillet	12	21	2.3	23	175	202	67*	85	117	122	99	9	12
Paste	1 tsp	7	14	1.4	14	106	123	41*	52	71	74	60	6	7
Bass, fried	1 lb	453	756	96	857	6513	7542	2485*	3171	4371	4542	3685	345	445
Cod, canned	1 lb	453	385	87	870	6609	7655	2523*	3216	4435	4611	3742	345	450
Flounder, baked	1 lb	453	915	135	1359	10,125	11,880	3915*	4995	6885	7155	5805	536	699
Haddock, fried	1 lb	453	742	88	888	6709	7762	2556*	3262	4530	4675	3793	350	456
Herring, pickled	1 lb	453	1003	91	924	6930	8040	2681*	3420	4711	4896	3973	367	478
Mackerel, canned	1 lb	453	789	87	957	7178	8326	2775*	3541	4785	5072	4115	385	497
Perch, yellow, raw	1 lb	453	412	87	883	6459	7773	2563*	3266	4502	4684	3796	351	457
Pike														
Blue and northern, flesh only	1 lb	453	403	82	830	6225	7304	2407*	3071	4223	4399	3569	334	431
Walleye, flesh only	1 lb	453	392	86	875	6562	7700	2538*	3238	4462	4638	3762	353	455
Salmon, pink, canned	1 lb	453	639	93	929	6967	8081	2695*	3433	4643	4919	3995	374	481
Shrimp														
Canned	1 lb	453	525	110	1098	8345	9662	3184*	4063	5600	5819	4721	442	571
Cooked	1 lb	453	989	92	821	6240	7225	2381*	3038	4187	4351	3530	331	427
Smelt, raw	4-5 med	100	98	18.6	186	1395	1637	539*	688	949	986	800	75	97
Swordfish, broiled	1 lb	453	764	129	1268	9513	11,161	3678*	4693	6469	6722	5454	504	657
Trout, rainbow, raw	1 lb	453	883	97	974	7302	8571	2827*	3606	6654	5164	4186	387	505
Tuna, canned in oil, drained	1 lb	453	892	130	1307	9804	11,504	3791*	4837	6667	6930	5621	527	679
FOOD SUBSTITUTES														
Cream substitute, liquid	1 tbsp	14	24	0.12	1	11	9	3*	6	8	8	5	1	1
FRUITS														
Apple, raw, whole	1 med	130	76	0.26	—*	17	14	5	12	19	12	10	—	—
Apricot, raw	1 med	38	19	0.38	—*	68	68	13	38	41	56	48	—	—
Avocado	1 lg	216	361	4.54	46	—*	240	38	—*	—*	—*	—*	—	—
Banana, raw	1 med	150	128	1.65	28	—*	82	16	—*	—*	—*	—*	—	—
Cantaloupe, raw	1/4	100	30	0.7	1	—*	18	2	—*	—*	—*	—*	—	—
Dates														
Dried	1 med	10	27	0.22	6	8	7	3*	6	7	9	6	1	1
Dried and pitted	1 cup	178	488	3.92	109	136	117	47*	113	133	168	109	7	8
Fig, raw	1 med	38	30	0.46	20	103	95	20*	57	72	91	76	3	4
Grapefruit:														
Canned	1 cup	250	175	1.5	1	—*	9	—*	—*	—*	—*	—*	—	—
Red flesh	1 med	260	180	1.3	1	—*	9	—*	—*	—*	—*	—*	—	—
Orange, fresh	1 med	180	88	1.8	5	—*	48	5	—*	—*	—*	—*	—	—

* Limiting amino acid.
† Percentages are based on Recommended Dietary Allowances for limiting amino acid of each particular food.

Table A.1   Continued
Essential Amino Acid Values in Typical American Foods

Food Item	Measure	Weight g	Calories	Protein g	TRP	LEU	LYS	MET	PHA	ISL	VAL	THR	Men (160 lb)	Women (124 lb)
								Essential Amino Acids, mg					Percent of Limiting Amino Acid Supplied†	
Papaya, raw	1 lg	400	156	2.4	16	—*	51	3	—*	—*	—*	—*	—	—
Peach, fresh	1 med	100	38	0.68	4*	29	30	31	18	13	40	27	1	2
Pear, Japanese	1 med	182	111	1.27	7	36	25	9*	21	25	36	23	1	1
Persimmon, raw	1 med	100	96	0.88	14	52	42	8*	38	36	38	49	1	1
Pineapple, canned in heavy syrup	1 slice	122	90	0.37	5	—*	9	1	—*	—*	—*	—*	—	—
Strawberries, raw	1 cup	149	55	1.04	13	63	48	1.5*	34	27	34	37	1	1
MEATS, POULTRY, AND GAME														
Beef														
Chuck roast	1 lb	453	1481	108	1154	7888	8369	2405*	3944	5002	5291	4233	334	431
Corned beef	1 lb	453	1685	72	836	5864	6254	1775*	2944	3746	3976	3160	247	318
Dried beef, uncooked	3 oz	85	173	29.1	341	2388	2547	723*	1199	1526	1618	1288	100	130
Heart, lean	1 lb	453	490	78	1009	6906	6363	1862*	3492	3880	4423	3570	259	334
Liver, fried	1 lb	453	635	120	1354	8398	6772	2167*	4515	3786	5689	4334	301	388
Rump roast	1 lb	453	1571	107	1176	8036	8526	1752*	4018	5096	5390	3084	243	314
Round steak	1 lb	453	856	141	1062	7257	7700	2212*	3628	4602	4868	3894	307	395
Short ribs	1 lb	453	1092	128	1148	7847	8326	2392*	3924	4976	4264	4211	332	429
Sirloin steak, broiled	1 lb	453	1848	101	1187	8110	8604	2472*	4055	5143	5440	4352	343	443
Beef and vegetable stew	1 lb	453	403	29	305	1936	2083	573*	1069	1281	1398	1096	80	103
Brains, cooked, all kinds	1 lb	453	566	47	625	3828	3443	997*	2292	2283	2428	2238	138	179
Calf														
Liver, fried	1 lb	453	1182	134	1306	8100	6532	2090*	4355	4529	5487	4181	290	315
Sweetbread (pancreas), braised	1 lb	453	760	87	1132	6794	6445	1568*	3658	4442	4703	4007	218	281
Lamb														
Leg, roast	1 lb	453	1264	80	1525	9075	9543	2824*	4832	6131	5768	5421	392	506
Shoulder	1 lb	453	1531	98	902	5413	5621	1666*	2845	3609	3401	3192	231	299
Pork														
Bacon, broiled, drained	1 lb	453	2767	137	381	3048	2476	610*	1829	1676	1829	1295	85	109
Canadian bacon, cooked, drained	1 lb	453	1255	125	907	7256	5896	1451*	4354	3991	4354	3084	202	260
Ham, cured, roasted	1 lb	453	1309	95	1238	7037	7807	2386*	3715	4847	4953	4379	331	428
Liver, fried	1 lb	453	594	93	1410	8686	7005	2242*	4670	4950	5884	4484	311	402
Spareribs, cooked	1 lb	453	1993	94	509	2901	3214	980*	1529	1999	2030	1803	136	176
Veal, rump roast	1 lb	453	1064	126	1150	6460	7346	2036*	3540	4690	4514	2806	283	365
NUTS AND SEEDS														
Almonds, dried	1 cup	133	760	25	234	1934	774	344*	1524	1161	1495	811	47	61
Brazil nuts, unsalted	1 cup	167	1079	23	312	1885	740	1571	1030	990	1374	705	85	110
Cashews, unsalted	1 cup	100	569	15	430	1410	740	327*	877	1135	1479	688	45	59
Coconut														
Fresh	1 cup	100	346	3.5	33	269	151	71*	174	180	212	129	10	13
Shredded	1 cup	62	344	2.2	21	175	98	46*	113	117	138	84	6	8
Hazelnuts	11 avg	15	97	1.6	27	118	53	18*	68	107	118	52	3	3
Peanuts														
Roasted with skin	1 cup	240	1397	60	800	4432	2592	640*	3680	2992	3616	1952	89	115
Salted, roasted	1 cup	240	1418	62	800	4800	2816	704*	4000	3248	3936	2128	98	126
Pecans, raw halves	1 cup	104	715	10	144	804	452	159*	587	575	546	405	22	28
Pistachios	1 cup	100	594	19	—*	1523	1080	367	1088	881	1344	613	—	—
Pumpkin and squash kernels	1 cup	230	1271	67	1201	5269	3068	1267*	3735	3735	3602	2001	176	227
Sesame seeds	1 cup	230	1339	42	711	3641	1256	1382*	3181	2052	1925	1548	192	248
Sunflower seeds, dry	1 cup	100	560	24	85	401	225	119*	278	267	317	230	17	21
Walnuts, English	1 cup	100	651	15	175	1228	441	306*	767	767	974	589	43	55
SAUSAGE, COLD CUTS, AND LUNCHEON MEATS														
Braunschweiger	1 lb	453	1447	67.1	738	5636	5234	1409*	3020	3288	4160	2885	196	253
Frankfurters, cooked	1 lb	453	1377	56	454	4026	4536	1191*	2041	2722	2835	2325	165	213

* Limiting amino acid.

† Percentages are based on Recommended Dietary Allowances for limiting amino acid of each particular food.

Table A.1   Continued
Essential Amino Acid Values in Typical American Foods

Food Item	Measure	Weight g	Calories	Protein g	TRP	LEU	LYS	MET	PHA	ISL	VAL	THR	Men (160 lb)	Women (124 lb)
													Percent of Limiting Amino Acid Supplied†	
Headcheese	1 lb	453	1216	70.3	351	4429	4288	1195*	2671	2390	2882	1968	166	214
Liverwurst	1 lb	453	1393	73.5	808	6174	5733	1544*	3381	3602	4557	3160	214	277
Salami	1 lb	453	1411	79.4	972	7776	8748	2268*	3996	5292	5400	4428	315	406
Sausage, bologna	1 lb	453	1379	54.9	439	3953	4447	1153*	1976	2690	2745	2251	160	207
Vienna sausage, canned	1 lb	453	1089	63.5	572	4572	5144	1334*	2286	3048	3175	2604	185	239
VEGETABLES														
Asparagus, raw	1 spear	16	44	2.9	5	18	20	6*	13	15	20	13	1	1
Beans														
Green, cooked	1 cup	125	31	2	28	116	104	30*	48	90	00	76	4	5
Lima, raw	1 cup	100	346	20	202	1628	1488	250	1212	992	1030	836	34	44
Yellow or wax, cooked	1 cup	100	22	1.4	20	81	73	21*	34	63	67	57	3	4
Bean sprouts (mung beans)	1 cup	100	28	3.2	22	291	218	35*	154	179	189	99	5	6
Broccoli	1 cup	150	39	4.65	45	202	181	61*	149	157	210	153	8	11
Cabbage														
Red, raw	1 cup	100	31	2.0	16	80	94	18*	42	78	60	56	3	3
Shredded	1 cup	105	25	1.4	11	55	64	13*	28	54	41	38	2	2
Carrots														
Diced, cooked	1 cup	150	47	1.35	11	77	62	11*	50	54	66	51	2	2
Raw	1 lg	100	42	1.1	9	59	48	9*	38	42	51	40	1	2
Cauliflower, raw	1 cup	100	27	2.7	35	181	151	54*	84	116	162	113	8	10
Celery, raw	1 lg													
	stalk	50	8	0.45	4	—*	6	5	—*	—*	—*	—*	—	—
Chick-peas (garbanzos), dry, raw	½ cup	100	360	20.5	164	1517	1415	266*	1004	1189	1004	738	37	48
Collards, leaves, steamed	1 cup	200	66	7.2	76	302	280	64*	172	168	270	156	9	11
Sweet corn														
Cream style	1 cup	200	164	4.2	32	572	192	98*	292	192	328	214	14	18
Whole kernel	1 cup	200	132	3.8	22	418	140	72*	212	140	240	156	10	13
Cucumber, raw	½ med	50	8	0.5	4	23	22	5*	12	16	17	14	1	1
Eggplant, cooked	1 cup	180	34	1.8	16	112	49	9*	79	92	106	63	1	2
Kale, raw w/stems	1 cup	125	47	5.25	57.5	341	162.5	47.5*	215	179	246	189	625	8.75
Lentils, dry, whole	1 cup	200	680	49.4	444	3508	3014	346*	2272	2618	2668	1728	48	60
cooked	1 cup	200	212	15.6	140	954	898	100†	654	540	626	496	13	17
Lettuce														
Iceberg	3½ oz	100	13	0.9	12	—*	70	4	—*	—*	—*	—*	—	—
Leaf	3½ oz	100	18	0.3	13	—*	75	4	—*	—*	—*	—*	—	—
Romaine	3½ oz	100	18	0.3	13	—*	75	4	—*	—*	—*	—*	—	—
Mushrooms, canned	1 cup	200	34	3.8	12	444	—*	266	—*	840	596	—*	—	—
Onions														
Cooked, mature	1 cup	210	61	2.5	38	65	116	23*	71	38	55	40	3	4
Dry, mature	1 med	100	38	1.5	22	39	69	14*	42	22	23	24	2	3
Flakes	1 oz	29	100	2.5	38	65	117	23*	71	38	55	40	3	4
Peas, green, cooked	1 cup	133	94	7.2	58	452	338	51*	281	330	294	114	6.65	7.98
Pepper, green, raw	1 lg	100	22	1.2	8	46	50	16*	55	46	32	50	2	3
Potato														
Baked with skin	1 med	100	93	2.6	26	130	138	31*	114	114	138	107	4	6
Mashed with butter and milk	1 cup	200	188	4.2	42	210	222	50*	184	184	222	172	7	9
Pan fried	1 cup	133	356	5.32	53	266	282	64*	235	235	282	217	8	11

* Limiting amino acid.

† Percentages are based on Recommended Dietary Allowances for limiting amino acid of each particular food.

Source: From John Krischmann, *Nutrition Almanac,* New York: McGraw-Hill, 1975. Used with the permission of McGraw-Hill Book Company.

Table A.2
Nutritive Values of the Edible Part of Foods

Food	Weight g	Approximate Measure	Energy Kcal	Protein g	Fat g	Total Carbohydrate g	Minerals Calcium mg	Phosphorus mg	Magnesium mg	Sodium mg	Potassium mg	Zinc mg	Copper mg	Iron mg	Vitamins Total Vitamin A Activity IU	Thiamin mg	Riboflavin mg	Niacin mg	Vitamin B-6 mg	Pantothenic Acid mg	Folacin (free) mcg	Vitamin B-12 mcg	Vitamin C mg
Almonds, chopped	15	12–15 nuts, 2 tbsp	90	3.0	8.0	3	35	75	40	1	115	0.2	0.1	0.7	0	0.04	0.1	0.5	0.02	0.07	5	0	tr
Apples, raw with skin	150	1 medium 3/lb	80	0.3	0.8	20	10	15	10	1	150	0.08	0.1	0.4	100	0.04	0.1	0.1	0.04	0.2	5	0	6
Apple juice, canned, no sugar added	125	½ c	60	0.1	tr	15	10	10	5	1	125	0.04	0.01	0.6	u	0.01	0.02	0.1	0.04	0.1	1	0	1
Applesauce, sweetened	125	½ c	120	0.3	0.1	30	5	5	5	3	100	0.1	0.01	0.6	50	0.03	0.01	tr	0.04	0.1	1	0	1
Apricots																							
Fresh	100	2–3 medium	50	1.0	0.2	13	15	25	10	1	280	0.04	0.1	0.5	2700	0.03	0.04	0.6	0.07	0.2	u	0	10
Canned, heavy syrup	120	4 halves, 2 tbsp juice	100	0.7	0.1	25	15	20	10	1	235	0.04	0.1	0.4	2000	0.02	0.02	0.5	0.06	0.1	u	0	5
water pack	100	4 halves, 2 tbsp juice	40	0.7	0.1	10	10	15	5	1	245	0.03	0.1	0.3	1800	0.02	0.06	0.4	0.06	0.1	u	0	4
Dried, sulfured, raw	30	4–6 medium halves	80	1.5	0.2	20	20	30	20	1	295	0.04	0.1	1.7	3300	tr	0.05	1.0	0.05	0.2	3	0	4
Apricot nectar, canned	125	½ c	70	0.4	0.1	18	10	15	5	tr	190	u	u	0.3	1200	0.01	0.01	0.3	0.04	0.10	u	0	4
Artichokes, French, boiled	120	1 large (300 g as purchased)	30	3.0	0.2	12	60	85	u	35	360	0.4	0.4	1.3	200	0.08	0.05	0.8	0.30	0.60	u	0	10
Asparagus																							
Fresh, green, cooked	100	½ c cut, 6–7 spears	20	2.0	0.2	4	20	50	15	1	185	0.3	0.1	0.6	900	0.2	0.2	1.5	0.2	0.6	60	0	25
Canned, salt added	100	½ c cut, 6–7 spears	20	2.0	0.4	3	20	50	15	235	165	0.8	0.1	1.9	800	0.06	0.1	0.8	0.06	0.2	25	0	15
Avocados	125	½ fruit, 4-in. long	190	2.0	18.0	7	10	45	55	5	680	0.5	0.5	0.7	350	0.1	0.2	2.0	0.4	1.1	40	0	15
Baby foods																							
Dinners																							
beef-noodle	130	Contents 4½ oz jar	60	3.5	1.5	9	15	35	u	150	205	u	0.1	0.6	790	0.03	0.06	0.6	0.04	0.2	u	0.3	3
beef-vegetable			110	9.5	4.5	8	15	35	u	115	145	u	0.1	1.5	1410	0.09	0.2	2.0	0.10	0.3	u	0.3	3
vegetable-beef-cereal			70	3.5	2.0	10	20	50	u	150	185	u	0.1	1.0	3580	0.04	0.05	1.0	0.05	0.2	u	0.2	1
Fruits and desserts																							
banana-pineapple	135	Contents 4¾ oz jar	110	0.5	0.1	30	30	15	u	10	100	u	0.1	0.3	40	0.01	0.01	0.1	0.06	0.2	1	0.05	3
custard pudding			130	3.0	2.5	25	80	80	u	80	120	u	0.06	0.4	130	0.03	0.2	0.1	0.02	0.3	u	0.2	1
fruit pudding			130	1.5	1.0	30	35	45	5	15	100	u	0.1	0.4	140	0.04	0.07	0.1	0.02	0.2	u	0.08	4
Bacon, broiled, drained	25	2 strips, thick	140	6.5	12.5	1	3	55	5	245	60	1.2	0.1	0.8	0	0.1	0.03	1.0	0.03	0.08	1	0.2	0
Bagels	60	4-in. diameter	180	6.5	2.0	30	10	50	u	u	u	0.6	0.2	1.3	30	0.15	0.11	1.3	u	u	u	u	0
Bamboo shoots	100	¾ c	25	2.5	0.3	6	13	60	u	u	630	u	u	0.5	20	0.15	0.07	0.6	u	u	u	u	4
Bananas	120	1 medium	100	1.5	0.2	25	10	30	55	1	440	0.3	0.2	0.8	250	0.06	0.07	0.8	0.6	0.3	25	0	10
Bean sprouts. See Sprouts																							
Beans																							
Canned, with pork and tomato sauce	130	½ c	160	8.0	3.5	25	70	115	35	590	270	1.0	0.2	2.3	150	0.10	0.04	0.8	0.4	0.1	10	0	3
Canned, with pork and sweet sauce	130	½ c	190	8.0	6.0	25	80	145	35	485	u	1.0	0.3	3.0	u	0.08	0.05	0.7	0.1	0.1	10	0	3
Lima, fresh or frozen, boiled	85	½ c	95	6.5	0.4	17	40	105	65	2	360	0.9	0.4	2.2	250	0.20	0.08	1.0	0.1	0.2	8	0	15
Red, canned	15	½ c	120	7.0	0.5	20	35	140	35	4	335	1.0	0.2	2.3	tr	0.06	0.05	0.8	0.4	0.1	10	0	0
Refried	120	½ c	230	8.5	12.5	25	50	165	35	340	360	1.0	0.2	2.3	tr	0.30	0.07	0.8	0.2	0.2	20	0	0
Snap, green, fresh or frozen, boiled	65	½ c	15	1.0	0.2	3	55	25	15	2	95	0.2	0.08	0.4	350	0.05	0.06	0.3	0.04	0.1	5	0	8
canned	65	½ c	15	1.0	0.2	3	55	25	15	150	60	0.2	0.08	1.0	300	0.02	0.04	0.2	0.03	tr	5	0	2
Soybeans, mature, dry, cooked	90	½ c (1 oz dry wt)	120	10.0	5.0	10	65	160	80	2	490	0.6	0.3	2.5	20	0.20	0.08	0.6	u	0.3	20	0	0
Beef																							
Corned, canned	80	2 slices each, 3 in. × 2 in. × ¼ in.	170	20.0	9.5	0	15	85	20	u	u	2.5	u	3.4	tr	0.02	0.20	3.0	0.08	0.5	2	1.5	0
hash, with potatoes	110	½ c	200	10.0	12.5	12	15	75	20	595	220	1.4	u	2.2	tr	0.01	0.10	2.5	0.08	0.6	u	0.8	0
Dried, creamed	120	½ c	190	10.0	12.5	9	130	170	40	880	190	1.8	u	1.0	450	0.08	0.20	0.8	0.60	0.7	u	u	1
Hamburger, broiled, lean, 21% fat	85	4/lb, raw wt	240	20.0	16.5	0	10	160	20	50	220	3.7	0.07	2.6	30	0.07	0.20	4.5	0.4	0.3	8	1.5	0
very lean, 10% fat	85	4/lb, raw wt	190	23.0	9.5	0	10	195	20	60	260	4.9	0.09	3.0	20	0.08	0.20	5.0	0.4	0.3	10	1.5	0
Roast, chuck, braised	85	3 oz	240	23.0	16.5	0	10	115	20	40	185	3.7	0.07	2.9	30	0.04	0.20	3.5	0.2	u	3	1.5	0
rib, U.S. choice	85	3 oz	380	17.0	33.5	0	10	160	20	40	190	3.1	0.07	2.2	70	0.05	0.10	3.0	0.3	0.3	3	1.5	0
Steak, broiled																							
round with fat	85	3 oz	220	24.5	13.0	0	10	215	25	60	270	5.0	0.09	3.0	20	0.07	0.20	5.0	0.3	0.4	3	2.2	0
sirloin with fat	85	3 oz	330	20.0	27.0	0	10	160	20	50	220	3.7	0.07	2.5	50	0.05	0.20	4.0	u	u	3	1.5	0
Beef stew, with vegetables	245	1 c	220	15.5	10.5	15	30	185	50	90	615	2.4	0.05	2.9	2400	0.15	0.15	4.7	0.3	0.2	7	1.6	15
Beer	360	12-oz bottle	150	1.0	0	14	20	110	35	25	90	0.1	0.2	tr	0	0.01	0.10	2.0	0.2	0.3	25	0	0
Beet greens, boiled	75	½ c	15	1.0	0.2	2	70	20	80	55	240	0.5	0.2	1.4	3700	0.05	0.10	0.2	0.08	0.2	*	0	10
Beets, sliced, canned	85	½ c	30	1.0	0.1	8	15	15	15	200	135	0.3	0.1	0.6	20	0.01	0.03	0.1	0.04	0.1	30	0	2
Beverages. See Carbonated beverages, individual entries.																							

Food	Measure	g																					
Biscuits, from mix, enriched	1 of 2-in. diameter	30	90	2.0	3.0	15	90	65	5	270	30	0.3	0.09	0.5	tr	0.08	0.07	0.6	0.01	0.1	2	0	0
Blackberries, boysenberries, etc., raw	1/2 c	70	40	0.8	0.6	9	25	15	20	1	120	0.05	0.1	0.5	150	0.02	0.03	0.3	0.04	0.2	2	0	15
Blueberries, raw	1/2 c	70	45	0.5	0.4	11	10	10	4	1	60	0.05	0.08	0.3	80	0.02	0.04	0.4	0.05	0.1	2	0	10
Bokchoy. See Pakchoy.																							
Brazil nuts, raw	6 large nuts	30	180	4.0	19.0	3	55	195	65	tr	205	1.4	0.4	1.3	tr	0.30	0.03	0.5	0.05	0.1	tr	0.1	0
Bread																							
Boston brown, canned	1 slice, 1/2 in. thick	45	95	2.5	0.6	20	40	70	u	115	130	u	u	0.9	30	0.05	0.3	0.5	tr	0.1	u	u	0
Corn, from mix	2 1/2 in. square	55	180	4.0	6.0	30	135	210	u	265	60	u	u	0.8	150	0.10	0.10	0.8	tr	0.2	u	u	0
Cracked wheat	1 slice	25	65	2.2	0.6	13	20	30	10	130	35	0.3	0.05	0.3	tr	0.03	0.02	0.3	0.02	0.2	3	0	0
French, Vienna, Italian, enriched	1 slice	25	70	2.3	0.8	14	10	20	5	145	20	0.5	0.09	0.5	0	0.07	0.06	0.6	0.02	0.1	3	0	0
Fry bread, Indian, enriched	1 piece, medium	60	200	4.0	7.5	28	80	50	u	305	35	u	u	1.0	0	0.10	0.09	1.3	0.02	0.2	10	0	0
Raisin, not enriched	1 slice	25	65	1.5	0.7	13	20	20	5	90	60	0.3	0.05	0.3	0	0.01	0.02	0.2	0.01	0.1	3	0	0
Rye, American	1 slice	25	65	2.5	0.3	13	15	40	10	140	35	0.4	0.05	0.4	0	0.05	0.02	0.4	0.02	0.1	2	0	0
White, not enriched	1 slice	25	70	2.2	0.8	13	20	25	5	130	25	0.2	0.05	0.2	tr	0.02	0.02	0.6	0.01	0.1	3	0	0
enriched	1 slice	25	70	2.2	0.8	13	20	25	5	130	25	0.6	0.05	0.6	tr	0.06	0.05	0.6	0.01	0.1	3	0	0
Whole wheat	1 slice	25	65	2.5	0.8	12	25	60	10	130	70	0.4	0.07	0.8	tr	0.06	0.03	0.7	0.04	0.2	9	0	0
Broccoli, fresh or frozen, boiled	1/2 c	85	20	2.5	0.2	4	70	50	15	8	205	0.2	0.07	0.6	1900	0.07	0.20	0.6	0.1	0.4	20	0	70
Brussels sprouts, fresh or frozen, boiled	4 large sprouts	85	30	3.5	0.3	5	25	60	15	8	230	0.3	0.08	0.9	440	0.07	0.12	0.7	1.1	15	0	70	
Butter, salted	1 tsp or pat (90/lb)	5	35	tr	4.0	tr	1	1	tr	40	1	tr	0	tr	150	tr	tr	tr	tr	0	0	tr	tr
	1 tbsp	15	100	0.1	11.5	0.1	3	3	tr	120	3	tr	0	tr	450	tr	tr	tr	tr	0	0	tr	tr
Cabbage, green, headed																							
Raw, shredded	1 c	70	17	0.9	0.1	4	35	20	10	15	165	0.3	0.08	0.3	90	0.04	0.04	0.2	0.1	0.1	20	0	35
Cooked, chopped	1/2 c	70	15	0.8	0.2	3	30	15	10	10	120	0.3	0.02	0.2	100	0.03	0.03	0.2	0.1	0.1	2	0	25
Cakes																							
Angel food	2-in. sector of 10-in. cake	40	105	2.5	0.1	25	40	50	10	60	25	0.1	0.02	0.1	0	tr	0.04	tr	tr	0.08	1	tr	0
Cheese cake, frozen	1/10 of cake	85	225	6.5	12.5	24	80	80	30	170	90	u	0.04	0.5	200	0.05	0.1	0.3	u	u	u	tr	
Chocolate, with chocolate icing	2-in. sector of 8-in. cake	90	310	4.0	11.5	55	55	95	20	240	120	1.1	0.3	0.7	150	0.03	0.07	0.3	0.4	3	0.1	0	
Gingerbread	2 3/8 in. square	65	170	2.0	4.5	30	55	65	u	190	175	u	u	1.0	tr	0.02	0.06	0.5	u	u	u	u	0
Cupcake, iced	1 medium	50	190	2.0	6.0	30	60	95	u	160	55	u	u	0.4	80	0.02	0.05	0.1	u	u	u	u	0
Pound cake	3 1/2 in. × 3 in. × 1/2 in.	30	140	1.5	9.0	14	6	25	5	35	20	0.2	0.02	0.2	80	0.01	0.03	0.1	0.09	2	u	0	
Yellow with chocolate icing	2-in. sector of 8-in. cake	70	230	3.0	8.0	40	65	125	15	160	75	0.3	0.07	0.4	100	0.01	0.06	0.1	0.2	2	u	0	
Candy																							
Caramels	1 oz	30	120	1.0	3.0	20	40	35	u	65	55	u	0.01	0.4	tr	0.01	0.05	0.1	0.1	u	tr	0	
Chocolate bar																							
plain milk chocolate	1 oz	30	140	2.0	9.0	16	65	65	20	25	110	0.1	0.3	0.3	80	0.02	0.10	0.1	0.2	1	tr	0.03	
with almonds	1 oz	30	150	2.5	10.0	14	65	75	u	25	125	0.1	u	0.5	70	0.02	0.10	0.2	0.1	1	u	0.1	
Fudge with nuts	1 oz	30	120	1.0	5.0	20	20	30	u	50	50	u	u	0.3	tr	0.01	0.03	0.1	u	tr	u	0	
Hard	1 oz	30	110	0	0.3	30	6	2	u	10	1	u	0.03	0.5	0	0	0	0	0	u	u	0	
Marshmallow	1 oz	30	90	0.6	tr	25	5	2	u	2	2	0.01	0.06	0.5	0	0	tr	0	u	0	u	0	
Peanut brittle	1 oz	30	120	1.5	3.0	25	10	25	5	10	45	u	u	0.7	0	0.05	0.01	1.0	tr	2	u	0	
Cantaloupe. See Melons.																							
Carbonated beverages, sweet	6 oz	170	65	0	0	17	0	0	0	0	0	0	0	0.4	0	0	0	0	0	0	0	0	0
Carrots																							
Raw	1 carrot, 7 1/2 in. × 1 1/8 in.	80	30	0.8	0.1	7	25	25	15	35	245	0.3	0.07	0.5	7900	0.04	0.04	0.4	0.2	10	0	6	
Boiled	1/2 c diced	70	20	0.5	0.1	5	25	20	4	25	160	0.2	0.07	0.4	7600	0.04	0.04	0.5	0.2	2	0	4	
Cashews, roasted	1 oz	30	160	5.0	13.0	8	10	105	80	60	130	1.3	0.2	1.1	30	0.1	0.07	0.5	0.4	2	0	0	
Cauliflower																							
Raw	1/2 c whole flower buds	50	15	1.5	0.1	3	10	30	12	5	150	0.5	0.1	0.6	60	0.1	0.1	0.7	0.5	15	0	75	
Boiled	1/2 c	60	15	1.5	0.2	3	15	25	8	10	130	0.1	0.1	0.4	40	0.06	0.05	0.4	0.5	2	0	35	
Celery																							
Raw	2 large stalks	80	15	0.8	0.1	3	30	20	17	100	270	0.09	0.09	0.2	200	0.02	0.02	0.3	0.3	5	0	8	
Boiled	1/2 c diced	75	10	0.6	0.1	2	25	15	u	65	180	0.08	0.08	0.2	200	0.02	0.02	0.3	0.3	u	0	4	

tr — trace amounts
u — unknown thought to be present
0 — Absent or below detection level

Source: Reproduced from C. F. Adams, *Nutritive Value of American Foods in Common Units,* USDA Agriculture Handbook No. 456, 1975, updated, as available, from revised USDA Handbook No. 8 (Vols. I and II, 1976).

Table A.2 Continued

Nutritive Values of the Edible Part of Foods

Food	Weight g	Approximate Measure	Energy Kcal	Protein g	Fat g	Total Carbohydrate g	Calcium mg	Phosphorus mg	Magnesium mg	Sodium mg	Potassium mg	Zinc mg	Copper mg	Iron mg	Total Vitamin A Activity IU	Thiamin mg	Riboflavin mg	Niacin mg	Vitamin B-6 mg	Pantothenic Acid mg	Folacin (free) mcg	Vitamin B-12 mcg	Vitamin C mg
Cereals, breakfast																							
Ready-to-eat																							
bran flakes, 40% enr.	35	1 c	100	3.5	0.6	30	20	125	u	205	135	1.3	0.4	12.4	0	0.4	0.5	4.0	0.1	0.3	6	0	0
corn flakes, enriched	25	1 c	95	2.0	0.1	20	4	10	4	250	30	0.07	0.03	0.6	0	0.4	0.4	3.0	0.02	0.05	3	0	0
granola	50	1/2 c	215	5.7	9.6	29	30	170	60	3	180	1.0	0.4	1.6	0	0.16	0.08	1.1	0.06	0.45	20	tr	0
rice, puffed, enriched	15	1 c	60	0.9	0.1	13	3	15	u	tr	15	0.2	0.03	0.3	0	0.07	0.01	0.7	0.01	0.06	1	0	0
wheat flakes, enriched	30	1 c	100	3.0	0.5	25	10	85	30	310	80	0.7	0.3	1.1	0	0.4	0.4	3.5	0.09	0.1	3	0	0
wheat, shredded	50	1 c of spn-sized	180	5.0	1.0	40	20	195	65	2	175	1.4	0.4	1.8	0	0.1	0.06	2.0	0.1	0.4	5	0	0
Cooked, 1 oz dry wt, salt added																							
cornmeal and grits																							
unenriched	120	1/2 c	60	1.5	0.2	13	1	15	10	130	20	0.1	0.06	0.2	70	0.02	0.01	0.1	0.04	0.2	2	0	0
enriched	120	1/2 c	60	1.5	0.2	13	1	15	10	130	20	0.1	0.06	0.5	70	0.07	0.05	0.6	0.04	0.2	2	0	0
oatmeal	120	1/2 c	65	2.5	1.0	12	10	70	30	260	75	0.6	0.04	0.7	0	0.10	0.02	0.1	0.04	0.4	5	0	0
wheat farina																							
light, enriched (e.g., Cream of Wheat)	120	1/2 c	50	1.5	0.1	10	5	15	4	175	10	0.07	0.04	0.4	0	0.05	0.04	0.5	0.02	0.1	5	0	0
whole-meal (e.g., Ralston)	120	1/2 c	55	2.0	0.4	12	10	65	35	260	60	0.6	0.3	0.6	0	0.08	0.02	0.8	0.1	0.2	10	0	0
Chard, Swiss, boiled	70	1/2 c	15	1.5	0.2	2	55	20	45	60	230	u	u	1.3	3900	0.03	0.08	0.3	u	0.1	u	0	0
Cheese																							
Natural																							
blue, Roquefort	30	1 oz	100	6.0	8.0	0.7	150	110	7	395	75	0.8	0.04	0.1	200	0.01	0.1	0.3	0.05	0.5	0.3	0.3	0
cheddar	30	1 oz	115	7.0	9.5	0.4	205	145	8	175	30	0.9	0.04	0.2	300	0.01	0.1	tr	0.02	0.1	0.3	0.2	0
cottage, creamed	110	1/2 c	120	14.0	5.0	3.0	70	150	6	455	95	0.4	0.02	0.2	180	0.02	0.2	0.1	0.2	0.15	15.0	0.7	0
cream	30	2 tbsp	100	2.0	10.0	0.8	25	30	2	85	35	0.2	0.01	0.3	400	tr	0.06	tr	0.01	0.1	0.2	0.1	0
Parmesan	30	1 oz	130	12.0	8.5	1.0	390	230	15	455	30	0.8	0.1	0.3	200	0.01	0.1	0.1	0.03	0.1	0.3	u	0
Swiss	30	1 oz	110	8.0	8.0	1.0	270	170	10	75	30	1.1	0.04	0.1	250	tr	0.1	tr	0.02	0.1	0.3	0.5	0
Pasteurized, processed																							
American	30	1 oz	110	6.0	9.0	0.5	175	210	6	405	45	0.8	0.05	0.1	350	0.01	0.1	tr	0.02	0.1	0.9	0.2	0
cheese spread	30	1 oz	80	4.5	6.0	2	160	200	8	380	70	0.7	u	0.1	200	0.01	0.1	tr	0.03	0.2	u	0.1	0
Cheese fondue	100	2/3 c	260	15.0	18.5	10	320	295	u	540	165	u	0.04	1.2	900	0.06	0.3	0.2	u	0.1	u	u	0
Cherries																							
Raw, sweet	75	10 cherries	45	0.9	0.2	12	15	15	10	1	130	0.1	0.1	0.3	70	0.03	0.04	0.3	0.02	0.2	4	0	7
Red, canned																							
heavy syrup	130	1/2 c with syrup	100	1.0	0.2	25	20	15	10	2	160	u	0.06	0.4	80	0.02	0.02	0.2	0.06	0.1	tr	0	4
water pack	120	1/2 c with juice	50	1.0	0.2	13	20	15	10	2	160	u	0.06	0.4	80	0.04	0.02	0.2	u	u	tr	0	4
Chicken																							
Canned, flesh only	100	1/2 c	200	22.5	12.0	0	20	255	20	u	140	2	0.2	1.6	250	0.04	0.1	4.5	0.3	0.8	2	0.8	0
Creamed	120	1/2 c	210	17.5	12.0	7	85	140	u	u	u	u	u	1.1	300	0.04	0.2	4.0	u	u	u	u	u
Fried																							
breast	95	1/2 breast	160	25.5	5.0	1	9	220	10	u	140	0.8	0.1	1.3	70	0.04	0.2	11.5	0.6	0.8	2	0.4	0
leg	55	1 medium	90	12.0	4.0	0.4	6	90	10	u	80	1.4	0.1	0.9	50	0.03	0.2	2.5	0.3	0.2	3	0.2	0
thigh	65	1 medium	120	15.0	6.0	1	7	120	10	u	160	1.6	0.1	1.2	100	0.03	0.2	3.5	0.4	0.5	3	0.3	0
Roasted, light meat, without skin	100	3 1/2 oz	170	31.5	3.0	0	12	265	u	65	410	0.9	0.1	1.4	60	0.04	0.1	11.5	0.7	0.8	3	0.4	0
Chickpeas or garbanzos, cooked without salt	125	1/2 c (30 g, dry wt)	110	6.0	1.0	18	45	106	u	10	240	2.7	u	2.1	15	0.1	0.03	0.6	0.2	0.4	7	0	tr
Chili con carne, with beans, canned	255	1 c	340	19.0	15.5	30	80	320	65	1355	595	4.2	0.8	4.3	150	0.08	0.20	3.3	0.3	0.4	10	u	tr
Chili powder, chilis. See peppers.																							
Chili relleno (stuffed pepper)	110	1 pepper	190	10.5	14.0	6	225	195	u	465	270	u	u	1.3	1600	0.08	0.2	0.8	0.1	0.7	15	1.0	55
Chocolate, bitter or baking	30	1 oz	140	3.0	15.0	8	20	110	u	1	235	0.7	0.8	1.9	20	0.01	0.07	0.4	0.01	0.06	4	0	0
Sweet, milk. See Candy.																							
Chow mein, canned, chicken without noodles	250	1 c	95	6.5	0.3	18	45	85	45	725	420	1.2	0.3	1.3	150	0.05	0.10	1.0	0.4	1.2	10	1.6	15
Clams, canned, with liquid	100	3 1/2 oz, 1/2 c	50	8.0	0.7	3	55	135	115	u	140	1.2	0	4.0	u	0.01	0.1	1.0	0.08	0.3	3	20	0
Cocoa, dry	5	1 tbsp	15	0.9	1.0	3	5	55	20	tr	80	0.3	0.2	0.6	tr	0.01	0.02	0.1	tr	tr	tr	u	tr
Coconut, dry, unsweetened	30	1 oz	180	2.0	17.5	6	5	50	u	u	160	u	0.2	0.9	0	0.02	0.01	0.2	0.01	0.06	u	u	0
Coffee, instant, regular dry powder	2.5	1 tbsp	3	tr	tr	0	4	10	10	2	80	0.01	0.02	0.1	0	0	0.08	0.08	0.02	u	u	u	0	0
Collards, boiled	70	1/2 c	20	2.0	0.4	4	110	30	30	35	170	0.5	0.2	0.4	3900	0.1	0.2	0.8	0.1	0.3	25	0	35
Cookies																							
Commercial assortment	35	4 cookies	170	1.5	7.0	25	10	55	5	125	25	0.2	0.05	0.2	30	0.01	0.02	0.1	0.02	0.1	1	0	0
Fig bar	55	4 cookies	200	2.0	3.0	40	45	35	15	140	110	0.6	0.1	0.6	60	0.02	0.04	0.2	0.05	0.2	2	0	tr
Oatmeal with raisins	50	4 cookies	235	3.0	8.0	40	10	55	u	85	190	0.6	0.06	1.5	30	0.06	0.04	0.3	u	u	2	u	tr

Corn, sweet, yellow																							
Fresh or frozen, boiled	80	½ c	70	2.5	0.8	15	2	75	25	tr	135	0.3	0.08	0.5	350	0.09	0.08	1.0	0.2	0.3	2	0	6
Canned, whole kernel	80	½ c	70	2.0	0.6	16	4	40	15	195	80	0.3	0.05	0.4	300	0.02	0.04	0.8	0.2	0.2	2	0	4
Cream style	130	4 c	110	2.5	0.8	25	4	70	25	300	125	0.6	0.08	0.8	400	0.04	0.06	1.5	0.3	0.4	2	0	6
Corn fritter	35	1 fritter 2 in. × 1½ in.	130	2.5	8.0	14	20	55	u	165	45	u	u	0.6	150	0.06	0.07	0.6	u	u	u	u	tr
Corn syrup	20	1 tbsp	60	0	0	15	10	3	u	15	1	u	0.07	u	0	0	0	0	0	0	0	0	0
Cowpeas or blackeye peas																							
Immature	80	½ c	90	7.0	0.6	15	20	120	15	1	310	0.6	0.2	1.7	300	0.2	0.09	1.0	0.04	0.2	20	0	15
Mature, dry, cooked	125	½ c (1 oz dry wt)	95	6.5	0.4	17	20	120	u	10	285	2.0	0.2	1.6	10	0.2	0.05	0.5	0.07	0.3	20	0	u
Crabmeat	100	½ c, packed	100	18.0	2.0	0.6	45	185	u	u	90	4.5	1.0	0.8	2300	0.2	0.08	3.0	0.3	0.6	2	10	2
Crackers																							
Butter (e.g., Ritz)	15	5 round	75	1.1	3.0	11	25	40	u	180	20	u	0.03	0.1	30	tr	tr	0.1	u	u	u	0	0
Graham	15	1 cracker 5 in. × 2½ in.	55	1.0	1.0	10	5	20	5	95	55	0.2	0.03	0.2	0	0.01	0.03	0.2	0.01	0.08	4	0	0
Rye wafer (e.g., Rykrisp)	5	2 wafers	40	1.5	0.2	10	5	50	u	110	u	u	0.04	0.5	0	0.04	0.03	0.2	u	u	u	0	0
Saltines	10	4 each, 2 in. square	50	1.0	1.5	8	2	10	3	125	15	0.05	0.02	0.1	0	tr	tr	0.1	0.01	0.05	2	0	0
Cranberry jelly, or sauce, canned	35	⅛ c	50	tr	tr	13	2	1	u	tr	10	tr	u	tr	10	tr	tr	tr	0.01	u	u	0	tr
Cream																							
half-and-half	60	¼ c or 4 tbsp	80	2.0	7.0	3	65	55	8	25	80	0.3	0.07	tr	300	0.02	0.08	0.02	0.02	0.2	1	0.2	tr
Heavy whipping	60	¼ c; ½ c whipped volume	210	1.0	22.0	2	45	35	4	20	45	0.1	0.06	tr	850	0.01	0.08	0.02	0.01	0.2	0.6	0.1	tr
Light, for coffee	60	¼ c, 4 tbsp	120	2.0	12.0	2	60	50	5	25	75	0.2	0.06	tr	450	0.02	0.08	tr	0.02	0.2	0.6	0.1	tr
Sour	60	¼ c, 4 tbsp	130	1.5	11.0	2	60	50	5	25	80	0.2	0.06	tr	450	0.02	0.09	0.05	0.01	0.2	7	0.1	tr
Cream substitutes																							
Coffee whitener	3	1 tsp or packet	15	0.1	0.8	2	1	12	tr	5	20	0.02	u	tr	5	0	0	0	0	0	0	0	0
Whipped topping, frozen	10	2 tbsp	30	0.1	2.5	2	1	1	tr	2	2	tr	u	tr	80	0	0	0	0	0	0	0	0
Cucumber, raw, peeled	80	½ small	10	0.4	0.1	2	15	15	5	4	125	0.08	0.04	0.2	tr	0.02	0.03	0.2	0.03	0.2	10	0	8
Custard, baked	130	½ c	150	7.0	7.5	15	150	155	u	105	195	u	0.1	0.6	450	0.06	0.2	0.2	u	u	4	u	0
Dandelion greens, boiled	50	½ c	20	1.0	0.3	3	75	20	20	25	120	u	u	1.0	6100	0.07	0.08	u	u	u	u	0	10
Dasheen (Japanese taro), raw	100	1⅓ corms	100	2.0	0.2	25	30	60	u	5	515	u	u	1.0	20	0.1	0.04	1.1	u	u	u	0	4
Dates, dried	30	10, pitted	220	2.0	0.4	60	45	50	45	1	520	u	0.2	2.4	40	0.07	0.08	2.0	0.1	0.6	10	0	0
Doughnuts																							
Cake type	40	1 average	160	2.0	8.0	20	15	80	5	210	40	0.2	0.04	0.6	30	0.07	0.07	0.5	0.02	0.2	3	0	0
Yeast, raised	40	1 average	180	2.5	11.0	16	15	30	5	100	35	0.3	0.04	0.6	30	0.07	0.07	0.6	0.02	0.2	4	0	0
Eggnog	250	1 c	340	9.5	19.0	34	330	275	45	140	420	1.1	u	0.6	900	0.08	0.5	0.3	0.1	1.1	2	1.1	3
Eggs, chicken																							
Whole, raw or hard cooked	50	1 large	80	6.0	5.5	0.6	30	90	6	60	65	0.7	0.05	1.0	300	0.04	0.15	tr	0.06	0.9	25	0.6	0
white	33	1 white	15	3.5	tr	0.4	4	4	3	50	45	tr	0.01	tr	0	tr	0.09	tr	tr	0.07	1	0.02	0
yolk	17	1 yolk	65	3.0	5.0	tr	25	85	3	10	15	0.6	0.05	0.9	300	0.04	0.07	tr	0.05	0.9	25	0.6	0
Scrambled	140	2 eggs	190	12.0	14.0	30	95	195	15	310	170	1.4	0.07	1.9	600	0.07	0.30	0.1	0.1	1.8	50	1.3	tr
Eggplant, boiled	100	½ c diced	20	1.0	0.2	4	10	20	15	1	150	u	0.1	0.6	10	0.05	0.04	0.5	0.08	0.2	2	0	3
Enchiladas, beef																							
Frozen, commercial	200	7-oz portion	240	15.0	8.5	25	20	190	u	725	155	u	u	2.5	600	0.1	0.2	3.0	u	u	u	u	u
Home recipe	190	2 enchiladas	365	32.0	16.7	22	450	480	u	510	585	u	u	5	6000	0.1	0.4	6.0	0.8	0.7	10	2	10
Fats, shortening, solid	100	½ c	880	0	100.0	0	0	0	0	0	0	0	0	0	0	0	0	0	0	0	0	0	0
or oil	12	1 tbsp	110	0	12.0	0	0	0	0	0	0	0	0	0	0	0	0	0	0	0	0	0	0
Figs, fresh	100	2 medium	80	1.0	0.4	20	35	20	20	2	195	u	0.07	0.6	80	0.06	0.06	0.4	0.1	0.3	u	0	2
Dried	30	2 small	80	1.5	0.4	20	40	25	20	u	190	u	0.08	0.6	20	0.03	0.03	0.2	0.05	0.1	1	0	0
Fish																							
Cod, steak, sautéed	110	4 oz	180	30.0	6.0	0	30	285	30	115	420	0.9	0.2	1.0	200	0.08	0.1	3.0	0.3	0.3	10	0.9	0
Fish sticks, breaded	110	4 sticks	200	19.0	10.0	7	10	190	20	u	u	0.3	0.2	0.4	0	0.04	0.08	2.0	0.06	0.3	10	1.1	0
Haddock, fried	110	4 oz	180	22.0	7.0	6	45	270	30	195	385	1.1	0.2	1.3	u	0.04	0.08	3.5	0.2	0.1	5	1.4	2
Mackerel, sautéed	105	3 average	250	23.0	17.0	0	5	295	30	u	u	1.0	0.2	1.3	550	0.2	0.3	8.0	0.7	0.9	5	9.4	0
Salmon,																							
steak, broiled	145	1 average 6 in. × 2 in.	230	35.0	9.0	0	u	630	60	150	565	2.4	1.2	1.5	200	0.2	0.08	12.5	1.0	1.9	6	5.8	0
canned, pink	110	½ c	160	23.0	6.0	0	215	315	30	425	395	1.0	0.3	0.9	80	0.04	0.2	9.0	0.3	0.6	10	7.6	0
red	110	½ c	190	22.0	10.0	0	285	380	30	575	380	1.0	0.3	1.3	250	0.04	0.2	8.0	0.3	0.6	10	7.6	0
Sardines																							
canned in oil	85	3 oz drained	170	20.5	9.0	0	370	425	35	700	500	2.4	0.03	2.4	200	0.03	0.2	4.5	0.2	0.7	10	8.5	0
Sole or flounder, fillet, baked	100	3 oz	200	30.0	8.0	0	25	345	30	235	585	1.0	0.07	1.4	u	0.07	0.08	2.5	0.2	0.8	10	1.2	2
Swordfish, broiled	100	3 oz	170	26.5	6.0	0	25	260	u	u	u	u	u	1.3	2000	0.04	0.05	10.5	u	0.2	u	1.0	0
Tuna, raw	100	½ c	135	27.5	3.0	0	5	175	30	35	180	0.5	0.5	1.3	50	0.02	0.05	6.6	0.9	0.5	3	3.0	7
canned in oil	100	½ c	200	28.0	8.0	0	10	230	25	u	u	1.0	0.1	1.9	80	0.05	0.1	12.0	0.4	0.3	8	2.2	0
in water	100	½ c	130	28.0	0.8	0	15	190	25	865	275	u	u	1.6	80	0.05	0.1	13.0	0.4	0.3	8	2.2	0

tr — trace amounts
u — unknown thought to be present
0 — Absent or below detection level

Table A.2   Continued
Nutritive Values of the Edible Part of Foods

Food	Weight g	Approximate Measure	Energy Kcal	Protein g	Fat g	Total Carbohydrate g	Calcium mg	Phosphorus mg	Magnesium mg	Sodium mg	Potassium mg	Zinc mg	Copper mg	Iron mg	Total Vitamin A Activity IU	Thiamin mg	Riboflavin mg	Niacin mg	Vitamin B-6 mg	Pantothenic Acid mg	Folacin (free) mcg	Vitamin B-12 mcg	Vitamin C mg
Flour, wheat																							
White, all purpose																							
unenriched	115	1 c	420	12.0	1.0	90	20	100	30	2	110	0.8	0.2	0.9	0	0.07	0.06	1.0	0.07	0.5	20	0	0
enriched	115	1 c	420	12.0	1.0	90	20	100	30	2	110	0.8	0.2	3.3	0	0.05	0.3	4.0	0.07	0.5	20	0	0
Whole-grain	120	1 c	400	16.0	2.5	85	50	445	135	4	445	2.9	0.6	4.0	0	0.7	0.1	5.0	0.4	1.3	35	0	0
French toast, frozen	65	1 slice	130	5.0	4.3	18	50	85	u	305	80	u	u	1.3	250	0.1	0.1	0.7	u	u	u	u	0
Frozen dinners																							
Chicken, fried, with potatoes, mixed vegetables	310	11-oz dinner	570	28.0	29.0	48	70	350	60	1075	350	3.0	0.4	3.2	1800	0.2	0.6	16.0	0.9	1.6	20	0.7	10
Meat loaf, with tomato sauce, potatoes, peas	310	11-oz dinner	410	25.0	21.0	30	60	365	60	1225	360	3.5	0.5	4.0	1300	0.3	0.4	5.5	0.7	0.9	20	1.1	10
Turkey with gravy, potatoes, peas	310	11-oz dinner	340	25.0	9.0	40	80	260	65	1200	530	3.0	0.4	3.3	400	0.2	0.3	7.0	0.8	1.8	30	0.6	10
Fruit cocktail	130	1/2 c	95	0.5	0.2	25	10	15	40	5	205	u	0.04	0.5	200	0.02	0.02	0.5	0.04	u	0	0	2
Gelatin, dry	8	1 tbsp or packet	30	7.0	0	0	u	u	2	1	u	u	0.1	u	0	0	0	0	0	0	0	0	0
Gelatin dessert, plain	120	1/2 c	70	2.0	0	17	u	u	2	1	u	0.02	0.03	u	0	0	0	0	0	0.03	0	0	0
Grapefruit, raw	100	1/2 medium	40	0.5	0.1	10	15	15	12	1	130	0.1	0.04	0.4	80	0.04	0.02	0.2	0.03	0.2	8	0	35
Grapefruit juice, canned																							
Unsweetened	180	3/4 c	75	0.9	0.2	18	15	25	22	2	300	u	0.02	0.7	20	0.06	0.04	0.4	0.02	0.2	15	0	65
Sweetened	180	3/4 c	100	0.9	0.2	25	15	25	20	2	300	u	0.02	0.7	20	0.06	0.04	0.4	0.02	u	15	0	60
Grapes, raw																							
Slip-skin	100	20 grapes	45	0.8	0.8	10	10	10	10	2	105	0.17	0.1	0.2	80	0.02	0.02	0.08	0.08	0.08	4	0	2
Adherent skin	100	20 grapes	70	0.6	0.4	17	10	20	6	4	175	0.3	0.1	0.4	100	0.06	0.04	0.4	0.08	0.08	4	0	4
Grape juice	190	3/4 c	120	0.4	tr	30	20	20	25	4	220	u	0.03	0.6	u	0.08	0.04	0.4	0.04	0.08	4	0	tr
Guacamole	120	1/2 c	140	2.1	12.8	7	15	40	u	165	565	u	0.3	0.7	550	0.10	0.2	1.6	0.4	0.9	30	0.4	35
Ham, baked	85	3 oz	250	18.0	19.0	0	10	145	15	635	200	3.4	0.3	2.2	0	0.4	0.2	3.0	0.3	0.3	1	0	0
Hominy grits. See Cereal, cooked.																							
Honey, strained	20	1 tbsp	65	0.1	0	17	1	1	1	1	10	0.02	0.03	0.1	0	tr	0.01	0.1	0.01	0.04	0	0	tr
Ice cream, vanilla																							
Plain, 10% fat	65	1/2 c	135	2.5	7.0	15	90	70	10	60	130	0.7	0.02	0.05	300	0.02	0.2	0.05	0.03	0.3	1	0.3	0
Rich, 16% fat	75	1/2 c	175	2.0	12.0	16	75	60	8	50	110	0.6	0.02	0.05	450	0.02	0.15	0.05	0.03	0.3	1	0.3	0
Ice milk, vanilla	65	1/2 c	90	2.5	3.0	15	90	65	10	50	130	0.3	u	0.09	100	0.04	0.2	0.04	0.04	0.3	0	0.4	0
Ices, water, lime	95	1/2 c	120	0.4	tr	30	tr	tr	u	3	20	u	u	tr	0	tr	tr	tr	u	0	0	0	0
Jams and jellies	20	1 tbsp	55	0.1	tr	14	4	2	1	2	20	0.1	0.02	0.2	tr	tr	0.01	tr	0.02	0	tr	0	tr
Kale, boiled without stems	55	1/2 c	20	2.5	0.4	3	105	30	18	25	120	u	u	0.9	4600	0.06	0.1	0.2	0.2	0.6	25	0	50
Kidney, braised	100	3 1/2 oz	250	33.0	12.0	0.8	20	240	20	250	320	2.4	0.1	13.0	1100	0.5	4.87	10.5	0.4	3.8	60	30	u
Kohlrabi, boiled	80	1/2 c, diced	20	1.5	0.1	4	25	35	30	5	215	u	u	0.2	15	0.05	0.02	0.2	0.1	0.5	u	u	35
Kumquat, raw	20	1 medium	10	0.2	tr	3	10	4	u	1	45	u	u	0.1	100	0.01	0.02	0.1	u	u	6	0	7
Lamb, choice grade																							
Chop, loin, broiled																							
lean and fat	95	1 average	340	21.0	28.0	0	10	165	15	50	235	u	0.1	1.2	u	0.1	0.2	5.0	0.3	0.5	1	2.0	0
lean only	65	1 average	120	18.0	5.0	0	10	140	15	45	205	3.0	0.1	1.3	u	0.1	0.2	4.0	0.2	0.4	1	1.4	0
Leg, roasted																							
lean only	85	3 oz	160	24.0	6.0	0	10	200	15	60	275	3.6	0.05	1.9	0	0.1	0.3	5.5	0.2	0.5	1	1.8	0
Shoulder, roasted																							
lean and fat	85	3 oz	280	18.5	23.0	0	10	145	15	45	205	u	0.1	1.0	tr	0.1	0.2	4.0	0.2	0.5	1	1.8	0
Lard, see Fats.																							
Lasagna, frozen	225	8-oz serving	380	27.0	12.4	43	310	470	55	1100	740	1.4	u	5.6	1300	0.4	0.4	4.5	u	0.6	u	u	15
Lemon juice, fresh	15	1 tbsp	5	0.1	tr	tr	1	2	1	tr	20	u	u	tr	tr	tr	tr	tr	0.02	0.02	u	0	7
Lemonade, from frozen concentrate	250	1 c	110	0.1	tr	30	2	3	2	1	40	0.02	0.02	tr	10	0.01	0.02	0.2	0.01	0.03	5	0	15
Lentils, dried, cooked	100	1/2 c	110	8.0	tr	19	25	120	20	u	250	1.0	0.3	2.1	20	0.07	0.06	0.6	u	u	6	0	0
Lettuce, raw																							
Head, solid (iceberg type)	90	1/6 head	10	0.8	0.1	3	20	20	10	10	160	0.4	0.08	0.5	300	0.05	0.05	0.3	0.05	0.2	30	0	5
Loose leaf, romaine, cos	55	1 c, chopped	10	0.7	0.2	2	35	15	10	5	145	0.2	0.05	0.8	1000	0.03	0.04	0.2	0.03	0.1	30	0	10
Liver																							
Beef, fried	85	3 oz	200	22.5	9.0	4	10	405	15	155	325	4.3	2.5	7.5	45,400	0.2	3.6	24.0	0.7	6.5	70	68.0	25
Calf, fried	85	3 oz	220	25.0	11.2	3	10	455	20	100	385	5.2	6.5	12.1	27,800	0.2	3.5	14.0	0.6	6.5	70	51.0	30
Chicken, simmered	70	1/2 c, chopped	120	18.5	3.0	2	10	110	u	40	105	2.4	0.2	6.0	8600	0.1	1.9	8.0	0.5	4.2	u	17.5	10
Lobster, northern, cooked	95	2/3 c meat	90	18.0	1.5	0.3	65	185	20	205	175	2.1	1.6	0.8	0	0.1	0.07	u	u	1.4	8	0.5	u
Lychee nuts, raw	150	10 nuts	60	0.8	0.3	15	5	40	3	3	155	u	u	0.4	0	u	0.05	u	u	u	u	u	40
Macaroni and other pastas, cooked																							
Unenriched	130	1 c	190	6.5	0.7	40	15	85	25	1	105	0.6	0.03	0.7	0	0.03	0.03	0.5	0.03	0.2	5	0	0
Enriched	130	1 c	190	6.5	0.7	40	15	85	25	1	105	0.6	0.03	1.4	0	0.2	0.1	2.0	0.03	0.2	5	0	0

Macaroni with cheese, casserole, baked	200	1 c	430	17.0	22.0	40	360	320	50	1085	240	1.3	0.08	1.8	850	0.2	0.4	2.0	0.09	0.4	10	0.8	0
Mangos, raw	165	1 c, diced	110	1.0	0.7	30	15	20	30	10	310	0.8	0.2	0.7	7900	0.08	0.08	2.0	u	0.3	u	u	60
Margarine	5	1 tsp, 1 pat (90/lb)	35	tr	4	tr	1	1	tr	50	1	0.01	tr	0	160	0	0	0	0	0	0	0	0
Melons																							
Cantaloupe	160	½ melon or 1 c, cubed	50	1.0	0.2	12	20	25	20	20	400	0.1	0.06	0.6	5400	0.06	0.05	1.0	0.1	0.4	50	0	5
Honeydew	170	⅛ melon or 1 c, cubed	55	1.4	0.5	13	25	25	u	20	425	0.1	0.06	0.7	70	0.07	0.05	1.0	u	u	u	0	40
Watermelon	425	¹⁄₁₆ melon (2 lb with rind)	110	2.0	0.9	25	30	45	35	5	425	u	0.3	2.1	2500	0.1	0.[illegible]	0.9	0.3	1.2	8	0	30
Milk, cow																							
Whole, fluid	245	1 c	155	8.0	8.5	11	290	225	30	120	370	1.0	0.08	0.1	350	0.09	0.4	0.2	0.1	0.8	10	0.9	2
2%, low-fat	245	1 c	140	10.0	5.0	14	350	275	40	145	450	1.1	0.08	0.1	200	0.1	0.5	0.2	0.1	0.9	15	1.0	2
Skim, nonfat, or buttermilk	245	1 c	90	8.5	0.4	12	300	245	3	125	400	1.0	0.08	0.1	10	0.09	0.4	0.2	0.1	0.8	15	1.0	2
Chocolate, low-fat	250	1 c	180	8.0	5.0	26	285	255	30	150	420	1.0	u	0.6	200	0.1	0.4	0.3	0.1	0.7	10	0.8	2
Dried, instant																							
whole	30	¼ c	160	8.5	8.5	12	290	250	25	120	425	1.0	0.06	0.1	300	0.09	0.4	0.2	0.09	0.7	10	1.0	2
nonfat	35	¼ c	125	12.0	0.2	13	445	345	40	190	600	1.5	0.1	0.1	10	0.09	0.5	0.3	0.1	1.1	15	1.4	2
Evaporated	250	1 c	340	17.5	20.0	25	660	510	60	265	765	1.9	0.2	0.4	600	0.1	0.8	0.5	0.1	1.6	20	0.4	3
Condensed, sweetened	40	1 fl oz	120	3.0	3.5	20	105	95	10	50	140	0.4	0.08	0.1	100	0.03	0.2	0.1	0.02	0.3	4	0.2	tr
Milk, human, U.S.	30	1 fl oz	21	0.3	1.3	2.1	10	4	1	5	16	0.05	0.01	0.01	70	.004	0.01	0.1	0.003	0.07	2	0.02	2
Milkshakes, commercial	270	10 fl oz	320	11.0	7.0	50	365	340	30	300	600	0.5	0.04	0.3	300	0.08	0.5	0.4	0.1	1.0	15	0.6	tr
Molasses																							
Light	20	1 tbsp	50	0	0	13	35	10	9	3	185	u	u	0.9	0	0.01	0.01	tr	u	u	u	0	0
Medium	20	1 tbsp	50	0	0	12	60	15	16	5	215	0.9	03	1.2	0	u	0.02	0.2	0.04	0.07	2	0	0
Blackstrap	20	1tbsp	45	tr	0	11	135	15	52	20	585	u	u	3.2	0	0.02	0.04	0.4	u	u	u	0	0
Muffins																							
Bran	40	1 muffin	100	3.0	4.0	15	55	160	u	180	170	u	u	1.5	100	0.06	0.[illegible]	1.5	u	u	u	u	0
Cornmeal	40	1 muffin	130	3.0	4.0	19	40	70	20	190	55	u	u	0.7	100	0.08	0.09	0.6	u	u	u	u	0
Plain or blueberry	40	1 muffin	120	3.0	4.0	17	40	60	10	175	50	0.5	0.09	0.6	50	0.07	0.09	0.6	0.02	0.2	3	0.1	0
Mushrooms, raw	35	½ c, sliced	10	1.0	0.1	2	2	40	5	5	145	0.1	0.04	0.3	tr	0.04	0.2	1.5	0.04	0.8	7	0	1
Mustard greens, boiled	70	½ c	15	1.5	0.3	3	95	20	10	10	155	0.2	0.06	1.2	4100	0.06	0.[illegible]	0.4	0.09	0.1	u	0	35
Mustard, prepared, yellow	5	1 tsp	4	0.2	0.2	0.3	4	4	2	65	5	0.03	0.02	0.1	0	u	u	u	u	u	u	0	0
Noodles, egg, cooked																							
Unenriched	105	⅔ c	130	4.5	1.5	25	10	65	25	2	45	0.6	0.02	0.6	70	0.03	0.02	0.4	0.02	0.2	2	tr	0
Enriched	105	⅔ c	130	4.5	1.5	25	10	65	25	2	45	0.6	0.02	0.9	70	0.10	0.09	1.3	0.02	0.2	2	tr	0
Oils. See *Fats*.																							
Okra, boiled	105	10 pods	30	2.0	0.3	6	100	45	40	2	185	u	0.1	0.5	500	0.1	0.2	1.0	0.08	0.2	10	0	20
Olives																							
Green	25	5 large	20	0.2	2.5	0.2	10	4	5	465	10	0.02	0.09	0.3	60	u	u	u	0.01	0	3	0	0
Ripe	25	5 large	35	0.2	4.0	0.6	20	4	u	150	5	0.07	0.09	0.4	20	tr	tr	u	tr	tr	u	0	0
Onions																							
Green, raw, bulb and top	25	¼ c, chopped or 3 onions	10	0.4	tr	2	15	10	3	1	60	0.07	0.01	0.3	500	0.01	0.01	0.1	u	0.4	10	0	8
Mature, dry	85	½ c, chopped	30	1.5	0.1	7	25	30	10	10	135	0.3	0.1	0.4	35	0.02	0.04	0.2	0.1	0.1	8	0	8
raw	10	1 tbsp, ⅛ onion	4	0.2	tr	0.9	3	4	1	1	15	0.03	0.01	0.1	tr	tr	tr	tr	0.01	0.01	1	0	1
boiled	105	½ c, sliced	30	1.0	0.1	7	25	30	10	10	115	0.6	0.08	0.4	40	0.03	0.03	0.2	0.1	0.1	10	0	8
Oranges, raw	140	1 medium	80	1.8	0.1	18	60	30	30	1	270	0.3	0.09	0.6	280	0.14	0.06	0.6	0.08	0.4	45	0	85
Orange juice, fresh or frozen	185	¾ c	85	1.5	0.4	19	20	30	20	2	370	0.04	0.09	0.4	400	0.2	0.05	0.8	0.07	0.4	65	0	95
Oysters, raw																							
Eastern	120	6 oysters	80	10.0	2.0	4	115	170	40	90	145	90.0	4.0	6.6	350	0.2	0.2	3.0	0.6	0.3	u	21.6	u
Pacific	120	6 oysters	110	12.5	2.5	8	100	185	30	u	u	10.8	4.0	8.6	u	0.1	u	1.6	u	u	u	u	35
Pakchoy, raw	100	⅔ c	15	1.0	0.1	3	165	45	u	25	305	u	u	0.8	3000	0.05	0.1	0.8	u	u	u	0	25
Pancakes, plain	110	4, ea. 4-in. diam	245	7.5	10.0	35	230	280	15	610	170	0.9	0.06	1.2	300	0.2	0.2	0.8	0.4	0.8	10	u	0
Papaya, raw	225	½ fruit or 1 c, cubed	60	0.9	0.2	15	30	25	u	4	355	u	0.02	0.4	2700	0.06	0.06	0.4	u	0.5	u	0	85
Parsley, raw	5	1 tbsp, chopped	2	0.1	tr	0.3	5	2	2	2	25	u	0.02	0.2	300	tr	0.01	tr	0.01	0.02	2	0	6
Peaches, without skin																							
Raw, yellow	115	1 medium	40	0.6	0.1	10	10	20	12	1	200	0.2	0.06	0.5	1300	0.02	0.05	1.0	0.03	0.2	2	0	7
Canned, heavy syrup	130	2 halves and 3 tbsp juice	120	0.6	0.2	30	5	20	9	4	200	0.1	0.1	0.4	650	0.02	0.04	1.0	0.03	0.08	u	0	4
water pack	135	2 halves and 3 tbsp juice	50	0.6	0.2	12	5	20	9	4	210	u	0.08	0.4	700	0.02	0.04	1.0	u	u	u	0	4
Dried, unsulfured, uncooked	65	5 halves	170	2.0	0.4	45	30	75	30	10	620	u	u	3.9	2500	tr	0.1	3.5	0.06,	u	u	0	10
Peanuts, roasted, salted	30	1 oz, 30 nuts	65	7.5	14.0	5	20	115	50	120	190	0.9	0.1	0.6	0	0.09	0.04	4.9	0.1	0.6	8	0	0
Peanut butter	15	1 tbsp	95	4.0	8.0	3	10	60	25	95	100	0.4	0.09	0.3	0	0.02	0.02	2.4	0.05	0.3	3	0	0

tr — trace amounts
u — unknown thought to be present
0 — Absent or below detection level

Table A.2 Continued
Nutritive Values of the Edible Part of Foods

Food	Weight g	Approximate Measure	Energy Kcal	Protein g	Fat g	Total Carbohydrate g	Calcium mg	Phosphorus mg	Magnesium mg	Sodium mg	Potassium mg	Zinc mg	Copper mg	Iron mg	Total Vitamin A Activity IU	Thiamin mg	Riboflavin mg	Niacin mg	Vitamin B-6 mg	Pantothenic Acid mg	Folacin (free) mcg	Vitamin B-12 mcg	Vitamin C mg
Pears																							
Raw, with skin	180	1, 3½ in. × 2½ in.	100	1.0	0.7	25	15	20	15	3	215	u	0.3	0.5	30	0.03	0.07	0.2	0.03	0.1	9	0	7
Canned syrup	150	2 halves and 3 tbsp juice	115	0.4	0.4	30	10	10	7	2	130	u	0.06	0.4	tr	0.02	0.04	0.2	0.02	0.3	9	0	2
water pack	155	2 halves and 3 tbsp juice	50	0.4	0.4	13	10	10	7	2	135	u	0.08	0.4	tr	0.02	0.04	0.2	u	u	u	0	2
Peas																							
Green, frozen, boiled	80	½ c	55	4.0	0.2	9	15	70	15	90	110	0.6	0.2	1.5	500	0.2	0.1	2.2	0.1	0.3	14	0	15
Canned, drained	85	½ c	75	4.0	0.4	14	20	65	10	200	80	0.7	0.1	1.6	500	0.08	0.05	0.7	0.04	0.1	5	0	7
Split, dry, cooked	100	½ c (1 oz, dry wt)	115	8.0	0.3	20	10	90	8	15	295	1.1	0.07	1.7	40	0.2	0.09	0.9	0.08	0.6	20	0	0
Peas and carrots, frozen, boiled	80	½ c	40	2.5	0.2	8	20	45	15	65	125	u	0.3	0.9	7400	0.2	0.05	1.0	0.04	0.2	u	0	6
Pecans	30	1 oz, 20 halves	200	2.5	20.0	4	20	80	40	tr	170	u	0.3	0.7	40	0.2	0.04	0.3	0.05	0.5	4	0	1
Peppers, hot (chili)																							
Green, canned sauce	15	1 tbsp	3	0.1	tr	1	1	2	u	u	u	u	u	0.1	100	tr	tr	0.1	u	u	u	0	10
Red, dry, chili powder	3	1 tsp	8	0.3	0.4	1	7	8	4	25	50	0.07	u	0.4	900	0.01	0.02	0.2	u	u	u	0	2
Peppers, sweet																							
Green, raw	75	½ c, chopped	15	0.9	0.1	4	5	15	15	10	155	0.2	0.07	0.5	300	0.06	0.06	0.4	0.2	0.2	5	0	95
Red, raw	90	1 medium	25	1.0	0.2	5	10	20	u	u	u	u	u	0.4	3300	0.06	0.06	0.4	u	0.2	20	0	150
Pickles, cucumber																							
Dill	135	1 large	15	0.9	0.3	3	35	30	1	1930	270	0.4	0.03	1.4	150	tr	0.03	tr	0.01	0.3	4	0	8
Sweet	35	1 medium	50	0.2	0.1	13	4	5	tr	u	u	0.05	0.07	0.4	30	tr	0.01	tr	u	0.07	1	0	2
Relish, sweet	15	1 tbsp	20	0.1	0.1	5	3	2	u	105	u	0.01	0.05	0.1	u	0	u	0	u	u	0	0	tr
Pies																							
Apple, berry, rhubarb	160	⅙ of 9-in. pie	400	3.5	17.5	60	15	35	5	475	125	0.1	0.1	0.5	50	0.03	0.03	0.6	0.06	0.2	3	0	2
Cherry, peach	160	⅙ of 9-in. pie	410	4.0	18.0	60	20	40	10	480	165	0.06	0.1	0.5	700	0.03	0.03	0.8	u	u	u	0	tr
Cream, pudding type with meringue	150	⅙ of 9-in. pie	380	7.5	18.0	50	105	150	u	390	210	u	u	1.1	300	0.05	0.20	0.3	u	1.4	u	u	tr
Custard	150	⅙ of 9-in. pie	330	9.5	17.0	35	145	170	u	u	u	u	u	0.9	350	0.08	0.30	0.5	u	u	3	u	0
Lemon meringue	140	⅙ of 9-in. pie	360	5.0	14.5	55	20	70	u	395	70	u	u	0.7	250	0.04	0.10	0.3	u	u	3	u	4
Mince	160	⅙ of 9-in. pie	430	4.0	18.0	65	45	60	u	710	280	u	0.1	1.6	tr	0.10	0.06	0.6	u	u	2	u	2
Pecan	140	⅙ of 9-in. pie	580	7.0	31.5	70	65	140	u	305	170	u	0.1	3.9	200	0.20	0.10	0.4	u	u	u	u	tr
Pumpkin	150	⅙ of 9-in. pie	320	6.0	17.0	35	80	105	10	325	245	0.6	0.08	0.8	3800	0.05	0.20	0.8	0.06	0.8	5	u	tr
Sweet potato	150	⅙ of 9-in. pie	325	7.0	17.0	36	105	130	u	330	250	u	u	0.8	3800	0.08	0.20	0.5	u	u	6	u	6
Pineapple, diced or crushed																							
Raw	155	1 c	80	0.6	0.3	20	25	10	20	2	225	0.3	0.1	0.8	100	0.1	0.05	0.3	0.1	0.2	15	0	25
Canned, in heavy syrup	130	½ c solids and liquid	95	0.4	0.2	25	15	6	10	2	120	0.3	0.2	0.4	60	0.1	0.02	0.2	0.1	0.1	3	0	9
in juice	125	½ c solids and liquid	70	0.4	0.2	17	15	8	15	1	180	0.3	0.1	0.6	80	0.1	0.04	0.2	0.1	0.2	u	0	15
water pack	125	½ c solids and liquid	50	0.4	0.1	13	15	5	u	1	120	u	u	0.4	60	0.1	0.02	0.2	u	u	u	0	8
Pineapple juice vv9,8190		¾ c	105	0.8	0.6	25	30	15	20	2	280	u	0.1	0.6	100	0.1	0.04	0.4	0.2	0.2	u	0	15
Pinenuts, piñon	30	1 oz, 4 tbsp	180	3.5	17.0	6	3	170	u	u	u	u	u	1.5	10	0.4	0.07	1.3	u	u	tr	0	tr
Pizza, cheese	65	⅛ of 14-in. pizza	150	8.0	6.5	18	145	125	20	455	85	0.8	0.2	0.7	400	0.04	0.1	0.7	u	u	u	u	5
Sausage	65	⅛ of 14-in. pizza	160	5.0	6.0	20	10	60	u	490	115	0.8	u	0.8	400	0.06	0.08	1.0	u	u	u	u	6
Plantain	265	1 banana 11 in. × 2 in.	310	3.0	1.0	82	20	80	u	15	1010	u	u	1.8	u	0.2	0.1	1.6	u	0.7	u	0	35
Plums, raw	70	1 medium	30	0.3	0.1	8	10	10	6	1	110	u	0.07	0.3	150	0.02	0.02	0.3	0.04	0.1	1	0	4
Canned, purple in heavy syrup	140	3 and 3 tbsp syrup	110	0.5	0.1	30	10	15	7	1	190	u	u	1.2	500	0.03	0.03	0.5	0.04	0.1	u	0	3
Popcorn with oil and salt	10	1 c	40	0.9	2.0	5	1	20	10	175	u	0.2	0.03	0.2	u	u	u	0.2	0.02	0.04	0	0	0
Pork																							
Chop, broiled																							
lean and fat	80	1 medium	300	19.5	24.5	0	10	210	15	45	215	u	u	2.7	0	0.8	0.2	4.5	0.3	0.5	3	0.4	0
lean only	50	1 medium	110	13.0	6.5	0	5	135	10	30	145	1.5	0.04	1.6	0	0.5	0.1	2.9	0.1	0.2	2	0.2	0
Loin, roasted																							
lean and fat	85	2½ in. × 2½ in. × ¾ in.	310	21.0	24.0	0	10	220	20	50	235	u	0.05	2.7	0	0.8	0.2	4.8	0.3	0.5	1	0.5	0
Spareribs, braised	90	yield from ½ lb, raw wt	400	18.5	35.0	0	15	220	u	65	300	u	u	4.7	0	0.8	0.4	6.1	u	u	u	0.6	0

Food composition table (values per measure indicated). Column key (left to right): weight (g); measure; food energy (cal); protein (g); fat (g); carbohydrate (g); and mineral/vitamin columns.

Food	g	Measure	Cal	Pro (g)	Fat (g)	CHO (g)	Ca	P	(7)	Na	K	(10)	(11)	Fe	Vit A	Thiamin	Riboflavin	Niacin	(17)	(18)	(19)	Vit C	(21)	(22)
Potatoes																								
Baked	200	1 large	140	4.0	0.2	35	15	100	45	5	780	0.4	0.3	1.1	tr	tr	0.2	C.07	2.7	0.5	0.8	20	0	30
Boiled, pared before cooking	135	1 medium	90	2.5	0.1	20	10	55	u	3	385	0.4	0.1	0.7	tr	tr	0.1	C.05	1.6	0.5	0.8	15	0	20
French-fried, commercial	70	1 "order"	220	3.0	10.2	28	9	70	20	120	u	u	u	0.4	tr	tr	0.1	C.04	2.4	0.2	u	5	0	9
French-fried, frozen, reheated	100	20 strips	220	3.5	8.4	35	10	90	30	4	660	0.3	0.3	0.8	tr	u	0.1	C.02	2.6	0.2	0.5	10	0	20
Mashed with milk	100	½ c	100	2.0	4.5	13	25	50	15	350	260	0.1	0.1	0.4	200	u	0.08	C.05	1.0	0.1	0.2	10	0	10
Potato chips	20	10 chips, 2-in. diameter each	115	1.0	8.0	10	10	30	10	200	225	0.2	0.04	0.4	tr	0	0.04	C.01	1.0	0.04	0.1	2	0	3
Potato salad. See salads.																								
Pretzels	30	10, 3-ring pretzels	120	3.0	1.5	25	5	40	u	500	80	0.3	0.04	0.5	0	tr	0.01	C.02	0.4	0.01	0.2	0	tr	0
Prunes, dried, raw	50	5	130	1.0	0.3	35	25	40	u	4	355	u	0.1	2.0	800	0.04	0.08	C.08	0.8	0.1	0.2	2	0	2
Cooked without sugar	125	½ c	120	1.0	0.3	35	25	40	u	4	350	u	0.2	1.9	800	0.04	0.08	C.08	0.8	u	u	tr	0	1
Prune juice, canned	190	¾ c	150	0.8	0.2	35	25	40	u	4	450	tr	0.04	2.0	800	0.02	0.02	C.02	0.8	u	u	u	0	4
Puddings																								
Almendrado	65	⅓ c and 2 tbsp sauce	100	2.7	4.3	14	35	50	u	35	50	u	0.3	0.3	250	0.02	0.08	C.08	0.03	0.02	0.3	0.4	8	tr
Apple Brown Betty	110	½ c	160	1.5	4.0	30	20	25	5	165	110	u	0.06	0.6	100	0.06	0.04	0.4	0.06	6	u	1		
Capirotada	385	½ c	385	10.8	14.0	58	230	200	5	335	355	u	0.10	2.5	250	0.10	0.20	3.0	4	0	0		
Chocolate, instant, packaged	155	½ c	160	5.0	3.0	30	185	120	u	160	170	u	0.04	0.4	150	0.04	0.20	0.2	u	0	0		
Custard	130	½ c	150	7.0	7.5	15	150	155	u	105	195	u	0.06	0.6	450	0.06	0.2	0.2	4	tr			
Rice with raisins	200	½ c	200	5.0	4.0	35	130	125	u	95	235	0.4	0.04	0.6	150	0.04	0.2	0.2	5	tr			
Tapioca	80	½ c	110	4.0	4.0	14	85	90	u	130	110	0.04	0.04	0.4	250	0.04	0.2	0.1	2	tr			
Vanilla, home recipe	130	½ c	140	4.5	5.0	20	150	115	u	85	175	0.05	0.04	tr	200	0.04	0.2	0.2	u	0			
Pumpkin, canned	245	1 c	80	2.5	0.7	19	60	65	30	5	560	0.3	1.0	15,700	0.07	0.1	1.5	0.1	10	10			
Radishes, raw	45	4 large	7	0.4	tr	1	10	10	7	10	130	0.1	0.4	10	0.01	0.01	0.4	0.03	0.08	4	10			
Raisins	35	¼ c	100	0.9	0.1	30	20	35	10	10	275	0.06	0.08	1.3	10	0.04	0.03	0.2	0.2	1	tr		
Rhubarb, cooked with sugar	135	½ c	190	0.7	0.2	50	105	20	20	2	275	0.1	0.1	0.8	100	0.02	0.07	0.4	0.03	0.09	10	8		
Rice cooked, salt added																								
Brown	130	⅔ c	130	3.5	0.8	35	15	95	40	370	90	0.8	0.1	0.7	0	0.1	0.03	1.8	0.2	0.5	10	0	0
White, enriched	135	⅔ c	150	3.0	0.1	35	15	85	10	515	40	0.5	0.07	1.2	0	0.2	0.01	1.4	0.05	0.3	1	0	0
Precooked, instant	110	⅔ c	120	2.5	tr	25	3	20	u	300	u	0.2	0.1	0.9	0	0.1	0.07	1.1	u	1	0	0	
Rolls and Buns																								
Danish pastry	85	1, of 4-in. diameter	270	5.0	15.5	30	35	70	15	240	75	0.2	0.1	0.6	200	0.04	0.1	0.5	0.1	5	tr		
Hamburger or frankfurter bun, enriched	40	1 average	120	3.5	2.0	20	30	35	10	200	40	0.08	0.07	0.8	tr	0.1	0.07	0.9	5	0	0		
Hard rolls, enriched	50	1 large	160	5.0	1.5	30	25	45	15	315	50	0.6	0.1	1.2	tr	0.1	0.1	1.4	6	0	0		
Plain pan rolls, white, enriched	30	1 small	85	2.5	1.5	15	20	25	10	140	25	0.4	0.08	0.5	tr	0.08	0.05	0.6	0.01	4	0	0
Rutabagas, boiled	85	½ c, cubed	30	0.8	0.1	7	50	25	12	4	140	u	0.05	0.2	500	0.05	0.05	0.7	0.08	0.1	20	20
Salads																								
Chef's (lettuce w/ham, cheese, dressing)	u	1 serving	285	13.0	24.0	3	150	185	u	u	u	u	u	2.2	1250	0.2	u	1.2	u	13			
Potato, home recipe	125	½ c	120	3.5	3.5	20	40	80	u	650	400	0.3	0.1	0.8	150	0.1	0.1	1.4	0.09	14			
Tuna fish	100	½ c	170	15.0	10.0	4	20	145	12	u	u	u	0.04	1.3	250	0.04	u	5.1	u	1			
Salad dressings																								
Blue cheese	15	1 tbsp	75	0.7	8.0	1	10	10	u	165	5	0.04	tr	tr	30	tr	0.02	tr	u	tr			
French, regular	15	1 tbsp	65	0.1	6.0	3	2	2	2	220	15	0.01	u	0.1	tr	tr	u	tr	0	u			
French, low-calorie	15	1 tbsp	15	0.1	0.7	3	2	2	1	125	15	u	u	0.1	tr	u	u	tr	0	0			
Italian, regular	15	1 tbsp	85	tr	9.0	1.0	2	1	1	315	2	0.02	0.1	tr	tr	u	u	tr	0	0			
Italian, low-calorie	15	1 tbsp	10	tr	0.7	0.4	tr	1	tr	120	2	u	u	tr	tr	u	u	tr	0	0			
Mayonnaise	15	1 tbsp	100	0.2	11.0	0.3	3	4	tr	85	5	u	0.02	0.1	40	tr	0.01	tr	0.02	0			
Salad dressing	15	1 tbsp	65	0.2	6.5	2.0	2	4	tr	90	1	0.8	0.02	tr	30	tr	u	tr	0.02	0			
Thousand Island, or Louis-type	15	1 tbsp	80	0.1	8.0	2.5	2	3	u	110	20	0.02	0.02	0.1	50	tr	u	tr	tr	0			
Salmon. See Fish.																								
Sandwiches																								
Bacon, lettuce, tomato on white bread	150	1 average	280	7.0	15.5	30	55	90	u	u	u	u	u	1.5	850	0.2	u	1.5	u	15			
Egg salad on white bread	140	1 average	280	10.5	12.5	30	70	155	u	u	u	u	u	2.4	600	0.2	0.02	1.0	0.2	2			
Fish fillet, fried on bun	135	1 average	410	15.0	21.5	37	95	235	20	760	u	u	u	1.6	80	0.2	0.4	2.9	0.1	20	2	0.8	
Ham and cheese on white bread	u	1 average	350	20.0	19.0	30	215	240	u	u	u	u	u	3.1	300	0.4	0.3	2.5	0.1	0			
Hamburger on bun	95	1 regular	250	13.0	9.6	28	50	120	15	540	u	u	u	2.6	160	0.2	0.4	3.7	0.1	20	0.8		
"Big Mac"	185	1 large	560	26.0	32.0	40	160	290	30	1060	u	u	u	3.8	200	0.8	0.6	6.5	0.2	30	1.5		
Tuna salad on white bread	105	1 average	280	11.0	14.0	25	50	135	u	u	u	u	u	1.2	250	0.1	0.1	4.0	u	1			
Sashimi. See Fish, tuna, raw.																								
Sardines. See Fish.																								

tr — trace amounts
u — unknown thought to be present
0 — Absent or below detection level

Table A.2 Continued
Nutritive Values of the Edible Part of Foods

Food	Weight g	Approximate Measure	Energy Kcal	Protein g	Fat g	Total Carbohydrate g	Calcium mg	Phosphorus mg	Magnesium mg	Sodium mg	Potassium mg	Zinc mg	Copper mg	Iron mg	Total Vitamin A Activity IU	Thiamin mg	Riboflavin mg	Niacin mg	Vitamin B-6 mg	Pantothenic Acid mg	Folacin (free) mcg	Vitamin B-12 mcg	Vitamin C mg
Sauces																							
Butterscotch	45	2 tbsp	200	0.5	7.0	35	40	25	u	u	u	u	u	1.4	300	tr	tr	tr	u	u	u	u	0
Cheese	40	2 tbsp	65	3.0	5.0	2	90	65	u	u	u	u	u	0.1	200	0.01	0.08	0.1	u	u	u	u	tr
Chocolate																							
thin syrup	40	2 tbsp	100	0.9	0.8	25	7	35	u	u	u	u	0.2	0.6	tr	0.01	0.03	0.2	u	u	u	u	0
fudge type	40	2 tbsp	125	2.0	5.0	20	50	60	u	35	105	u	u	0.5	60	0.02	0.08	0.2	u	u	u	tr	0
Custard	70	¼ c	85	3.5	4.0	10	80	80	u	u	u	u	u	0.4	250	0.04	0.2	0.1	u	u	u	tr	tr
Hard sauce	20	2 tbsp	95	0.1	5.5	12	2	1	u	u	u	u	u	tr	250	tr	tr	tr	0	0	0	0	tr
Hollandaise	50	¼ c scant	180	2.0	18.5	0.4	25	80	u	u	u	u	u	0.9	1000	0.03	0.04	tr	u	u	u	u	0
Soy	35	2 tbsp	25	2.0	0.5	4	30	40	u	2665	135	u	u	1.7	0	0.01	0.09	0.1	u	u	u	u	0
Tartar	15	1 tbsp	75	0.2	8.0	0.6	3	4	u	100	10	u	u	0.1	30	tr	tr	tr	u	u	tr	u	tr
Tomato catsup	15	1 tbsp	15	0.3	0.1	4	3	10	3	155	55	0.04	0.09	0.1	200	0.01	0.01	0.2	0.02	tr	tr	0	2
White, medium	125	½ c	200	5.0	15.5	11	145	115	20	475	175	0.5	0.05	0.2	600	0.05	0.2	0.2	0.06	0.8	1	0.2	tr
Sauerkraut, canned	120	½ c	20	1.0	0.2	5	40	20	u	880	165	1.0	0.1	0.6	60	0.04	0.04	0.2	0.2	0.1	u	0	16
Sausages																							
Bologna	30	1 slice, 4½ in. × ¼ in.	85	3.5	8.0	0.3	2	35	u	370	65	0.5	tr	0.5	0	0.05	0.06	0.7	0.03	u	1	u	0
Frankfurter (all-meat)	45	1 average	135	5.5	12.0	0.7	2	45	2	u	u	0.7	0.04	0.7	0	0.07	0.09	1.1	0.06	0.2	1	0.6	0
Liverwurst	30	1 oz	85	4.5	7.0	0.5	3	70	5	u	u	2.2	0.9	1.5	1800	0.06	0.4	1.6	0.06	0.8	6	4.2	tr
Luncheon meat, pork, cured	30	1 oz	85	4.5	7.0	0.4	3	30	u	350	65	u	0.02	0.6	0	0.09	0.06	0.9	u	0.2	1	u	0
Pork sausage, links	40	3 links	185	7.0	17.0	0.1	3	60	5	375	105	0.2	0.06	0.9	0	0.3	0.1	1.5	0.07	0.3	1	0.2	0
Salami, dry	30	3 small slices	130	6.5	11.0	0.3	4	80	u	u	u	u	u	1.0	0	0.1	0.07	1.5	0.04	u	1	u	0
Vienna, canned	50	3 sausages	115	6.5	9.5	0.1	3	75	u	u	u	u	u	0.9	0	0.03	0.06	1.2	0.04	u	1	u	0
Scallops																							
Breaded, fried	95	3½ oz	180	17.0	8.0	10	u	u	u	u	u	u	u	2.8	0	u	u	u	u	0.1	15	u	u
Steamed	95	3½ oz	105	22.0	1.5	3	110	320	u	250	455	0.1	0.1	2.8	0	u	0.06	1.3	u	u	18	1.1	u
Sesame seeds, hulled	40	¼ c	220	7.0	20.0	7	40	220	7	u	100	0.6	0.6	0.9	90	0.07	0.05	2.0	0.01	tr	25	0	2
Sherbet, orange	95	½ c	135	1.0	2.0	30	50	75	8	45	105	0.6	0.02	0.1	90	0.01	0.04	tr	0.01	tr	7	0.1	2
Shrimp, canned	85	3 oz	100	20.5	0.9	0.6	100	225	45	u	105	1.8	0.1	2.7	60	0.01	0.03	1.5	0.05	0.2	6	0.1	0
French-fried	85	3 oz	190	17.5	9.5	8	60	160	40	160	195	0.8	0.3	1.8	u	0.03	0.06	2.5	0.05	0.3	5	0.6	0
Soups																							
Albondiga (meatballs in tomato broth)	240	1 c with 4 meatballs	340	18.5	21.4	17	25	175	u	180	460	u	u	3.6	500	0.2	0.2	5.0	0.6	0.7	10	1.2	8
Bean, with pork	250	1 c	170	8.0	6.0	22	65	130	u	1010	395	u	u	2.3	650	0.1	0.08	1.0	u	u	u	u	3
Bouillon, broth, consomme	240	1 c	30	5.0	0	3	tr	30	u	780	130	u	0.02	0.5	tr	tr	0.02	1.0	u	u	u	u	0
Cream soups, canned,																							
diluted with water	240	1 c	65	2.5	1.5	10	25	40	u	985	120	u	u	0.7	300	0.05	0.1	0.7	u	u	u	u	u
diluted with milk	245	1 c	150	7.0	6.0	17	175	160	u	1070	300	u	u	0.7	500	0.07	0.3	0.7	u	u	10	u	tr
Chicken noodle, from dry mix	240	1 c	55	2.0	1.5	8	7	20	u	580	20	0.1	u	0.2	50	0.07	0.05	0.5	u	u	u	u	0
Clam chowder, Manhattan	245	1 c	80	2.0	2.5	12	35	45	u	940	185	1.4	0.1	1.0	900	0.02	0.02	1.0	u	u	8	u	u
Onion	240	1 c	35	1.5	1.0	6	10	10	u	690	60	0.07	u	0.2	tr	tr	tr	tr	u	u	u	u	2
Split pea	245	1 c	140	8.5	3.0	20	30	150	15	940	270	1.0	0.2	1.5	450	0.2	0.2	1.5	0.1	0.2	2	0.4	tr
Tomato	245	1 c	90	2.0	2.5	16	15	35	15	970	230	0.2	0.2	0.7	1000	0.05	0.05	1.0	0.05	0.2	5	0	10
Vegetable beef	245	1 c	80	5.0	2.0	10	10	50	25	1050	160	0.4	0.1	0.7	2700	0.05	0.05	1.0	0.07	0.2	5	u	u
Spaghetti																							
Canned, with tomato sauce and meatballs	210	1 can, 7½ oz	250	10.4	12.8	23	20	120	u	1035	375	u	0.3	2.2	1030	0.15	0.2	3.4	u	u	10	u	u
Home recipe, with tomato sauce																							
with cheese	250	1 c	260	9.0	9.0	35	80	135	30	955	410	0.2	0.3	2.3	1100	0.2	0.2	2.5	0.1	0.8	2	0.6	15
with meatballs	250	1 c	330	18.5	11.5	40	125	235	40	1010	665	3.5	0.4	3.7	1600	0.2	0.3	4.0	0.4	0.5	15	0.6	20
Spinach, fresh or frozen, boiled	90	½ c	20	2.5	0.2	3	90	40	60	50	300	0.5	0.1	2.0	7300	0.06	0.1	0.4	0.2	0.2	60	0	20
Sprouts, raw																							
Alfalfa	100	1 c, packed	40	5.0	0.6	5	30	u	u	u	u	1.0	u	1.4	20	0.1	0.2	1.5	u	u	u	0	15
Mung bean	100	1 c	35	4.0	0.2	7	20	65	u	5	235	0.9	u	1.4	20	0.1	0.1	0.8	u	u	u	0	20
Soybean	100	1 c	50	6.5	1.5	6	50	70	u	u	u	1.6	u	1.1	80	0.2	0.2	0.8	u	u	u	0	15
Squash																							
Summer, boiled	90	½ c	10	0.8	0.1	3	20	20	15	1	125	0.2	0.07	0.4	350	0.04	0.07	0.7	0.2	0.1	2	0	9
Winter																							
baked	100	½ c	65	2.0	0.4	15	30	50	17	1	470	u	u	0.8	430	0.05	0.1	0.7	0.09	0.3	u	0	15
boiled	120	½ c	45	1.5	0.4	10	25	40	17	1	315	u	u	0.6	4300	0.05	0.1	0.5	0.1	0.3	u	0	10

Strawberries																							
Fresh	100	⅔ c chole	35	0.7	0.5	8	20	20	12	1	165	0.08	u	1.0	60	0.03	0.07	0.6	0.06	0.3	15	0	60
Frozen, sweetened	170	⅔ c	160	0.7	0.3	40	20	25	14	2	180	u	u	1.0	50	0.03	0.1	0.9	0.07	0.2	15	0	95
Sugar																							
Brown	220	1 c, packed	820	0	0	210	185	40	u	65	765	u	0.7	7.5	0	0.02	0.07	0.4	u	u	u	0	0
White																							
granulated	200	1 c	770	0	0	200	0	0	0	2	5	0.1	0.04	0.2	0	0	0	0	0	0	0	0	0
	4	1 tsp	15	0	0	4	0	0	0	tr	tr	tr	tr	tr	0	0	0	0	0	0	0	0	0
powdered	8	1 tbsp	30	0	0	8	0	0	0	tr	tr	tr	tr	tr	0	0	0	0	0	0	0	0	0
Sunflower seeds, hulled	36	¼ c	200	8.5	17.0	7	45	305	13	10	335	u	0.6	2.6	20	0.7	0.08	2.0	0.4	0.5	u	0	0
Sweet potatoes																							
Baked in skin	145	1 potato, 5 in. × 2 in.	160	2.5	0.6	35	45	65	45	15	340	1.0	0.2	1.0	9200	0.1	0.08	0.8	0.05	1.0	10	0	25
Boiled in skin	130	½ c mashed	150	2.0	0.5	35	40	60	u	15	620	u	0.2	0.9	9200	0.1	0.08	0.8	0.3	1.0	9	0	20
Candied	105	½ medium	180	1.5	3.5	35	40	45	u	45	200	u	0.06	0.9	6600	0.06	0.04	0.4	u	u	7	0	10
Syrup, maple-flavored, artificial	20	1 tbsp	50	0	0	13	20	2	u	2	35	tr	0.08	0.2	0	0	0	0	0	0	0	0	0
Tacos, beef	80	1 taco	160	11.0	8.5	9	135	160	u	200	210	u	u	2.0	530	0.07	0.1	2.3	0.3	0.3	25	0.7	3
Tamales, canned	100	3½ oz	140	4.5	7.0	14	20	40	10	665	u	0.9	0.05	1.2	u	u	u	u	u	u	u	u	u
Home recipe, chicken	130	2 tamales	275	8.3	23.7	8	100	60	u	60	90	u	u	0.9	2800	0.05	0.1	2.7	0.2	0.3	1	0.1	7
Tea, instant	1	½ tsp	3	0	0	1	tr	u	4	u	45	u	u	tr	0	0	tr	tr	u	u	u	0	0
Tofu, soybean curd	120	1 piece, 2½ in. × 2¾ in. × 1 in.	85	9.5	5.0	3	155	150	130	10	50	u	u	2.3	0	0.07	0.04	0.1	u	u	u	0	0
Tomatoes, raw	135	1 medium	25	1.5	0.2	6	15	35	20	4	300	0.3	0.1	0.6	1100	0.07	0.05	0.9	0.1	0.4	25	0	30
Canned	120	½ c	25	1.0	0.2	5	5	25	15	155	260	0.2	0.2	0.6	1100	0.06	0.04	0.8	0.1	0.3	10	0	20
Tomato juice, canned	180	¾ c	35	1.5	0.2	8	15	35	20	365	415	u	0.1	1.6	1500	0.09	0.05	1.5	0.3	0.4	18	0	30
Tomato paste	130	½ c	110	4.5	0.5	25	35	90	25	50	1120	u	0.9	4.6	4300	0.3	0.2	4.0	0.5	0.6	25	0	65
Tongue, beef, braised	100	3½ oz	250	21.5	17.0	0.4	5	120	16	60	165	u	0.07	2.2	0	0.05	0.3	3.5	0.1	2.0	u	u	0
Tortillas																							
Corn, lime-treated	30	1, of 6-in. diameter	65	1.5	0.6	14	60	40	30	u	u	0.03	0.06	0.9	tr	0.04	0.02	0.3	0.02	0.03	tr	0	0
White flour	30	1, of 6-in. diameter	110	3.0	1.0	20	4	50	15	250	30	u	u	1.0	0	0.08	0.04	0.5	0.02	0.03	5	0	0
Tostada with beans and small portion of cheese	210	1 tostada	335	11.6	17.6	35	195	245	u	350	425	u	u	3.2	1650	0.3	0.2	1.3	0.2	0.4	10	0.2	10
Tune. See *Fish*.																							
Turkey, roasted																							
Light meat	85	2 slices, each 4 in. × 2 in. × ¼ in.	150	28.0	3.5	0	7	200	20	70	350	1.8	0.2	1.0	u	0.04	0.1	9.5	0.3	0.5	3	0.4	0
Dark meat	85	4 slices, each 2½ in. × 1½ in. × ¼ in.	170	25.5	7.0	0	7	200	20	85	340	3.7	0.2	2.0	u	0.03	0.2	3.5	0.3	1.0	7	0.4	0
Turnips, boiled	80	½ c, cubed	20	0.6	0.2	4	25	20	10	25	145	0.07	0.03	0.3	tr	0.03	0.04	0.2	0.06	0.08	u	0	15
Turnip greens, boiled	70	½ c	15	1.5	0.2	3	135	25	20	u	u	u	u	0.8	4600	0.1	0.2	0.4	0.7	0.1	u	0	50
Veal cutlet, broiled	85	3 oz	180	23.0	9.5	0	10	195	20	55	260	4.1	0.04	2.7	0	0.06	0.2	4.5	0.3	0.8	15	1.6	0
Vinegar cider	15	1 tbsp	2	tr	0	1	1	1	u	tr	15	0.02	0.01	0.1	0	0	0	0	0	0	0	0	0
Waffles																							
Made from mix	75	1, of 7-in. diameter	210	6.5	8.0	25	180	260	20	515	145	u	u	1.0	200	0.1	0.2	0.7	u	0.5	u	u	0
Frozen	45	2 sections	120	3.0	4.0	16	130	195	u	340	u	u	u	0.5	u	0.04	0.05	0.5	u	u	u	u	0
Walnuts, English	100	1 c halves	650	15.0	64.0	16	100	380	135	2	450	2.8	0.9	3.1	30	0.3	0.1	0.9	0.7	0.9	45[16]	0	2
	15	2 tbsp, chopped	100	2.5	10.0	3	15	60	20	tr	70	0.4	0.1	0.4	10	0.06	0.02	0.2	0.1	0.1	5[16]	0	tr
Watercress, raw	35	10 sprigs	5	0.8	0.1	1	55	20	5	20	100	u	0.03	0.6	1700	0.03	0.06	0.3	0.04	0.1	70	0	30
Wheat bran, crude	30	1 oz	60	4.5	1.0	17	35	355	135	3	315	2.7	0.4	4.2	0	0.2	0.1	6.0	0.2	0.1	u	0	0
Wheat germ, raw	30	1 oz	100	7.5	3.0	13	20	315	90	tr	230	1.7	0.7	2.6	u	0.6	0.2	1.0	0.3	0.9	80	0	0
Toasted	30	1 oz	120	9.0	3.5	15	15	350	90	tr	285	1.7	0.7	2.5	50	0.5	0.2	1.5	0.3	0.4	u	0	0
Wine, dessert (18.8%)	105	3½ fl oz	140	0.1	0	8	10	u	5	4	75	0.1	0.08	0.4	u	0.01	0.02	0.2	0.04	0	0	0	0
Table (12.2%)	100	3½ fl oz	85	0.1	0	4	10	10	10	5	95	0.1	0.01	0.4	u	tr	0.01	0.1	0.04	0	0	0	0
Yeast																							
Dry, active	5	1 tbsp	20	2.5	0.1	3	3	90	3	4	140	u	0.2	1.1	tr	0.2	0.4	2.5	0.1	0.6	7	0	0
Brewer's, debittered	5	1 tbsp	25	3.0	0.1	3	15	140	10	10	150	u	u	1.4	tr	1.2	0.3	3.0	0.1	0.6	9	0	0
Yogurt																							
Low-fat																							
plain	230	8 fl oz carton	145	12.0	3.5	16	415	325	40	160	530	2.0	u	0.2	150	0.1	0.5	0.3	0.1	1.3	25	1.3	2
fruit, sweetened	230	8 fl oz carton	225	9.0	2.6	42	315	245	30	120	400	1.5	u	0.[illegible]	110	0.08	0.4	0.2	0.1	1.0	20	1.0	1
Regular																							
plain	230	8 fl oz carton	140	8.0	7.5	11	275	215	25	105	350	1.3	u	0.[illegible]	280	0.07	0.3	0.2	0.1	0.9	20	0.8	2

tr — trace amounts
u — unknown thought to be present
0 — Absent or below detection level

Chapter 1

1. Cadwalader, Mary H., "Early Warnings of Future Disaster," *Smithsonian Magazine,* May 1974, pp. 27–29.

2. Dubos, Rene, "Health and Creative Adaptation," *Human Nature,* January 1978, pp. 74–82.

3. Dubos, Rene, *Mirage of Health,* Garden City, N.Y.: Doubleday, 1961.

4. Dunn, H. L., *High Level Wellness,* Washington, D.C.: Mt. Vernon Printing Co., 1961.

5. Dunn, H. L., "Points of Attack for Raising the Levels of Wellness," *Journal of the American Medical Association,* July 1957.

6. Glasser, William, *Reality Therapy,* New York: Harper & Row, 1965.

7. Haggerty, Robert J., "Changing Life Styles to Improve Health," *Preventive Medicine* 6, 1977, pp. 276–289.

8. Hoyman, H. S., "Our Modern Concepts of Health," *Journal of School Health,* September 1962, p. 253.

9. Illich, Ivan, *Limits to Medicine,* Toronto, McClelland & Stewart, 1976.

10. Johnson, Donald D., "Listen to Your Body," Newsletter, *Society of Prospective Medicine* 1:3, May 1978.

11. Kahn, Carol, "If I Die Tomorrow It Ain't Going to be My Fault," *Family Health,* February 1978, pp. 43–45.

12. Kluger, Mathew J., "The Importance of Being Feverish," *Natural History Magazine,* January 1976, pp. 147–150.

13. Knox, E. G., "Foods and Diseases," *British Journal of Preventive and Social Medicine* 31, 1977, pp. 71–80.

14. Kugler, Hans J., *Dr. Kugler's Seven Keys to a Longer Life,* New York: Stein and Day Publishers, 1978.

15. Lalonde, Marc, *A New Perspective on the Health of Canadians,* Ottawa, Canada: The Queen's Printer, 1974.

16. Maslow, Abraham H., "A Theory of Metamotivation: The Biological Routing of the Value Life," *Journal of Humanistic Psychology,* Fall 1967.

17. Maslow, Abraham H., *Eupsychian Management,* Homewood, Ill.: Dorsey Press, 1965.

18. Maslow, Abraham H., *Religions, Values and Peak Experiences,* Columbus: Ohio State Univ. Press, 1964.

19. Maslow, Abraham H., *Toward a Psychology of Being,* New York: Van Nostrand Reinhold, 1968.

20. Mayo, Rollo, *Man's Search for Himself,* New York: American Library, 1967.

21. Mathison, David A., "On Hay Fever and Other Bedeviling Allergies," *Executive Health,* July 1977, 6 pp.

22. McCamy, John C., and James Presley, *Human Life Styling: Keep Whole in the Twentieth Century,* New York: Harper & Row, 1975.

23. McKeown, Thomas, "Determinants of Health," *Human Nature,* April 1978, pp. 60–67.

24. McLuhan, Marshall, "Playboy Interview: Marshall McLuhan," *Playboy,* March 1969.

25. Reisfeld, Ralph A., and Barry D. Kahan, "Markers of Individuality," *Scientific American,* June 1972, pp. 208–217.

26. Rogers, E. S., *Human Ecology and Health,* New York: MacMillan, 1960.

27. Rosen, G., *A History of Public Health,* New York: M. D. Publications, 1958.

28. Selye, Hans, *The Stress of Life,* New York: McGraw-Hill, 1959.

29. Sorochan, Walter D., "Health Concepts as a Basis for Orthobiosis," *The Journal of School Health,* December 1968, pp. 673–682.

30. Sorochan, Walter D., "Life Style as an Approach to Health," *California School Health,* July 1974, pp. 36–38.

31. Toffler, Alvin, *Future Shock,* New York: Random House, 1970.

32. Will, George F., "A Right to Health?", *Newsweek,* August 7, 1978, p. 88.

33. Williams, Roger, "On Your Startling Biochemical Individuality," *Executive Health,* May 1976, 8 pp.

34. Williams, Roger, *Nutrition Against Disease,* New York: Bantam Books, 1973.

Chapter 2

1. American Heart Association, *Recommendations for Human Blood Pressure Determination by Sphygmomanometers* (Pamphlet), New York: American Heart Association, 1967.

2. Bland, Jeffrey, "Warning System Within Your Hair," *Let's Live,* February 1978, pp. 51–52.

3. Cadwalader, Mary H., "Early Warnings of Future Disaster," *Smithsonian Magazine,* 1974, pp. 27–29.

4. Chattapadhgay, Amares, T. Michael Roberts, and Robert E. Jervis, "Scalp Hair as a Monitor of Community Exposure to Lead," *Archives of Environmental Health,* September-October 1973, pp. 226–236.

5. Creason, J. P., et al., "Trace Elements in Hair, as Related to Exposure in Metropolitan New York," *Clinical Chemistry,* 1975, pp. 603.

6. Davis, Dean F., "Progress Toward the Assessment of Health Status," *Preventive Medicine* 4, 1975, pp. 282–295

7. Davies, Dean F., and James B. Tchobanoff, *Health Evaluation,* New York: Intercontinental Medical Book Corporation, 1973.

8. _____, *Diagnostics,* Minneapolis: Lufkin Medical Laboratories.

9. _____, "Do-It-Yourself Blood-Pressure Devices," *Consumer Reports,* October 1974, pp. 740–743.

10. Douglas, Bruce E., "Predicting Disease — Is It Possible?", *Executive Health* 8:7, 5 pp.

11. _____, *Focal Points,* Atlanta: Center for Disease Control, March 1978.

12. French, Ruth M., *The Nurse's Guide to Diagnostic Procedures,* New York: McGraw-Hill, 1971.

13. Garb, Solomon, *Laboratory Tests in Common Use,* New York: Springer Publishing Co., 1971.

14. Ganong, William F., *Review of Medical Physiology,* Los Altos: Longe Medical Publications, 1963.

15. Gordus, A., "Factors Affecting the Trace Metal Content of Human Hair," *Journal of Radioanalytical Chemistry* 15, 1973, pp. 229–243.

16. Greger, J., et al., "Nutritional Status of Adolescent Girls in Regard to Zinc, Copper, and Iron," *American Journal of Clinical Nutrition,* February 1978, pp. 269–275.

17. _____, *Health Hazards* (Pamphlet), Bellevue, Ohio: Medical Datamation, 1976, 23 pp.

18. _____, "High Blood Pressure: What to Do When Your Numbers Are Up," *Consumer Reports,* October 1974, pp. 735–739.

19. Kuhne, P., "High Blood Pressure," *Home Medical Encyclopedia,* New York: Fawcett, 1960, pp. 57–58.

20. _____, "Laboratory Testing," *Patient Care,* September 30, 1969, pp. 10–121.

21. Louria, D. B., et al., "Program for Risk Factor Modification and Selective Screening for Ostensibly Healthy Adults," *The Journal of the Medical Society of New Jersey,* September 1977, pp. 759–766.

22. Linne, Jean J., and Karen M. Ringsreed, *Basic Laboratory Techniques for the Medical Laboratory Technician,* New York: McGraw-Hill, 1970.

23. Mark, Donald D., and Arthur Zimmer, *Atlas of Clinical Laboratory Procedures,* New York: McGraw-Hill, 1967.

24. Morales, Betty Lee, "What's Your Problem," *Let's Live,* April 1978, pp. 48.

25. National Heart Institute, *Hypertension* (Bulletin No. 1714), Washington, D.C.: U.S. Government Printing Office, 1969.

26. Omran, Abdel R., "A Century of Epidemiological Transition in the United States," *Preventative Medicine* 6, 1977, pp. 30–51.

27. Pihl, R., and M. Parkes, "Hair Element Content in Learning Disabled Children," *Science,* October 14, 1977, pp. 204–206.

28. _____, *Prospective Medicine: Before Illness Strikes* (Pamphlet), San Diego: Interhealth, 1975.

29. _____, *The Remedco Laboratory Handbook,* Van Nuys, Remedco Analytical Laboratory, 1977.

30. Robbins, Lew and Robert Hall, *How to Practice Prospective Medicine* (Manual), Indianapolis, Ind.: Methodist Hospital, 1970.

31. Rudolph, C., "Trace Element Patterning in Degenerative Diseases," *Journal of the International Academy of Preventative Medicine,* July 1977.

32. Strain, William H., et al., "Trace Element Nutriture and Metabolism Through Head Hair and Analysis," Reprint from *Trace Substance in Environmental Health V:A Symposium at the University of Missouri,* Columbia, 1972.

33. *Technician Charts,* Technician Instruments Corporation, Tarrytown, N.Y., 1968.

34. Widmann, Frances K., *Govdale's Clinical Interpretation of Laboratory Tests,* Philadelphia: F. A. Davis Co., 1973.

Chapter 3

1. Adams, Ruth and Frank Murray, *Minerals: Ill or Cure?,* New York: Larchmont Books, 1977.

2. Arehart-Treichel, Joan, "Mental Patterns of Disease," *Human Behavior,* January 1976, pp. 24–27.

3. Berkman, Paul L., "Life Stress and Psychological Well-Being: A Replication of Longner's Analysis in the Midtown Manhattan Study," *Journal of Health and Social Behavior,* March 1971, pp. 35–45.

4. Bloomfield, Harold H., and Robert B. Kory, *Happiness,* New York: Pocket Books, 1977.

5. Brenner, Meyer Harvey, *Mental Illness and the Economy,* Cambridge: Harvard University Press, 1973.

6. Brill, Norman Q., "Social Problems and Psychiatric Illness," *Mili-*

tary Medicine, February 1975, pp. 98–107.

7. _____, "Can't Get a Good Night's Sleep," *Changing Times,* pp. 82–84.

8. Challem, Jack J., "Dr. Harvey Ross, M.D.—Fighting Depression," *Bestways,* February 1978, pp. 77–78.

9. Cheraskin, E., and W. M. Ringsdorf, *Psychodietetics,* New York: Bantam Books, 1976.

10. Colligan, Douglas, "The Dangers of Stress: That Helpless Feeling," *New York Magazine,* July 14, 1975, pp. 80–81.

11. _____, "Coping with Life's Strains," *U. S. News & World Report, Inc.,* May 1, 1978, pp. 80–81.

12. Covi, Lino, et al., "Drug Psychotherapy Interactions in Depression," *American Journal of Psychiatry,* May 1976, pp. 502–509.

13. deCastro, Fernando, J., et al., "Hypertension in Adolescents," *Clinical Pediatrics,* January 1976, pp. 24–26.

14. _____, "Depression: When the Blues Become Serious," *Changing Times,* March 1978, pp. 37–39.

15. Dingman, Paul R., "Work and Psychological Well-being: A Theoretical Framework," *Paper Presented at APHA Meeting,* Chicago: November 18, 1975, 10 pp.

16. Draper, Edgar, "A Developmental Theory of Suicide," *Comprehensive Psychiatry,* January-February 1976, pp. 63–80.

17. Dressler, David, James M. Donovan, and Ruth A. Geller, "Life Stress and Emotional Crisis—the Idiosyncratic Interpretation of Life Events," *Comprehensive Psychiatry,* July-August 1976, pp. 549–558.

18. Dubos, Rene, *So Human an Animal,* New York: Scribner, 1968.

19. Duffy, William, *Sugar Blues,* New York: Warner Books, 1975.

20. Dunham, H. Warren, "Society, Culture and Mental Disorder," *Archives of General Psychiatry,* February 1976, pp. 147–156.

21. Dunn, H. L., *High Level Wellness,* Washington, D.C.: Mt. Vernon Printing Co., 1961.

22. Dupuy, Harold J., "Self-representations of General Psychological Well-being of American Adults," a paper presented at the American Public Health Association meeting in Los Angeles, on October 17, 1978, 12 pp.

23. Ebon, Martin, *Which Vitamins Do You Need?,* New York: Bantam Books, 1976.

24. Erikson, Erik, *Identity, Youth and Crisis,* New York: W. W. Norton, 1968.

25. Foulds, G. A., and A. Bedford, "The Relationship Between Anxiety—Depression and the Neuroses," *British Journal of Psychiatry* 128, 1976, pp. 166–168.

26. Freeman, Howard., et al., "Relations Between Nutrition and Cognition in Rural Guatemala," *AJPH,* March 1977, pp. 233–239.

27. Gaitz, Charles M., and Judith Scott, "Age and the Measurement of Mental Health," *Journal of Health and Social Behavior,* March 1972, pp. 55–67.

28. Gladstone, William, *Test Your Own Mental Health,* New York: Arco Publishing Co., 1978.

29. Glasser, William, *Positive Addiction,* New York: Harper & Row, 1976.

30. _____, "Help for Your Headaches," *Changing Times,* pp. 85–87.

31. Hountras, Peter T., *Mental Hygiene,* Columbus: Charles E. Merrill, 1961.

32. Howard, R., and Martha E. Lewis, "Does Your Personality Invite Disease?", *Science Digest,* December 1972, pp. 30–32.

33. Kety, Seymour S., "It's Not All in Your Head," *Saturday Review,* February 21, 1976, pp. 68–71.

34. Kohopka, Gisela, "Mental Depression, a Serious Disease," *San Diego Union,* October 6, 1975.

35. Lakein, Alan, *How to Get Control of Your Time and Your Life,* New York: Signet Books, 1974.

36. Loevinger, Jane, *Ego Development,* San Francisco: Jossey-Bass Publishers, 1976.

37. Maltz, Maxwell, *Psycho-eybernetics and Self-fulfillment,* New York: Bantam Books, 1976.

38. Mandino, Og, *A Treasury of Success Unlimited,* New York: Pocket Books, 1976.

39. Maslow, Abraham H., *Toward a Psychology of Being,* New York: Van Nostrand Reinhold, 1968.

40. Mayo, Rollo, *Man's Search for Himself,* New York: Signet Books, 1967.

41. McCoy, James T., *The Management of Time,* Englewood Cliffs, N.J.: Prentice-Hall, 1959.

42. McLuhan, Marshall, "Playboy Interview: Marshall McLuhan," *Playboy,* March 1969, pp. 53–158.

43. McPheeters, Harold L., "Primary Prevention and Health Promotion in Mental Health," *Preventive Medicine* 5, 1976, pp. 187–198.

44. Mead, Margaret, "Mental Health in Our Changing Culture," *Mental Hygiene,* Summer 1972, pp. 6–8.

45. _____, *Menninger Quarterly* 22:2–3, 1966.

46. _____, "Mentally Ill Americans," *Parade Magazine,* October 30, 1977, p. 12.

47. Menninger, Karl, *The Vital Balance,* New York: Penguin Books, 1977.

48. Mishara, Brian L., Harvey A. Baker, and Janju T. Mishara, "The Frequency of Suicide Attempts: A Retrospective Approach Applied to College Students," *American Journal of Psychiatry,* July 1976, pp. 841–843.

49. Mueller, William Behr, "Hypoglycemia," *Bestways,* February 1978, pp. 44–45.

50. Musa, Kathleen E., and Mary Ellen Roach, "Adolescent Appearance and Self-concept," *Adolescence,* Fall 1973, pp. 385–394.

51. Myers, Jerome K., et al., "Life Events and Mental Status: A Longi-

tudinal Study," *Journal of Health and Social Behavior,* December 1972, pp. 398–405.

52. O'Neill, Nena, and George O'Neill, *Shifting Gears,* New York: Avon Books, 1975.

53. Palm, J. Daniel, *Diet Away Your Stress, Tension and Anxiety,* New York: Pocket Books, 1977.

54. Palmore, Erdman, and Clark Luikart, "Health and Social Factors Related to Life Satisfaction," *Journal of Health and Social Behavior,* March 1972, pp. 68–80.

55. Passwater, Richard A., *Super-nutrition,* New York: Pocket Books, 1976.

56. Pauling, Linus, "Orthomolecular Psychiatry," *Science,* April 19, 1968, pp. 265–271.

57. Proctor, Pam, "The Big Resurgence of Positive Thinking," *Parade,* May 21, 1978, pp. 24–25.

58. Rahe, Richard, et al., "Psychosocial Predictors of Illness Behavior and Failure in Stressful Training," *Journal of Health and Social Behavior,* December 1972, pp. 393–397.

59. Remsberg, Charles, and Bonnie Remsberg, "Exercises to Help You Relax," *Reader's Digest,* May 1978, pp. 65–71.

60. Renshaw, Domeena C., "Depression in the 1970's," *Diseases of the Nervous System,* June 1973, pp. 241–245.

61. Ringer, Robert J., *Winning Through Intimidation,* Greenwich, Conn.: Fawcett Crest Book, 1974.

62. Rippere, Vicky, "What's the Thing to Do When You're Feeling Depressed?—A Pilot Study," *Behavioral Research and Therapy* 15, 1977, pp. 185–191.

63. Rosenberg, Harold, *The Book of Vitamin Therapy,* New York: Berkley Windhover Books, 1975.

64. Ross, Harvey M., *Fighting Depression,* New York: Larchmont Books, 1976.

65. Ruben, Harvey L., *C.I.: Crisis Intervention,* New York: Popular Library, 1976.

66. Rucker, W. Ray, et al., *Human Values in Education,* Dubuque, Iowa: Wm. C. Brown Co., 1969.

67. Selye, Hans, *The Stress of Life,* New York: McGraw-Hill, 1959.

68. Select Committee on Nutrition and Human Needs of the United States Senate, *Diet Related to Killer Disease: Mental Health and Mental Development,* Washington: U.S. Government Printing Office, June 22, 1977.

69. Sheehy, Gail, *Passages,* New York: Bantam Books, 1977.

70. Snaith, R. P., G. W. K. Bridge, and Max Hamilton, "The Leeds Scales for the Self-Assessment of Anxiety and Depression," *British Journal of Psychiatry* 128, 1976, pp. 156–165.

71. Sorochan, Walter, *Personal Health Appraisal,* New York: Wiley, 1976.

72. Tanner, Ogden, and editors, *Stress,* Alexandria, Va.: Time-life Books, 1976.

73. Thommen, George S., *Is This Your Day?,* New York: Avon Books, 1976.

74. Toffler, Alvin, *Future Shock,* New York: Random House, 1970.

75. USDHEW, *A Concurrent Validation Study of the NCHS General Well-being Schedule,* (No. 78-1347), Washington, D.C.: U.S. Government Printing Press, September 1977.

76. Vaillant, George E., "Natural History of Male Psychological Health," *Archives of General Psychiatry,* May 1976, pp. 535–545.

77. VanBuren, Abigail, "Dear Abby: Rx for Depression: Kindness by You," *Los Angeles Times,* March 12, 1978, Part II, p. 6.

78. Ware, John E., Jr., et al., *Associations Among Psychological Well-being and Other Health Status Constructs* (Rand Paper P-6213), Santa Monica: The Rand Corporation, November 1978.

79. Watson, George, *Nutrition and Your Mind,* New York: Bantam Books, 1974.

80. Weinberg, George, *Self-Creation,* New York: St. Martin's Press, 1978.

81. Williams, Roger J., *Nutrition Against Disease,* New York: Bantam Books, 1973.

Chapter 4

1. Benet, Sula, "Why They Live to Be 100 or Even Older in Abkhasia," *The New York Times Magazine* (Reprint), December 26, 1971.

2. Bosco, Dominick, "Friends Are Your Best Medicine," *Prevention,* September 1978, pp. 155–163.

3. Bradburn, Norm M., *The Structure of Psychological Well-being,* Chicago: Aldine Publishing Co., 1969.

4. Brill, Norman Q., "Social Problems and Psychiatric Illness," *Military Medicine,* February 1975, pp. 98–100.

5. Butler, Robert N., and Myrna I. Lewis, *Aging and Mental Health,* St. Louis: C. V. Mosby, 1977.

6. Coplan, Gerald, "Opportunities for School Psychologists in the Primary Prevention of Mental Disorders in Children," in *The Protection and Promotion of Mental Health in Schools,* Publication No. 1226, Washington, D.C.: U.S. Government Printing Office, 1965, pp. 9–22.

7. Cutler, Stephen J., "Voluntary Association Participation and Life Satisfaction: A Cautionary Research Note," *Journal of Gerontology,* 1973, pp. 96–100.

8. Donald, C. A., et al., *Conceptualization and Measurement of Health for Adults in the Health Insurance Study,* Vol. IV, *Social Health,* Santa Monica: The Rand Corporation, 1978.

9. Dubos, Rene, *Mirage of Health,* Garden City, N.Y.: Anchor Books, 1959.

10. Douvan, Elizabeth, "Commitment and Social Contract in Adolescence," *Psychiatry,* February 1974, pp. 22–35.

11. Dunham, H. Warren, "Society, Culture, and Mental Disorder," *Archives of General Psychiatry,* February 1976, pp. 147–156.

12. Dunn, Halbert L., *High Level Wellness,* Washington, D.C.: Mt. Vernon Printing Co., 1967.

13. Erikson, Erik H., *Childhood and Society,* New York: W. W. Norton & Co., 1963.

14. Erikson, Erik H., "Identity and the Life Cycle," *Psychological Issues I,* 1959.

15. Fromm, Erich, *The Revolution of Hope,* New York: Bantam Books, 1968.

16. Foot, Hugh C., Antony J. Chapman, and Jean R. Smith, "Friendship and Social Responsiveness in Boys and Girls," *Journal of Personality and Social Psychology* 35:6, 1977, pp. 401–411.

17. Gardner, Lytt I., "Depression Dwarfism," *Scientific American,* July 1972, p. 7.

18. Gladstone, William, *Test Your Own Mental Health,* New York: Arco Publishing Co., 1978.

19. Glasser, William, *Schools Without Failure,* New York: Harper & Row, 1969.

20. Goldman, William, and Philip Lewis, "Beautiful Is Good: Evidence That the Physically Attractive Are More Socially Skillful," *Journal of Experimental Social Psychology* 13, 1977, pp. 125–130.

21. Gruenberg, Ernest M., et al., "Social Breakdown Syndrome: Environmental and Host Factors Associated with Chronicity," *American Journal of Public Health,* January 1972, pp. 91–94.

22. Hountras, Peter T., *Mental Hygiene,* Columbus: Charles C. Merrill, 1961.

23. Kimmel, Douglas C., *Adulthood and Aging,* New York: Wiley, 1974.

24. Leaf, Alexander, "Everyday Is a Gift When You Are Over 100," *National Geographic,* January 1973, pp. 93–118.

25. Levinson, Daniel J., "The Mid-life Transition: A Period of Adult Psychosocial Development," *Psychiatry,* May 1977, pp. 99–112.

26. Maslow, Abraham H., "A Theory of Metamotivation: The Biological Routing of the Value Life," *Journal of Humanistic Psychology,* Fall 1967.

27. Maslow, Abraham H., *Toward a Psychology of Being,* New York: Van Nostrand Reinhold, 1968.

28. Merrill, Francis E., "The Self and the Other: An Emerging Field of Social Problems," pp. 79–90 in *Social Environment and Behavior,* edited by Harold Greenberg, Cambridge, Mass.: Schenkman Publishing Co., 1971.

29. Miller, P., and J. G. Ingham, "Friends, Confidants, and Symptoms," *Social Psychiatry* 11, 1976, pp. 51–58.

30. Portigal, Alan H., ed., *Measuring the Quality of Working Life,* Ottawa, Canada: Imprimerie Jacques-Cartier, 1974.

31. Rahe, Richard H., et al., "Psychosocial Predictors of Illness Behavior and Failure in Stressful Training, *Journal of Health and Social Behavior,* December 1972, pp. 393–397.

32. *Science News,* August 1, 1970, p. 100.

33. *Science News,* April 29, 1972, p. 281.

34. *Science News,* May 13, 1972, p. 311.

35. Shubin, Seymour, "People Who Need People," April, 1978 *Family Health.*

36. Toffler, Alvin, *Future Shock,* New York: Random House, 1970.

37. Trotter, Robert J., "The Biological Depths of Loneliness," *Science News,* March 3, 1973.

38. Ware, John E., Jr., et al., *Associations Among Psychological Well-being and Other Health Status Constructs,* Santa Monica: The Rand Corporation, November 1978, pp. 6–13.

39. Zimbardo, Philip G., *Shyness: What It Is, What to Do About It,* Reading, Mass.: Addison-Wesley, 1977.

Chapter 5

1. American Association for Health, Physical Education and Recreation, *Weight Training in Sports and Physical Education,* Washington, D.C.: National Education Association, 1962.

2. Boyer, John L., "What Exercise Can and Cannot Do," *Consultants,* September 1975, pp. 110–112.

3. Castelli, William, and Irving M. Levitas, "New Look at Lipids— Why They're Not All Bad," *Current Prescribing,* June 1973, pp. 39–43.

4. Cooper, Kenneth H., *Aerobics,* New York: M. Evans & Co., 1968.

5. ———, *The New Aerobics,* New York: M. Evans & Co., 1970.

6. ———, *The Aerobics Way,* New York: M. Evans & Co., 1978.

7. Cooper, Mildred, and Kenneth H. Cooper, *Aerobics for Women,* New York: M. Evans & Co., 1972.

8. Department of Health and Welfare, *Physical Activity in Canada,* Paper 78-1, Ottawa, Canada: July 1978, 102 pp.

9. Fleishman, Edwin A., *The Structure and Measurement of Physical Fitness,* Englewood Cliffs, N.J.: Prentice-Hall, 1964.

10. Getchell, Bud, *Physical Fitness—A Way of Life,* New York: Wiley, 1976.

11. Howell, Maxwell L., and W. R. Morford, *Fitness Training Methods,* Toronto, Canada: Canadian Association for Health, Physical Education, and Recreation, 1966.

12. Karpovich, Peter V., and Wayne E. Sinning, *Physiology of Muscular Activity,* Philadelphia: Saunders, 1971.

13. Leaf, Alexander, "On the Physical Fitness of Men Who Live to a Great Age," *Executive Health,* August 1977, 8 pp.

14. Mathews, Donald K., and Edward L. Fox, *The Physiological Basis of*

Physical Education and Athletics, Philadelphia: Saunders, 1971.

15. Morehouse, Lawrence E., and Leonard Gross, *Total Fitness in 30 Minutes a Week,* New York: Pocket Books, 1975.

16. President's Council on Physical Fitness, *Adult Physical Fitness,* Washington, D.C.: U.S. Government Printing Office, 1977.

17. Williams, Melvin H., *Nutritional Aspects of Human Physical Athletic Performance,* Springfield, Ill.: Charles C Thomas, 1976.

Chapter 6

1. *A Bircher-Benner Way to Positive Health and Vitality,* Bircher-Benner Verlag, Zurich, Switzerland. Also, Kraut, H. T., Max Planck Institute for Nutrition Research, Der Wendepunkt, Vol. 52, p. 443, 1975.

2. Adams, Ruth, and Frank Murray, *Minerals: Kill or Cure?,* New York: Larchmont Books, 1977

3. Ahrens, R. A., "Sucrose, Hypertension and Heart Disease: An Historical Perspective," *American Journal of Clinical Nutrition* 27, 1974; pp. 403–422.

4. Airola, Paavo, *Hypoglycemia,* Phoenix: Health Plus Publishers, 1977.

5. Anderson, R. K., et al., "Nutrition Appraisal in Mexico," *American Journal of Public Health* 38, 1948, p. 1126.

6. Asimov, Isaac, *The Chemicals of Life,* New York: Mento Books, 1954.

7. Benarde, Melvin A., *The Chemicals We Eat,* New York: McGraw-Hill, 1975.

8. Berland, Theodore, and editors, *Rating the Diets,* Skokie, Ill.: Consumer Guide, 1974.

9. Borsook, Henry, *Vitamins,* New York: Pyramid Books, 1977.

10. Brewster, Letitia, and Michael F. Jacobson, *The Changing American Diet,* Washington, D.C.: Center for Science in the Public Interest, 1978.

11. Bricker, M., et al., "The Protein Requirements of Adult Human Subjects in Terms of the Protein Contained in Individual Foods and Food Combinations," *Journal of Nutrition* 30, 1945, p. 269.

12. Briggs, George M., and Doris H. Calloway, *Bogert's Nutrition and Physical Fitness,* Philadelphia: Saunders, 1979.

13. Burkitt, Denis P., "The Link Between Low-fat Diets and Disease," *Human Nature,* December 1978, pp. 34–41.

14. Castelli, William, and Irving M. Levitas, "New Look at Lipids— Why They're Not All Bad," *Current Prescribing,* June 1973, pp. 39–43.

15. Cheraskin, Emanuel, and William Ringsdorf, *Psychodietetics,* New York: Bantam Books, 1976.

16. Clark, Linda, *Know Your Nutrition,* New Canaan, Conn.: Keats Publishing, 1973.

17. _____, *Consumer Report,* January 1976.

18. Deutsch, Ronald M., *Realities of Nutrition,* Palo Alto: Bull Publishing Co., 1976.

19. Deutsch, Ronald M., *The New Nuts Among the Berries,* Palo Alto: Bull Publishing Co., 1977.

20. DiCyan, Erwin, *Vitamins in Your Life,* New York: Simon & Schuster, 1974.

21. Duffy, William, *Sugar Blues,* New York: Warner Books, 1976.

22. Ebon, Martin, *Which Vitamins Do You Need,* New York: Bantam Books, 1976.

23. Eckholm, Erik, and Frank Record, "The Affluent Diet: A Worldwide Health Hazards," *The Futurist,* February 1977, pp. 32–42.

24. Editorial, "Food Additives," *Lancet,* August 16, 1969, p. 361.

25. Franklin, Getty, "An M.D. Reveals the Power in Minerals," *Let's Live,* January 1978, pp. 30–38.

26. Fredericks, Carlton, *High-Fiber Way to Total Health,* New York: Pocket Books, 1976.

27. Fremes, Ruth, and Zak, Sabry, *Nutriscore: The Rate-Yourself Plan for*

Better Nutrition, New York: Methuen, 1976.

28. Gershoff, Stanley N., et al., "Studies of the Elderly in Boston: The Effects of Iron Fortification on Moderately Anemic People," *The American Journal of Clinical Nutrition,* February 1977, pp. 226–234.

29. _____, "GOOD vs. BAD Cholesterol," *Time,* November 24, 1977, p. 119.

30. Groen, J. J., et al., "Nutrition of the Bedouins in the Negel Desert," *American Journal of Clinical Nutrition* 14:37, 1968.

31. Hall, Ross Hume, *Food for Naught,* New York: Random House, 1974.

32. Hegsted, D. M., et al., "Protein Requirements of Adults," *Journal of Laboratory and Clinical Medicine* 31, 1946, p. 261.

33. Hindhede, M., "The Effects of Food Restriction During War on Mortality in Copenhagen," *JAMA* 74, 1920, p. 381.

34. Hulley, Stephen B., et al., "Plasma High Density Lipoprotein Cholesterol Level," *JAMA,* November 21, 1977, pp. 2269–2271.

35. Keen, Sam, "Eating Our Way to Enlightenment," *Psychology Today,* October 19, 1978, p. 62+.

36. Keen, Sam, "The Pure, the Impure, and the Paranoid," *Psychology Today,* October, 1978, p. 67+.

37. Keusch, Gerald T., "Malnutrition and Infection: Deadly Allies," *Natural History Magazine,* November 1975, 6 pp.

38. Keys, A., F. Grande, and J. Anderson, "Bias and Misrepresentation—Perspective on Saturated Fat," *American Journal of Clinical Nutrition* 27, 1974, pp. 188–212.

39. Kiehm, Tae, G., Jones W. Anderson, and Kyleen Ward, "Beneficial Effects of a High Carbohydrate, High Fiber Diet on Hyperglycemic Diabetic Men," *The American Journal of Clinical Nutrition,* August 1976, pp. 895–899.

40. Kirkeby, K., "Blood Lipids, Lipoproteins, and Proteins in Vege-

tarians," *Acta, Med. Scandinivia,* vol. 179, supp. 443, 1966, pp. 56–60.

41. Knox, E. G., "Foods and Diseases," *British Journal of Preventive and Social Medicine,* 1977, pp. 71–80.

42. Labuza, Theodore P., *The Nutrition Crises: A Reader,* St. Paul: West Publishing, 1975.

43. Lappe, Frances Moore, *Diet for a Small Planet,* New York: Ballantine Books, 1975.

44. Leonard, Jon N., J. L. Hofer, and N. Pritikin, *Live Longer Now,* New York: Grosset & Dunlap, 1977.

45. Kritchevsky, D., and J. A. Storey, "Binding of Biosalts in Vitro by Nonnutritive Fiber," *Journal of Nutrition* 104, 1974, pp. 458–462.

46. Mann, George V., "A Factor in Yogurt Which Lowers Cholesteremia in Man," *Atherosclerosis* 26, 1977, pp. 335–340.

47. Mayer, Jean, *A Diet for Living,* New York: Pocket Books, 1977.

48. Morris, J. N., Jean W. Marr, and D. G. Clayton, "Diet and Heart: a Postscript," *British Medical Journal,* November 19, 1977, pp. 1307–1314.

49. National Academy of Sciences, *Recommended Daily Allowances,* Washington, D.C.: National Academy of Science, 1974.

50. Norgay, T., and J. R. Ullman, *Tiger of the Snows,* New York: G. P. Putnam's Sons, 1955, p. 14.

51. Nutrition Research, Inc., *Nutrition Almanac,* New York: McGraw-Hill, 1975.

52. Ohlson, M. A., "Dietary Patterns and Effects on Nutrient Intake," *World Review of Nutrition and Dietetics* 10, 1969, p. 13.

53. Palm, J. Daniel, *Diet Away Your Stress, Tension, and Anxiety,* New York: Pocket Books, 1977.

54. Passwater, Richard A., *Supernutrition,* New York: Pocket Books, 1976.

55. Pauling, Linus, "Orthomolecular Psychiatry," *Science,* April 19, 1968, pp. 265–271.

56. Pauling, Linus, *Vitamin C: The Common Cold and the Flu,* San Francisco: W. H. Freemand and Co., 1976.

57. Pierre, Clara, "The Nutrition Dilemma," *Saturday Review World,* May 18, 1974, 3 pp.

58. Proxmiere, William, "Why Title IV—The Vitamin Title of 5.988 Should Be Passed," Washington, D.C.: *U.S. Senate Congressional Record,* no. 183, December 11, 1975.

59. Reiser, R., "Saturated Fat in the Diet and Serum Cholesterol Concentration: A Critical Examination of the Literature," *American Journal of Clinical Nutrition* 26, 1973, pp. 524–555.

60. Rosenberg, Harold, and Feldzaman, A. N., *The Book of Vitamin Therapy,* New York: Berkley Windhover Books, 1975.

61. Scheer, James F., "The Awesome Ascorbates," *Let's Live,* January 1978, pp. 57–62.

62. Schlierf, G., et al., "Acute Dietary Effects on Diurnal Plasma Lipids in Normal Subjects," *Atherosclerosis* 26, 1977, pp. 525–533.

63. Stare, Frederick J., and Elizabeth M. Whelan, "The Best Diet for You and Your Health," *Health Values: Achieving High Level Wellness,* January/February 1977, pp. 27–33.

64. Steiner, P. E., "Necropsies on Okinawans: Anatomic and Pathologic Observations," *Archives of Pathology,* October 1946, pp. 359–380.

65. Toomey, E. G., and P. W. White, "A Brief Survey on the Health of Aged Hunzas," *Journal of the American Heart Association* 69, 1964 p. 842.

66. Trowell, Hugh, "Ischemic Heart Disease and Dietary Fiber," *The American Journal of Clinical Nutrition,* September 1972, pp. 926–931.

67. U.S. Select Senate Committee on Nutrition and Human Needs, *Dietary Goals for the United States,* Washington, D.C.: December 1977.

68. _____, March 31, 1977.

69. _____, November 1977.

70. _____, February 1977.

71. Weisner, Roland L., "Salt and the Development of Essential Hypertension," *Preventive Medicine* 5, 1976, pp. 7–14.

72. Whitney, Eleanor, and May Hamilton, *Understanding Nutrition,* New York: West Publishing, 1977.

73. Williams, Roger J., *Nutrition Against Disease,* New York: Bantam Books, 1973.

74. Williams, Roger J., and Dwight K. Kalita, *A Physician's Handbook on Orthomolecular Medicine,* New York: Pergamon Press, August 1978.

75. Winikoff, Beverly, "Changing Public Diet," *Human Nature,* January 1978, pp. 60–65.

76. Young, Eleanor A., Ellen H. Brennan, and Gaynell L. Irving, "Prospectives on Fast Foods," *Public Health Currents,* January/February 1979, pp. 2–15.

Chapter 7

1. Atkins, Robert C., *Dr. Atkins Diet Revolution,* New York: B. McKay Company, 1972.

2. Berland, Theodore, and Editors, *Rating the Diets,* Skokie, Ill.: Consumer Guide, 1974.

3. Briggs, George M., and Doris Howes Calloway, *Bogert's Nutrition and Physical Fitness,* Philadelphia: Saunders, 1979.

4. Cheraskin, Emanuel, and William Ringsdorf, *Psychodietetics,* New York: Bantam Books, 1976.

5. Gilmore, C. P., "The One Way to Lose Weight Without Dieting," *Reader's Digest,* July 1979, pp. 67–70.

6. Mayer, Jean, *A Diet for Living,* New York: Pocket Books, 1977.

7. Pierce, Carol, "Time: A New Key to Weight Loss," *Woman's Day,* No. 7, 1979, p. 29.

8. Seltzer, C. C., and Jean Mayer, "A Simple Criterion of Obesity," *Postgraduate Medicine* 38:2, 1965.

9. Shannon, Ira L., *Brand Name Guide to Sugar* (Sucrose content of over 1000 common foods and beverages), Chicago: Nelson-Hall, 1977.

10. Vanltallie, Theodore, "Conspiracy Against Fatness," *Psychology Today,* October 1978, pp. 97–107.

11. Williams, Roger J., *Nutrition Against Disease,* New York: Bantam Books, 1973.

Chapter 8

1. "Alcohol I.D. Guidelines," *Alcohol and Alcohol Education,* January 27, 1978, pp. 8–9.

2. Baker, Susan P., and Russell S. Fisher, "Alcohol and Motorcycle Fatalities," *AJPH,* March 1977, pp. 246–249.

3. Beauchamp, D. E., "Blaming the Alcoholic: The Concept of Alcoholism as Ideology," Papers Presented at the 20th International Council on Alcohol and Addictions. Phoenix: Do It Now Foundation, P. O. Box 5115, 1974, p. 96.

4. Editorial, "The Fetal Alcohol Syndrome," *Alcoholism: Clinical and Experimental Research,* July 1977, pp. 191–192.

5. Estes, Nada J., and M. Edith Heinemann, *Alcoholism: Development, Consequences, and Interventions,* St. Louis: C. V. Mosby, 1977.

6. Fillmore, Kaye M., and Philip W. Marden, "Longitudinal Research at the Rutgers Center of Alcohol Studies," *Alcoholism: Clinical and Experimental Research,* July 1977, pp. 251–257.

7. Hafen, Brent Q., *Alcohol: The Crutch That Cripples,* New York: West Publishing Co., 1977.

8. Girdano, Dorothy Dusek, and Daniel A. Girdano, *Drugs — A Factual Account,* Reading, Mass.: Addison-Wesley, 1973.

9. Jacobson, George R., *The Alcoholisms: Detection, Diagnosis and Assessment,* New York: Human Sciences Press, 1976.

10. Manson, Morse P., "A Psychometric Determination of Alcoholic Addiction," *American Journal of Psychiatry,* June 1949, pp. 199–205.

11. Martin, Joan, et al., "Maternal Alcohol Ingestion and Cigarette Smoking and Their Effects on Newborn Conditioning," *Alcoholism: Clinical and Experimental Research,* July 1977, pp. 293–247.

12. Oakley S., *Drugs, Society, and Human Behavior,* St. Louis: C. V. Mosby, 1972.

13. Seixas, Frank A., ed., "The Fatal Alcohol Syndrome: A Seminar," *Alcoholism: Clinical and Experimental Research,* July 1977, p. 217.

14. Straus, Robert, *Alcohol and Society, Psychiatric Annals* (Reprint), October 1973.

15. USDHEW, *Alcohol and Alcoholism: Problems, Programs, and Progress,* Washington, D.C.: U.S. Government Printing Office, 1972.

16. USDHEW, *Alcohol and Health,* Second Special Report to the U.S. Congress, Washington, D.C.: U.S. Government Printing Office, June 1974.

17. USDHEW, "Social Drinking Affects Behavior of Newborns," *National Institute on Alcohol Abuse and Alcoholism* (No. 78-151), March 3, 1978, p. 3.

18. Zinberg, "Alcoholics Anonymous and the Treatment and Prevention of Alcoholism," *Alcoholism: Clinical and Experimental Research,* January 1977, pp. 91–102.

Chapter 9

1. Brook, M., and J. J. Grimshaw, "Vitamin C Concentration of Plasma and Leukocytes as Related to Smoking Habit, Age, and Sex of Humans," *The American Journal of Clinical Nutrition,* November 1968, pp. 1254–1258.

2. Califano, Joseph A., Jr., "Remarks on Smoking and Health," Presented to the Youth Conference of the National Interagency Council on Smoking and Health, San Francisco, April 26, 1979.

3. Girdano, Dorothy Dusek, and Daniel A. Girdano, *Drugs — A Factual Account,* Reading, Mass.: Addison-Wesley, 1973.

4. Gonzalez, Nicholas, "Preventing Cancer," *Family Health,* May 1976.

5. Hilliard, Sheryl, "How Not to Gain Weight When You Stop Smoking," *Woman's Day,* November 7, 1978, p. 91.

6. Hauser, Norm W., *About You and Smoking,* Glenview, Ill.: Scott, Foresman and Co., 1971.

7. Kaplan, Ervin, and Lewis W. Mayron, "Evaluation on Perfusion the ^{81}Rb-^{81m}Kr Generator," reprint from *Seminars in Nuclear Medicine,* April 1976, pp. 163–192.

8. McCormick, W. J., "Ascorbic Acid as a Chemotherapeutic Agent," *Archives of Pediatrics,* April 1952, pp. 151–155.

9. Miller, William, "Smoking and Health: A Commentary," *Texas Medicine,* January 1978, pp. 83–88.

10. Oakley, Ray S., *Drugs, Society and Human Behavior,* St. Louis: C. V. Mosby, 1972.

11. Ochsner, Alton, *Smoking: Your Choice Between Life and Death,* New York: Simon & Schuster, 1970.

12. Olshavsky, Richard W., *No More Butts,* A Psychologist's Approach to Quitting Cigarettes, Bloomington: Indiana University Press, 1978.

13. Pelletier, Omer, "Smoking and Vitamin C Levels in Humans," *The American Journal of Clinical Nutrition,* November 1968, pp. 1259–1267.

14. Ross, Walter S., "Cigarettes: Who Do the Smoke Signals Say?", *Reader's Digest,* April 1978, pp. 95–99.

15. Ross, Walter S., "Do You Know

What Happens When You Smoke?'', *Reader's Digest* (Reprint), 1972, 6 pp.

16. Schmeltz, Irwin, Dietrich Hoffman, and Ernest L. Wynber, ''The Influence of Tobacco Smoke on Indoor Atmosphere,'' *Preventive Medicine* 4, 1975, pp. 66–82.

17. Sebben, John, Peter Pimm, and Roy J. Shephard, ''Cigarette Smoke in Enclosed Public Facilities,'' *Archives of Environmental Health,* March/April 1977, pp. 53–57.

18. _____, ''Smoke-filled Wombs,'' *Health Digest,* January 1978, p. 3.

19. _____, ''So Show Me,'' *Current Health* 2, March 1978.

20. Surgeon General's Report, *The Health Consequences of Smoking,* Washington, D.C.: U.S. Government Printing Office, 1972.

21. Wood, Curtis, *Overfed but Undernourished,* New York: Tower Publications, 1971.

Chapter 10

1. Airola, Paavo, *Hypoglycemia,* Phoenix: Health Plus Publishers, 1977.

2. Bellet, Samuel, et al., ''Effect of Coffee Ingestion in Catecholamine Release,'' *Metabolism,* April 1969, pp. 288–291.

3. Brecher, Edward M., and editors, ''Marijuana: The Health Questions,'' *Consumer Reports,* Mt. Vernon, N.Y., 1975, pp. 160–166.

4. Burns, Stanley, et al., ''Phencyclidine—States of Acute Intoxication and Fatalities,'' *The Western Journal of Medicine,* November 1975, pp. 345–349.

5. Cheraskin, Emanuel, and William Ringsdorf, *Psychodietetics,* New York: Bantam Books, 1976.

6. DeBakey, Lois, ''Happiness Is Only a Pill Away: Madison Avenue Rhetoric Without Reason,'' *Addictive Diseases* 3:2, 1977, pp. 273–286.

7. Duffy, William, *Sugar Blues,* New York: Warner Books, 1976.

8. Editorial, ''A Two-Edged Sword,''

The Lancet, September 6, 1975, pp. 441–443.

9. Editorial, ''Chronic Insomnia Provokes More Prescriptions Than Diagnosis,'' *Journal of the American Medical Association,* April 11, 1977, p. 1569.

10. Editorial, ''The Archaic Barbiturate Hypnotics,'' *New England Journal of Medicine,* October 10, 1974, pp. 790–791.

11. Fort, Joel, *The Pleasure Seekers,* New York: Bobbs-Merrill, 1969.

12. Franklin, Betty, ''Is Smoking Pot Really Harmless,'' *Let's Live,* February 1978, pp. 65–68.

13. Franks, H. M., et al., ''The Effect of Caffeine on Human Performance, Alone and in Combination with Ethanol,'' *Psychopharmacologia* 45, 1975, pp. 177–181.

14. Fredricks, Carlton, *High-Fiber Way to Total Health,* New York: Pocket Books, 1976.

15. Girdano, Dorothy Dusek, and Daniel A. Girdano, *Drugs—A Factual Account,* Reading, Mass.: Addison-Wesley, 1973.

16. Hennekens, Charles H., et al., ''Coffee Drinking and Death Due to Coronary Heart Disease,'' *New England Journal of Medicine,* March 18, 1976, pp. 633–636.

17. Heyden, S., et al., ''Coffee Consumption and Mortality in a Community Study—Evans Co., GA.'', *Z. Ernahrungswiss* 15, 1976, pp. 143–150.

18. _____, ''High on PCP,'' *Emergency Medicine* (Reprint), April 1977, pp. 264–267.

19. Institute of Criminal Justice and Criminology, ''Sociocultural Factors in Nonmedical Drug Use,'' *Proceedings of International Seminar Convened at the University of Maryland,* University of Maryland Press, September 1976.

20. Jick, Hershel, et al., ''Coffee and Myocardial Infarction,'' *The New England Journal of Medicine,* July 12, 1973, pp. 63–67.

21. Kales, Anthony, et al., ''Chronic Hypnotic-Drug Use,'' *Journal of*

the American Medical Association, February 1974, pp. 513–517.

22. Kolton, Marilyn, et al., *Innovative Approaches to Youth Services,* Madison, Wis.: Stash Press, 1973.

23. Leonard, Jon N., J. L. Hofer, and N. Pritikin, *Live Longer Now,* New York: Grosset & Dunlap, 1977.

24. Nahas, Gabriel G., *Marihuana—Deceptive Weed,* New York: Raven Press, 1975.

25. National Institute on Drug Abuse, *Alternative Pursuits for America's 3rd Century: A Resource Book on Alternatives to Drugs* (No. 75-241), Washington, D.C.: U.S. Government Printing Office, 1975.

26. National Institute on Drug Abuse, *Recommendations for Future Federal Activities in Drug Abuse Prevention* (No. 77-498), Washington, D.C.: U.S. Government Printing Office, 1977.

27. Nightingale, Stuart L., ''Treatment for Drug Abusers in the United States,'' *Addictive Diseases* 3:1, 1977, pp. 11–20.

28. _____, ''On the Drug Scene: New Rival for Heroin,'' *U.S. News & World Report,* August 8, 1977, p. 65.

29. Passwater, Richard A., *Supernutrition,* New York: Pocket Books, 1976.

30. Perkins, Robin, and Williams, Melvin H., ''Effect of Caffeine upon Maximal Muscular Endurance of Females,'' *Medicine and Science in Sports* 7:3, 1975, pp. 221–224.

31. Ray, Oakley S., *Drugs, Society and Human Behavior,* St. Louis: C. V. Mosby, 1972.

32. Riely, Caroline A., ''Drugs and What They Do to the Liver,'' *Medical Times,* January 1978, pp. 87–92.

33. Rosenberg, Harold, and A. N. Feldzamen, *The Book of Vitamin Therapy,* New York: Berkley Windhover Book, 1975.

34. Select Committee on Nutrition and Human Needs of the United States Senate, *Dietary Goals for the United States,* Washington, D.C.:

U.S. Government Printing Office, December, 1977.

35. Simon, David, Stella Yen, and Philip Cole, "Coffee Drinking and Cancer of the Lower Urinary Tract," *Journal of the National Cancer Institute,* March 1975, pp. 587–590.

36. Seifert, "Public Enemies in Our Private Lives," *Let's Live,* February 1978, pp. 43–47.

37. Smart, Reginal G., "Drug Abuse and Its Treatment in Canada," *Addictive Diseases* 3:1, 1977, pp. 5–10.

38. Tennant, Forest S., Jr., and Roger Detels, "Relationship of Alcohol, Cigarette, and Drug Abuse in Adulthood with Alcohol, Cigarette and Coffee Consumption in Childhood," *Preventive Medicine* 5, 1976, pp. 70–77.

39. _____, "The Deadly 'Angel Dust' ", *Newsweek,* March 13, 1978.

40. _____, "Too Much Sugar?", *Consumer Reports,* Consumer Union, March 1978, pp. 136–142.

41. USDHEW, *Drugs and Attitude Change* (No. 76-185), Washington, D.C.: U.S. Government Printing Office, November 1974.

42. USDHEW, *Drugs and Family/Peer Influence* (No. 76-186), Washington, D.C.: U.S. Government Printing Office, November 1974.

43. USDHEW, *Drug Abuse Instrument Handbook* (No. 271-75-3071), Washington, D.C.: U.S. Government Printing Office, 1976.

44. USDHEW, *Drug Abuse Prevention* (No. 78-588), Washington, D.C.: U.S. Government Printing Office, 1977.

45. USDHEW, *Marihuana and Health,* Fifth Annual Report to the U.S. Congress (No. 76-314), Washington, D.C.: U.S. Government Printing Office, 1976.

46. USDHEW, *Marihuana and Health,* Sixth Annual Report to the U.S. Congress (No. 77-443), Washington, D.C.: U.S. Government Printing Office, 1977.

47. USDHEW, *The Epidemiology of Drug Abuse, Research Monograph Series* (No. 77-432), Washington, D.C.: U.S. Government Printing Office, 1977.

48. USDHEW, *Sedative-Hypnotic Drugs: Risks and Benefits* (Prepublication copy), Washington, D.C.: U.S. Government Printing Office, August 1977.

49. USDHEW, *White Paper on Drug Abuse: A Report to the President from the Domestic Council Drug Abuse Task Force,* Washington, D.C.: U.S. Government Printing Office, September 1975.

50. Young, Lawrence A., et al., *Recreational Drugs,* New York: Collier Books, 1977.

51. Wallace, T. D., "The Moral Duty of the Profession in the Tranquilizer-on-demand Syndrome," *Canadian Medical Association Journal,* August 23, 1975, p. 317.

52. Weathersbee, Paul S., Larry K. Olsen, and J. Robert Lodge, "Caffeine and Pregnancy," *Postgraduate Medicine,* September 1977, pp. 64–69.

53. Williams, Roger J., *Nutrition Against Disease,* New York: A Bantam Book, 1973.

Chapter 11

1. *Accident Facts: 1977 Edition,* Chicago: National Safety Council, 1977.

2. Cline, Foster W., "Adolescent Suicide," *Nurse-Practitioner,* September-October 1978, pp. 44–53.

3. Draper, Edgar, "A Developmental Theory of Suicide," *Comprehensive Psychiatry,* January-February 1976, pp. 63–78.

4. Foote, Carol, "Getting Tough About Rape," *Human Behavior,* December 1978, pp. 24–26.

5. Freudenheim, Betty, "Rape Evidence Kits Boost Chances for Successful Prosecution," *The San Diego Union,* December 10, 1978.

6. Hafen, Brent Q., and Eugene J. Faux, *Self-Destructive Behavior,*

Minneapolis: Burgess Publishing Co., 1972.

7. Hoiberg, Anne, and Arthur D. Garfein, "Predicting Suicide Gestures in a Naval Recruit Population," *Military Medicine,* May 1976, pp. 327–331.

8. Hotchkiss, Sandy, "The Realities of Rape," *Human Behavior,* December 1978, pp. 18–23.

9. Iskrant, Albert P., and Paul V. Joliet, *Accidents and Homicide,* Cambridge, Mass.: Harvard Univ. Press, 1968.

10. Kiev, Ari, "Cluster Analysis Profiles of Suicide Attempters," *American Journal of Psychiatry,* February 1976, pp. 150–153.

11. Kovacs, Maria, Aaron T. Beck, and Arlene Weissman, "The Communication of Suicidal Intent," *Archives of General Psychiatry,* February 1976, pp. 198–201.

12. Mishara, Brian L., A. Harvey Baker, and Tanju T. Mishara, "The Frequency of Suicide Attempts: A Retrospective Approach Applied to College Students," *American Journal of Psychiatry,* July 1976, pp. 841–843.

13. _____, *Self-Defense for Women: A Simple Method,* Ventura, Calif.: Thor Publishing Co., 1973.

14. Shinar, David, *Psychology on the Road,* New York: Wiley, 1978.

15. Singer, Richard G., and Irving J. Blumenthal, "Suicide Clues in Psychotic Patients," *Mental Hygiene,* July 1969.

16. Storaska, Frederic, *How to Say No to a Rapist and Survive,* New York: Random House, 1975.

17. _____, "Suicide," *Health Tips,* San Francisco: California Medical Education and Research Foundation, January 1976, 2 pp.

18. Tegner, Bruce, and Alice McGrath, *Self-defense for Girls and Women: A Physical Education Course,* Ventura, Calif.: Thor Publishing Co., 1973.

19. Thygerson, Alton L., *Accidents and Disasters,* Englewood Cliffs, N.J.: Prentice-Hall, 1977.

20. _____, *Traffic Safety '76*, Washington, D.C.: U.S. Department of Transportation, 1976.

Chapter 12

1. Adams, Ruth, and Frank Murray, *Minerals: Kill or Cure?*, New York: Larchmont Books, 1977.
2. Berland, T., "Periodontal Diseases: Hidden Threat to Grown-ups Teeth," *Today's Health*, August 1969, pp. 28–30.
3. Braham, Raymond L., et al., "Nutrition and Its Importance in Dental Health," *The Journal of Family Practice* 6:1, 1978, pp. 49–58.
4. Caldwell, R. C., and D. E. Hunt, "A Comparison of the Antimicrobial Activity of Disclosing Agents," *Journal of Dental Research*, September/October 1969, pp. 913–915.
5. Challem, Jack Joseph, "Skin Problems—What You Can Do," *Bestways*, February 1978, pp. 35–38.
6. Cheraskin, E., *Predictive Medicine*, Mountain View, Calif.: Pacific Press Publishing Association, 1973.
7. Duffy, William, *Sugar Blues*, New York: Warner Books, 1975.
8. _____, "Feminine Hygiene in the Age of Advertising," *Health Tips*, San Francisco, July/August 1978.
9. Guyton, Arthur C., *Textbook of Medical Physiology*, Philadelphia: Saunders, 1966.
10. Haldelman, Stanley L., and Charles Hess, "Bacterial Populations of Selected Tooth Surface Sites," *Journal of Dental Research*, February 1969, pp. 67–70.
11. Heenan, Jane, "If You're Coloring Your Hair," *FDA Consumer*, November 1974.
12. Hopkins, Harold C., "And Now a Word About Your Shampoo," *FDA Consumer*, March 1975.
13. Horowitz, Herschel S., "A Review of Systemic and Topical Fluorides for the Prevention of Dental Caries," *Community Dental Oral Epidemiology* 1, 1973, pp. 103–114.
14. Marples, M. J., *The Ecology of Human Skin*, Springfield, Ill.: Charles C Thomas, 1965.
15. Martins, Leslie V., and Lawrence H. Meskin, "An Innovative Technique for Assessing Oral Hygiene," *ASDC Journal of Dentistry for Children*, January/February 1972.
16. McGuire, Thomas, *The Tooth Trip*, Berkeley: Random House, 1972.
17. Michaelsson, Gerd, Lennart Juhlin, and Anders Vahlquist, "Effects of Oral Zinc and Vitamin A in Acne," *Archives of Dematology*, January 1977, pp. 31–37.
18. Morrison, Margaret, "Cosmetics," *FDA Consumer*, April 1977.
19. Niklas, Mata K., "Prevention in Oral Health Problems: Social Behavioral Aspects," *Preventive Medicine* 5, 1976, pp. 149–164.
20. _____, "On Zinc . . . the Amazing Metal So Essential to Your Health," *Executive Health*, December 1978, p. 6.
21. Ratcliff, Perry A., *For 9 Out of 10 Adults Only* (Pamphlet), School of Dentistry, University of California, San Francisco.
22. Ronsard, Nicole, *Cellulite*, New York: Bantam Books, 1978.
23. Select committee on Nutrition and Human needs of the U.S. Senate, *Diet Related to Killer Diseases*, v. Nutrition and Mental Health, U.S. Government Printing Office, June 22, 1977, p. 282.
24. The Joy of Living Library, *Feel Younger, Live Longer*, New York: Rand McNally, 1978.
25. _____, "Weathered Skin—Too Much Sun," *Health Tips*, San Francisco: California Medical Association, July/August 1978.
26. _____, "What To Do About Bad Breath," *Health Tips*, San Francisco: California Medical Association, February 1978.
27. Williams, Roger J., *Nutrition Against Disease*, New York: Bantam Books, 1973.
28. Wood, Curtis, *Overfed but Undernourished*, New York: Tower Publications, 1971.
29. _____, "Your Skin . . . How Much Do You Know About It That Isn't So?", Rancho Sante Fe, Calif., *Executive Health*, 7:11.
30. Private communication with Dr. George A. Bray, Professor of Medicine at UCLA School of Medicine. "The basic observation is that the rate at which fat depots are removed from some regions of the body is faster than others. Moreover, the influence of various hormones on fat mobilization differs with fat from different parts of the body. Thus, today, I have to conclude that there are important regional metabolic differences in fat, which might be called cellulite," January 29, 1979.

Chapter 13

1. Abramson, J. H., and C. Hopp, "The Control of Cardiovascular Risk Factors in the Elderly," *Preventive Medicine* 5, 1976, pp. 32–47.
2. Ball, Keith P., and Richard Turner, "Realism in the Prevention of Coronary Heart Disease," *Preventive Medicine* 4, 1975, pp. 390–397
3. Benditt, Earl P., "The Origin of Atherosclerosis," *Diet Related to Killer Diseases, III*, Hearings before the Select Committee on Nutrition and Human Needs of the United States Senate, Washington, D.C.: U.S. Government Printing Office, March 24, 1977, p. 384+.
4. Bortner, Rayman W., "A Short Rating Scale as a Potential Measure of Pattern A Behavior," *Journal of Chronic Diseases* 22, 1969, pp. 87–91.
5. Bortner, Rayman W., Ray H. Rosenman, and Meyer Friedman, "Familial Similarity in Pattern A Behavior," *Journal of Chronic Diseases* 23, 1970, pp. 39–43.
6. Burton, Alan C., *Physiology and Biophysics of the Circulation*,

Chicago: Year Book Medical Publishers, 1965.

7. Castelli, William P., "CHD Rich Factors in the Elderly," *Hospital Practice,* October 1976, pp. 113–121.

8. Corday, Eliot, and Stephen Richard Corday, "Prevention of Heart Disease by Control of Risk Factors: The Time Has Come to Face the Facts," *Diet Related to Killer Diseases,* III, Hearings before the Select Committee on Nutrition and Human Needs of the United States Senate, Washington, D.C.: U.S. Government Printing Office, March 24, 1977,, pp. 100–105.

9. _____, "Do-it-Yourself Blood Pressure Devices," *Consumer Reports,* October 1974, pp. 740–743.

10. Editorial, "The Economic Impact of Arteriosclerotic Disease," *Hospital Practice,* December 1972.

11. Dudley, Eugene F., Richard A. Beldin, and Benjamin C. Johnson, "Climate, Water Hardness, and Coronary Heart Disease," *Journal of Chronic Diseases* 22, 1969, pp. 25–48.

12. Elek, Stephen R., "Emotional Tension as a Factor in Coronary Disease," *Hospital Medicine,* February 1970, pp. 115–129.

13. Epstein, Frederick H., "Preventive Trials and the Diet-heart Question —Wait for Results or Act Now?", *Atherosclerosis* 26, 1977, pp. 515–523.
Trials and the Diet-heart Question —Wait for Results or Act Now?", *Atherosclerosis* 26, 1977, pp. 515–523.

14. Froelicher, Victor F., "Dietary Prevention of Atherosclerosis," *AFP,* March 1973, pp. 79–85.

15. Ganong, William F., *Review of Medical Physiology,* Los Altos: Lange Medical Publications, 1963.

16. Gottlieb, Bill, "Fiber Fights Middle-age Health Enemies," *Prevention,* March 1978, pp. 84–88.

17. Hatch, Frederick T., "Interactions Between Nutrition and Heredity in Coronary Heart Diseases," pp. 393–412, in *The Nutrition Crisis* by Theodore P. Labuza, New York: West Publishing, 1975.

18. _____, *Heart Facts, 1978,* New York: American Heart Association, 1978.

19. Hurt, H. D., "Heart Disease — Is Diet a Factor?", pp. 323–339, in *The Nutrition Crisis* by Theodore P. Labuza, New York: West Publishing, 1975.

20. Johnson, Harry J., "Low Cholesterol Diet: It Won't Prevent Heart Attacks," *Diet Related to Killer Diseases, III,* Hearings before the Select Committee on Nutrition and Human Needs of the United States Senate, Washington, D.C.: U.S. Government Printing Office, March 24, 1977, pp. 232+.

21. Kannel, William B., "The Role of Cholesterol in Coronary Atherogenesis," pp. 355–373, in *The Nutrition Crisis* by Theodore P. Labuza, New York: West Publishing, 1975.

22. Kuhne, P., "High Blood Pressure," *Home Medical Encyclopedia,* New York: Fawcett, 1960, pp. 57–58.

23. _____, "Latest in Fight Against Heart Attacks," *U.S.. News & World Report,* February 3, 1975, pp. 139–140.

24. Leonard, Jon N., J. L. Hofer, and N. Pritikin, *Live Longer Now,* New York: Grosset & Dunlap, 1977.

25. Lyon, Nancy, "Cholesterol," *Diet Related to Killer Diseases, III,* Hearings before the Select Committee on Nutrition and Human Needs of the United States Senate, March 1977, pp. 376–383.

26. Maccoby, Nathan, et al., "Effects of a Community-Based Campaign on Knowledge and Behavior," *Journal of Community Health,* Winter 1977, pp. 100–114.

27. MacCornack, Frederick A., "The Effects of Coffee Drinking on the Cardiovascular System: Experimental and Epidemiological Research," *Preventive Medicine* 6, 1977, pp. 104–119.

28. Mann, George V., "The Saturated vs. Unsaturated Fat Controversy," *Diet Related to Killer Diseases, III,* Hearings before the Select Committee on Nutrition and Human Needs of the United States Senate, Washington, D.C.: U.S. Government Printing Office, March 24, 1977, pp. 256–265.

29. Mason, Harold L., and Ralph D. Ellefson, "Chemical Screening and Evaluation of Coronary and Coronary-Prone Patients," *Geriatrics,* January 1974, pp. 109–114.

30. Mathews, Karen A., et al., "Competitive Drive, Pattern A, and Coronary Heart Disease: A Further Analysis of Some Data from the Western Collaborative Group Study," *Journal of Chronic Diseases* 30, 1977, pp. 489–498.

31. Menoti, A., et al., "Identifying Subsets of Major Risk Factors in Multivariate Estimation of Coronary Risk," *Journal of Chronic Diseases* 30, 1977, pp. 557–565.

32. Metzner, Helen Low, Ernest Harburg, and Donald E. Lamphiear, "Early Life Social Incongruities, Health Risk Factors and Chronic Disease," *Journal of Chronic Diseases* 30, 1977, pp. 225–245.

33. Meyer, Anthony J., and Judith B. Henderson, "Multiple Risk Factor Reduction in the Prevention of Cardiovascular Disease," *Preventive Medicine* 3, 1974.

34. Nager, Norman R., "Apathetic Hearts," *Human Behavior,* February 1976, pp. 12–13.

35. Nolan, William A., "New Ways to Control High Blood Pressure," *McCalls Magazine,* February 1978, p. 94.

36. Ochsner, Alton, "How to Cut One's Risk of Dying from Heart Disease or a Stroke," *Executive Health,* April 1978.

37. Peacock, Peter B., "Atherosclerotic Heart Disease and the Environment," pp. 413–419, in *The Nutrition Crisis,* by Theodore P. Labuza, New York: West Publishing Co., 1975.

38. Pilowsky, I., et al., "Hypertension and Personality," *Psychosomatic Medicine,* January-February 1973, pp. 50–55.

39. _____, "Prevention of Coronary Heart Disease Starts in Childhood," *Archives of Disease in Childhood* 52, 1977, pp. 904–906.

40. _____, *Recommendations for Human Blood Pressure Determination by Sphygmomanometers* (Pamphlet), New York: American Heart Association, 1967.

41. Rosenberg, Harold, *The Book of Vitamin Therapy,* New York: A Berkley Windhover Book, 1975.

42. _____, "Salt and Blood Pressure," *Health Digest* (Newsletter), January 1978.

43. Sales, Stephen M., and James Hause, "Job Dissatisfaction as a Possible Risk Factor in Coronary Heart Disease," *Journal of Chronic Diseases* 23, 1971, pp. 861–873.

44. Schroeder, Henry A., "The Role of Trace elements in Cardiovascular Diseases," pp. 374–392, in *The Nutrition Crisis,* by Theodore P. Labuza, New York: West Publishing Co., 1975.

45. Segall, Jeffrey J., "Is Milk a Coronary Health Hazard?", *British Journal of Preventive and Social Medicine* 31, 1977, pp. 81–85.

46. Shorey, Rose Ann L., Bennett Sewell, and Michael O'Brien, "Efficiency of Diet and Exercise in the Reduction of Serum Cholesterol and Triglyceride in Free-living Adult Males," *The American Journal of Clinical Nutrition,* May 1976, pp. 512–521.

47. Shute, Wilfrid E., and Harold J. Taub, *Vitamin E for Ailing and Healthy Hearts,* New York: Pyramid Books, 1974.

48. Simborg, Donald W., "The Status of Risk Factors and Coronary Heart Disease," *Journal of Chronic Diseases* 22, 1970, pp. 515–552.

49. Spain, David M., "Atherosclerosis," pp. 29–37, *Human Physiology and the Environments in Health and Disease (Readings from Scientific American),* San Francisco: W. H. Freeman and Co., 1976.

50. Theorell, Tores, and Richard H. Rahe, "Behavior and Life Satisfaction Characteristics of Swedish Subjects with Myocardial Infarction," *Journal of Chronic Diseases* 25, 1972, pp. 139–147.

51. USDHEW, *Hypertension: High Blood Pressure,* Washington, D.C.: U.S. Government Printing Office, 1969.

52. _____, "Vitamin E Lubricates the Circulation," *Prevention,* April 1978, pp. 91–100.

53. Weinsier, Roland L., "Overview: Salt and the Development of Essential Hypertension," *Preventive Medicine* 5, 1976, pp. 7–14.

54. Williams, Christine L., Charles B. Arnold, and Ernest L. Wynder, "Primary Prevention of Chronic Disease Beginning in Childhood" *Preventive Medicine* 6, 1977, pp. 344–357.

55. Williams, Roger, *Nutrition Against Disease,* New York: Bantam Books, 1973.

56. Williams, Roger J., and Dwight K. Kalita, *A Physician's Handbook on Orthomolecular Medicine,* New York: Pergamon Press, 1978.

57. Wilmore, Jack H., *Athletic Training and Physical Fitness,* Boston: Allyn and Bacon, 1977.

58. Zohman, Burton L., "Emotional Factors in Coronary Disease," *Geriatrics,* February 1973, pp. 110–119.

Chapter 14

1. Adams, Ruth, and Frank Murray, *Minerals: Kill or Cure?,* New York: Larchmont Books, 1977.

2. Adler, Richard, "'111.2° Super-Heat Treatment Kills 99% of Cancer Cells," *Pageant,* January 1966, pp. 75–80.

3. Anderson, M. R., and R. Nayak, "Epidemiology of Hodgkin's Disease," *Journal of Chronic Disease* 25, 1972, pp. 253–259.

4. Arthur, Thelma E., "Morphologic Changes and Kinetics of Leukocytes as a Detection Test for Early Cancer," *Journal of American Pathology* 78:1, 1975, p. 65.

5. Bjeklke, E., "Dietary vitamin A and human lung cancer," *American Journal of Cancer* 15, 1975, pp. 561–565.

6. _____, *Cancer Facts and Figures: 1978,* New York: American Cancer Society, 1977.

7. _____, *Nutrition and Cancer,* New York: American Cancer Society, 1972.

8. Chowka, Peter Barry, "Laetrile at Sloan-Kettering, Part 1 — The Medical World's Watergate," *New Age,* July 1978, pp. 40–44.

9. Corbett, Bob, "Skin Test Seen as Cancer Cure," *San Diego Union,* April 4, 1978, p. A–10.

10. Cullin, J. W., B. H. Fox, and R. N. Isom, *Cancer: The Behavioral Dimensions,* New York: Raven Press, 1976.

11. Dawson, C. H., and T. E. Arthur, "A Possible Screening Test for the Detection of Malignancy in Untreated Patients Based on White Blood Analysis," *Journal of American Pathology* 78:1, 1975, p. 66.

12. Fox, Bernard H., and John R. Goldsmith, "Behavioral Issues in Prevention of Cancer," *Preventive Medicine* 5, 1976, pp. 106–121.

13. Fredericks, Carlton, *High-Fiber Way to Total Health,* New York: Pocket Books, 1976, p. 43.

14. Germann, Donald R., and Margaret Danbrot, "The Diet That Reduces Cancer Risk," *Woman's Day,* March 27, 1978, pp. 54–56.

15. Gerson, Max, *A Cancer Therapy,* Del Mar, CA; Totality Books, 1975.

16. Gori, Gio B., and James A. Peters, "Etiology and Prevention of Cancer," *Preventive Medicine* 4, 1975, pp. 239–246.

17. Gottlieb, Bill, "Fiber Fights Middle-Age Health Enemies," *Prevention,* March 1978, pp. 84–88.

18. Hellstrom, Karl E., and Ingegerd

Hellstrom, "Immunologic Defenses Against Cancer," *Hospital Practice,* January 1970, pp. 45–61.

19. Homberger, F., ed., *The Physio-pathology of Cancer,* New York: S. Karger, 1976.

20. Kelly, William, *One Answer to Cancer,* North Berendo, CA: Cancer Book House, 1969.

21. Kirschmann, John D., *Nutrition Almanac,* New York: McGraw-Hill, 1975.

22. Kittler, Glenn D., *Control for Cancer (Laetrile),* New York: Warner Books, 1976.

23. Livingston, Virginia, *Cancer: A New Breakthrough,* San Diego: Production House Publishers, 1972.

24. Newell, Guy R., and William Rawlings, "Evidence for Environmental Factors in the Etiology of Hodgkin's Disease," *Journal of Chronic Disease* 25, 1972, pp. 261–267.

25. ———, "New Test for Breast Cancer," *Health Digest,* February 1978, p. 6.

26. ———, *Nutrition and Cancer,* Hearings before the Select Committee on Nutrition and Human Needs of the United States Senate, Washington, D.C.: U.S. Government Printing Office, July 27, 28, 1976.

27. O'Donnell, Walter E., et al., *Early Detection and Diagnosis of Cancer,* St. Louis: C. V. Mosby, 1962.

28. Pauling, Linus, "On Vitamin C and Cancer," *Executive Health* 13:4, January 1976, 5 pp.

29. Roggenbuck, Peggy, "A Guide to Cancer Care," *New Age,* July 1978, pp. 48–51.

30. Rosenfeld, Claude, and Walter Davis, eds., *Environmental Pollution and Carcinogenic Risks,* Paris: Inserm, 1976.

31. Schamberger, Raymond J., "On Your Risk of Stomach Cancer from Untreated Beef," *Executive Health* 14:12, September 1978, 4 pp.

32. Schrauzer, G. N., *Inorganic Nutritional Aspects of Cancer,* New York: Plenum Press, 1978.

33.. Schrauzer, Gerhard N., and Debra Ishmael, "Effects of Selenium and of Arsenic on the Genesis of Spontaneous Mammary Tumors in Inbred C_3H mice," *Annals of Clinical and Laboratory Science* 4:6, 1974, pp. 441–447.

34. Simonton, Carl O., *Getting Well Again,* Los Angeles: J. P. Tarcher, 1978.

35. Sobel, Dava, "Do You Have a Cancer Personality?", *Science Digest,* July 1976, pp. 66–71.

36. Stauth, Cameron, "Alternative Cancer Therapies," *New Age,* July 1978, pp. 28–35.

37. Stauth, Cameron, "The Preventive Life Style," *New Age,* July 1978, pp. 45–47.

38. Sweeney, James P., "High-fiber Diet," *Bestways,* February 1978, pp. 59–60.

39. ———, "The Life-saving Banned Vitamin," *Prevention,* May 1968, pp. 75–78.

40. ———, "What Causes Cancer?", *Newsweek,* January 26, 1976, pp. 141–146.

41. ———, "Will Cancer Become America's Top Political Issue?", *New Age,* July 1978, pp. 18–19.

42. Williams, Roger J., *Nutrition Against Disease,* New York: Bantam Books, 1973.

43. Williams, Roger J., and Dwight K. Kalita, *A Physician's Handbook on Orthomolecular Medicine,* New York: Pergamon Press, 1978.

44. Winchester, A. M., "Can You Inherit Cancer?", *Life and Health,* May 1979, pp. 10–12.

45. Winter, Ruth, "New, Promising Developments in Some Cancer Treatments," *Science Digest,* December 1978, pp. 19–23.

46. Wynder, Ernest L., "Overview: Nutrition and Cancer," *Preventive Medicine* 4, 1975, pp. 322–327.

47. Laetrile's use has been made legal in 17 states: Alaska, Arizona, Delaware, Florida, Idaho, Illinois, Indiana, Kansas, Louisiana, Maryland, Nevada, New Hampshire, New Jersey, Oklahoma, Oregon, Texas, and Washington, as reported in: "Malpractice Alert" *Current Prescribing,* November 1978, p. 42.

Chapter 15

1. ———, *Arthritis: The Basic Facts,* Atlanta: The Arthritis Foundation, 1976.

2. Bender, Stephen J., *Venereal Diseases,* Dubuque, Iowa: Wm. C. Brown, 1971.

3. Cherniak, Donna, and Allan Feingold, *V.D. Handbook,* Montreal: Montreal Health Press, June 1975.

4. ———, "Cold Related to Life Styles," *San Diego Union,* February 24, 1974.

5. Crook, William G., *Are You Allergic: A Guide to Normal Living for Allergic Adults and Children,* Jackson, Tenn.: Professional Books, 1974.

6. Frazer, D. W., et al., "Field Investigation Team: Legionnaire's Diseases, Description of an Epidemic of Pneumonia," *New England Journal of Medicine* 297, 1977, pp. 1189–1197.

7. Gudmond-Hoyer, E., and K. Simony, "Individual Sensitivity to Lactose in Lactose Malabsorption," *Digestive Diseases,* March 1977, pp. 177–181.

8. Jones, Kenneth L., Louis W. Shainberg, and Curtis O. Byer, *V.D.,* New York: Harper & Row, 1974.

9. ———, "Legionnaire's Disease—United States," *Morbidity and Mortality Weekly Report,* November 10, 1978, pp. 439–441.

10. ———, "Legionnaire's Disease Germ has Long Life," *Evening Tribune,* San Diego, November 15, 1978, p. A–25.

11. Limbeck, George, "Juvenile Rheumatoid Arthritis," *AFP,* May 1970, pp. 88–89.

12. Kolata, Gina Bari, "Strategies for

the Control of Gonorrhea," *Science,* April 16, 1976, p. 245.

13. Mandell, Marshall, "Cerebral Reactions in Allergic Patients: Illustration Case Histories and Comments," in *A Physician's Handbook on Orthomolecular Medicine,* pp. 130–139, edited by Roger J. Williams and Dwight K. Kalita, New York: Pergamon Press, 1978.

14. Philpott, William H., "Maladaptive Reactions to Frequently Used Food and Commonly Met Chemicals as Precipitating Factors in Many Chronic Physical and Chronic Emotional Illnesses," in *A Physician's Handbook on Orthomolecular Medicine,* pp. 140–150, edited by Roger J. Williams and Dwight K. Kalita, New York: Pergamon Press, 1978.

15. Rapaport, Howard, and Shirley Linde, *The Complete Allergy Guide,* New York: M. S. Simon & Schuster, 1971.

16. Subak-Sharpe, Genell, "The Venereal Disease of the New Morality," *Today's Health Magazine,* March 1975, pp. 155–156.

17. The Student Committee on Sexuality at Syracuse University, *Sex in a Plain Brown Wrapper,* Syracuse, N.Y.: The Institute for Family Research and Education, 1973.

18. _____, "The Venereal Diseases," *Health Tips* (CMA) (D-374), San Francisco, 1974.

19. Travis, Luther B., *An Instructional Aid on Juvenile Diabetes Mellitus,* E. R. Squibb and Sons, 1969.

20. _____, *Understanding Diabetes,* New York: Pfizer, 1972.

21. _____, "Vaginitis," *Health Tips,* San Francisco: California Medical Education and Research Foundation, April 1974.

22. _____, "V.D. Alarm," *Parade Magazine,* November 12, 1978, p. 19.

23. _____, "V.D. Update" (Supplement), *Current Health 2,* Curriculum Innovations, March 1978.

24. Warner, Rebecca, Sidney M. Wolfe, and Rebecca Rich, *Off Diabetes Pills: A Diabetic's Guide to Longer Life,* Washington: Public Citizens Health Research Group, 1978.

25. Williams, Ralph C., "Osteoarthritis and Rheumatic Disease," *Postgraduate Medicine,* October 1967, pp. 334–338.

Chapter 16

1. _____, "A Second Look at the Sexual Revolution," *Time,* November 21, 1977, and condensed in *The Readers Digest,* June 1978, pp. 117–119.

2. Bell, Robert R., *Marriage and Family Interaction,* Homewood, Ill.: Dorsey Press, 1967.

3. Belliveau, Fred, and Lin Richter, *Understanding Human Sexual Inadequacy,* New York: Bantam Books, 1970.

4. Bieber, I., et al., *Homosexuality: A Psychoanalytic Study,* New York: Basic Books, 1962.

5. Bing, Elizabeth, *Six Practical Lessons for an Easier Childbirth,* New York: Bantam Books, 1977.

6. Brecher, Arline, "Marriage Is Not Dying," *National Enquirer,* April 4, 1978, p. 42.

7. Brecher, Jeremy, and Brecher, Edward M., "Sex Is Good for Your Health," *P/A Magazine,* June 1976.

8. Colman, Libby, and Arthur Colman, *Pregnancy,* New York: Bantam Books, 1977.

9. Comfort, Alex, *The Joy of Sex,* New York: Crown Publishers, 1972.

10. Deutsch, Ronald M., *The Key to Feminine Response in Marriage,* New York: Random House, 1968.

11. Duvall, Evelyn Millis, *Family Development,* New York: J. B. Lippincott, 1967.

12. _____, *Love and the Facts of Life,* New York: Association Press, 1966.

13. Fromme, Eric, *The Art of Loving,* New York: Harper & Row, 1974.

14. Gerard, Alice, *Please Breast Feed Your Baby,* New York: Signet Books, 1971.

15. Group for the Advancement of Psychiatry, *Sex and the College Student,* New York: Antheneum, 1966.

16. Guttmacher, Alan F., *Pregnancy and Birth,* New York: Signet Books, 1962.

17. Hite, Shere, *The Hite Report,* New York: Dell Publishing, 1976.

18. Kirkendall, Lester A., *Marriage and Family Relations,* Dubuque, Iowa: Wm. C. Brown, 1968.

19. Kranteler, Mel, *Creative Divorce,* New York: Signet Books, 1973.

20. Lantz, Herman R., and Eloise C. Snyder, *Marriage,* New York: Wiley, 1962.

21. Masters, William H., and Virginia E. Johnson, *Human Sexual Response,* Boston: Little, Brown, 1966.

22. McCrary, James L., *Human Sexuality,* New York: D. Van Nostrand Co., 1967.

23. McLennan, Holly, "10 Ways to Improve Your Marriage," *Sexology,* February 1970, pp. 4–8.

24. O'Reilly, Jane, "Why Liberated Women Are Getting Married," *McCall's Magazine,* April 1978, pp. 109+.

25. Schnall, Maxine, *Your Marriage,* New York: Pyramid Books, 1976.

26. Schumacher, Warren F., "What Is Healthy Sex?", *Sexology,* November 1969.

27. _____, *Sex Education,* Minneapolis: Sacred Design Associates, 1968.

28. Sheehy, Gail, *Passages: Predictable Crises of Adult Life,* New York: Bantam Books, 1977.

29. Singleton, Mary Ann, *Life After Marriage* (Divorce as a new beginning), New York: Dell Publishing, 1974.

30. Slater, Philip E., "Sexual Adequacy in America," *Intellectual Digest,* November 1973.

31. Switzer, Ellen, "Female Sexuality," *Family Health,* March 1974.

32. Toffler, Alvin, *Future Shock,* New York: Random House, 1970.

33. The Child Study Association of America, *What to Tell Your Children About Sex,* New York: Pocket Books, 1968.

34. Vahanian, Tillan, and Sally Wendkas Olds, "How Good Is Your Marriage?", *Reader's Digest,* May 1978, pp. 136–139.

35. Woods, Marjorie Binford, *Your Wedding: How to Plan and Enjoy It,* New York: Pyramid Books, 1960.

Chapter 17

1. Apgar, Virginia, and Joan Beck, "A Perfect Baby," *Is My Baby All Right?,* New York: Simon & Schuster, 1972, pp. 134–138.

2. Arms, Suzanne, "How Hospitals Complicate Childbirth," *Immaculate Deception: A New Look at Women and Childbirth in America,* New York: Houghton Mifflin, 1975, pp. 235–239.

3. Braun, Jonathan, "The Struggle for Acceptance of a New Birth Technique," *Parade Magazine,* November 23, 1975, pp. 17–19.

4. Bylinsky, Gene, "What Science Can Do about Hereditary Diseases," *Fortune Magazine,* September 1974, pp. 111–118.

5. Department of Medical and Public Affairs, *Population Reports* (Population Information Program), Washington, D.C.: The George Washington University Medical Center, March 1977.

6. Editorial, "The Ethnic Distribution of Disease in the United States," *Journal of Chronic Diseases* 20, 1967, pp. 115–118.

7. Editors of Consumer Reports, *Family Planning,* Mt. Vernon, N.Y.: Consumer's Union, 1966.

8. Gerard, Alice, *Please Breast-feed Your Baby,* New York: Signet Books, 1970.

9. Goldstein, Philip, *Genetics Is Easy,* New York: Viking Press, 1967.

10. Grant, Lillian, "Our Precious Health Heritage," *Bestways Magazine,* February 1978, pp. 40–43.

11. Guthrie, Obert, "Mass Screening for Genetic Disease," *Hospital Practice,* June 1972, pp. 93–100.

12. Guttmacher, Alan F., *Pregnancy and Birth: A Book for Expectant Parents,* New York: Signet Books, 1962.

13. Holmes, Lewis, "How Fathers Can Cause the Down's Syndrome," *Natural Science,* Oct. 1978, pp. 70–72.

14. Horowitz, Charles A., and C. Y. Lee, "Pregnancy Testing," *Postgraduate Medicine,* June 1978, pp. 145–150.

15. House, Aline, "What Contraceptive Type Are You?", *Ms. Magazine,* March 1973, pp. 7–14.

16. Leboyer, Frederick, *Birth Without Violence,* New York: Alfred A. Knopf, 1975.

17. Marx, Jean L., "Drugs During Pregnancy: Do They Affect the Unborn Child?", *Science,* April 1973 pp. 174–175.

18. McCary, James Leslie, *Human Sexuality,* New York: D. Van Nostrand Co., 1967.

19. Medical Department, *Pregnancy: In Anatomical Illustrations,* Los Angeles: Carnation Company, 1965.

20. Montreal Health Press, *Birth Control Handbook,* Montreal Health Press, 1975.

21. Nakashima, Ida I., "Teenage Pregnancy—Its Causes, Costs, and Consequences," *Nurse Practitioner,* September/October, 1977.

22. *Am I Parent Material?* (Pamphlet), Baltimore: National Organization for NonParents.

23. Omran, Abdel R., "Health Benefits for Mother and Child," *World Health* (Reprint), January 1974.

24. ———, *Daughters of DES Mothers* (Pamphlet), New York: Planned Parenthood Federation of America, 1977.

25. ———, *Voluntary Sterilization for Men and Women* (Pamphlet), New York: Planned Parenthood World Population, 1976.

26. ———, *Ways to Chart Your Fertility Pattern* (Pamphlet), New York: Planned Parenthood Federation of America, 1977.

27. ———, *Intercom: The International Newsletter on Population,* Washington, D.C.: Population Reference Bureau, June 1977, p. 3.

28. Riccardi, Vincent, and Arthur Robinson, "Preventive Medicine Through Genetic Counseling," *Preventive Medicine* 4, 1975, pp. 126–134.

29. ———, "Self-help Pregnancy Test," *McCalls Magazine,* March 1978, p. 46.

30. Smithells, R. W., et al., "Maternal Nutrition in Early Pregnancy," *British Journal of Nutrition* 38 1977, pp. 497–506.

31. Sutton, H. Eldon, *An Introduction to Human Genetics,* New York: Holt, Rinehart & Winston, 1975.

32. Rosenberg, Harold, *The Book of Vitamin Therapy,* New York: Berkley Windhover Books, 1975.

33. The Diagram Group, *Woman's Body,* New York: Paddington Press, 1977.

34. The National Foundation, *Genetic Counseling* (Pamphlet), New York: The National Foundation/March of Dimes.

35. USHEW, *The Extra Advantages of Family Planning* (Pamphlet), Washington, D.C.: U.S. Government Printing Office, 1975.

36. ———, *Family Planning and Health* (Pamphlet), Washington, D.C.: U.S. Government Printing Office, 1975.

37. ———, *Women and Estrogens* (Pamphlet), Washington, D.C.: U.S. Government Printing Office, 1977.

38. ———, *Women and the Pill* (Pamphlet), Washington, D.C.: U.S. Government Printing Office, 1976.

39. Westoff, Charles F., and Elise F. Jones, "Contraception and Sterilization in the United States, 1965–

1975," *Perspectives*, July/August 1977, pp. 153–157.

40. Williams, Rogert J., *Nutrition Against Disease*, New York: Bantam Books, 1971.

Chapter 18

1. Brier, Judith, and Dan Rubenstein, "Sex for the Elderly? Why Not?", Parts I and I, pp. 65–74, in *Health Aspects of Aging*, edited by Geraldene Marr Burdman and Ruth Brewer. Portland: A Continuing Education Publication, 1978.

2. Bylinsky, Gene, "Science Is on the Trail of the Fountain of Youth," *Fortune*, July 1976.

3. Golden, Charles, "How Long You Will Live—the 38 Factors That Determine It," *National Enquirer*, December 1971

4. Hayflick, Leonard, "Human Cells and Aging," *Human Physiology and the Environment in Health and Disease (readings from Scientific American)*, San Francisco: W. H. Freeman, 1976, pp. 252–257.

5. Hayflick, Leonard, "On the Facts of Life," *Executive Health*, June 1978.

6. Harris, J. A., *The Measurement of Man* (organ growth curves of different parts and tissues of the body), Minneapolis: University of Minnesota Press, 1930.

7. Kugler, Hans J., *Slowing Down the Aging Process*, New York: Pyramid Books, 1976.

8. Leaf, Alexander, "Every Day Is a Gift When You Are Over 100," *National Geographic*, January 1973, pp. 93–118.

9. Leaf, Alexander, "Getting Old," *Human Physiology and the Environment in Health and Disease (Readings from Scientific American)*, San Francisco: W. H. Freeman, 1976, pp. 235–242.

10. Leonard, Jon N., J. L. Hoffer, and N. Pritikin, *Live Longer Now*, New York: Grosset & Dunlap, 1974.

11. Mayer, Jean, "Aging and Nutri-

tion," *Geriatrics*, May 1974, pp. 57–59.

12. Mapleton, Alexander J., "Factors of Human Longevity—Mystery, Myth or Truth?", *Gerontology Quarterly*, Fall 1973, pp. 11–21.

13. Oschsner, Alton, "Aging," *Journal of the American Geriatrics Society* 24:9, pp. 385–393.

14. Palmore, Erdman, and Francis C. Jeffers, *Prediction of Life Span*, Lexington, Mass.: D. C. Heath, 1971.

15. Palmore, Erdman, and Clark Luikart, "Health and Social Factors Related to Life Satisfaction," *Journal of Health and Social Behavior*, March 1972, pp. 68–80.

16. Palmore, Erdman B., and Virginia Stone, "Predictors of Longevity: A Follow-up of the Aged in Chapel Hill," *The Gerontologist*, Spring, 1973, pp. 88–90.

17. Patterson, Robert, Ruby Abrahams, and Frank Baker, "Preventing Self-destructive Behavior," *Geriatrics*, November 1974, pp. 115–121.

18. Prehoda, Robert W., "Our Children May Live to Be 200 Years Old," *The Futurist*, February 1969.

19. Rosenberg, Harold, *The Book of Vitamin Therapy*, New York: Berkley Windhover Books, 1975.

20. Rosenfeld, Albert, "Are We Programmed To Die?", *Saturday Review*, October 2, 1976, pp. 17–21.

21. Rothenberg, Robert E., *Health in the Later Years*, New York: Signet Books, 1972.

22. Salvador, Miquel, and Associates, *Vilcabamba, Tierra de Longevos*, Quito: Cultural Publishing House, 1972.

23. Select Committee on Nutrition and Human Needs of the United States Senate, *Nutrition: Aging and the Elderly: Diet Related to Killer Diseases, VII*, Washington, D.C.: U.S. Government Printing Office, September 23, 1977.

24. Shock, Nathan W., "The Physiology of Aging," *Human Physiology and the Environment in Health and Disease (Readings from Scientific*

American)*, San Francisco: W. H. Freeman, 1976, pp. 243–251.

25. Sorochan, Walter D., "Life Style as an Approach to Health," *Journal of California School Health*, Summer 1974, pp. 36–38.

26. Tappel, Al, "On Antioxidant Nutrients," *Executive Health*, March 6, 1980, 6 pp.

27. Weg, Ruth B., "Changing Physiology of Aging: Normal and Pathological," pp. 229–256, in *Aging: Scientific Perspectives and Social Issues*, by Diana S. Woodruff and James E. Birren, New York: D. Van Nostrand Co., 1975.

28. Woodruff, Diana S., and Birren, James E., *Aging: Scientific Perspectives and Social Issues*, New York: D. Van Nostrand Co., 1975.

Chapter 19

1. Bensley, Lorne, *Death Education as a Learning Experience*, Washington, D.C.: Eric Clearinghouse on Teacher Education, November 1975.

2. Kubler-Ross, Elisabeth, *Death: The Final Stage of Growth*, Englewood Cliffs, N.J.: Prentice-Hall, 1975.

3. Kubler-Ross, Elisabeth, "Facing up to Death," *Today's Education*, January 1972, pp. 69–71.

4. Engel, George, "Can Your Emotions Kill You?", *Psychology Today*, November 1977.

5. Johnson, Laurie, "Stricken Artist's Final Work Is Her Own Ritual Suicide," *San Diego Union*, June 17, 1979.

6. Klein, Norman, "Is There a Right Way to Die?", *Psychology Today*, October 1978, pp. 122–123.

7. Mitford, Jessica, *The American Way of Death*, New York: Simon & Schuster, 1963.

8. Morison, Robert S., "Dying," *Scientific American, Life and Death and Medicine*, September 1973, pp. 55–62.

9. Rosenfeld, Albert, "Are We Programmed to Die?", *Saturday Review*, October 2, 1976.

10. Sage, Wayne, "Choosing the Good Death," *Human Behavior,* June 1974.

11. Stoddard, Sandol, *The Hospice Movement,* New York: The Hospice Movement, 1978.

12. United States Senate Special Committee on Aging, *Death with Dignity,* Washington, D.C.: U.S. Government Printing Office, 1972.

13. White, Robert B., and Leroy T. Gathman, "The Syndrome of Ordinary Grief," *American Family Physician,* August 1973, p. 97.

Chapter 20

1. _____, "Acid Rains Pose Threat to Man," *San Diego Union,* November 19, 1978.

2. _____, "A Nuclear Nightmare," *Time,* April 19, 1979, pp. 8–18.

3. Asimov, Isaac, and Theodosius Dobzhansky, *The Genetic Effects of Radiation,* Oak Ridge, Tenn., U.S. Atomic Energy Commission, 1966.

4. Bartlett, Donald L., and James B. Steele, "Oil Shortage Myth—Oil, the Created Crisis," *The Philadelphia Inquirer,* July 22, 1973.

5. Bernarde, Melvin A., *Our Precarious Habitat,* New York: W. W. Norton and Company, 1973.

6. Borchardt, J. A., "Eutrophication," *Journal of AWWA,* June 1969, p. 272.

7. Carmon, Richard, *Our Endangered Hearing,* Emmaus, Penn.: Rodale Press, 1977.

8. Chew, T. J., and J. L. Earl, "Lead Aerosols in the Atmosphere: Increasing Concentrations," *Science,* 1970, pp. 577–580.

9. Corliss, William R., *Space Radiation,* Oak Ridge, Tenn.: U.S. Atomic Energy Commission, 1968.

10. Cralley, Lester, ed., *Industrial Environmental Health,* New York: Academic Press, 1972.

11. Dasmann, Raymond F., *Environmental Conservation,* New York: Wiley, 1976.

12. Eckholm, Erik, and Lester R. Brown, "The Deserts are Coming," *The Futurist,* December 1977, pp. 361–369.

13. Ehrlich, Paul R., *The Population Bomb,* New York: Sierra Club, Ballantine, 1971.

14. Eyl, Thomas B., "Methyl Mercury Poisoning in Fish and Human Beings," *Modern Medicine,* November 16, 1970, pp. 135–141.

15. Fox, Charles H., *Radioactive Wastes,* Oak Ridge, Tenn.: U.S. Atomic Energy Commission, 1969.

16. Galbraith, John Kenneth, "Economics and the Quality of Life," *Science,* July 1964, pp. 117–123.

17. Goldsmith, John R., "Air Pollution and Disease," *Hospital Practice,* May 1970, pp. 61–71.

18. Gwynne, Peter, "How Do You Get Rid of 3.5 Billion Tons of Waste a Year?", *California Geology,* May 1972.

19. Holdren, John, and Herrera, Philip, *Energy,* New York: Sierra Club, 1971.

20. Kastner, Jacob, *The Natural Radiation Environment,* Oak Ridge, Tenn.: U.S. Atomic Energy Commission, 1968.

21. Kennedy, Edward M., "U.S. in Grip of a Concrete Octapus," *Los Angeles Times,* December 3, 1972.

22. Kinsman, Simon, "The Irradiated Man," *California's Health,* July-August 1970, pp. 8–9.

23. Kormondy, Edward J., *Concepts of Ecology,* Englewood Cliffs, N.J.: Prentice-Hall, 1976.

24. Krehl, Willard A., "Mercury, the Slippery Metal," *Nutrition Today,* November/December 1972.

25. Nader, Ralph, *The Menace of Atomic Power,* New York, Norton, 1979.

26. Nelson, Nancy L., "Asbestos, Airborne Danger," *Safety Standards,* Washington, D.C.: U.S. Department of Labor, May-June 1972.

27. _____, "Nuclear Accident," *Newsweek,* April 9, 1979, pp. 24–45.

28. Peterson, A. P. G., and E. E. Gross, Jr., *Handbook of Noise Measurement,* West Concord, Mass.: General Radio Co., 1967.

29. Powers, Charles F., and Andrew Robertson, "The Aging Great Lakes," *Scientific American,* November 1966, p. 29.

30. Purdom, P. Walton, *Environmental Health,* New York: Academic Press, 1971.

31. Schiff, Maurice, "Nonauditory Effects of Noise," *Transactions,* September/October 1973.

32. Stephans, Edgar R., "Photochemistry of Smog," *California Air Environment.*

33. Tchobanoglaus, George, Hilary Theisen, and Rolf Eliassen, *Solid Wastes,* New York: McGraw-Hill, 1977.

34. Wagner, Richard H., *Environment and Man,* New York: W. W. Norton and Co., 1978.

35. Waldbott, George, *Health Effects on Environmental Pollutants,* St. Louis, C. V. Mobley, 1973.

36. Xintaras, Charles, Barry L. Johnson, and Ido deGroot, *Behavioral Toxicology: Early Detection of Occupational Hazards,* Washington, D.C.: U.S. Government Printing Office, 1974.

37. _____, "Zoology: Man Exterminates One Animal Species Each Year," *Futurist,* December 1973, p. 242.

Chapter 21

1. Asimov, Isaac, "The Computer Revolution," *Modern Maturity,* August/September 1974.

2. _____, "At the Interface: Technology and Mysticism," *Playboy,* December 1971, pp. 130–274.

3. Bell, Daniel, *The Coming of Post-Industrial Society,* New York, Basic Books, 1973.

4. Cole, H. S. D., et al., *Models of Doom: A Critique to the Limits of Growth,* New York: Universe Books, 1973.

5. Commoner, Barry, *The Closing Circle,* New York: Bantam Books, 1974.

6. Congdon, R. J., ed., *Introduction to Appropriate Technology,* Emmaus, Pa.: Rodale Press, 1977.

7. Crawford, Berry A., "Energy Crisis: A Blessing in Disguise," *The Futurist,* August 1976, pp. 198–203.

8. Dubos, Rene, *Mirage of Health,* New York: Doubleday, 1961.

9. _____, *So Human an Animal,* New York: Scribner, 1968.

10. Elgin, Duane S., and Arnold Mitchell, "Voluntary Simplicity: Life Style of the Future?", *The Futurist,* August 1977, pp. 200–206.

11. Harman, Willis W., "The Coming Transformation," *The Futurist,* February 1977, pp. 5–7.

12. Koff, Richard M., "And End to All This" (Review of Meadows, *The Limits to Growth*), *Playboy,* July 1971, pp. 112+.

13. Little, Dennis, "Post-Industrial Society and What It May Mean," *The Futurist,* December 1973, pp. 259–262.

14. Meadows, Dennis L., *The Limits to Growth,* New York: Universe Books, 1972.

15. Price, T., "Low Technology Solar Homes That Work with Nature," *Popular Science,* December 1976, pp. 94–98.

16. Schumacher, E. F., *A Guide for the Perplexed,* New York: Harper & Row, 1977.

17. Schumacher, E. F., *Small Is Beautiful: Economics as if People Mattered,* New York: Harper & Row, 1973.

18. Sherrill, Robert, "Power Play," *Playboy,* May 1971, p. 113.

19. Skurka, Norma, and Jon Naar, *Design for a Limited Planet,* New York: Ballantine Books, 1976.

20. Stellman, Jeanne M., and Susan M. Daum, *Work Is Dangerous to Your Health,* New York: Vintage Books, 1973.

21. Stoner, Carol H., *Producing Your Own Power,* Emmaus, Pa.: Rodale Press, 1974.

22. Wakefield, Rowan A., and Patricia Stafford, "Appropriate Technology: What Is It and Where It Is

Going," *The Futurist,* April 1977, pp. 72–76.

23. Watts, Kenneth E. F., "A Tragedy of Errors," *Science Review,* November 25, 1972, pp. 56–60.

24. _____, "Winona: The New Vision," *The Futurist,* April 1977, pp. 81–82.

Chapter 22

1. _____, "Battle Begins over National Health Insurance," *U.S. News & World Report,* June 25, 1979, pp. 62–63.

2. Blue Cross of Southern California, *Manual for Physicians: 1977 Edition,* Publication M-4532, Los Angeles.

3. _____, "Carter Announces National Health Plan," *Congressional Quarterly Weekly Report,* June 16, 1979, pp. 4–9.

4. Chisari, Francis, Robert Nakamura, and Lorena Thorup, *The Consumer's Guide to Health Care,* Boston: Little, Brown, 1976.

5. Conniff, James C. G., "How to Tell a Good Hospital from a Bad One," *Today's Health,* November 1973, pp. 42–45.

6. Conrad, Fran, "Society May Be Dangerous to Your Health," *Science for the People,* March/April 1979, pp. 14–17.

7. Consumer's Union, "Health Maintenance Organizations: Are HMO's the Answer to Your Medical Needs?" (reprint), Mount Vernon, N.Y.: October 1974, 8 pp.

8. Consumer's Union, "Medical Malpractice," Mount Vernon, N.Y.: September 1977, pp. 544–548.

9. Department of HEW, *Health: United States 1978,* Publication No. 78-1232, Washington, D.C.: U.S. Government Printing Office, December 1978.

10. Eckholm, Erik P., *The Picture of Health,* New York: W. W. Norton and Co., 1977.

11. Ehrenreich, Barbara, and John Ehrenreich, *The American Health

Empire,* New York: Vintage Books, 1971.

12. Feldstein, Martin S., "The Medical Economy," *Life and Death and Medicine,* San Francisco: W. H. Freeman and Co., 1973, pp. 112–118.

13. Fisher, Peter, *Prescription for National Health Insurance,* Croton-on-Hudson, N.Y.: North River Press, 1972.

14. Ferguson, Tom, ed., *Medical Self-Care Magazine,* Box 718, Inverness Co., 94937, 1977–1979.

15. Goddard, James L., "The Medical Business," *Life and Death and Medicine,* San Francisco: W. H. Freeman and Co., 1973, pp. 120–125.

16. _____, "Health-Care Battle," *Newsweek,* May 28, 1979, pp. 23–38.

17. _____, Health Costs: What Limit?", *Time,* May 28, 1979, pp. 60–68.

18. _____, "How to Tell When You're Getting a Good Physical," by Editors in *99 New Ideas on Your Money, Job and Living: The Changing Times Family Success Book,* Washington, D.C.: The Kiplinger Washington Editors, 1977, pp. 74–77.

19. _____, "Inside Our Hospitals," *U.S. News & World Report,* March 5, 1979, pp. 33–41.

20. Illich, Ivan, *Limits to Medicine,* Toronto: McClelland and Stewart, 1976.

21. Ingelfinger, Franz J., "Can You Survive a Medical Diagnosis," *Human Nature,* November 1978, pp. 38–39.

22. Jacobs, Paul, "Prepaid Health Plans Line Up for San Diego Patients," *Los Angeles Times,* January 7, 1979.

23. Kaiser Foundation, *Kaiser Foundation Medical Care Program 1970,* Oakland, Calif., 1970.

24. Kaiser Foundation, *Kaiser Foundation Medical Care Program: 1978,* Oakland, Calif., 1978.

25. _____, "Kennedy, Labor Coali-

tion Outline Comprehensive National Health Plan," *Congressional Quarterly Weekly Report,* May 19, 1979, pp. 970–972.

26. Kleinman, Arthur, "The Failure of Western Medicine," *Human Nature,* November 1978, pp. 63–68.

27. Kristein, M., Charles B. Arnold, and Ernest L. Wynder, "Health Economics and Preventive Care," *Science,* February 1977, pp. 457–461.

28. Lake, Alice, "How and When to Be Your Own Doctor," *McCall's,* September 1979, pp. 129–136.

29. Lalonde, Marc, *A New Perspective on the Health of Canadians,* Ottawa, Canada: Department of National Health and Welfare, April 1974.

30. Lee, Tsun-Nin, "Chinese Medicine: A Paragon of Holistic Medicine," *Journal of Holistic Health 3,* San Diego: The Word Shop, Mondala Holistic Health, 1978, pp. 61–65.

31. Leninger, Medeleine, *Barriers and Facilitator to Quality Health Care,* Philadelphia: F. A. David Co., 1975.

32. Margolis, Richard J., "National Health Insurance — The Dream Whose Time has Come," *The New York Times Magazine,* January 9, 1977.

33. McKeown, Thomas, "Determinants of Health," *Human Nature,* April 1978, pp. 60–67.

34. McTaggart, Aubrey, C., *The Health Care Dilemma,* Boston: Halbrook Press, 1978.

35. Mechanic, David, *Future Issues in Health Care,* New York: Free Press, 1979.

36. Mechanic, David, *Medical Sociology,* New York: Free Press, 1978.

37. Peterson, Osler L., "Medical Care in the U.S.," *Scientific American,* August 1973, pp. 19–27.

38. _____, "Prepaid Plans Proliferating," *MD Medical News Magazine,* November 1978, pp. 55–58.

39. Richie, Nicholas D., "Health Planning — an Overview," *Journal of Health Planning,* April 1978, pp. 36–42.

40. Russell, Harry J., and Mary V. Wells, "Care Beyond Acute General Hospital," *Journal of the American Hospital Association,* April 1, 1970, pp. 56–59.

41. Schadewald, Robert, "Take Before Necessary," *The Ambassador,* June 1979, 77-83.

42. Sehnert, Keith W., and Howard Eisenberg, *How to Be Your own Doctor — Sometimes,* New York: Grosset & Dunlap, 1975.

43. _____, "Soaring Cost of Medical Care," *U.S. News & World Report,* June 15, 1975.

44. The Regents of the University of California, *Health Plan Grading System: A System for Evaluation of Health Insurance Plans.*

45. Travis, Jon W., "Wellness Education and Holistic Health — How They're Related," *Journal of Holistic Health 3,* San Diego: The Word Shop, Mandala Holistic Health, 1978, pp. 25–32.

46. Vayda, Eugene, "Keeping People Well: A New Approach to Medicine," *Human Nature,* July 1978, pp. 64–71.

47. Vickery, Donald M., and James F. Fries, *Take Care of Yourself: A Consumer's Guide to Medical Care,* Reading, Mass.: Addison-Wesley, 1977.

48. White, Kerr L., "International Comparisons of Medical Care," *Scientific American,* August 1975, pp. 17–25.

49. White, Robert Lanon, *Right to Health: The Evolution of an Idea,* Iowa City: Univ. of Iowa Press, 1971.

50. Winter, Ruth, *How to Reduce Your Medical Bills,* New York: Crown Publishers, 1970.

51. Yarmon, Morton, "Facing the Unthinkable," *Parade,* February 4, 1979, pp. 24–26.

abortion removal of the embryo or premature fetus from a pregnant woman's uterus at any early point in pregnancy.

accident an unplanned happening or circumstance that causes body injury, death, or property damage.

acupuncture healing illnesses by puncturing the skin at different places in the body with special needles. The idea of acupuncture is to restore the energy flows throughout the body.

adultery sexual intercourse between a married person and someone other than his or her marriage partner.

aerobics exercises that demand large amounts of oxygen and last long enough to produce a definite training effect on the cardiovascular, respiratory, and muscular systems.

alcoholism chronic, long-term drinking wherein the person has lost control of his or her drinking. This affects the lives of others, and the care and maintenance of body health is neglected.

allergy hypersensitivity to a specific substance.

amniocentesis a medical technique—inserting a hollow needle through the abdominal wall and uterus of a pregnant female to obtain amniotic fluid to assess the sex or health of a fetus.

anemia a deficiency in the oxygen-carrying capacity in the blood.

angina pectoris a condition in which the heart muscle does not receive enough blood, causing severe pain in the chest and often in the left arm and shoulder.

angiogram X-ray viewing of a blood vessel following injection of a dye.

anorexia nervosa loss of appetite due to lack of love, affection, or emotional support.

antibody a protein substance produced in and by the body that protects against specific disease infections and allergies. Antibodies neutralize foreign proteins, producing immunity from them.

anxiety what we feel when our existence is threatened. One feels tense and uneasy and worries about a social situation or stressful circumstances.

appestat a center in the brain that controls hunger, appetite, thirst, and emotions. It is also referred to as the hypothalamus.

appropriate technology using inexpensive methods and equipment to employ people in meaningful work that is nonpolluting and energy independent. Opposite of inappropriate technology.

arteriosclerosis arteries harden and lose their elasticity and therefore become blocked, causing high blood pressure. This disorder is a consequence of atherosclerosis.

arthritis inflammation of a joint.

asymptomatic absence of any evidence of a disease (symptoms).

atherosclerosis deposits of fat plaques on the inner lining of arteries.

autogenic training a process of learning general body relaxation through the use of imagery and the feeling of heaviness and warmth in the body's limbs.

autoimmune disease a disease resulting when the body's immune system turns against the body and attacks one of its own organs.

autopsy examination of surgically removed tissue from a victim after death to determine cause of death.

BAC blood alcohol concentration.

basal metabolism the least amount of energy required to maintain vital functions in an organism at rest.

behavior modification psychological and social techniques used to modify deleterious behaviors.

benign tumor tumor that does not form metastases and does not invade or destroy adjacent tissue.

beriberi a disease caused by absence in diet of thiamine (vitamin B_1). Symptoms include loss of coordination, numbness or tingling in toes and feet, loss of appetite, depression, irritability, inability to concentrate, fatigue, and loss of morale.

biochemical individuality each person is different biochemically from all other persons. For example, one's appearance, finger prints, blood type, voice, and metabolic endowments are unique and distinguish one from all others. This concept of Roger Williams also implies that because our bodies are unique, we may need different amounts and kinds of nutrients as compared to others.

biofeedback use of machines that feed back tones and visual readouts of body processes—like brainwave activity, muscle activity, and skin temperature. Feedback information is used to change poor habits and reinforce positive health behaviors.

bioflavonoids or vitamin P various pigments and related compounds—such as the white peel in citrus fruits and other plants—that complement the function of vitamin C in the body.

biopsy a procedure for taking a sample of tissue from a living organism.

biorhythms three biological rhythms concerned with variations in physical, emotional, and intellectual capacities.

bronchitis inflammation of the mucous membrane of the bronchial tubes.

Caesarean section a surgical incision performed through the abdominal wall and uterus to give birth to a fetus.

calculus (dental) dental (bacterial) plaque accumulating over a long period of time and hardening to become tartar or calculus.

cancer uncontrolled and abnormal growth of cells; thereby changing their normal body functions.

carbohydrates substances made up of carbon, hydrogen, and oxygen, with hydrogen and oxygen almost always present in a 2:1 proportion. Food carbohydrates are made up of simple sugars or monosaccharides, two sugar chains or dissacharides, or many sugar units referred to as polysaccharides.

carcinogen substance that initiates uncontrolled growth or cancer.

carcinoma a cancer of the tissue near the skin surface, such as the lungs, breast, and skin.

cellulite unattractive, dimpled, rippling masses of flabby skin. Purported to be a disorder of the lymphatic and circulatory systems.

cervix neck of the uterus joining the vagina.

chancre a sore that appears on the spot where spirochete infection took place.

chiropractic a system of healing that emphasizes the manipulation of the spinal column.

choline a B-complex vitamin essential for growth of animals, prevention of accumulation of excess fat in the liver, and metabolism of fats and proteins.

cirrhosis liver cells being replaced by fat cells usually caused by lack of adequate nutrition, causing hardening of the liver and destruction of the liver cells, as in chronic alcoholics.

coitus sexual intercourse.

cold turkey sudden stoppage of taking a drug.

collagen a fibrous, protein-like connective tissue that holds tissues and bones together. Vitamin C is essential for body synthesis of collagen.

colostomy surgical removal of a cancerous rectum.

condon or rubber a thin rubber sheath, shaped like a finger of a glove, that is worn over the penis during sexual intercourse to prevent spermatozoa from entering the vagina.

contraception prevention of conception or birth by any means.

cremation the incineration of dead bodies.

cultural well-being interacting with the community. It includes giving or contributing (as a performer or artist) to the community, as well as receiving, taking, or appreciating (as a spectator or audience). Cultural well-being establishes roots in the community and gives one a sense of belonging to a place.

curettage scraping of the uterus to remove the embryo.

CVD cardiovascular disorders.

cystitis an inflammation of the bladder, usually in women.

death end of the life cycle. When the vital life support organs (brain, heart, liver, kidneys) stop functioning and rigor mortis sets in.

defecation the discharge of fecal material from the intestines. Process of having a bowel movement.

dental caries tooth decay or teeth that have decay.

dental plaque large colonies of many bacteria on surfaces of teeth or gums.

depression an emotional feeling of sadness, discouragement, emptiness, and hopelessness, resulting in chronic fatigue, exhaustion, ineptitude, and inability to perform or function in society.

dermatitis irritation of the skin.

DES—diethylstilbestrol a strong artificial estrogen that can cause cancer and other disorders in future offspring.

desertification erosion of soil in a region resulting in climatic changes, drought, and loss of vegetation.

detoxification the metabolic breakdown of drugs and chemicals, and their elimination from the body.

diabetes inability of the body to regulate the supply of glucose at all times to body cells.

diaphragm a soft rubber cup about 3 inches in diameter. It is placed over the cervix to block spermatozoa from entering the uterus.

digestion process of breaking down foods in the gastrointestinal tract into compounds that can pass into the bloodstream and be used for energy, growth, and repair.

disaccharide a carbohydrate composed of two molecules of sugar that must be broken down by digestion into simple sugars before being absorbed and used by the body.

diuretic an agent that promotes the excretion of urine.

diverticulosis an inflammation of and ballooning of the intestinal wall in the lower colon. Symptoms include fever, abdominal pain, and constipation or diarrhea.

Down's syndrome a mongoloid abnormality suspected of being caused by a defective egg or sperm.

drug any chemical substance that, when taken into the body, produces physiological, emotional, and/or behavioral changes.

dying that period of time between chronic illness and death when the person is dependent on care from others and is nonfunctioning in society. This is a psychological-spiritual, as well as physiological, change in the life of a person.

dysmenorrhea painful or uncomfortable menstruation.

dyspaveunia painful intercourse.

ecosystem study of relationship patterns between different organisms and their environment.

electrocardiogram (EKG or ECG) a graphic picture on a tape that records the electrical action of the heart muscle.

emotional well-being feeling good about self and others, being able to successfully resolve problems and to cope with the stresses and crises of living in socially acceptable ways, so as to be able to function successfully within a culture. It reflects a person's subjective emotional or feeling states, thoughts, behaviors, body image, and self-identities.

emphysema nonfunctioning air sacs caused by rupture of air sacs or alveoli.

endorphin an opiate-like body chemical that is produced when one exercises or meditates, which gives one relaxed, good feelings or a natural high.

episiotomy surgical cutting of the vaginal opening to enlarge it during childbirth.

EPT early pregnancy test.

euthanasia pulling the plug or mercy killing—painless allowing of death.

eutrophication aging of a lake or ocean.

fats mixtures of compounds of glycerol and fatty acids, at least one of which, linolenic acid, is an essential fatty acid.

fellatio the act of taking the penis into the mouth for purposes of sexual stimulation.

fiber (roughage) substance that cannot be digested because the human digestive system lacks the enzymes to do so.

flatus gas or air in the stomach or intestines.

food intoxication or food poisoning ingestion of bacterial toxins that paralyze the ability of the large intestine to absorb fluids, causing diarrhea, fatigue, and nausea.

fossil fuels fuels such as crude oil, coal, and gas that were formed over millions of years of pressure from vegetation and other living things.

frigidity lack of interest in sex on the part of a woman.

gastritis inflammation of the stomach.

genitalia the sex organs of males and females.

geriatrics study of diseases and disabilities of older people.

gigolo male prostitute.

gingivitis inflammation of the gums.

glucose a simple molecule of sugar or hexose from which starches are made and that as a single molecule or unit requires no digestion.

grief emotional pain or suffering accompanying death or separation of a loved one.

hemotacrit the percentage of blood cells (mostly red blood cells) comprising the total blood volume.

hepatitis inflammation of the liver.

high blood pressure see hypertension.

HMO—health maintenance organization an alternative group insurance approach to traditional private medical-hospital insurance, which focuses on prevention instead of treatment of diseases.

Hodgkin's disease a swelling of the lymph glands in many parts of the body, resulting in cancer.

holistic (wholistic) health a preventive medicine viewpoint that perceives a person functioning as a whole entity. This includes an interrelated balance of the physical, emotional, social, spiritual, and cultural dimensions of well-being. Holistic approaches to treatment of illness and disease often include unconventional medical practices—like faith healing and iridology.

homicide death of a person resulting from violence, such as being knifed or shot with a gun by another person.

homosexuality having physical contact and sexual arousal with a person of the same sex.

hospice a home for dying patients where no life-saving techniques are used and the dying person dies in pleasant and caring circumstances.

hypoglycemia a sudden rise and drop in blood glucose levels within the first one to three hours, causing anxiety, insomnia, fatigue, mental confusion, depression, acute hunger, and a craving for sweets and alcoholic beverages.

hysterectomy surgical removal of the uterus.

iatrogenic an illness or disease caused by medical treatment or intervention.

identify crisis (identity confusion) a delay in structuring a mature identity resulting in psychological distress—such as confusion, lack of morals and values by which to live, rebellion, and inability to function. An identity is made up of numerous commitments, which need to be fulfilled at various stages of life.

impotence inability of a male to attain or maintain an erection long enough to have sexual intercourse.

inositol a sugarlike substance included among the B-complex vitamins which is an important growth factor for certain yeasts and lower organisms.

insomnia inability to sleep.

iridology diagnosis of disease based on observations of the iris.

ischemia disruption or cutting off of the blood supply (oxygen) to a body part.

IUD—intrauterine device a small object placed inside the uterus to prevent pregnancy.

jaundice a disease symptom that causes the skin and the whites of the eyes to turn yellow.

keratosis small skin thickening, swelling, or lump that may be a precursor to cancer.

lactation breast-feeding a baby.

lesbian a woman having physical contact and sexual arousal with another woman.

linoleic acid the only essential fat that the body needs and from which it can make all other body fats.

lipoprotein fat molecules combining with protein molecules in the bloodstream.

lymphatic system a circulatory system of small vessels that collects tissue fluid (lymph) and transports it to the veins. This is also the immune system.

malnutrition faulty or poor nutrition in all of its aspects, whether from inadequate intake of nutrients or overconsumption of foods.

mammography radiological examination of the female breast, used most often to detect evidence of breast cancer.

masturbation self-stimulation of the

sex organs or other parts of the body for sexual pleasure.

menopause a time when a woman stops ovulating, when menstruation stops, marking the end of the child-bearing period—"a change of life."

menstruation shedding of the inner lining (endometrium) of the uterus approximately once a month.

metabolism chemical changes taking place in the body cells, such as the breakdown of fats, carbohydrates, and proteins and the release of energy, heat, water, and carbon dioxide.

metastasis spread of disease (cancer) within the body.

miscarriage a natural abortion or expulsion of the embryo or fetus from the uterus.

mourning expressing and releasing one's grief and emotions.

myocardium heart muscle.

mysectomy (radial) a controversial surgical operation removing the lymph nodes of a cancerous breast and adjacent lymph nodes as in the shoulder joint.

nephritis inflammation and malfunction of the kidney.

noise unwanted, garbled sound that causes chemical-hormonal changes that are similar to stress adaptation.

nomogram a series of graphs that interpolate human data and predict degree of body fat, metabolic rate, and desirable caloric intake.

nutrition the science of food as it relates to optimal health and performance.

nymphomania abnormal and uncontrollable sexual desire in women.

orgasm climax or peak of sexual response.

orthobiosis right or proper style of living that fulfills one's basic health needs, promotes optimal well-being and prolongs life. It is made up of positive constructive habits, behaviors, and health practices.

osteoporosis loss of minerals in the bones of elderly persons, causing bones to be brittle and soft.

OTC—over-the-counter ingesting drugs that may be purchased without a medical prescription.

oxidant a common term used to describe chemical substances having an oxygen molecule that is a by-product of photochemical smog.

PABA—para-aminobenzoic acid a vitamin-like substance that is a growth factor and serves as a sparing factor in the diet for folacin.

pathogen disease-producing organism.

pellegra a niacin vitamin deficiency causing sore tongue and mouth, skin eruptions, digestive disturbances, general weakness, and emotional depression.

phagocytes white blood cells that specialize in ingesting and digesting undesirable bacteria and other matter.

phenylketonuria (PKU) an inherited amino acid enzyme (phenylalanine) deficiency that can cause mental retardation because of the body's inability to metabolize the amino acid phenylalanine.

placenta an organ connecting the umbilical cord to the wall of the uterus. It is the organ through which the fetus receives nourishment from and empties waste into the circulatory system of the mother. Following birth, the placenta is expelled.

plaque fatty deposits on inner lining of arteries.

pollution degradation of the environment; disruption of the ecosystem(s) occurs when the wastes of one organism cannot be scavenged by another.

polydrug use using more than one drug at a time.

polygamy multiple marriage involving more than one man and one woman. Polyandry refers to a marriage of one woman to two or more men, while polygyny refers to one man married to two or more women.

precursor those behaviors, habits, and factors of living that are asymptomatic and may eventually contribute to chronic disease, illness, or premature death.

prostitution having sexual intercourse with another for financial reward.

proteins large nitrogen-containing molecules that also contain mineral molecules. A large molecule is made up of many small simple units called amino acids.

psychedelic drug a drug that produces hallucinations and that alters perception, mood, time sense, and thought processes.

pyorrhea or periodontal disease an infection of the gums and supporting structures of teeth, causing the gums to feel tender, weak, and to give off a highly offensive breath. If not treated, this infection may cause loss of teeth.

pyrolysis a process using high temperature and pressures to convert garbage and wastes into oil and other substances.

rape occurs when one person forces another to have sexual intercourse without consent or with violent physical assault.

RDA recommended daily allowances of nutrients. RMDA refers to recommended minimum daily allowances of nutrients purported essential to sustain life.

rem a unit of the absorbed dose of ionizing radiation that accounts for biological effectiveness.

salpingitis infection and inflammation of the Fallopian tubes.

sarcoma cancer of the deeper tissues of the body, such as bones, muscles, and ligaments.

saturated fats compounds of fatty acids and glycerol that cannot accept more hydrogen atoms.

self-actualization developing and utilizing one's full creative, mental or psychic, and intellectual abilities and talents to the highest level possible.

semen a viscous, whitish fluid expelled from the penis during ejaculation. It is composed of seminal fluid, secretions of the prostate gland, Cowper's gland, and spermatozoa.

shiatsu finger pressure massage used to relieve muscular tension.

sickle-cell anemia a painful blood disorder common among blacks.

sigmoidoscopy examination of the colon immediately above the rectum by a sigmoidoscope or scoping device.

SMAC—sequential multiple analysis computer analysis of biochemicals in blood by computer.

smegma a white, cheesy substance secreted by the skin, especially in the genital areas of the human body.

smog (photochemical) automobile exhausts are changed, in the presence of ultraviolet rays and warm temperatures, into gases—ozone, PAN, and other chemical pollutants that irritate the skin, eyes, and lungs.

social drinking a person drinks moderately and socially and has control of his or her drinking habit.

social well-being interacting and becoming involved with others. This includes intimate relationships with family members, relatives, co-workers, and acquaintances.

sphygmomanometer an instrument used to measure blood pressure.

spiritual well-being that inner strength or energy that includes aspirations, ideals, and the energy to direct our everyday life.

starch made up of glucose units that always break down into glucose.

stress any action or situation that places physiological, social, or psychological demands on a person. Stress can be either bad (distress) or good (eustress).

stroke a blood clot or obstruction in a blood vessel. A stroke usually refers to a blood clot obstruction in a brain vessel, although such an obstruction could occur anywhere in the body.

sucrose a disaccharide made up of a molecule of the simple sugars, fructose and glucose. Refined white sugar is sucrose.

sugar addiction eating more refined sugar or sucrose than the body needs, contributing to the possibility of mild hypoglycemia.

suicide death of a person from self-inflicted causes.

supernutrition a nutrition plan that allows one to attain optimal well-being. This plan suggests ingesting vitamins and minerals in megadose levels far in excess of RDA.

synergistic a situation in which two causes work together and have a greater total effect than the sum of their individual effects.

Tay-Sachs an enzyme deficiency disease among Jews.

technology application of new chemical, biological, and physical information to industry; this replaces manual human effort with fossil and electrical forms of energy through organization of factories into mass assembly lines and computer check stations, resulting in mass production of many varieties of products for human consumption.

THC—tetrahydrocannabinol the chemical in marijuana capable of altering mental perceptions and causing hallucinations.

thermography photographic portrayal of the surface temperature of soft tissues of the body produced by measuring naturally occurring infrared radiation. It is used to diagnose cancer and other diseases that cause local changes in temperature.

tolerance (drug) the body's gradual adaptation to a drug over prolonged use, so that more and more of the drug is required to obtain the desired effect.

toxin a waste product of bacteria that often causes allergic reactions and illness in people.

toxoplasmosis an infection of the fetus and pregnant women during pregnancy that may be caused by exposure of pregnant women to infected pets, such as cats.

tranquilizer depressant drugs whose effects are milder than those of sedative hypnotics and with less potential for addiction or overdose.

transcendental meditation (TM) developing will power and control of the psychic or mind so that the whole body can function in a more integrated and orderly manner, resulting in a self-induced hypnosis or trance and bringing on a natural body high.

transsexualism reconstruction through surgery and hormone therapy of external sexual organs to help a person feel more emotionally and physically compatible with a desired sex role.

transvestite a male who dresses in feminine clothes and impersonates a woman.

triglyceride (a true fat) is formed by a chemical combination of three fatty acids with glycerol, containing large amounts of carbon and hydrogen.

tubal ligation—"tying the tubes" a surgical operation cutting both Fallopian tubes, tying the cut ends, and thereby preventing eggs from traveling to the uterus.

unsaturated fats compounds of fatty acids and glycerol that can accept more hydrogen atoms (polysaturated).

urbanization development of industries, commerce, and housing, and concentrating these in cities and metropolitan centers.

urinalysis a chemical analysis of the composition of urine.

vaginismus an involuntary tightening of the muscles in the vagina so that the penis may not enter—or, if it does, only with a good deal of pain.

vaginitis inflammation of the vagina.

vasectomy surgical excision of the vas deferens, which prevents spermatozoa from being ejaculated.

VDRL veneral disease research laboratory; test to measure syphilis antibodies or reagin. A test to detect syphilis infection.

vitamin organic compounds other than fats, carbohydrates, proteins, and minerals that are essential to human life.

voyeurism practice of getting sexual satisfaction by watching others who are nude or engaging in sexual activities.

withdrawal or coitus interruptus withdrawal of penis from vagina to prevent ejaculation of semen into the vagina.

xerophthalmia a disease of the eyes due to a deficiency of vitamin A in which the conjunctiva becomes inflamed and atrophied.

Photo credit list
Chapter Opening photographs and collages by ©
Menschenfreund.

Chapter 1
Fig. 1.4   (a) Steve Eagle/Nancy Palmer. (b) Alon Rein-
            inger/Design Photographers International.
Fig. 1.8   Terence Lennon.

Chapter 2
Fig. 2.4   © Joel Gordon 1980.

Chapter 3
Fig. 3.1   The Sunday Times, London. Artwork courtesy
            The Plain Truth.
Fig. 3.4   Ken Heyman, page 74; Leeanne Schmidt/DPI,
            page 75 top left; Elihu Blotnick/Omni-Photo
            Communications, page 75 top right; Chester
            Higgins Jr./Rapho-Photo Researchers, page 75
            bottom left; Jim Anderson/Woodfin Camp, page
            75 bottom right.
Fig. 3.6   Lorinda Morris.

Chapter 4
Fig. 4.1   (a) Joel Gordon/DPI. (b) Joan Menschenfreund.
Fig. 4.2   Sylvia Johnson/Woodfin Camp.
Fig. 4.3   Daniel S. Brody/Stock, Boston.
Fig. 4.4   (a) Larry P. Trone/DPI. (b) Emilio A. Mercado/
            Jeroboam. (c) Frank Siteman/Stock, Boston.
Fig. 4.5   Peter Menzel/Stock, Boston.
Fig. 4.6   (a) Craig Aurness/Woodfin Camp. (b) Werner
            Stoy/Camera Hawaii/DPI. (c) Lionel Delevingne/
            Stock, Boston. (d) Peter Miller/Photo Re-
            searchers.
Fig. 4.7   Craig Aurness/Woodfin Camp.

Chapter 5
Fig. 5.7   Ira Berger.
Fig. 5.8   Robert A. Isaacs/Photo Researchers.
Fig. 5.9   Arthur Grace/Stock, Boston.

Chapter 6
Fig. 6.2   Gret Manheim/DPI.
Fig. 6.4   Henry Monroe/DPI.
Fig. 6.12   Transworld Feature Syndicate, Inc.
Fig. 6.14   Joel Gordon/DPI.

Chapter 7
Page 178   Sidney Harris.
Fig. 7.7   Lorinda Morris.
Fig. 7.11   Union-Tribune Publishing Company.

Chapter 8
Fig. 8.1   Hanson, J. W., Jones, K. L., Smith, D. W.;
            J.A.M.A. 235:1458-1460, 1976 copyright Ameri-
            can Medical Association.
Fig. 8.2   Christa Armstrong/Photo Researchers.
Fig. 8.5   Lorinda Morris.
Fig. 8.9   Jim Anderson/Woodfin Camp, top; Joel Gordon/
            DPI, bottom.
Fig. 8.12   Omni-Photo Communications.

Chapter 9
Fig. 9.4   (a) American Cancer Society. (b) Picture Library
            Society.

Fig. 9.5   Rohn Engh/Photo Researchers.
Fig. 9.6   American Cancer Society.
Fig. 9.8   Michael C. Hayman/Photo Researchers.

Chapter 10
Fig. 10.2   Joel Gordon/DPI.
Fig. 10.3   "Courtesy of the New York Historical Society",
            New York City.
Fig. 10-4   Lorinda Morris.
Fig. 10.5   Maxwell Coplan/DPI.
Fig. 10.6   Courtesy U.S. Drug Enforcement.
Fig. 10.7   Kathy Bendo.

Chapter 11
Fig. 11.4   (a) Wide World. (b) J. Berndt/Stock, Boston.
Fig. 11.7   Terence Lennon.

Chapter 12
Fig. 12.5   Lorinda Morris.
Fig. 12.7   Kent Reno/Jeroboam.
Fig. 12.8   From Cellulite: *Those Lumps, Bumps, and Bulges
            You Couldn't Lose Before* by Nicole Ronsard.
            Copyright © 1973 by Beauty and Health Pub-
            lishing Corp. By permission of Bantam Books,
            Inc. All rights reserved.

Chapter 13
Fig. 13.1   Bruce Roberts/Rapho-Photo Researchers.
Fig. 13.14 Joel Gordon/DPI.

Chapter 14
Fig. 14.5   Bruce Roberts/Rapho-Photo Researchers.

Chapter 15
Fig. 15.1   Courtesy Mission Bay Hospital Newsletter, April
            1978.

Chapter 16
Fig. 16.2   Joanne Leonard/Woodfin Camp.
Fig. 16.3   Joel Gordon/DPI.
Fig. 16.4   Sylvia Johnson/Woodfin Camp.
Fig. 16.5   Bonnie Freer/Photo Researchers.
Fig. 16.6   Globe Photos.

Chapter 17
Fig. 17.4   Inger McAbe/Rapho-Photo Researchers.
Fig. 17.12 Kathy Bendo.
Fig. 17.13 Bruce Roberts/Rapho-Photo Researchers.
Page 409   Sidney Harris.
Fig. 17.14 Al Kaplan/DPI.
Fig. 17.15 Al Kaplan/DPI.

Chapter 18
Fig. 18.1   Wide World.
Fig. 18.6   Julie Jensen.
Fig. 18.7   Karen R. Preuss/Jeroboam.
Fig. 18.8   Sylvia Johnson/Woodfin Camp, left; Richard
            Frieman/Photo Researchers, right.
Fig. 18.9   Kenn Goldblatt/DPI.
Fig. 18.11 Wide World, top; Copyright © 1979 by Warner
            Brothers, Inc./Movie Star News, bottom left;
            Wide World, bottom right.
Fig. 18.12 Reprinted with permission from Clive Cocking
            "The Legendary Gordon Shrum," *UBC Alumni
            Chronicle,* Autumn, 1978.

Chapter 19

Fig. 19.1   Karen R. Preuss/Jeroboam.
Fig. 19.2   Joan Liftin/Woodfin Camp.
Fig. 19.3   Sepp Seitz/Woodfin Camp, top; Barbara Paup/ Jeroboum, bottom.
Fig. 19.4   Sylvia Johnson/Woodfin Camp.
Fig. 19.5   Mark & Dan Jury, left; Mark Jury, right.

Chapter 20

Fig. 20.3   Charles Rotkin/P.F.I.
Fig. 20.4   Library of Congress, left; Bill Ganzel, right.
Fig. 20.5   Robert W. Young/DPI.
Fig. 20.6   Elihu Blotnick/Omni Photo.
Fig. 20.7   Grant Heilman.
Fig. 20.10   Bill Gillette/EPA-Documerica.
Fig. 20.12   Hal Fay/DPI.
Fig. 20.13   (a) Alain deJean/Sygma. (b) Tom McHugh/Photo Researchers.
Fig. 20.14   Herman Emmet/Photo Researchers.
Fig. 20.19   Courtesy of Amana Refrigerator, Inc.

Fig. 20.23   Jean-Louis Atlan/Sygma.
Fig. 20.25   Grant Heilman.
Fig. 20.26   Franken/Sygma; Columbia Pictures/Movie Star News, insert.
Fig. 20.27   Wide World.
Fig. 20.28   Wide World.

Chapter 21

Fig. 21.1   Grant Heilman.
Fig. 21.2   Grant Heilman.
Fig. 21.6   United Nations/Muddon, left; Grant Heilman, right.
Fig. 21.7   United Nations.
Fig. 21.8   Brace Research Institute, MacDonald College of McGill University.
Fig. 21.9   Daniel S. Brody/Stock, Boston.

Chapter 22

Fig. 22.3   (a) Steve Hansen/Stock, Boston. (b) Timothy Eagan/Woodfin Camp.